AF449192

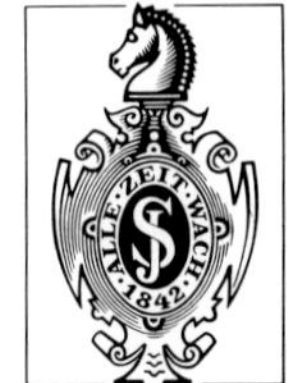

M.-C. Marti   J.-C. Givel (Eds.)

Surgery of Anorectal Diseases

With Pre- and Postoperative Management

With Contributions by
P. Aeberhard A. Akovbiantz R. Auckenthaler
P. Buchmann A. Forster A. Froidevaux
E. Gemsenjäger J.-C. Givel P. Graber R. Gumener
B. Hammer M. Harms A. Huber M.-C. Marti
P. Meyer D. Mirescu D. Montandon G. Pipard
A. A. Poltera A. Rohner F. Sadry A. F. Schärli
H. Wehrli S. Widgren

Foreword by J. Nicholls

With 184 Figures in 414 Separate Illustrations
and 92 Tables

Springer-Verlag Berlin Heidelberg New York
London Paris Tokyo Hong Kong

Prof. Dr. Marc-Claude Marti
Département de Chirurgie, Hôpital Cantonal Universitaire de Genève,
CH-1211 Genève 4

PD Dr. Jean-Claude Givel
Service de Chirurgie A, Centre Hospitalier Universitaire Vaudois,
CH-1011 Lausanne

Drawings by Alain Fasel
Hôpital Cantonal Universitaire de Genève, CH-1211 Genève 4

ISBN 3-540-50928-3 Springer-Verlag Berlin Heidelberg New York
ISBN 0-387-50928-3 Springer-Verlag New York Berlin Heidelberg

Typesetting, Printing and Binding: Appl, Wemding
2124/3140-543210 – Printed on acid-free paper

Foreword

Understanding of the pathology and causation of anorectal diseases is constantly increasing. This has led to changes in how treatment is chosen. There is almost no anorectal condition for which some new therapeutic approach has not been recently tried, and several of these do not involve surgery at all. In any developing field it is important to maintain contact with change. *Surgery of Anorectal Diseases* does this in abundance by its very breadth and by the detailed and up-to-date manner in which it deals with each condition. Beautifully illustrated and clearly written, it is a reference text of major importance.
The editors have managed to achieve uniformity of style without stifling the individuality of the various contributing authors. The book will appeal both to surgeons and physicians and must be one of the most complete and all-encompassing works in the field. Besides the standard topics, which themselves are dealt with excellently, there are welcome contributions on microbiology, physiology, dermatology as well as on aspects of paediatrics and gynaecology. The reader will find informed comment on any subject, combined with a current bibliography. More could not be wished from any reference book.

London, November 1989   John Nicholls

Preface

Proctology is no more a minor speciality. Better knowledge of colo-rec-
to-anal anatomy and of physio-pathology, progress in clinical, imaging
and bacteriological investigations have resulted in numerous and more
complex therapies.
The aim of this book is to provide the practitioner as well as the proctologist, the surgeon or the gastroenterologue with updated knowl-
edges in medical and surgical management of the various colo-recto-
anal diseases.
Illustrations and drawings should help in understanding clinical conditions and detailed surgical procedures. Extensive bibliography will
provide the lecturer with references.
We wish to thank all the authors for their contribution. A debt of grati-
tude is owed to John Nicholls for writing the Foreword.

Genève, December 1989   M.-C. Marti
                                                         J.-C. Givel

Contents

4   Microbiological Examinations

R. Auckenthaler 25

5   Management of Biopsies and Operation Specimens of the Anorectal Region

S. Widgren 31

6   Radiological Investigations

D. Mirescu and F. Sadry 35

7   *Manometry and Electromyography*

M.-C. Marti 46

8   *Positioning and Anesthesia for Anorectal Surgery*

A. Forster and M.-C. Marti 49

9 *Hemorrhoids*

M.-C. Marti 56

10 Anal Fissure

M.-C. Marti 76

11 Anorectal Abscesses and Fistulas

M.-C. Marti 84

12 Pilonidal Sinus

A. Froidevaux 99

13 Anorectal Crohn's Disease

P. Buchmann 102

14 Ulcerative Colitis

H. Wehrli and A. Akovbiantz 112

18 Polyps

19 Malignant Anal Tumors

23 Rectal Prolapse, Solitary Rectal Ulcer Syndrome, Descending Perianal Syndrome

E. Gemsenjäger 218

List of Contributors

Aeberhard, P., Prof. Dr.
Departement Chirurgie, Chirurgische Klinik, Kantonsspital Aarau,
CH-5001 Aarau

Akovbiantz, A., Prof. Dr.
Chirurgische Klinik, Stadtspital Waid Zürich, Tièchestrasse 99,
CH-8037 Zürich 10

Auckenthaler, R., Dr.
Laboratoire Central de Bactériologie, Hôpital Cantonal Universitaire
de Genève, 24, rue Micheli-du-Crest, CH-1211 Genève 4

Buchmann, P., PD Dr.
Klinik für Viszeralchirurgie, Departement Chirurgie, Universitätsspital
Zürich, Rämistrasse 100, CH-8091 Zürich

Forster, A., Dr.
Département d'Anesthésiologie, Hôpital Cantonal Universitaire
de Genève, CH-1211 Genève 4

Froidevaux, A., Dr.
Service de Chirurgie, Hôpital de la Gruyère, CH-1632 Riaz

Gemsenjäger, E., PD Dr.
Chirurgische Klinik, Spital Neumünster, CH-8125 Zollikerberg-Zürich

Givel, J.-C., PD Dr.
Service de Chirurgie A, Centre Hospitalier Universitaire Vaudois,
CH-1011 Lausanne

Graber, P., Prof. Dr.
Clinique d'Urologie, Département de Chirurgie, Hôpital Cantonal
Universitaire de Genève, CH-1211 Genève 4

Gumener, R., Dr.
Unité de Chirurgie Plastique et Reconstructive, Division de Chirurgie
Réparatrice, Département de Chirurgie, Hôpital Cantonal Universitaire
de Genève, CH-1211 Genève 4

Hammer, B., Dr.
Gastroenterologische Abteilung, Medizinische Klinik C, Kantonsspital
St. Gallen, CH-9007 St. Gallen

Harms, M., Dr.
Policlinique de Dermatologie, Hôpital Cantonal Universitaire
de Genève, CH-1211 Genève 4

Huber, A., PD Dr.
Chirurgische Klinik, Kantonsspital Luzern, CH-6004 Luzern

Marti, M.-C., Prof. Dr.
Département de Chirurgie, Hôpital Cantonal Universitaire de Genève,
CH-1211 Genève 4

Meyer, P., Dr.
Clinique Universitaire de Chirurgie Digestive, Département
de Chirurgie, Hôpital Cantonal Universitaire de Genève,
CH-1211 Genève 4

Mirescu, D., Dr.
Département de Radiologie, Hôpital Cantonal Universitaire de Genève,
CH-1211 Genève 4

Montandon, D., PD Dr.
Unité de Chirurgie Plastique et Reconstructive, Division de Chirurgie
Réparatrice, Département de Chirurgie, Hôpital Cantonal Universitaire
de Genève, CH-1211 Genève 4

Pipard, G., Dr.
Département de Radiologie, Service de Radiothérapie, Hôpital Cantonal
Universitaire de Genève, 21, rue Alcide-Jentzer, CH-1211 Genève 4

Poltera, A. A., PD Dr.
CIBA-GEIGY, Pharma International, K 121.3.02, Postfach,
CH-4002 Basel

Rohner, A., Prof. Dr.
Clinique Universitaire de Chirurgie Digestive, Département
de Chirurgie, Hôpital Cantonal Universitaire de Genève,
CH-1211 Genève 4

Sadry, F., Dr.
Département de Radiologie, Hôpital Cantonal Universitaire de Genève,
CH-1211 Genève 4

Schärli, A. F., Prof. Dr.
Kinderchirurgische Klinik, Kinderspital Luzern, CH-6000 Luzern 16

Wehrli, H., Dr.
Chirurgische Klinik, Stadtspital Waid Zürich, Tièchestrasse 99,
CH-8037 Zürich 10

Widgren, S., Prof. Dr.
Départment de Pathologie, Centre Médical Universitaire,
Hôpital Cantonal Universitaire de Genève, 1, rue Michel Servet,
CH-1211 Genève 4

1 Surgical Anatomy of the Rectum, Anal Canal, and Perineum

A. Huber

Pelvic Floor, Levator Ani Muscle, and Sphincters
(Figs. 1.1–1.6)

The two levator ani muscles form a funnel whose outlet begins at the level of the puborectalis sling and there forms a sharp angle – about 90° – backward. The medial fibers of the levator ani form a muscular sling which arises from the pubic bone and encircles the anorectal flexure. This muscle sling, called the "puborectalis sling", plays a crucial role in maintaining fecal continence. The sphincter ani externus muscle forms the lower part of the funnel of the pelvic floor. It consists of three parts (subcutaneous, superficial, and deep) which cannot be distinguished clearly but merge into each other. Muscle fibers running from the tip of the coccyx to the external sphincters are called the anococcygeal ligament. Cranial to this ligament are the left and right ischiorectal spaces, which are located caudal to the pelvic floor. The levator ani and sphincter externus ani muscles are supplied with blood by branches of the pudendal artery.

Alcock's canal is traversed by the pudendal nerve and pudendal vessels after they have left the lesser pelvis and looped around the ischial spine and sacrospinous ligament. The sphincters are divided in the posterior midline, and the pelvic floor is divided by a left parasacral incision. Division of the longitudinal muscle coat of the rectum shows the exposure of the circular muscle layer, which thickens caudally to form the sphincter ani internus. It is apparent that the inner fibers of the levator ani muscle take mainly a longitudinal course in the posterior and caudal portions, blending with the longitudinal muscle coat of the rectum. Both intraoperatively and in anatomical specimens, one is struck by the variability in the mass and arrangement of the levator ani fibers, and the two telescoping layers that are customarily depicted for this muscle cannot always be distinguished clearly, especially in the elderly. In the specimen used for the current investigation, an internal layer with longitudinal fibers and an external layer with a more circular fiber pattern could be demonstrated, but only after painstaking dissection.

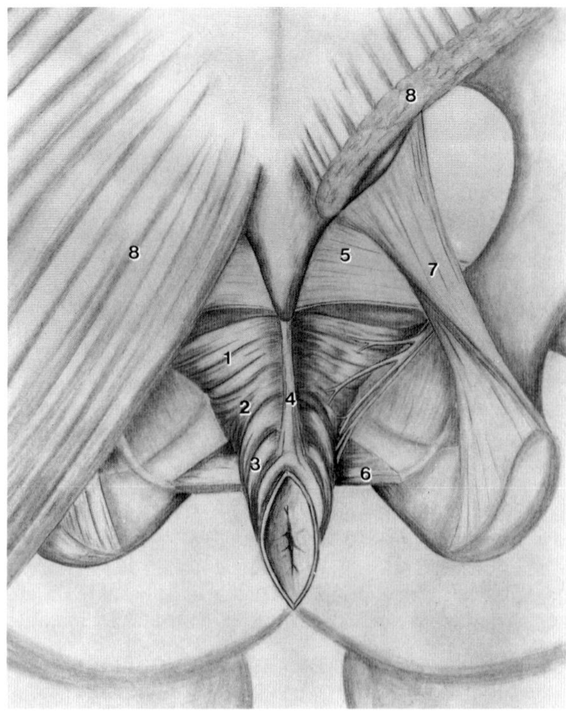

Fig. 1.1. *1,* Levator ani muscle; *2,* puborectalis sling; *3,* sphincter ani externus muscle; *4,* anococcygeal ligament; *5,* coccygeal muscle; *6,* perineus muscle; *7,* tuberous (sacrospinus) ligament; *8,* gluteus maximus muscle. (Adapted from [7])

Mesorecta (Fig. 1.7)

The pars pelvina recti is surrounded by the perirectal fat and a fascial capsule. The term "Waldeyer's fascia" actually refers only to the posterior part of the rectal capsule. On either side the fascial capsule is extended to form lateral wings or the so-called mesorecta which is continuous with the pelvic wall. Waldeyer's [16] fascia is incised longitudinally to demonstrate the local nerves and blood vessels supplying the rectum. The superior rectal artery enters the fascial capsule of the rectum, accompanied by its veins and the hypogastric nerves. Passing through the lateral wings, the middle rectal artery,

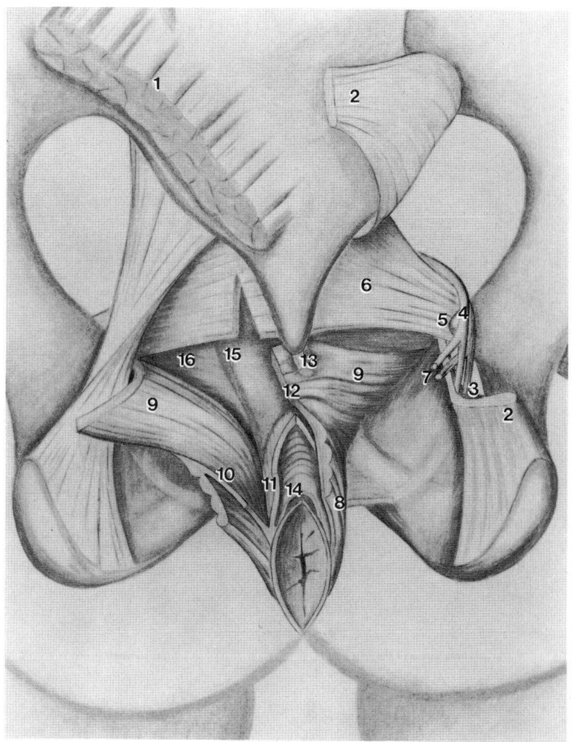

Fig. 1.2. *1*, Gluteus maximus muscle; *2*, sacrotuberous ligament (cut); *3*, canalis of Alcock; *4*, pudendal vessels and nerve; *5*, ischiadic spine; *6*, sacrospinous ligament; *7*, inferior rectal artery, inferior rectal nerve (cut); *8*, external sphincter; *9*, pelvic floor (levator ani muscle); *10*, inner, longitudinal fibers of levator ani muscle; *11*, longitudinal fibers of external muscle layer of rectum; *12*, raphe anococcygica; *13*, anococcygeal ligament; *14*, sphincter ani internus muscle; *15*, Waldeyer's fascia; *16*, lateral wing of the rectum. (Adapted from [7])

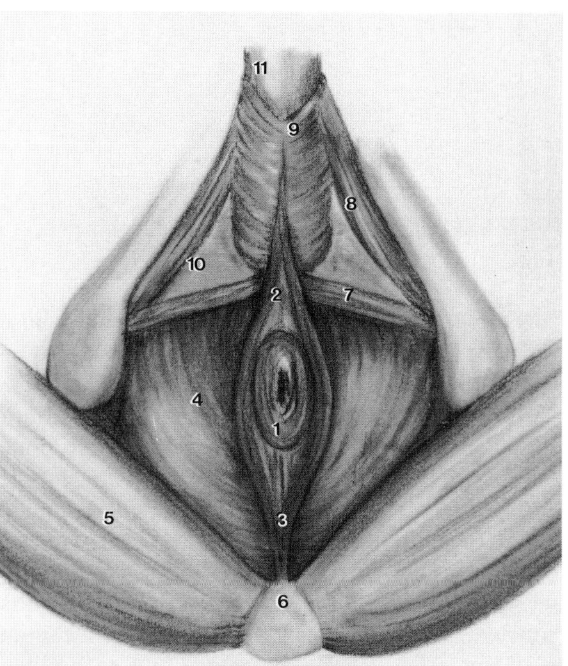

Fig. 1.3. Anatomy in male. *1*, External sphincter ani muscle; *2*, central point of perineum; *3*, anococcygeal ligament; *4*, levator ani muscle; *5*, gluteus maximus muscle; *6*, tip of coccyx; *7*, superficial transverse perineal muscle; *8*, ischiocavernous muscle; *9*, bulbocavernous muscle; *10*, urogenital diaphragm; *11*, corpora cavernosa

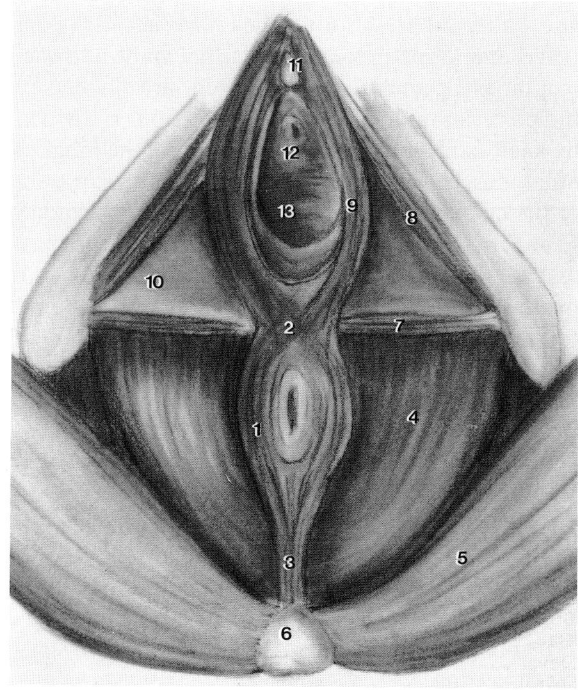

Fig. 1.4. Anatomy in female. *1*, External sphincter ani muscle; *2*, central point of perineum; *3*, anococcygeal ligament; *4*, levator ani muscle; *5*, gluteus maximus muscle; *6*, tip of coccyx; *7*, superficial transverse perineal muscle; *8*, ischiocavernous muscle; *9*, bulbocavernous muscle; *10*, urogenital diaphragm; *11*, clitoris; *12*, urethra; *13*, vagina

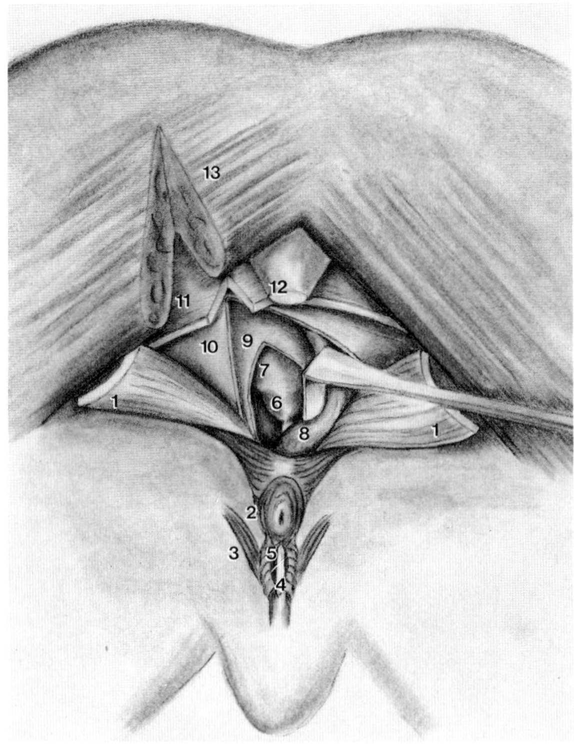

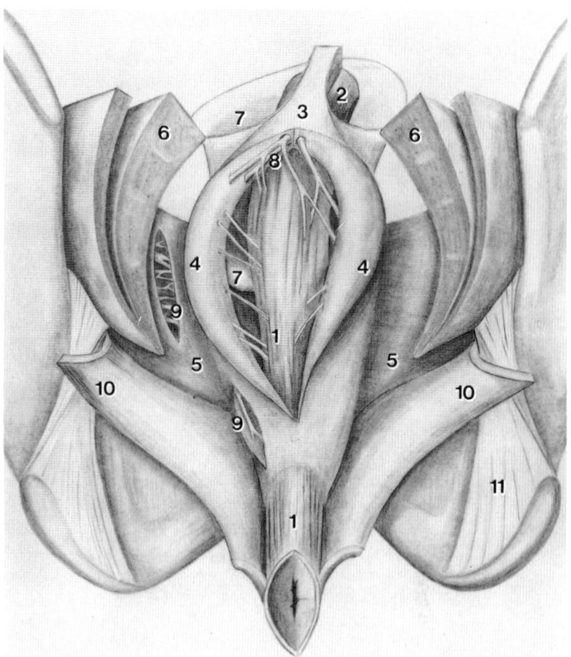

Fig. 1.5. *1*, Levator ani muscle; *2*, sphincter ani externus muscle; *3*, ischiocavernous muscle; *4*, bulbocavernous muscle; *5*, urethra; *6*, prostate; *7*, urinary bladder; *8*, rectum; *9*, Denonvilliers' fascia; *10*, Waldeyer's fascia; *11*, sacrospinous ligament; *12*, tip of coccyx resected; *13*, gluteus maximus muscle

Fig. 1.7. *1*, Rectum; *2*, sigmoid; *3*, mesosigmoid; *4*, Waldeyer's fascia; *5*, lateral wings (mesorecta); *6*, split sacrum; *7*, excavatio rectovesicalis/-uterina (Douglas); *8*, superior rectal artery and vein; *9*, middle rectal artery and vein; *10*, split levator ani muscle; *11*, sacrotuberous ligament. (Adapted from [7])

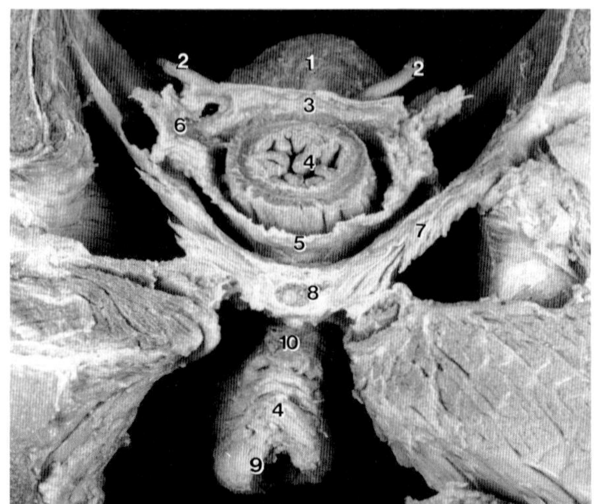

Fig. 1.6. *1*, Urinary bladder; *2*, ureters; *3*, Denonvilliers' fascia; *4*, rectum; *5*, Waldeyer's fascia; *6*, left lateral wing; *7*, levator ani muscle; *8*, tip of coccyx; *9*, anus; *10*, anorectal flexure

venous plexuses, pelvic splanchnic nerves, and communicating branches of the pelvic sympathetic trunk reach the interior of the rectal capsule.

Rectum, Anal Canal (Figs. 1.8–1.10)

The rectum arises from the sigmoid colon either at the point where the free sigmoid mesocolon terminates or at about the level of the third sacral vertebra. The approximately 15-cm long segment of the rectum located above the rectal diaphragm is known as the pars pelvina or as the rectal ampulla when dilated. Below the rectal diaphragm is the pars perinealis of the rectum, which terminates at the anus. This subdivision is justified on ontogenetic grounds, among others, since the pars pelvina develops from the embryonic gut while the pars perinealis is derived from the cloaca.

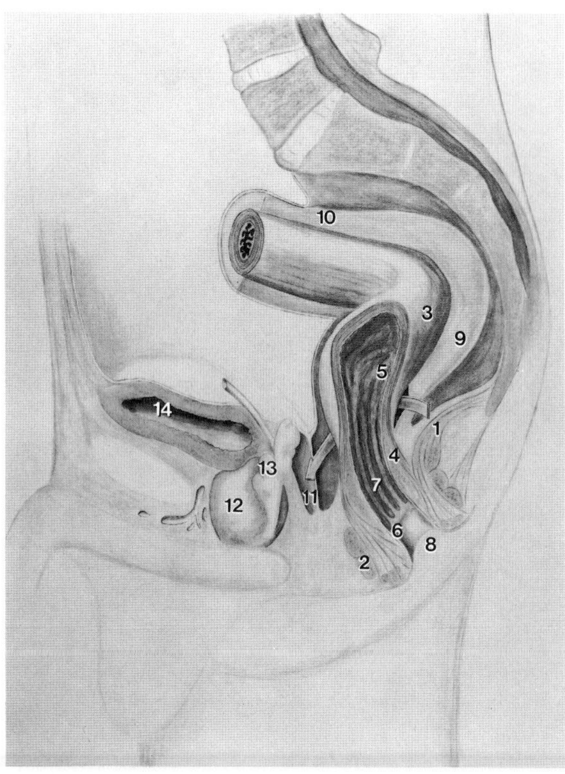

Fig. 1.8. Anatomy in male. *1,* Levator ani muscle; *2,* sphincter ani externus muscle; *3,* pars pelvina of rectum; *4,* pars perinealis of rectum; *5,* transverse fold of Houston (Kohlrausch); *6,* pectinate line; *7,* anal columns of Morgagni; *8,* anocutaneous line of Hilton; *9,* fascial capsule of rectum; *10,* connective tissue of sigmoid mesocolon; *11,* prostatoperineal fascia (Denonvilliers); *12,* prostate; *13,* seminal vesicles; *14,* bladder. (Adapted from [7])

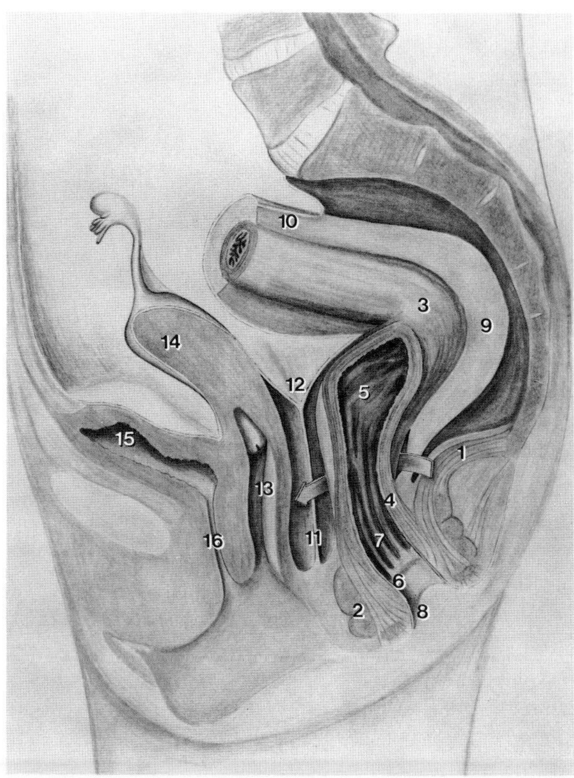

Fig. 1.9. Anatomy in female. *1,* Levator ani muscle; *2,* sphincter ani externus muscle; *3,* pars pelvina of rectum; *4,* pars perinealis of rectum; *5,* transverse fold of Houston (Kohlrausch); *6,* pectinate line; *7,* anal columns of Morgagni; *8,* anocutaneous line of Hilton; *9,* fascial capsule of rectum; *10,* connective tissue of sigmoid mesocolon; *11,* rectovaginal fascia; *12,* rectouterine pouch; *13,* vagina; *14,* uterus; *15,* bladder; *16,* urethra. (Adapted from [7])

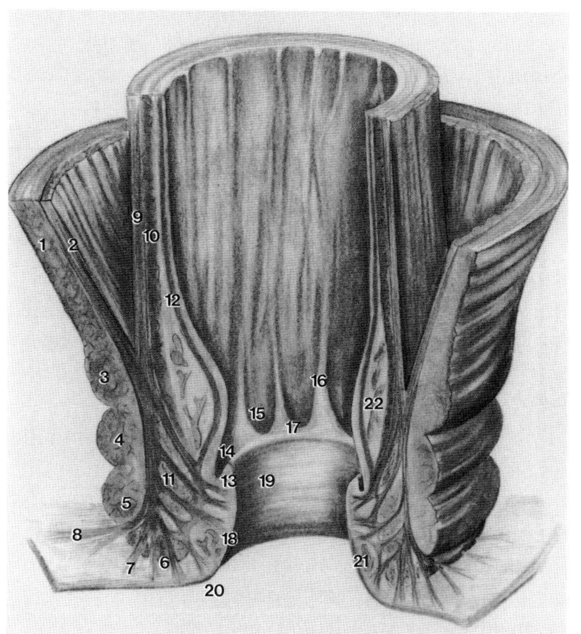

◁

Fig. 1.10. *1,* Levator ani muscle, circular layer; *2,* levator ani muscle, longitudinal layer; *3,* puborectalis muscle; *4,* external sphincter, deep portion; *5,* external sphincter, superficial portion; *6,* external sphincter, subcutaneous portion; *7,* corrugator cutis ani muscle; *8,* transverse septum of ischiorectal fossa; *9,* longitudinal muscle layer of rectum; *10,* circular muscle layer of rectum; *11,* internal sphincter; *12,* muscularis mucosae; *13,* anal valve; *14,* anal crypt; *15,* rectal sinus; *16,* rectal column of Morgagni; *17,* pectinate (dentate) line (2.5–3 cm above anal verge); *18,* intermuscular groove (white line of Hilton); *19,* pecten; *20,* anal verge; *21,* external hemorrhoidal plexus; *22,* internal hemorrhoidal plexus

The cranial half of the pars pelvina is intra-abdominal and retroperitoneal in location, while the caudal half is situated completely outside the abdominal cavity. The pars pelvina forms multiple curves: in the sagittal plane, the sacral flexure is formed as the rectum follows the concavity of the sacrum, and the perineal flexure is formed by the pull of the levator sling. The "anorectal angle" of the perineal flexure measures about 90°. In the frontal plane, the rectum typically curves first to the right and then to the left as it descends. These curves produce folds in the mucosa known as the transverse folds (of Houston).

Three transverse folds can be distinguished: an upper and a lower fold which protrude into the lumen from the left side, and a middle fold which projects from the right wall. The middle fold, also known as Kohlrausch's fold, is situated at the level of the peritoneal reflection. In the drawings (Figs. 1.8 and 1.9), the uppermost fold is hidden from view by the closed rectum, and the lowest fold has been cut away with the left half. The pars perinealis of the rectum is an alternate name for the anal canal; it commences below the pelvic diaphragm. At the upper border of the approximately 4-cm long canal is the pectinate line. Cords of muscle tissue, blood vessels, and lymphatic channels at the end of the pars pelvina create permanent vertical folds in the mucosa which are called the anal columns of Morgagni. The recesses between the columns, into which the proctodeal glands open, are known as the anal sinuses of crypts. The distal edges of the anal columns and sinuses form a circular, lobed margin (anal valves or pectinate line). The anocutaneous line (of Hilton) marks the lowermost egde of the anal canal.

The pars pelvina of the rectum is enclosed within a fascial capsule. The posterior surface of this capsule is known as Waldeyer's fascia. At the sides, the capsule is attached to the pelvic wall by two fascial expansions, called the lateral wings, which are continuous with the internal parietal pelvic fascia. These wings are traversed by the blood vessels and nerve plexuses which supply the organs of the lesser pelvis. Cranially, Waldeyer's fascia becomes lost in the retroperitoneal connective tissue of the sigmoid mesocolon; distally it is reflected onto the parietal pelvic fascia. In the female the anterior surface of the fascial capsule is formed by the rectovaginal fascia, and in the male by the prostatoperineal fascia of Denonvilliers. In embryonic life the peritoneal pocket extends down to the pelvic floor in front of the rectum. As the deep portions of this serosal pouch become obliterated through adhesion, the frontal fascial sheet of Denonvilliers is formed. There are occasional reports in the literature that this fascia is lacking in the female, being represented only by loose connective tissue. However, we have found a thick fascial sheet in several female preparations. All that remains of the original serosal pocket extending to the pelvic floor is the rectouterine pouch (of Douglas) or the rectovesical pouch. In this deep portion of the peritoneal sac, the peritoneum in the female is reflected onto the uterus behind the posterosuperior part of the vaginal fornix, and in the male onto the urinary bladder level with the upper part of the seminal vesicles.

Remarks on Continence

Continence refers to the voluntary and involuntary control of the defecation. A distinction may be made between gross and fine continence, where gross continence is the ability to control the voiding of large, solid feces, and fine continence is the control of small fecal masses, liquid feces, and flatus. Thus, varying degrees of fecal incontinence may be present. Incontinence is said to be complete when the patient has no control whatsoever over the expulsion of feces or flatus.

Continence is maintained by a complex organ system comprised of the following elements:

- The rectum, the pelvic floor muscles (most notably the puborectalis sling), and the internal and external sphincters
- The sensory and motor functions of these organs
- Reflexes and central nervous mechanisms

The following factors in this system contribute to continence. The curvatures of the rectum in the frontal and sagittal planes and its transverse folds (Houston, Kohlrausch) retard progression of the fecal mass. Of particular importance is the anorectal angulation, whose function can be likened to that of a flutter valve or the phenomenon of a kinked garden hose. The anorectal angle is maintained by the pull of the puborectalis sling and by the anococcygeal ligament. The stellate cross-section of the anal canal mucosa and its corpus cavernosum-like elements (hemorrhoidal plexus) are believed to exercise a sealing function.

The pressure that can be measured within the anal canal at rest results from the resting tone of the internal and external sphincters and the puborectalis muscle. It normally ranges between 30 cm H_2O (2.94 kPa) and 50 cm H_2O (4.9 kPa). With this pressure, the anal canal creates an effective barrier against the pressure of 10–30 cm H_2O (0.98–2.94 kPa) that resides within the rectum. Reflex distension of the rectum triggers a transitory relaxation of the internal sphincter, accompanied by a measurable pressure fall within the anal canal. This makes possible the "sampling response" which enables rectal contents to be discriminated and their elimination controlled. Voluntary contraction of the external sphincters can strengthen the barrier effect by increasing the pressure in the anal canal. This voluntary "squeeze pressure" can be sustained for only about 1 min, however.

A rise of intra-abdominal pressure stimulates an increase in the tone of the external sphincters and puborectalis. This mechanism helps to maintain continence during coughing, sneezing, and laughing. A gradual increase in rectal distension produces a corresponding rise of pressure within the anal canal up to level of 80–130 cm H_2O (7.84–12.74 kPa) (the "resting yield pressure"). Further distension of the rectum stimulates a voluntary contraction of the sphincters, raising the pressure to as high as 400 cm H_2O (39.2 kPa) (the "augmented yield pressure"). One function of this reflex increase in voluntary sphincter contraction may be to preserve continence during sleep. At the same time, the compliant walls of the rectum expand in response to the elevated pressure or increasing mass, thus performing a reservoir function which also contributes to continence. This adaptive response is abolished by low rectal resections, but apparently it can be acquired to some degree by the bowel segment above the anastomosis. It is dependent, moreover, on functionally sound sphincter apparatus. Stretching of the external sphincters and the puborectalis sling excites the urge to defecate and triggers a voluntary contraction of these muscles. Two empirical facts are of great interest in this regard:

1. Loss of the voluntary sphincter muscles, especially the puborectalis, results in complete incontinence.
2. In children with severe anorectal malformations, an acceptable degree of continence can be achieved, even in the absence of the rectum, anal canal, and internal and external sphincters, by pulling the bowel through a functional puborectalis sling [1–3, 5, 8–10, 14, 18].

Nerve Supply (Fig. 1.11)

Levator Ani and Coccygeus

The levator ani and coccygeus muscles are supplied with nerve branches from the sacral plexus. These branches arise from S3 and S4 (occasionally from S2–4) and take a posterior-to-anterior course, passing close to the cranial and lateral muscle origins. The nerves generally run along the inner, cranial surface of the muscles, but individual fibers occasionally pierce the levator ani muscle and course a short distance on its inferior surface before passing back through the muscle to its inner surface. In some cases the levator ani is supplied by an accessory nerve which arises from the same sacral segments but which courses on the outer surface of the muscle sheet.

Puborectalis

The puborectalis muscle derives its nerve supply from S2–4. Reports vary as to whether the nerve

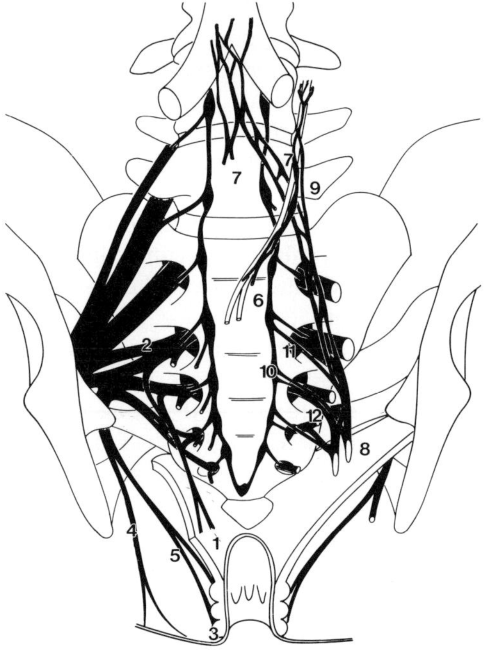

Fig. 1.11. Nerve supply. *1,* Nerves of levator ani muscle; *2,* sacral plexus; *3,* nerves of sphincter ani externus muscle; *4,* pudendal nerve; *5,* inferior rectal nerves; *6,* inferior mesenteric plexus; *7,* superior hypogastric plexus (hypogastric nerves); *8,* inferior hypogastric plexus (pelvic plexus); *9,* connecting nerves of inferior hypogastric plexus and inferior mesenteric plexus; *10,* sympathetic trunk; *11,* branches of sympathetic trunk to inferior hypogastric plexus; *12,* pelvic splanchnic nerves (nervi erigentes)

branches supplying the puborectalis arise from the pudendal nerve or directly from the sacral nerve roots, i. e., whether they course on the outer surface of levator ani or on its inner, pelvic surface. Shepherd [13] describes a pudendal innervation of the puborectalis, while Percy et al. [12] found that the puborectalis sling was supplied by pelvic branches from S 3,4. Ontogenically the puborectalis, like the external sphincters, is derived from the cloacal sphincter muscles which is supplied by the pudendal nerve. Lawson [11], drawing on the work of Uhlenhuth [15], Holl [6] and Gorsch [4], divides the muscle into the cranial part and a caudal part, with the cranial part supplied by pelvic nerves and the caudal part by branches of the pudendal. We cannot furnish a definitive answer to this question based on our work on anatomical preparations. We have found variable ascending and descending nerve branches at the junction of the puborectalis and external sphincter.

Sphincter Ani Externus

The sphincter ani externus is supplied by branches from the pudendal nerve. The corresponding fibers arise from S 2-4 (the sacral plexus). The branches to the sphincter ani externus leave Alcock's canal to reach their muscles as the inferior rectal nerves.

Sphincter Ani Internus

Being a smooth, visceral muscle, the sphincter ani internus derives its nerve supply from the inferior hypogastric plexus. It should be stressed that there are no intramural ganglia of Auerbach's plexus in the sphincter ani internus, and that the question of whether cholinergic nerves have an excitatory action and adrenergic nerves have an inhibitory action, or vice versa, has not yet been resolved.

Rectum

The rectum derives its innervation from both the sympathetic and parasympathetic systems and from afferent pathways. The nerve fibers reach the rectum via the superior rectal plexus and inferior hypogastric plexus.

Sympathetic Nerve Supply

The sympathetic fibers to the rectum are derived from the first two lumbar segments of the spinal cord. From the upper lumbar ganglia of the sympathetic trunk, the fibers pass to the abdominal aortic plexus. From there some pass to the rectum via the inferior mesenteric plexus, accompanied by the artery of the same name. Others pass through the superior hypogastric plexus (hypogastric nerves) to the inferior hypogastric (pelvic) plexus before reaching the rectum. The hypogastric nerves also receive fibers from the inferior mesenteric plexus. Fibers from the sacral ganglia of the sympathetic trunk radiate into the inferior hypogastric plexus and supply the rectum.

At present it is believed that the most important sympathetic pathway to the pelvis and rectum is that which passes through the inferior hypogastric plexus. Modern theory holds that the sympathetic nerves of the rectum are devoid of afferent fibers. A sympathectomy of the rectum, in any case, has no obvious physiological effects.

Parasympathetic Nerve Supply

The second, third, and fourth segments of the sacral parasympathetic center supply the rectum. The parasympathetic fibers branch off from the corresponding sacral nerves as the pelvic splanchnic nerves (nervi erigentes) which enter the inferior hypogastric plexus and from there pass to the rectum. A portion of the fibers ascends from the inferior hypogastric plexus via the hypogastric nerves to enter the inferior mesenteric plexus, from which they are distributed to the sigmoid colon and descending colon. The sacral parasympathetic fibers are followed in their course by the visceral afferent fibers.

Visceral Afferent Fibers

The rectum and anal canal are both supplied by afferent fibers from S 2-4. The visceral afferent fibers of the rectum and upper anal canal arise from the sacral nerves just outside the sacral foramina and pass with the parasympathetic fibers in the pelvic splanchnic (nervi erigentes) to the inferior hypogastric plexus. From here they supply the anorectum as far cranially as the rectosigmoid junction and as far caudally as the pectinate line.

The visceral afferent fibers of the anal canal and the afferent fibers of the perineal skin course within the

8   A. Huber

pudendal nerve before branching off as the inferior rectal nerves, accompanied by the voluntary motor fibers of the external sphincter. These inferior rectal branches course along the lower surface of the levator ani muscle to reach the lower anal canal and perineal skin.

The skin of the anal canal, like that of the body in general, is sensitive to touch, heat, cold, and pain. The rectal mucosa, on the other hand, lacks sensation. The boundary of sensation, i. e., of somatic and visceral afferent innervation, is situated at the pectinate line or about 1 cm above it. As in the remainder of the bowel, wall tension and ischemia can produce pain in the rectum. But while the pain fibers in the rest of the bowel are a part of the sympathetic system, those of the rectum follow parasympathetic pathways. It appears, in fact, that all afferent fibers of the rectum belong to the parasympathetic system.

Muscular Afferent Fibers

Various authors have reported finding stretch receptors in the sphincter ani externus and levator ani muscles [9, 10]. The interaction of these receptors with the visceral afferent fibers, reflex arcs, and the motor nerve supply of the external sphincter and levator are responsible for neuromuscular continence. It should be remembered, however, that the pars pelvina of the rectum with its visceral afferent fibers can be completely resected without causing significant disturbances of defecation and continence. It may be concluded then that the pars pelvina and particularly its visceral afferent fibers are not essential for defecation and continence. As mentioned earlier, the puborectalis muscle appears to play a crucial role in maintaining continence. Even in the absence of a normal anal canal, and internal and external sphincter, the sensory and motor capabilities of an intact puborectalis sling are sufficient to provide an acceptable degree of continence in conjunction with the reservoir function of the neorectum.

Blood Supply (Fig. 1.12)

Blood is supplied to the rectum at three levels, all of which interconnect through functional anastomoses. The upper level is formed by the unpaired superior rectal artery, a large terminal branch of the inferior mesenteric. At the middle level, the rectum is supplied by the left and right middle rectal arter-

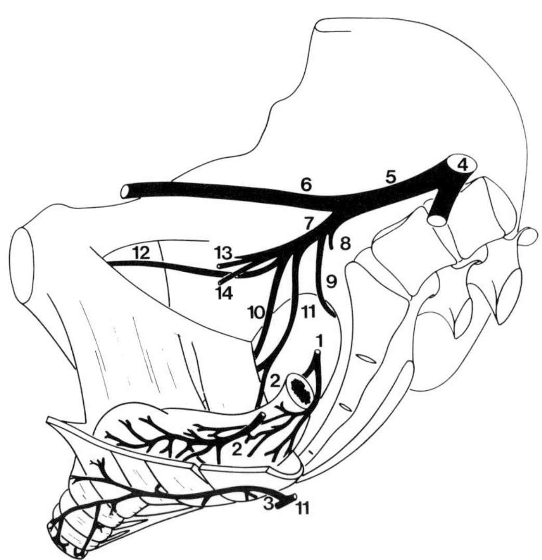

Fig. 1.12. Blood supply. *1,* Superior rectal artery; *2,* middle rectal artery; *3,* inferior rectal artery; *4,* aorta; *5,* common iliac artery; *6,* external iliac artery; *7,* internal iliac artery; *8,* lateral sacral artery; *9,* superior gluteal artery; *10,* inferior gluteal artery; *11,* internal pudendal artery; *12,* obdurator artery; *13,* superior vesical artery with obliterated umbilical ligament; *14,* inferior vesical artery

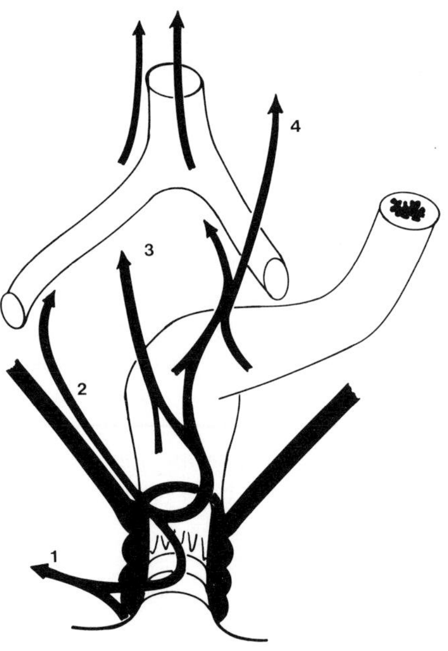

Fig. 1.13. Lymphatic drainage. *1,* To ischiorectal and inguinal nodes; *2,* to nodes of lateral zone of Miles and iliac nodes; *3,* to iliac and para-aortal/caval nodes; *4,* to inferior mesenteric and para-aortal/caval nodes

ies. At the lower level, the inferior rectal artery supplies the rectum, the anal region, the external sphincters, and the levator ani.

Lymphatic Drainage (Fig. 1.13)

The lymphatic vessels of the rectum form an expansive, coherent network. Lymph from the region of the anus drains to the inguinal lymph nodes. Lymph drainage from the pars perinealis of the anal canal occurs mainly along the inferior rectal and pudendal vessels, while lymph from the lower portion of the pars pelvina drains mainly along the middle rectal vessels to the internal iliac nodes. Lymph from the upper parts of the rectum drains along the superior rectal vessel to the para-aortic lymph nodes.

Anatomical Specimens and Drawings. All the illustrations are based upon specimens prepared at the Institute of Topographic and Clinical Anatomy of the Department of Surgery of the University of Basel. Working with A. von Hochstetter, specimens were selected, prepared, and then utilized to work out the relevant details. The illustrations were drawn by the author.

References

1. Deucher F (1976) Rund um den Sphinkter: Kontinenzprobleme in der Dickdarmchirurgie. Schweiz Med Wochenschr 106: 273–281
2. Dickinson VA (1978) Maintenance of anal continence: a review of pelvic floor physiology. Gut 19: 1163–1174
3. Goligher JC (1980) Surgery of the anus, colon and rectum, 4th edn. Baillière Tindall, London
4. Gorsch RV (1941) Perineopelvic anatomy from the proctologist's viewpoint. Tilgman, New York
5. Harris LD, Winans CS, Pope CE (1966) Determination of yield pressure: a method for measuring anal sphincter competence, Gastroenterology 50: 754
6. Holl M (1897) Die Muskeln und Faszien des Beckenausganges. In: Bardeleben K (ed) Handbuch der Anatomie des Menschen, vol 7. Fischer, Jena
7. Huber A, Allgöwer M, von Hochstetter A (1984) Transsphincteric surgery of the rectum. Springer, Berlin Heidelberg New York
8. Ihre T (1974) Studies of anal function in continent and incontinent patients. Scand J Gastroenterol 9: 1–64
9. Kerremans R (1969) Morphological and physiological aspects of anal continence and defaecation. Arscia, Brussel
10. Lane R, Parks AG (1977) Function of the anal sphincters following colo-anal anastomosis. Br J Surg 64: 596–599
11. Lawson J (1981) Motor nerve supply of pelvic floor. Lancet: 999
12. Percy J et al. (1981) Electrophysiological study of motor nerve supply of the pelvic floor. Lancet: 16–17
13. Shepherd JJ (1980) Anorectal function. In: Sircus W, Smith AN (eds) Scientific foundations of gastroenterology. Heinemann, London
14. Stephens FD, Smith ED (1971) Ano-rectal malformations in children. Chicago Year Book, Chicago
15. Uhlenhuth E (1953) Problems in the anatomy of the pelvis. Lippincott, Philadelphia
16. Waldeyer W (1899) Das Becken. Cohen, Bonn
17. Walls EW (1959) Recent observations on the anatomy of the anal canal. Proc R Soc Med (Suppl) 52: 85–87
18. Wilson PM (1977) Anorectal closing mechanisms. S Afr Med J 51: 802–808
19. Winckler G (1958) Remarques sur la morphologie et l'inervation du muscle releveur de l'anus. Arch Anat Histol Embryol (Strasb) 41: 77–95

2 Symptomatology of Anorectal Diseases

J.-C. Givel

Introduction

Patients suffering from anorectal disorders often complain of vague symptoms. A detailed description of these symptoms must therefore be obtained so that they may be associated with a precise anatomic location to provide a basis for appropriate examinations and a reliable diagnosis. Even without a specific association with a particular location, numerous symptoms nevertheless suggest a probable site of origin. The proctologic history is therefore of great importance (see Chapter 3). The circumstances in which a symptom appears, its localisation, its development, the appearance of secondary associated complaints, and their exact characteristics should all be ascertained in detail.

A distinction must be made between general symptoms and specifically proctologic disorders. Only the latter will be treated in this chapter. There are a total of eight principal symptoms due to anorectal disorders:

- Rectal bleeding
- Pruritus ani
- Pain
- Discharge
- Incontinence
- Diarrhea
- Constipation
- False need to defecate

Rectal Bleeding

A symptom found most frequently in conjunction with pruritus, rectal bleeding is also the least specific. Most lesions of the anorectal region and the alimentary canal may bleed at some time (Table 2.1). The phenomenon may be occult, appearing without the patient's knowledge, or apparent and symptomatic.

Bleeding of less than 50 ml/24 h originating from a source proximal to the splenic flexure cannot be detected macroscopically. It comes to light when examining the feces for occult blood. This complaint can be identified outside the clinical environment

Table 2.1. Most common causes of rectal bleeding

1. General	
Disorders of hematic origin	Blood disorders
	Medication
	Hepatic/renal insufficiency
	Malabsorption
2. Local	
Perianal	Cutaneous lesion
	Fissure
	Prolapse
	Condyloma
	Tumor
	Traumatic lesion
Anal canal	Hemorrhoids
	Prolapse
	Ulceration
	Tumor
	Traumatic lesion
Colorectal	Polyps
	Angiodysplasia
	Inflammatory colitis:
	Ischemic colitis
	Infectious and parasitic colitis
	Postactinic colitis
	Diverticulitis
	Tumor
	Traumatic lesion
Small bowel	Crohn's disease
	Meckel's diverticulum
	Ischemic lesion
	Tumor
	Traumatic lesion
Gastroduodenal	Mucosal erosion
	Ulcer
	Tumor
	Traumatic lesion

by a simple examination that patients may perform themselves (the Hemoccult test).

The rectal bleeding may be of variable intensity, a characteristic which provides valuable information on the origin of the hemorrhage. The duration of the phenomenon, the color of the blood, its quantity, frequency of emission, and possible relationship to defecation should be precisely determined. Slight bleeding, isolated or repeated, is often encountered in adults of all ages. Many do not initially consult a physician and mention this symptom only during a systematic anamnesis. In contrast, major hemorrhages, sometimes accompanied by shock, present urgent problems and oblige the physician to resort to complementary methods of diagnosis.

In most cases, blood mixed with stools originates from a tumor of the rectosigmoid region. In general, blood which precedes defecation or is spontaneously discharged has accumulated in the rectal ampulla; a phenomenon of this kind is found in ulcerative colitis, for example. Rectal bleeding with pain in the left iliac fossa is often due to a sigmoidal lesion, which may be segmental colitis, diverticulitis, or a tumor. Bleeding associated with diarrhea is encountered in ulcerative colitis, Crohn's disease, and tumors of the rectosigmoid junction; bleeding diarrhea indicates ulcerative colitis or Crohn's disease located in the colon. A dysentery-like syndrome associated with elimination of fragments of the colon wall may accompany cancer, sigmoiditis, or acute dysentery. Dark blood indicates a lesion situated in the colon or upper rectum, especially if it is mixed with the stools. The dark color in general indicates not only the localization of the hemorrhage but also the duration of its passage.

Massive hemorrhage of the distal gastrointestinal tract may be due to angiodysplasia or a diverticular disorder. It may also be caused by inflammatory conditions, tumors, or an ischemic lesion of the colon. Melena, characterized by the discharge of liquid, blackish, and putrid motions, is due to partially digested blood which has been in the bowel for at least 8 h. It usually originates from a site proximal to the hepatic flexure of the colon.

Bleeding associated with perianal pain appearing during or after defecation, especially when the region is washed, is due to perianal infections involving erosions or rhagades. A traumatic lesion of the rectum may give rise to isolated hemorrhages which are usually extensive, sometimes starting during a motion and subsequently repeated with the emission of pure blood without any fecal evacuation. Injury due to an endorectal thermometer or postactinic proctitis are two examples of such lesions.

Blood originating from the lower rectum or anus is clearer, not mixed with the stools but covering them, suggesting blood from a wound. It can be observed in the toilet bowl after defecation. Although it generally originates from internal hemorrhoids, this origin can be determined with some certainly only after other possible causes have been eliminated. Diffuse proctitis may show similar symptoms.

A polyp, an adenoma, a villous tumor with slight secretion, and a minor slowly growing cancer are examples of secreting lesions which, when of small volume and at a sufficiently low location, may be the origin of blood observed in striae around the stools. It is rare, but not impossible, for an anal fissure to present a similar clinical picture.

Blood observed on toilet paper or the underclothes originates from a distal site below the sphincter, except where incontinence is present. It generally indicates a lesion of the anal verge or perianal region such as erosion, rhagade, prolapsed hemorrhoids, punctured perianal hematoma, fistula, fissure, or tumor. When associated with intense pain occurring during defecation or a few hours afterwards, the presence of blood presents a picture typical of an anal fissure. Traces of blood and pain occurring after a certain time has elapsed are sometimes due to an incomplete fistula. Intermittent hemorrhagic prolapses of which the patient is unaware, with spontaneous remission, may also be encountered. An external open hemorrhoidal thrombosis, lesions due to scratching, pruritus ani, ulcerations with various causes, and marginal ulcerated tumors may also bleed.

The indications presented so far are by no means absolute; there are exceptions. Thus a lesion at a high location may be responsible for an issue of blood not mixed with stools, whereas a disorder of the lower tract may produce dark blood. Blackish coagulates may originate from a rectal lesion with prolonged discharge, while fresh blood may, if the passage is accelerated, be of colonic origin. The age of the patient also plays a role and must be taken into account when investigating the cause of rectal bleeding.

The general symptoms associated with bleeding, such as a modification of the habitual motions, abdominal pain, and disturbance of the general state of health (anorexia and loss of weight) suggest a systemic disorder in which an anal origin is highly unlikely. A discharge of mucus may be encountered in both anal and systemic conditions. An extensive discharge of phlegm often accompanies a villous tumor.

A perineal examination, rectal palpation, and a procto- or sigmoidoscopy should always be performed in the case of any rectal bleeding. A rigid rectoscope is used for systematic examinations, a flexible sigmoidoscope being reserved for situations in which a left colonic lesion, in particular a neoplastic one, is suspected. Colonoscopy allows diagnosis of small or superficial lesions, such as an inflammatory condition or angiodysplasia. A barium enema is performed as a matter of routine for inflammatory and neoplastic conditions. In the case of massive hemorrhage when colonoscopy proves negative, angiography should be considered. This examination, in addition to scintigraphy with red marker globules, allows the origin of a severe hemorrhage to be localized in most cases. After an origin in the upper digestive tract has been ruled out, the most probable diagnosis is angiodysplasia or possibly some other vascular malformations. A barium enema constitutes the examination of choice when a colonoscopy proves negative in the presence of minor hemorrhage.

Pruritus Ani

A symptom more frequently dermatologic or psychogenic rather than truly proctologic, pruritus is nevertheless characteristic of numerous anorectal disorders. Distinct from pain and of variable intensity, it may be intermittent. It may occur at night and not infrequently disturbs sleep. The primary cause of pruritus ani may be local or secondary to incontinence. It may also be the manifestation of a systemic condition (Table 2.2).

The fecal bacteria produce irritant metabolites. Transpiration or insufficient anal hygiene may thus result in maceration and cutaneous excoriations. Once the skin of the perianal region is damaged, a vicious circle is established. Itching gives rise to excessive scratching which in turn aggravates the epithelial lesions. As soon as the natural resistance of the perianal skin to infection is lowered, it is vulnerable to attack by saprophytic bacteria and cutaneous fungi, resulting in dermatitis. A detailed description of the pathogenesis and pathological physiology of pruritus ani can be found in Chap. 30.

Dermatoses, contact dermatitis, and various perianal lesions represent the most frequent causes of anal pruritus. The majority of cases are due to inadequate anal cleanliness, in particular after defecation. All conditions producing permanent perianal wetting may be a cause: hirsutism, excessive sweating, vaginal discharge, urinary incontinence, third-degree hemorrhoids, mucous prolapse, purulent discharge from a fistula or para-anal abscess, and frequent defecation, particularly with diarrheic stools. Excessive cleansing of the perianal region may also result in dermatitis leading to pruritus. Tightly fitting or synthetic clothing is sometimes responsible for this condition. In a number of cases, however, no causal factor can be found. Even though systemic disorders causing secondary cu-

taneous lesions rarely lead to anal pruritus, an attempt should be made to look for diabetes, intestinal helminthiasis, lice, anogenital herpes, molluscum contagiosum, a tendency to eczema, fungus infection, icterus, myelopathy, and blood disorders.

Pruritus occurring at night suggests parasitic infestation due to worms. These are sometimes found in other members of the family. A history of anogenital contact may provide relevant indications. Pruritus and a burning sensation associated with discharge are typical of humid eczema, a fistula, anusitis with hypersecretion of the anal glands, or ulcerative colitis. Pruritus, a burning sensation, and secretions combined with pain and the sensation of a foreign body are typical of a strangulated prolapse.

In evaluating the condition of a patient presenting with anal pruritus, any possible allergies should be identified. The physician will look into the use of suppositories or the application of local preparations. Local steroids affect the long-term natural re-

Table 2.2. Most common causes of pruritus ani

1. Primary	
Dermatosis	Eczema
	Psoriasis
	Lichen planus
	Allergic eruption
Perianal lesion	
Contact dermatitis	Local anesthetic
	Antibiotic ointment
Local	Fissure
	Crohn's disease
	Tumor
Infection	Fungus
	Worms
	Sexually transmitted disease
2. Secondary	
Irritative cutaneous lesion	
Transpiration	Inadequate anal hygiene
	Hirsutism
Mucus	Excessive production
	Prolapse
Pus	Anal fistula
Stools	Diarrhea
	Incontinence
	Inadequate anal hygiene
Systemic disorder	Diabetes
	Infectious disease
	Obstructive jaundice
	Myeloproliferative disorder
	Lymphoma
Idiopathic origin	
Psychogenic origin	

sistance of the skin to fungus infections. Local antibiotics and anesthetics increase skin sensitivity. The most serious perianal dermitites can result from abuse of such preparations.

The general examination will rule out dermatosis or systemic disorders. During an anal inspection, the physician will look particularly for cutaneous irritation, wetting, eruption, discharge, soiling, maceration, excoriation or eruption, excrescence, prolapse, or pain suggesting a fissure or fistula. Fecal soiling may be brought to light by wiping the region with a white tampon. The presence of worms is determined by microscopic examination of a biopsy taken from the perianal skin, which will reveal any eggs. Rectal palpation and endoscopic examinations may show sphincteric insufficiency, fistula, and hemorrhoids, as well as rectal lesions producing mucus. Biopsies should be taken after examination for bacteria and fungus, and serological tests made if a sexually transmitted disease is suspected. A microbiologic examination of the stools should be performed if there is diarrhea; a biopsy is taken from a rectal lesion and the anorectal physiology examined in patients with sphincter disorder.

Pain

Perineal pain is a complaint often encountered in proctologic practice. It is an expression of a disorder of the anus, rectum, or a pelvic structure. Its precise localization, whether superficial or deep, sometimes presents difficult problems of evaluation which may lead to errors of diagnosis and treatment.

The patient often has difficulty in stating the location and character of perineal pain with precision. An in-depth examination alone permits the exact site of its origin to be determined. The term "pain" is necessarily subjective and has a very wide range of meanings for different individuals. It is thus of great importance to obtain a detailed description, in particular of factors such as its periodicity, intensity, possible aggravating or alleviating circumstances, the duration of the symptoms, and all relationships to defecation and sexual intercourse.

Severe pain, generally aggravated by defecation, is most commonly due to an acute fissure, an anorectal abscess possibly complicated by a fistula, a perianal hematoma, a thrombosed perianal varix, or thrombosed and prolapsed internal hemorrhoids. The pain caused by a hematoma is very acute. If it becomes progressively worse, it indicates an abscess. A fissure is classically characterized by rhyth-

mic pain in three phases during the passage of stools: the absence of pain prior to evacuation, painful defecation, followed by the progressive disappearance of the pain after the motion. Less common causes of pain are condylomata acuminata, herpes, Crohn's disease, or a tumor. In all these cases, an ulcerated lesion, inflammation, infection, or invasion of nervous tissues may give rise to severe pain. Solitary ulcers of the rectum and proctalgia fugax may also be the origin of perineal pain not easily associated to a specific part of the system. Finally, certain patients suffer from persistent pain of the anus or the deep perineum without any apparent cause being found. Perineal pain can sometimes last for many years and be accompanied by major personality disorders or symptoms such as irritable colon.

A burning pain is characteristic of an inflammatory process such as dermatosis or anusitis. Constant or intermittent pain associated with a stinging sensation is encountered in infections of the anal canal, such as cryptitis, abscess, carcinoma, or thrombosis of internal hemorrhoids, and these lesions may produce a feeling of harboring a painful foreign body. Acute searing pain occurring during or after defecation is typical of a fissure. Dull pain in the anal canal, aggravated by defecation, is characteristic of cryptitis. A tension pain associated with a swelling in the anus indicates hemorrhoidal thrombosis or para-anal abscess. Painful defecation with tenesmus is typical of sphincter spasms. Very violent cramping pains originating from deep within the rectum, which may occur at any time but mainly at night, are typical of proctalgia fugax.

Apart from a local examination and endoscopy, investigation of perineal pain will include examination of the adjacent nonanorectal structures. In the absence of any apparent pathology, it is important to obtain information about the patient's medical history relating to a possible trauma, pelvic operation, or prior treatment of an anal lesion (Table 2.3).

Discharge

Discharge or a sensation of wetness in the perianal region is associated with a local cutaneous or mucosal inflammation. The most common cause is an organic disorder, but inadequate anal hygiene is often at the root of the problem in many inividuals. The unpleasant smell due to discharge often represents the main reason for consultation.

The precise nature of the discharge must be determined, as well as its site of origin and the presence

Table 2.3. Most common causes of perineal pain

Perianal region	Thrombosed varix
	Hematoma
	Fissure
	Condylomata acuminata
	Tumor
	Herpes
Anus	Cryptitis
	Acute abscess
	Chronic abscess
	Thrombosed and prolapsed hemorrhoids
	Crohn's disease
	Tumor
Rectum	Solitary ulcer
	Tumor
	Invagination
Pelvic floor	Proctalgia fugax
	Idiopathic pain
Nonproctologic origin	Gynecologic
	Urologic
	Musculoskeletal
	Neurologic

Table 2.4. Most common causes of discharge

Perianal	Transpiration
	Inadequate anal hygiene
	Cutaneous excoriation
	Eczema
	Fissure
	Condylomata acuminata
	Tumor
	Abscess
	Fistula
	Furuncle
Anal	Condylomata acuminata
	Hemorrhoids
	Mucosal prolapse
	Fistula
	Abscess
	Incontinence
Colorectal	Prolapse of the rectum
	Inflammatory disease
	Solitary ulcer
	Adenoma
	Irritable colon

of any associated symptoms such as pruritus, rectal bleeding, pain, or prolapse. Discharge may be aqueous, mucoid, purulent, or fecal. It may originate from the anal verge, the anal canal, or the rectum.

Direct examination, a complete anorectal inspection possibly including the colon, as well as serologic or microbiologic examinations generally reveal the origin of the discharge. In certain cases, however, this may be difficult to find or may remain obscure. Fecal soiling of the underclothes, for example, the most banal discharge possible, may have no apparent origin.

There may be various causes of discharge (Table 2.4):

- *Medical:* cutaneous lesion, fistula, inflammatory disease of the rectum, infectious anorectitis, hemorrhoidal prolapse, rectal prolapse
- *Surgical:* complications arising from interventions in the rectum and anus

An aqueous discharge indicates an irritation of the anal glands associated with anusitis or a villous adenoma. A clear, viscous discharge issues from the rectal epithelium when a prolapse or a solitary ulcer is present. A brownish discharge mixed with stools is found mainly in cases of sphincter incontinence. A purulent discharge originates from a fistula. A partially bloody mucopurulent discharge indicates colitis. A discharge tinged with blood is found in the presence of prolapsed hemorrhoids, a mucous or intestinal prolapse, and in ulcerative colitis. Ooz-

ing from a bleeding wound is frequently seen after the Whitehead operation with protrusion of the rectal mucosa, as well as after a hemorrhoidectomy performed by the Milligan-Morgan method. After this type of intervention, cicatrization may take a long time. A bloody discharge associated with pruritis, a burning feeling associated with the sensation of a foreign body, and pain indicate a strangulated prolapse.

Among less common organic causes are small abscesses of the posterior end of the anal canal with no perceptible track toward the anal verge, as well as excessive secretion of the subpectineal anal glands. Both phenomena are difficult to determine. The secretion of these glands may explain why a patient complains of minor oozing producing a sensation of constant wetness. In parting the folds of the anal verge, a minuscule orifice may be found in the subpectinal mucous zone within the anal canal. Distal pressure of the finger at this point produces a drop of pus, or more frequently a clear liquid like a drop of dew. The secretion is minimal and does not occur again during the same examination. Another rare cause of discharge is represented by voluminous internal nonprolapsing hemorrhoids. Finally, fecal oozing often occurs in the absence of any organic cause. It is a functional problem indicating a mini-incontinence. Clinical or electromanometric examination will often show a minor sphincter deficiency in patients whose anal verge is slightly soiled, often without their knowledge.

Incontinence

Anal incontinence is a very debilitating symptom to which sufferers do not readily admit, as it could lead to rejection by the family and society in general. By questioning the patient, a precise determination can be made of the severity of this defect, the consistency of the stools, the presence of any associated diarrhea as well as the patient's previous surgical history, in particular operations for anal fistulas or obstetric lesions. Any medication taken, radiotherapy, as well as indications of spinal or perineal trauma are also investigated. This information may permit the physician to differentiate between discharge and fecal incontinence. Patients frequently confuse the two symptoms. The severity of the phenomenon can be evaluated from the frequency of incontinence and the consistency of the discharged matter, which may range from simple oozing, emission of gas, or occasional soiling of underclothes to the involuntary emission of a fecal bolus several times per day. The consistency of the stools – aqueous, semi-solid, or firm – is of importance. The frequency and urgency of defecation may also be due to certain types of diarrhea. Finally, the physician will investigate the possibility of voluntary defecation and the circumstances under which uncontrolled evacuation may occur.

Diarrhea represents the most frequent cause of incontinence. This problem may even be found in a patient with intact sphincteric function when urgent need to defecate results in the passage of a liquid motion. Incontinence may thus complicate any condition at all associated with diarrhea.

Anal incontinence may have various causes (Table 2.5). Sphincteric deficiency may be due to muscular weakness, such as the dystrophy observed in association with a generalized neurologic disorder. Progressive dystrophy of the anal sphincter represents a normal consequence of aging and speeds up after the age of 70 years. A similar type of diffuse dystrophy may also be observed among younger patients suffering from low motor neuropathy affecting the muscles of the pelvic floor, for example in diabetics. Anal incontinence may also complicate fecal impaction when the distension of the rectum produces a reflex relaxation of the internal sphincter.

The sphincter mechanism may be damaged during trauma or surgical intervention. Surgery for an anal fissure represents the most frequent cause of traumatic incontinence. Incontinence is also observed when the anal sphincter is bypassed by a fistula from the rectum opening to the outside above the

Table 2.5. Most common causes of incontinence

Diarrhea	Inflammatory disease
	Infectious disease
	Solitary ulcer of the rectum
	Tumor
Neurologic disorder	Psychiatric disorder
	Senility
	Generalized neuropathy
	Localized neuropathy
	(pelvic floor)
	Diabetes
	Descended perineum
	Spinal trauma
Prolapse of the rectum	
Fecal impaction	
Fistula	Rectovaginal
	Anorectal
Trauma	Injury
	Surgical sequela
	Obstetric sequela

anorectal junction. Rectovaginal or extrarectal fistulas in contact with the perineum may be congenital or acquired, in the latter case resulting from a trauma or from specific disorders, or as a result of radiotherapy for carcinoma of the uterine cervix. Anal incontinence is also observed after medullary trauma with lesion of the cauda equina.

An examination will include inspection of any perianal soiling, any orifice, deformation, prolapse, or perineal scar. Absence of the radiating folds in a quadrant of the anal circumference is of great interest. Voluntary contraction of the perineum allows the strength of the skeletal muscles to be evaluated. By asking the patient to strain, an abnormal perineal descent or even a prolapse may be observed. A digital examination begins by palpation of the pelvic muscles. The tonus of the sphincters and the anal levator is determined and the response to voluntary contraction and to the coughing reflex also tested. Finally, any persistent gaping of the anus after removal of the finger is noted. An investigation of incontinence will inevitably include an examination of the anorectal physiology, in particular by manometry and electromyography.

Diarrhea

In general, the various types of diarrhea are due to an infectious or functional disorder of the gastrointestinal tract. They may, however, also accompany a specific colorectal disease. Symptoms of this kind may stem from an inflammatory disorder or an obstruction. Excessive production of mucus by a tumor or a solitary ulcer of the rectum may also produce diarrhea.

The term "diarrhea" is often used incorrectly by patients who give it various meanings: increased frequency of defecation, reduction of the consistency of the stools, an urgent need to defecate, or incontinence. Each of the associated symptoms must consequently be distinguished and precisely defined. Frequent passage of urine or stools may be due to diarrhea, but could equally well be caused by the elimination of an excessive quantity of mucus or pus. A solitary ulcer of the rectum sometimes gives rise to episodes of a false need to defecate. An urgent need to defecate often cannot be controlled and is accompanied by incontinence. Finally, we should not forget that fecal impaction represents a classical association of diarrhea and an episode of constipation (Table 2.6).

The patient's medical history allows the character of the diarrhea, any triggering factor or contamination, as well as the previous medical, surgical, or radiologic history to be precisely defined. Other associated signs or symptoms such as the presence of blood or mucus in the stools, a modification of the general state of health, or pain should also be sought.

Constipation

The term "constipation" is also understood somewhat differently by different individuals. Most of the time, it indicates poor bowel function. It may describe the regular elimination of hard stools or irregular passage of stools of normal consistency. Patients sometimes suffer from headaches; flatulence and anorexia are occasionally ascribed to constipation.

Constipation is generally due to a localized lesion producing an obstruction or a functional anomaly of the bowel and slowing the passage of fecal matter. The proctologic origins generally relate to bowel obstruction. More rarely, patients may have normal times of bowel passage but a functional disorder of rectal evacuation. Some constipated patients develop a perineal descent syndrome and a solitary ulcer of the rectum.

Patients suffering from constipation due to obstruction generally have a short medical history, whereas those with a problem of functional origin require a longer anamnesis.

Difficulty in defecation with a prolonged need to strain is frequently due to megarectum. A history of this kind will often have its origins in childhood

Table 2.6. Most common causes of diarrhea

Inflammatory
  Infectious
  Noninfectious
Excessive production of mucus
Digestive insufficiency
Malabsorption
Metabolic disease
Functional disorder
Medication
Psychologic cause
Mechanical obstacle

and is associated with frequent episodes of fecal impaction and soiling. Many patients suffering from defecation problems show an absence or rectal or colonic distension coupled with an excessive need to strain when passing motions. Several attempts to defecate generally end in incomplete evacuation. The number of daily sessions on the toilet and their duration should be precisely determined.

Consideration should also be given to any changes in lifestyle or dietary habits, pregnancy, general or psychiatric complaints, as well as ingestion of certain medicaments (Table 2.7).

False Need to Defecate

The false need to defecate is a symptom which produces pathologic evacuation instead of true defecation. It therefore indicates a need which is not totally false, but is both urgent and repeated. The patient often feels the need to evacuate gas. He or she may additionally produce a phlegmatic or phlegmatic-bloody evacuation or even pass pure blood.

Table 2.7. Most common causes of constipation

Local lesions	Tumor
	Diverticulitis
	Crohn's disease
	Stenosis
	Intussusception
	Rectocele
Functional disorder of the bowel	Megacolon
	Irritable colon
	Psychologic disorder
	Pregnancy
	Medication
	Systemic disorder
	Immobilization
	Dyschezia

Defined in this way, the false need to defecate represents a specific organic symptom. It may be due to a local or diffuse lesion of the rectum or the rectosigmoid, classically a rectal tumor.

Conclusion

Depending on their presence or absence, the characteristic signs or symptoms of anorectal disorders allow the examining physician to determine one or more specific sites of origin. These symptoms are listed together in Table 2.8 as a function of three relevant localizations: the anal verge, the anal canal, and the rectosigmoid junction.

Table 2.8. Most common locations of anorectal symptoms

	Anal verge	Anal canal	Recto-sigmoid
Rectal bleeding	×	×	×
Discharge	×	×	
Wetting	×		
Incontinence		×	
Pruritus ani	×		
Pain	×	×	×
Diarrhea			×
Constipation			×
False need to defecate			×
Burning	×		
Spasm (tenesmus)		×	×
Incomplete evacuation			×
Sensation of a foreign body	×		

3 The Proctological Examination

J.-C. Givel

Introduction

"More is missed by not looking than by not knowing." This statement by Thomas McCrae (1870–1935) underlines the paramount importance of clinical examination in protological diagnosis. Although a proctological consultation may well represent a routine professional activity for the doctor, it is quite otherwise for the patient. He or she often finds a procedure of this kind difficult to cope with, particularly if it is the first time. There are various personal, psychological, and social reasons for the interval of time, which may be quite long, elapsing between the appearance of the first symptoms and the proctological consultation. Likewise it is not uncommon, even at the present time, for patients to be subjected to a prolonged treatment for a proctological complaint without any prior local examination being made. This is why advanced lesions may sometimes be discovered at the specialist's initial consultation.

A proctological consultation is much like any other medical work-up comprising a record of the patient's medical history, general and local examination, and various supplementary examinations. Numerous proctological diagnoses may be made on the basis of the medical history and local findings without the need for any complex or time-consuming procedures.

Medical History

The first step is to have the patient describe the exact nature of the complaint, in particular the circumstances in which it occurred and the nature of the symptoms which have led him or her to seek treatment. It is important to question the patient about any loss of blood, discharge, incontinence, anal irritation, perineal pain, diarrhea, constipation, or a false need the defecate. Personal habits or unusual sexual practices may be relevant in some cases. Information on the patient's personal history, together with any earlier proctological or general conditions with possible effects in the anorectal region complete the record. Medication and obstetrical histories are often relevant too. Finally, a note should be made of the family medical history with the aim of determining the presence of any hereditary conditions.

General Examination

All proctological examinations start with a quick inspection aimed at determining any changes in the patient's general state of health or any associated symptoms. Particular attention is given to the digestive system, the skin, the mucosa, and the urogenital system. Examination of the nervous system may be indicated, for instance, in patients with continence problems.

Proctological Examination

It is absolutely essential to explain to the patient beforehand all the aspects of the proctological examination. This comprises the following phases:

- Inspection and palpation
- Rectal examination
- Endoscopy

Position of the Patient

Several positions may be used for a proctological examination. The choice of position depends on the equipment available, the age of the patient, and his or her state of health, als well as the doctor's preferences. The position adopted should be comfortable for the patient and the examining doctor, allowing him or her to carry out an effective inspection and to perform certain diagnostic activities, possibly therapeutic ones as well.

In a nonspecialist's consulting room, in the absence of suitable equipment, the examination is carried out in the left lateral or genucubital position. The left lateral (Sims's) position is comfortable for the patient. Since it avoids undue embarrassment, it is also the position of choice for older patients. Lying on the left side, the patient is positioned so that the trunk crosses the top of the couch obliquely at a 45° angle. The buttocks project slightly beyond the edge of the table, and the thighs are flexed so as to form an angle of about 90° with the trunk. This position allows the perianal and sacral regions to be comfortably examined, whereas the anterior perineum is masked from view. It allows an excellent proctological examination as well as certain endoscopic and therapeutic interventions (Fig. 3.1).

The genucubital position allows an excellent inspection of the perineal, sacral, and posterior perineal regions without any specialized aids. The patient kneels, the trunk leaning forward and supported by the forearms. This is a convenient position for the examining doctor, who parts the buttocks in a manner allowing complete observation of the anus and perianal region. This position is equally convenient for performing a rigid sigmoidoscopy, in which case the rectosigmoid junction is approached via the anteroinferior ptosis of the sigmoid flexure (Fig. 3.2). This position is easily tolerated by young patients, but is not recommended for older patients or those suffering from cardiac or respiratory failure.

If the doctor has an adequate examination couch available, as in a specialized surgery or in a hospital, the lithotomy or genupectoral positions may be considered. The lithotomy or gynecological position requires the use of a table with supports for the lower limbs. The patient lies on his or her back with the buttocks projecting beyond the end of the table and the lower limbs raised above the trunk. This position, which is generally easily tolerated by the patient, allows a convenient examination of the perineum and the perianal region. The proctological investigation is performed under excellent conditions, with most diagnostic and therapeutic interventions being feasible. This is the position used for most surgical interventions in proctology, in particular with an anesthetized patient. Less convenient for an ingress via the rectosigmoid junction than an anterior position, it nevertheless allows sigmoidoscopy with a rigid tube (Fig. 3.3).

A proctological lesion is conventionally localized by reference to a "clock face" surrounding the perineum with the patient in the lithotomy position. Twelve o'clock is the anterior direction, 6 o'clock posterior, while 3 and 9 o'clock are situated, respectively, to the patient's right and left (Fig. 3.4).

The genupectoral position requires a special examination table. The patient lies on his or her chest

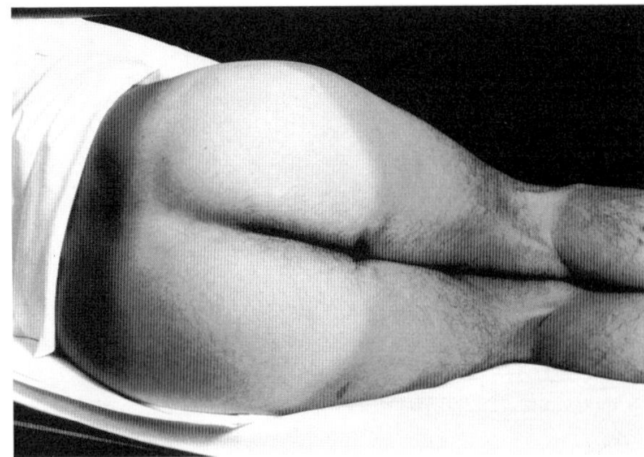

Fig. 3.1. Left lateral position

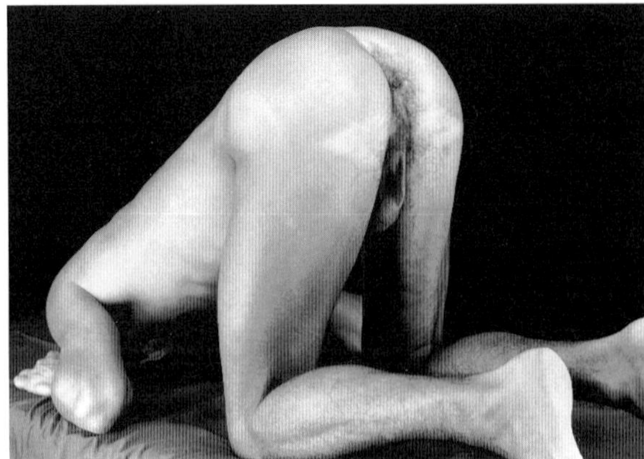

Fig. 3.2. Genucubital position

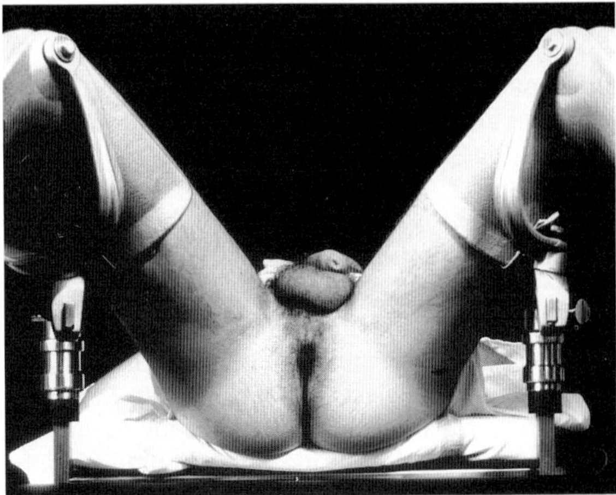

Fig. 3.3. Lithotomy or gynecological position

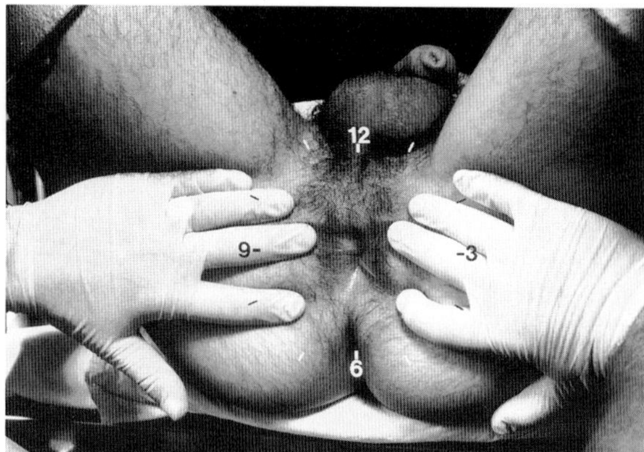

Fig. 3.4. Localisation of a proctological lesion

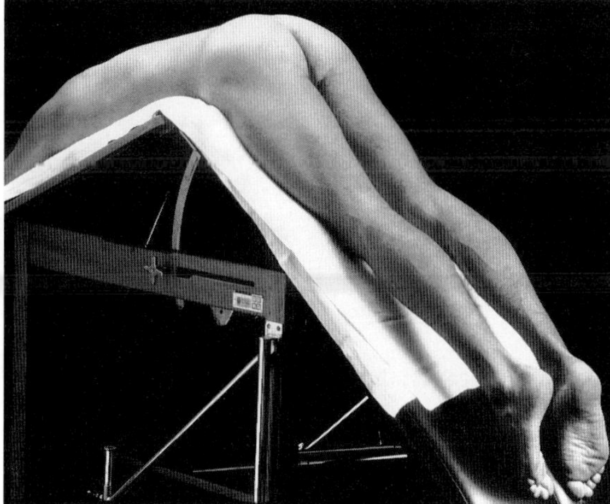

Fig. 3.5. Genupectoral position

(face down), the legs are supported, and there is a mechanism to ensure a 90° angle between the trunk and thighs. The perianal region is thus easy to observe, and examinations and treatments may be performed in conditions similar to those permitted by the genucubital position. This position is also indicated for anorectal surgery requiring a posterior approach (Fig. 3.5).

Inspection and Palpation

The proctological examination starts with a quick but complete inspection of the anus, the perianal region, and the adjacent perineum. All anomalies are noted, in particular the presence of scar tissue, any abnormal orifices, ulcerations, cutaneous lesions, swellings, or prolapses.

A scar generally indicates a previous operation or trauma. Often fibrous, this sequella causes a retraction of the adjacent tissues with a consequent modification or disappearance of the radiating folds of the anal margin. The entire anus may thus be drawn sideways toward a paramedian position. A scar should alert the physician to obtain a more precise proctological history and lead to a careful search for the nature of the pathological condition that caused it.

A para-anal orifice, solitary or multiple, generally represents the cutaneous end of a fistulous track. It is thus the external opening of a tract whose internal component can extend proximally as far as the pectinate line. Such a fistula, which may be simple or complex, represents the natural evolution of a trivial para-anal abscess. A lesion of this type, especially if present at several locations in the perianal region, should prompt a search for an inflammatory condition, particularly Crohn's disease of which it may sometimes be the first or sole apparent manifestation.

An ulceration is a break in the anal mucosa. Such a lesion, which may be shallow or deep, is often not initially apparent, being concealed under the radiating mucous folds. It can be clearly seen only by drawing back the skin of the perianal region. The most common type of ulceration is a fissure. Generally of a small dimension, solitary or multiple, a fissure may be acute or chronic. If acute, it is generally shallow and shaped like a segment of an orange, with a normal mucous lining. A history of acute pain, exacerbated by defecation, is usually diagnostic. A chronic lesion is deeper, showing the sphincterial muscle fibers at the base of a crater lined by a slightly fibrotic cicatricial mucosa. Sentinel piles or a skin tag frequently cover fissures of this kind.

Various dermatological lesions can be observed in the mucosa and the skin of the perianal region. Ranging from simple erythema to pseudotumoral growths, these may represent lesions specific to this region or, more frequently, a perianal localization of a systemic dermatological condition. Numerous proctological complaints are accompanied by cutaneous lesions, generally due to irritation. In practice, the underlying complaint often prevents correct perianal hygiene or gives rise to slight incontinence involving the discharge of irritating substances. Lesions due to scratching then invariably occur, adding to the basic problem.

A para-anal swelling is frequently encountered. It is the classic sign of a collection of fluid or a growth and is easy to recognize. If accompanied by inflammation, it indicates the presence of an abscess or a para-anal phlegmon which are both common and painful lesions. Benign or malignant tumors can be found at the anal margin or in the adjacent skin and may cause swelling.

A prolapse can occur when the patient is at rest or exerting an effort such as straining during defecation or coughing. It may be a superficial and exclusively mucosal phenomenon due to excessively abundant tissue. A prolapse may also occur due to growths such as internal hemorrhoids or neoplastic lesions of the rectum which have slipped through the anus. A complete, musculo-mucosal parietal prolapse may also be present, for example, in association with a rectal procidentia. It is not uncommon to observe an edematous component in conjunction with these lesions, especially when certain purplish zones represent thrombotic regions.

In contrast to inspection, palpation of the anal margin and the anterior and posterior poles does not involve drawing back the radiating folds. The induration of a sensitive fistulous track, which may be suspected by its exterior orifice or may even be totally blind, may thus be determined solely by feeling with the examining finger. The induration can generally be assumed to lie above the lesion, at least in part. At the posterior pole, a small infiltration may represent a prolongation of an infected fissure to the skin. In the anterior region, care must be taken not to confuse a fistulous track with the linear induration of the median raphe of the base of the scrotum.

Rectal Examination

Rectal examination is a simple examination requiring no more than a finger cot or a glove and a lubricant gel. It should always be performed when investigating a proctological problem. An effective examination provides information of the first order regarding both the morphology and content of the anus or rectum and the condition of the adjacent organs. It also permits the function of the neuromuscular structures involved in the mechanism of continence to be examined. Its only contraindications are, in some cases, certain acutely painful lesions of the anus.

The covered and lubricated index finger is inserted gently into the anus following the anatomical direction of the anal canal, advancing cranially along an axis toward the umbilicus in the lithotomy position. Six locations should be distinguished during rectal examination (Fig. 3.6):

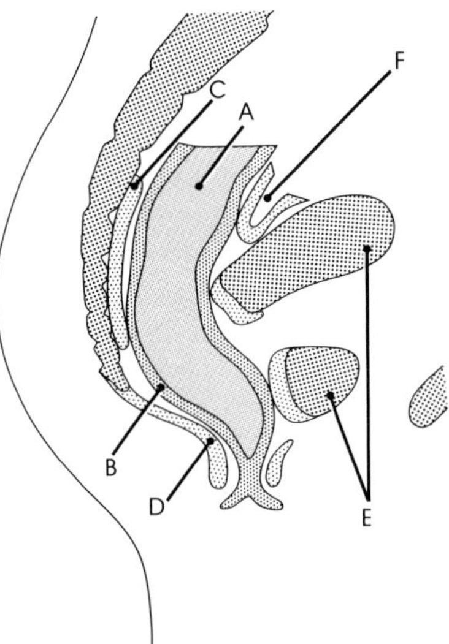

Fig. 3.6. Sites to be investigated during rectal examination (see text for details)

A. *Intestinal lumen* (anal and rectal): possible presence of feces, blood, or a foreign body.
B. *Wall* (mucosa and entire wall): palpable lesions, such as a polyp, a tumor, a diffuse inflammation of the mucosa, an ulceration, or an indurated zone, which may represent the thrombosis or sclerosis of old hemorrhoids.
C. *Behind the rectum:* through the rectal wall it is possible to feel the sacral concavity and coccyx and thus discover bone anomalies, adenopathies located in the perirectal fat, or occasionally tumors.
D. *Pelvic floor:* anal incontinence depends on the proper function of a dual mechanism: the puborectal sling, which maintains an adequate anorectal angulation, and the sphincter apparatus. The latter comprises two distinct muscles: a smooth internal one representing the caudal thickening of the intrinsic circular layer of the rectal muscles, and a striated external one capable of voluntary contraction. The morphology and function of these two structures can be checked during rectal examination. The puborectal sling can be palpated by a bidigital examination, the index finger pushing the puborectal muscle while the thumb is brought to meet it by an external route. Voluntary contraction may be tested by asking the patient to tense the anal muscles. The transition between internal and external sphincter muscles may also be palpated with the index finger when withdrawing it after completing the rectal examination. This exami-

nation therefore permits the doctor to note the tonus at rest, the presence or absence of voluntary contractions, and the coughing reflex. The function of these muscles may be tested by asking the patient to contract them. In this way it is sometimes possible to reveal indurations or swellings which are generally due to abscesses.

E. *In front of the rectum* (the region of the uterine cervix in females and the prostate in males: the presence, consistency, and morphology of any suspected tumoral abscesses or lesions of these two organs can be inspected through the rectal wall.

F. *Above the rectum:* palpation of the pouch of Douglas allows direct contact with the contents of the peritoneum, which are painful in certain circumstances, as well as with internal genital organs in females. An intestinal segment, for example, a colonic swelling associated with diverticulitis or Crohn's disease, may also be palpated.

Endoscopy

The proctological examination should be completed by an endoscopic investigation. This should include three procedures:

- Anuscopy
- Rectoscopy
- Sigmoidoscopy

Anuscopy allows the anal canal and the distal rectum to be examined. It does not require a specialist's knowledge and is within the capability of every general practitioner. Various anuscope models exist, made of both metal or disposable plastic and of various calibers and lengths. The light is provided by a cold lamp or by distal illumination located outside or inside the scope (Fig. 3.7).

The anuscope and its obturator are smeared with lubricant and introduced into the anal canal along an axis running from the anal margin to the umbilicus. This manipulation should not normally cause any pain and can be performed easily except when there is a strong reflex contraction of the sphincter due to a painful lesion of the anal canal (a fissure, for example). When the anuscope has reached the end of the rectum, its oburator is withdrawn and the light source adjusted. The last 8 cm of the alimentary canal are examined during the progressive withdrawal of this instrument. By twisting it in various directions, the walls and the anorectal lumen can be examined in detail. The rectum is characterized by fleshly mucous folds and a lumen which remains distended after the endoscope has been withdrawn. The pronounced parietal tonicity of the anal canal tends to expel the anuscope. The presence of the three venous plexuses corresponding to the sites of formation of internal hemorrhoids are observed at this point (at 3, 7, and 11 o'clock). The pectinate line, site of possible hypertrophied anal papillae, marks the transition between the rectal and anal mucosae.

Rectoscopy permits examination of the rectum and often of the distal part of the sigmoid. Metal or plastic (disposable) rigid rectoscopes usually have a diameter of 20 mm and a length of 20–25 cm. In

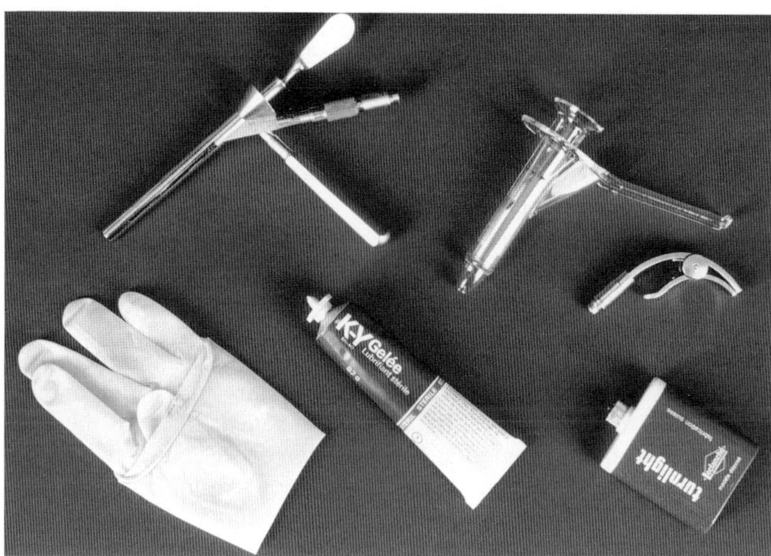

Fig. 3.7. Anuscopy equipment

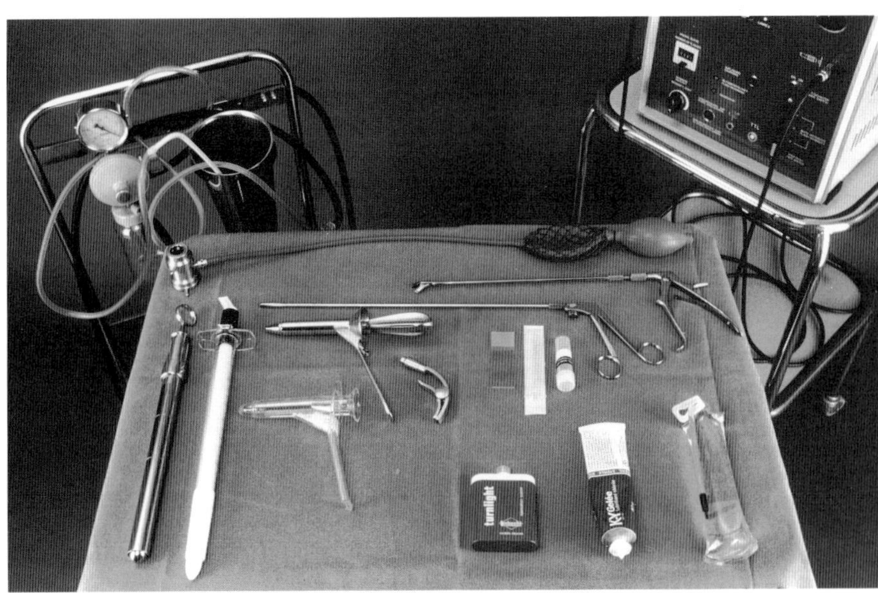

Fig. 3.8. Rectoscopy equipment

some cases, the rectosigmoid junction and certain constrictions can be traversed only by using a tube of smaller diameter. Illumination is provided by a cold light source and there is a lens attached to the external orifice of the rectoscope. Bellows connected to this orifice allow air to be insufflated so that the rectum can be distended to facilitate the passage of the instrument or to reveal certain regions which are not easily visible. A suction tube allows any endoluminal residues to be sucked out (Fig. 3.8).

The preparation for this examination varies according to individual preference. Some regard it as being contraindicated as it may mask important signs such as blood or mucus originating from a level higher than the one observed. It may also modify the nature of feces or any biopsies to be taken for bacteriological examination. For many, the routine preparation consists of a small enema of a hypertonic solution (120 ml sodium phosphate, for example) administered a few moments before the investigation.

The tube and its obturator are lubricated and gently inserted 5–8 cm through the sphincter of the anal canal, in the same direction as for anuscopy. When the instrument strikes a wall, the obturator is withdrawn, and the light and lens are installed. The tube is then advanced while examining the lumen and walls with small side-to-side movements, sometimes after insufflation of air. As little air as possible should be insufflated, and the advance must always be carefully controlled, never forcing against resistance at the risk of perforating the rectal wall. Simi-

larly, the advance must be interrupted if the patient complains of increasing pain. Houston's valves can be traversed by successively pressing them down. It may be necessary to retrace the path taken and to examine the crescent formed by the free edge of the valve to know in what direction to insert the tube.

At about 15 cm from the anal margin, the flexure of the rectosigmoid junction stops the advance of the rectoscope. One then looks for the small passage masked by a valve which is crossed under visual control. This is often a difficult moment and can cause extreme pain to the patient. In numerous subjects, this passage cannot be made with a rigid instrument. The walls of the rectal ampulla are sufficiently wide to form a cavity and contrast with those of the deeper-lying sigmoid, which is a portion of the colon folded back upon itself and not easy to illuminate.

The advance into the sigmoid must not be forced; if necassary, a fiber-optic sigmoidoscope may be used to explore this organ more extensively. The mean depth investigated during a rectoscopy is around 20 cm. The principal examination takes place during the withdrawal of the tube: an efficient retrograde helicoidal exploration will leave no mucosal surface unexamined. When examining a lesion during this procedure with the aim of performing a surgical excision for example, it should be remembered that the size of these structures is naturally increased by the bowel distension caused by the endoscope.

The examining doctor must have biopsy forceps available, allowing him or her to take mucosal and

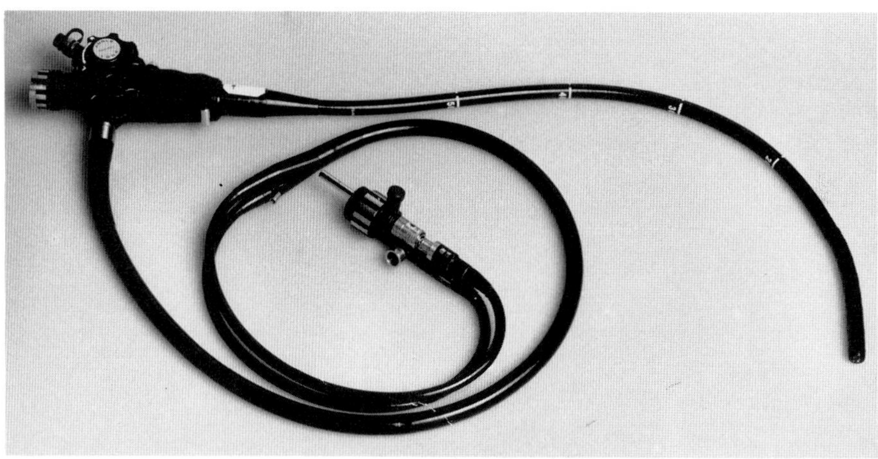

Fig. 3.9. Sigmoidoscope

submucosal samples. The tips of the forceps should not be too sharp, to avoid the risk of perforation. Several biopsies are taken during the investigation of a diffuse lesion. Problems of hemostasis and vascular lesions are contraindications to biopsy. After any biopsy, the bowel wall must be allowed to heal before performing a barium enema. This usually takes approximately 10 days. The two classic complications of biopsy are hemorrhage and perforation, but they are rare. Benign tumors, and sometimes small localized malignant ones, can be either excised or destroyed by endoscopic resection or electrocoagulation. Polyps in particular are usually treated in this manner.

Sigmoidoscopy using the fibroscope, a short variety of colonoscope (60 cm), permits the sigmoid as well as the entire left colon to be investigated. Sigmoidoscopes provide powerful suction and are designed to perform both wash-out and air insufflation, as well as allowing the use of biopsy forceps. These instruments are easy to handle and light. Preoperative preparation is identical to that for rectoscopy. Sigmoidoscopy therefore allows routine examinations to be made on an out-patient basis (Fig. 3.9).

Four times more neoplasms are discovered by sigmoidoscopy with a flexible tube than with a rigid one. The indication for this technique of investigation is thus very broad, particularly for patients over 40 years of age being investigated for a colorectal problem for the first time. The patient is placed in a left lateral position with the hips flexed slightly. The lubricated instrument is introduced into the anus by the right hand, while the left hand manipulates the controls. The technique of introducing the instrument and the examination are described in detail in the specialized literature on colonoscopy and requires practical instruction (see [1, 2]).

Complementary Examinations

Subsequent to clinical examination, various complementary examinations may be ordered. These are described in detail in Chaps. 4-7).

References

1. Cotton PB, Williams CB (1982) Practical gastrointestinal endoscopy, 2nd edn. Blackwell Scientific, Oxford
2. Pearl RK (1984) Gastrointestinal endoscopy for surgeons, 1st edn. Little, Brown, Boston

4 Microbiological Examinations

R. Auckenthaler

Introduction

Clinical Considerations. The anorectal region is exposed to regular bowel movements containing 10^{12} microorganisms per gram, so it seems extraordinary that it is not infected more frequently. The mechanical barrier of the mucosa seems to be essential for protection as, once there is a rupture and poor drainage, infection can readily occur. The anorectal region is not only exposed to fecal flora, but, since mankind has existed, also to sexually transmitted diseases. In the future the anorectal region might be increasingly protected from this type of infection, as one possibility of breaking the epidemiological chain of the AIDS pandemia is to change sexual practices and to use condoms.

Microbiological Considerations. As a rule, specimens to establish a diagnosis should be obtained before initiating or changing antibiotic therapy. In order to obtain reliable results, specimens must be collected in a manner that minimizes or avoids contamination. Collection with a swab contaminated with resident flora is generally less satisfactory than needle or catheter aspiration with a syringe: any pus of an abscess punctured in the perineal region will in general be due to one single microorganism, whereas a mixture of microorganisms points to an existing fistula. Specimens should be collected in sterile containers, and transfer or contact with anesthetic products or disinfectants sould be avoided [1, 3].
Direct examination with a Gram stain is often very useful for patient managment: however, it is only as reliable as the observer. As other more sensitive and precise diagnostic methods can be performed by the microbiologist, rapid transport to the microbiology laboratory is always recommended. Correctly labeled specimens and adequate information about the specimen and the clinical situation are mandatory to initiate the examination and culture procedures. Since the anorectal region is colonized by anaerobic bacteria, only abscess contents, deep-wounded aspirates, or surgical biopsy specimens should be processed for anaerobic culturing. Blood cultures should be limited to suspicion of systemic infection.

Gonococcal Infections

Clinical Manifestations. Infection caused by *Neisseria gonorrhoeae* remains a frequent sexually transmitted disease. Clinical manifestations vary according to the primary sites and the following entities can be distinguished: *asymptomatic carriers* are common in both sexes and represent the major source of disease transmission. *Urethritis* ist the most common form of gonococcal infection in men, whereas in women it is in general associated with *endocervicitis*. *Anorectal infections* are seen mainly among young homosexual men after rectal intercourse. In the female this type of infection is observed less frequently and is either due to a contiguous genitourinary source or to sexual intercourse. *Oropharyngeal infection* can be either symptomatic with inflammation and exudate or asymptomatic with a simple carriage. Specimens from this site in homosexual men should be routinely cultured. *Disseminated gonococcal infection* is characterized by typical skin lesions, tenosynovitis, and arthritis. Endocarditis or meningitis are rare in cases of dissemination [4].

Anorectal Infections. In general the infection is asymptomatic, but severe proctitis can occur. Even though the symptoms vary from nonspecific complaints such as pruritus to rectal pain with tenesmus and mucopurulent discharge, the infection is always limited to the rectum. A careful sexual history is mandatory in the case of proctitis.

Microbiology. *Neisseria gonorrhoeae* ist a Gram-negative, kidney-shaped diplococcus with flattened opposed margins which only grows at $35°-37°C$ in an atmosphere containing 5%–10% carbon dioxide.

Specimens and Transport. Clinical specimens from the pharynx, urethra, cervix, or rectum should be either directly inoculated on selective media such as Thayer-Martin medium or, if seeding is possible within 6 h after collection, sent to a laboratory in a transport medium such as Amies or Stuart medium. If the rectal swab is contaminated with feces, another "clean" specimen should be obtained. Acceptable urethral specimens must be taken at least 2 h after the last voiding. Optionally a second swab can be used to prepare a glass slide for direct microscopic examination (Gram stain or immunofluorescence). Blood cultures can be attempted, but are in general negative if conventional media are used [2, 3].

Direct Examination. Direct examination of gram-stains is only diagnostic in urethral specimens and as long as intracellular organisms are seen. All other specimens can be contaminated by other *Neisseria species,* and the direct examination must be confirmed by culture. More recently, immunological-enzymatic tests have been used for the detection of gonococcal antigens. They can be recommended only for urethral or cervical specimens. Even if used correctly, false-negative or false-positive results occur because of low antigen concentration or cross reactions with other *Neisseria.*

Culture. The positive culture remains the method of choice for the reliable detection of *Neisseria gonorrhoeae.* This is particularly true for pharyngeal or rectal specimens. In addition, sensitivity tests can be performed. They are particularly important for the detection of beta-lactamase-producing strains and for correct therapy.

Serology. Serological tests are not useful for the diagnosis of gonococcal infections. Even in the case of chronic infections or complications, such as perihepatitis or Fitz-Hugh-Curtis syndrome, the value of serology is questionable.

Chlamydia

Clinical Manifestations. Chlamydia trachomatis is the most frequent microorganism responsible for nongonococcal urethritis. Even though clinical manifestations resemble the syndromes known with *Neisseria gonorrhoeae,* uretheritis is in general less purulent. Clinically *Chlamydia trachomatis* infections can be divided into three categories: the *classic trachoma* occurring in endemic countries; the *sexually transmitted genital infections* including lymphogranuloma venereum (LGV) encountered in developing countries and the non-LGV infections in developed countries; and finally the *perinatal infant eye and respiratory infections* which are acquired from the mother's cervix during birth [4, 5].

Anorectal Infections. Non-LGV strains of *Chlamydia trachomatis* are observed among homosexual men with proctitis, while LGV strains are associated with either proctitis or proctocolitis. Mild to moderate rectal discharge, mild anorectal pain, tenesmus, constipation, and an erythematous or slightly friable rectal mucosa are the hallmarks of the non-LGV infection. In contrast, the infection due to LGV is more severe with a very friable, hemorrhagic, and ulcerated mucosa involving the sigmoid colon and the anorectum; fever, and inguinal lymphadenopathy. Chronic disease may result in rectovaginal or rectovesical fistulas, rectal or urethral strictures, and lymphedema from lymphatic obstruction.

Microbiology.Chlamydiae are Gram-negative bacteria which cannot synthesize adenosine triphosphate (ATP) and therefore are obligate energy parasites of eukaryotic cells. *Chlamydia trachomatis* is more frequently responsible for genital infections than *Chlamydia psittaci.* In a complicated life cycle, both species develop into elementary bodies adapted for extracellular survival without replication and into metabolically active reticulate bodies dividing continuously by binary fission. Therefore tissue cultures are necessary for the culture of *Chlamydiae. Chlamydia trachomatis* can be typed by microimmunofluorescence, where types A–K cause the usual infections, whereas types L1, L2, and L3 cause the systemic disease lymphogranuloma venereum [5].

Specimens and Transport. To obtain valid specimens epithelial cells must be obtained by vigorous swabbing or scraping. Urethral, cervical, and rectal specimens can be obtained with a swab, but fecal contamination must be avoided. Vaginal specimens or prostatic secretions and semen are inadequate because of their toxicity for the cell culture. Pus is inadequate because it contains no epithelial cells and should therefore be replaced by a biopsy of mucosa. The material should be immediately introduced into a special transport medium at 4 °C and transported to the laboratory. For direct examination clinical material can also be applied to two glass slides by rolling the swab over a small marked surface and air drying before transport [3, 5].

Direct Examination. The microscopic examination with stains such as Giemsa, Papanicolaou, etc. is not recommended and should be replaced by immunofluorescence (Microtrak, Syva Co., Palo Alto, California) or enzyme immunoassay (Chlamydiazyme, Abbott, North Chicago). In any case, this preliminary result should be confirmed by culture because of false-positive or false-negative results.

Culture. The culture is the only method which detects both *Chlamydia trachomatis* and *Chlamydia psittaci* and takes about 3–7 days. Typing and susceptibility testing are not performed routinely.

Serology. The complement fixation test is still used but yields positive results only in cases of lymphogranuloma venereum or perihepatitis. The indirect immunofluorescence test is more sensitive: in acute local infections elevated antibody titers are occasionally observed. A low titer of complement fixation combined with a high titer of immunofluorescence suggests the presence of a chronic local infection or a complication.

Syphilis

Clinical Manifestations. Primary syphilis is characterized by the *chancre* which appears at the primary infection site. *Secondary syphilis* is characterized either by constitutional symptoms or *skin manifestations* mimicking almost any dermatological disease including erythematous macular rash, mucous patches, and *condyloma latum. Tertiary syphilis* includes *gumma,* a solitary or multiple granulomatous lesion which may involve almost any organ system, *cardiovascular syphilis,* and *neurosyphilis* [3, 4].

Anorectal Infections. Primary chancre is a painless ulcer, usually indurated, with a sharply defined border and little or no exudative response. It may be multiple and accompanied by regional, painless, firm adenopathy. Depending on the sexual practice, it can be anywhere: external genitalia, oral cavity, lips, and anorectal area. *Condyloma latum* is a broad-based moist, reddish-brown or grayish, granulomatous, superficial, coalescent papular lesion in intertriginous areas such as the perianal area, vulva, inner thighs, axillae, or scrotum. It is highly infectious, and microorganisms can be readily seen if examined with dark-field microscopy.

Microbiology. Treponema pallidum is a slender spirochetal organism measuring 5–15 μm in length and less than 0.5 μm in width. Direct examination is only possible with a dark-field microscope. *Treponema pallidum* cannot be cultivated in vitro.

Specimens and Transport. The examiner should use gloves when obtaining specimens for dark-field examination. Crusts or debris must be removed with nonbacteriostatic saline before examination. Once dried the suspicious area is abraded and the expressed serum placed on a slide with a coverslip for immediate dark-field examination. If this facility is not available, the slide may be dried without a coverslip and sent to a laboratory for examination by immunofluorescence. In addition, blood should be sent to the laboratory for serological examination.

Direct Examination. As serology might be negative early after infection, a positive dark-field examination performed by an experienced observer is specific to initiate therapy.

Serology. Two types of tests can be distinguished. *Nonspecific antibodies or reagins* can be detected by the Venereal Disease Research Laboratory test (VDRL) or the rapid plasma reagin (RPR). They are based on a cardiolipin-lecithin antigen which can cross-react with normal host tissue and initiate false-positive results. This is particularly true in conjunction with infections due to viruses, *Mycoplasma pneumoniae,* malaria, and chlamydia, or in patients with narcotic addiction, age over 65, various autoimmune diseases, and leprosy. They are used for screening as they are positive 4–6 weeks after infection, for monitoring therapy as they should show a tendancy to turn negative, and for the diagnosis of neurosyphilis. *Specific antitreponemal antibody* tests include the fluorescent treponema antibody absorption test (FTA-ABS) and the *Treponema pallidum* hemagglutination test (TPHA). Both methods are able to detect antibodies against *Treponema pallidum:* however, cross-reactions with other treponemas occur (pian, pinta, bejel). They become positive 1–2 weeks after the reagins and once positive usually remain positive indefinetely, either with or without adequate therapy. Therefore these tests cannot be used to evaluate the adequacy of the therapy or the activity of the disease [3, 4].

Chancroid (Hemophilus Ducreyi)

*Clinical Manifestations.*Infections caused by *Hemophilus ducreyi* has a worldwide distribution and is associated with poor socioeconomic and hygenic conditions. A few days after exposure a papulopustular lesion develops primarily on the external genitalia or perianal areas of both sexes and rapidly becomes ulcerative. Tender unilateral inguinal lymphadenopathy becomes suppurative and can drain spontaneously. The diagnosis of chancroid is commonly made on clinical grounds alone. This is often inaccurate since primary syphilis, herpes genitalis, and lymphogranuloma venereum may be confused with chancroid [4].

Microbiology. *Hemophilus ducreyi* is a small Gram-negative coccobacillus which requires special culture media for isolation.

Specimens and Transport. The ulcer should be cleaned with sterile saline and dried with sterile gauze. Exudate from the ulcer should be obtained with a swab or wire loop or the involved lymph node should be aspirated the exudate should then be rolled carfully onto a glass slide in order to preserve the bacteriological characteristics. For culturing the laboratory should be contacted first.

Direct Examination. Gram stains should reveal large numbers of Gram-negative coccobacilli, which may be in chains or in a "school of fish" pattern. Dark-field examination should be performed simultaneously and, if necessary, repeatedly in conjunction with serology to exclude syphilis.

Culture. Cultures are performed only exceptionally as special media are required. If positive, the test is diagnostic.

Serology. No serological tests exist.

Herpes Simplex Virus

Clinical Manifestations. Infections caused by herpes simplex virus (HSV) type 2 or even type 1 are the most common cause of *vesiculoulcerative lesions* in the genital area. Tender vesicles or ulcers involve genitalia, anorectum, or oropharynx depending on the sexual practices. *Herpetic urethritis or cervicitis* causing a dysuria-pyuria syndrome is frequent in women. During primary infection a *flu-like syndrome* is due to a transient viremia. Primary genital lesions heal without scarring in general within 3–4 weeks. Once infected the patients suffer from *recurrences* occurring typically 5–8 times a year [4].

Anorectal Infection. Typical lesions include painful vesicles or ulcers and a history of recurrences. Particularly in patients with the acquired immunodeficiency syndrome, herpetic proctitis may be chronic and relentlessly destructive.

Microbiology. Herpes simplex is a virus with double-stranded DNA enveloped by a capsule. It can be seen by electron microscopy, detected by immunofluorescence or enzyme-linked immunosorbent assay (ELISA) or cultured on tissue.

Specimen and Transport. With any test, sensitivity is greatest in the vesicular stage and fall rapidly as the lesions progress. Vesicles should be punctured with a nonsiliconated needle which is submitted to the laboratory without refrigeration [3].

Direct Examination. Direct examination of Papanicolaou preparations revealing typical intracellular inclusions is specific but not very sensitive. The same holds true for immunofluorescence or ELISA.

Culture Viral isolation is the most sensitive test. It takes 3–8 days to obtain definitive results.

Serology. Serological examinations prove only that a seroconversion has occurred after a primary infection. Because titers are not modified by recurrent infections, serology is in general of limited use.

Condyloma Acuminatum

Clinical Manifestations. Verrucous papules or venereal warts are usually multiple and surrounded by smaller satellite lesions. Stalked or sessile, they may become elongated if located in moist areas. Perianal lesions in women are related to genital infection, whereas in men they are associated with receptive anal intercourse. Even if typical lesions suggest condyloma acuminatum they must be differentiated from syphilitic lesions [4].

Microbiology. Condyloma acuminatum is induced by the human papilloma virus, a double-stranded DNA virus. Papilloma virus cannot be multiplied in cell cultures. Therefore diagnostic proof of infection must be performed with hybridization techniques performed on tissue biopsies.

Specimen and Transport. Differential diagnosis with syphilitic lesions is best made by carefully abrading and performing an immediate dark-field examination.

Direct Examination. Visible spirochetes on dark-field examination do not definitely eliminate the possibility of condyloma acuminatum because this lesion can be superinfected with anaerobic spirochetes. As papilloma virus can induce intraepithelial neoplasia, a biopsy with histological examinations is always recommended.

Candida

Clinical Manifestations. Infections due to *Candida albicans* can cause mucocutaneous lesions such as thrush, esophagitis, gastrointestinal candidiasis, vaginitis, chronic mucocutaneous candidiasis, or cutaneous manifestations including perianal candidiasis. In addition, almost any organ can be attained by a deep infection [4].

Anorectal Manifestations. The infection is marked by intense pruritus and erythema which can progress to maceration. Occasionally the anal canal is involved, and the lesions progress over the perineum.

Microbiology. *Candida albicans* is the most frequently isolated yeast. It is made up of small (4–6 μm) thin-walled Gram-positive ovoid cells that reproduce by budding and grow easily in a variety of media. Yeast forms, hyphae, and pseudohyphae can be observed in tissue.

Specimens and Transport. Suspicious areas should first be cleaned with saline to eliminate crusts and debris, then vigorously swabbed or scraped. Not only anorectal specimens but also specimens from the vagina or preputium should be analyzed. In cases of chronic infection, culture of hair follicles can be diagnostic. Ideally, the material should be transported to the laboratory in an Amies or Stuart medium. No special attention to temperature is necessary.

Direct Examination. Gram-stained air-dried slides or preparations with 10% potassium hydroxide reveal characteristic cells and hyphae which are diagnostic for fungi, but not necessarily for *Candida species*. Negative results do not exclude a fungal infection.

Culture. In general, a culture is not necessary if characteristic microorganisms are seen by direct examination. It should be limited to cases where the organism must be precisely identified, when fungi are suspected, or when susceptibility tests are requested.

Serology. Serological tests are not useful because of frequent false-positive and -negative results.

Sexually Transmitted Enteric Disease

Clinical Aspects. Until the epidemy of the human immunodeficiency virus (HIV) became sufficiently known, sexual practices among homosexuals resulted in the transmission of several enteric diseases. Culturing stools for microorganisms, such as shigella, salmonella, campylobacter, or examinations for protozoa and ova becomes an integral part of the evaluation of anorectal complaints in male homosexuals [4].

Specimens and Transport. Fresh mucopurulent or hemorrhagic stool specimens can be sent to the laboratory in a clean container for routine bacteriological examination including shigella, salmonella, and campylobacter. Transport media are not requested as long as the specimens are refrigerated at 4 °C and analyzed within 24 h. The laboratory must be notified if a culture and toxin detection are requested for *Clostridium difficile*. Freshly passed liquid stool or biopsy material obtained from the periphery of an ulcer during sigmoidoscopy is necessary for the detection of motile trophozoites of *Entamoeba histolytica* or *Giardia lamblia*. In formed stool only cysts of *Entamoeba histolytica* can be observed. The ova of *Enterobius vermicularis* can be detected by microscopic examination of a transparent adhesive tape applied to the perianal skin overnight and then fixed onto a glass slide.

Direct Examination. Direct examination is only used for the detection of ova and parasites where it allows definitive diagnosis. Examination for bacteria is useless.

Culture. Bacteriological culture results for the microorganisms described above are definitive. Exceptionally cultures for *Entamoeba histolytica* can be performed on special media.

Serology. Serology for enteric bacteria used to be performed but should be abandoned because of totally unspecific results. In contrast, serological studies may be helpful for the diagnosis of invasive amebiasis.

Diarrhea Related to HIV Infections

Clinical Manifestations. Severe and prolonged diarrhea related to infection with HIV are frequent. Beside the organisms mentioned in the previous section, several other infections are characteristic bacteria including *Salmonella typhimurium, Salmonella species,* and *Mycobacterium avium-intracellulare;* parasites such as *Cryptosporidium species, Isospora belli,* and *Strongyloides stercoralis,* or cytomegalovirus.

Microbiology. Mycobacterium avium-intracellulare belongs to the atypical mycobacteria and has the same growth requirements as all tuberculous bacteria *Cryptosporidium species* and *Isospora belli* are tiny protozoan organisms found on the mucosal surface of the intestine. *Strongyloides stercoralis* are intestinal parasites which can persist for years in the intestinal tract without causing disease, but inducing diarrhea in immunocompromised hosts.

Specimens and Transport. Fresh stools should be examined for bacteria and parasites, indicating the various microorganisms suspected. For viral cultures the specimen should be carried in a special transport medium provided by the laboratory.

Direct Examination. Special staining, such as Giemsa, modified Ziehl-Neelsen, modified Kinyoun, Auramin, etc., allow a microscopic diagnosis of the *Mycobacterium avium-intracellulare* or parasites in stool specimens. Gramstains are not diagnostic for any bacteria and are therefore not recommended.

Culture. Parasites cannot be cultured. Bacteriological or viral culture results are diagnostic.

Serology. At the moment no routine serological tools are available.

References

1. Isenberg HD, Schoenknecht FD, von Graevenitz A (1979) Collection and processing of bacteriological specimens. American Society for Microbiology, Washington DC. (Cumulative Techniques and Procedures in Clinical Microbiology, vol 9)
2. Kellogg DS Jr, Holmes KK, Hill GA (1976) Laboratory diagnosis of gonorrhea. American Society for Microbiology, Washington DC. (Cumulative Techniques and Procedures in Clinical Microbiology, vol 4)
3. Lennete EH, Balows A, William J, Hausler JR, Shadomy HJ (1985) Manual of clinical microbiology, 4th edn. American Society for Microbiology, Washington DC
4. Mandell GL, Douglas RG, Bennett JE (1985) Principles and practice of infectious diseases, 2nd edn. Wiley, New York
5. Wallace AC Jr, George EK, Schachter J (1984) Laboratory diagnosis of chlamydial and mycoplasmal infections. American Society for Microbiology, Washington DC. (Cumulative Techniques and Procedures in Clinical Microbiology, vol 19)

5 Management of Biopsies and Operation Specimens of the Anorectal Region

S. Widgren

Introduction

As a member of the medical team responsible for the patient's health, the pathologist is a consultant whose duty is to give important advice on the diagnosis, the treatment, and the prognosis of the disease. It is not useless to emphasize that he will not be able to accomplish this task in a satisfactory manner unless he is given a minimum of clinical information on the one hand, and material of good quality and adequate quantity on the other [5, 10, 12]. *Clinical information* should be given to the pathologist either in writing on the request form or by oral communication. It should include the following features:

- Sufficient clinical data
- The endoscopic appearance of the lesions
- The site of the biopsy or biopsies
- The type of operation

Problems pertinent to the patient's case or specific questions should be clearly formulated and forwarded together with the biopsy or the operation specimen. This should be done immediately and not days or weeks later. Otherwise there is the risk that important questions may remain unanswered once the material has been modified by technical manipulations or by cutting the specimen. It is obvious that communication should be easier to establish when the surgical department and the pathology laboratory are located in the same hospital or in close proximity.

Biopsies

Biopsies must be performed under visual control (endoscopy or laparotomy) or with a needle puncture with the aid of an imaging system (CAT scan). In order to provide optimal results, *immediate fixation* of the specimen is *essential*. In our experience, formaline sublimate is a good and quick fixative for specimens which are not larger than 5 mm. For bigger specimens, buffered 10% formaldehyde is recommended. These fluids are indicated only as a suggestion, since individual laboratories might prefer other ones according to their experience or idiosyncrasies.

It is important to place the specimens on a piece of filter paper or ground glass with the mucosa facing upwards in order to prevent them rolling up due to the retraction produced by the fixation medium. Therefore, in order to avoid crushing artefacts, it is useful to handle the specimens gently with needles rather than with a forceps and with visual control under a dissecting microscope or, at least, a magnifying glass. When multiple biopsies are taken from lesions of various appearances, e. g., in cases of inflammatory bowel disease or multiple tumors, it is necessary to place them into separate containers. On certain occasions fresh biopsies may be useful, especially for immunohistochemical techniques. Such specimens should be taken immediately to the pathology laboratory. Especially in these cases, communication with the pathologist is important to avoid technical hazards. Finally, containers should be adequately labeled (name of the patient, type and location of biopsy).

For *frozen sections,* it seems quite unnecessary to recall that fresh material must be brought without delay to the pathology laboratory. If the time of transport exceeds a few minutes, it is useful to put the specimens on a compress soaked with saline serum in order to avoid dessication artefacts which are harmful for a good technique and interpretation.

Operation Specimens

Operation specimens should be sent directly to the pathology laboratory, when possible in a fresh state. Unnecessary handling (especially by untrained nonmedical staff) should be avoided in order not to alter the specimen to such an extent that the pathologist is no longer able to evaluate its macroscopic appearance (which is an important element of the diagnosis) or might prevent taking adequate blocks for histology. Undue incisions of the specimen are to be proscribed. Dividing the specimen into several pieces and sending these to several pathologists, under the pretence of securing an optimal diagnosis, often produces the opposite effect and is considered by the author as contrary to medical ethics.

Should the surgical and the pathology departments be far apart, requiring transportation by mail, it may be necessary to cut open an anorectal specimen on the anterior face, and to rinse it gently with serum saline in order to evacuate remnants of feces or blood, then to fix it flat on a piece of cork or polyurethane for 24 or 48 h in an adequate volume of 10% buffered formaldehyde. A specimen should never be immersed unopened in fixation fluid, particularly as the mucosa, which in the majority of cases is the site of the principal anatomic lesion, might become autolysed by the time the specimen reaches the pathologist due to the slow penetration of the fixation fluid through the wall. Finally the specimens must be put into a container of sufficient size to avoid the risk of unremediable deformations.

Before sending the specimen, the surgeon should take care to place that *thread markers* of various lengths and colors in order to indicate to the pathologist the superior vascular ligation (e. g., the inferior mesenteric artery or one of its branches) or any particular feature which might be important (e. g., lymph nodes), interesting, or intriguing. Any peculiar lesion that the surgeon has separated should be forwarded in a separate container. All these technical indications, which might seem fastidious to the busy surgeon but are vital for correct diagnosis and a good clinicopathological correlation, are given in order to render the *pathologist's work* easier. His task is to give the surgeon a confirmation of his clinical diagnosis or to throw some light on an unknown lesion. It seems useful to recall to the pathologist that all lesions should be thoroughly described and, when necessary, documented by a photograph or a drawing, and that blocks should be taken from representative lesions.

Special attention must be given to the *search for lymph nodes,* especially in cases of carcinoma. Various methods have been published, e. g., dissecting and collecting all lymph nodes along the vascular tree [10]; identification by specimen radiography [8], or the clearance technique with xylol-alcohol [2]. These various methods are unfortunately rather time-consuming and are more easily performed in specialized centers. They seem somewhat difficult to apply in an "all-round" pathology laboratory. In our experience, accurate pathological staging can be achieved by careful palpation and serial inci-

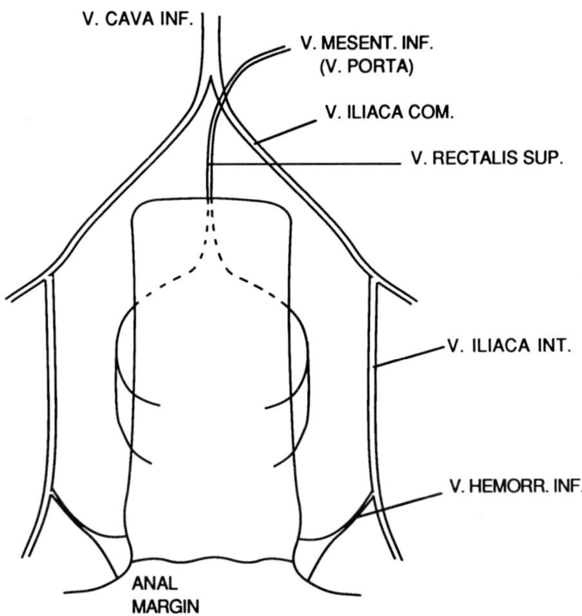

Fig. 5.1. Venous drainage of the rectum, anal canal, and anal margin. The lymph nodes to be examined are situated along these veins

sions of the mesorectum, dividing the lymph nodes into two or three groups. The first group comprises the distal lymph nodes, i. e., those situated near the tumor, within an area of 3 cm. The second group is constituted by the proximal nodes, located on the vascular ligature as identified by the surgeon. If necessary, a third group would include the nodes situated between the two former groups (Fig. 5.1).

Classification and Prognosis of Tumors

Colorectal Tumors

The prognostic classification of colorectal cancers has been the subject of numerous proposals which have not clarified the situation, but have brought confusion in the minds of the members of the medical community, and more so among the public. There was good example of such confusion a few years ago on the occasion of the operation performed on the President of the United States [9]. Zinkin [14] made a good critical review of various classifications, giving his preference to the TNM system of the Union Internationale Contre le Cancer (UICC; International Union Against Cancer) and to that of Dukes (1958 modification [4]). In the writer's opinion the TNM classification is difficult to manage for several reasons. First, it comprises in-

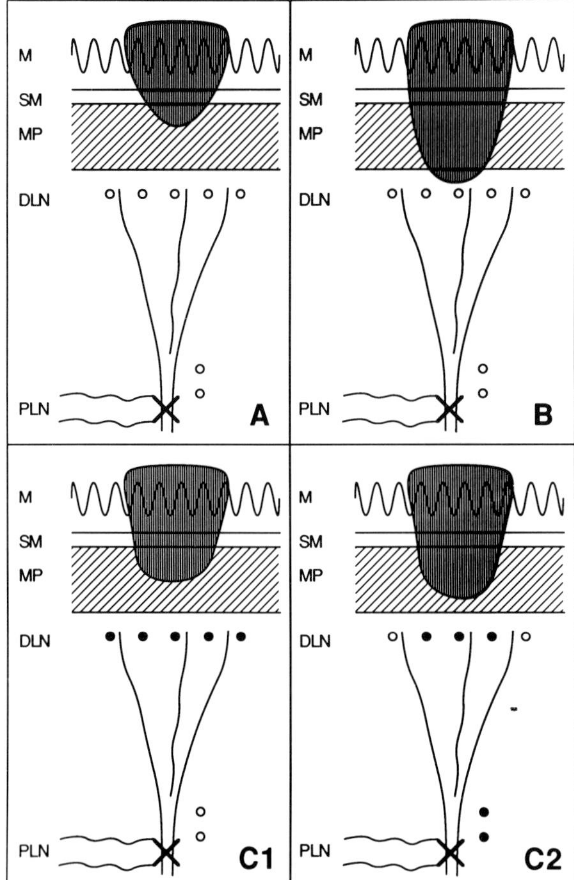

Fig. 5.2. Dukes' classification of tumor invasion and metastases. The stage is indicated by *A, B, C1,* and *C2.* Tumor invasion is shown by the *shaded area. Black dots* represent lymph node metastases. *X,* proximal vascular ligature; *M,* mucosa; *S* submucosa; *MP,* muscularis propria; *DLN,* distal lymph nodes; *PLN,* proximal lymph nodes

modification of Dukes' classification which is shown in Fig. 5.2.

Tumors of the Anal Canal

Classification of cancers of the anal canal is more difficult to perform due to the peculiar lymphatic drainage of this region – either to the inferior hemorrhoidal veins, satellites of the internal iliac veins, or to the inguinal nodes. Here again, the TNM system is not quite satisfactory because it does not take these two lymph node regions into consideration.

Essential Points of the Pathologist's Report

Several good papers have been published on the recording of colorectal tumors [1, 11]. The essential data are the following:

– Macroscopic appearance of the tumor with its dimensions, extension in depth and in circumference, distance to the closest surgical margin
– Histological type and degree of differentiation
– Site of lymph node metastases (if possible, the number of nodes involved compared to the total examined)
– Venous invasion

These indications will permit to produce an accurate pathological staging, the importance of which is obvious, so that the prognosis of the disease can be evaluated, and to determine, when necessary, whether further treatment is mandatory.

dications which the pathologist is often not aware of (presence of distant metastases). Secondly, it unduly simplifies lymph node metastases [13], the proximal and distal ones not being distinguished. Long-term results will have to confirm the promising preliminary data of the Australian Clinico-Pathological Staging system (ACPS) [3]. Another recent classification, providing a score range giving four prognostic groups based on four histological variables (local tumor spread, character of invasive margin, presence or absence of peritumoral lymphocytic infiltrate, number of lymph nodes with metastases) seems to provide an improvement on the Dukes' classification [6, 7]. This will also need comparison with similar data from other centers. In the meantime, we continue to employ the 1958

References

1. Buckwalter JA Jr, Kent TH (1973) Colonic cancer. Essential information for a pathologic report. Arch Pathol 95: 366–370
2. Cawthorn SJ, Gibbs NM, Marks CG (1984) A clearance technique for the detection of lymph nodes in colorectal cancer. Gut 25: A 1150
3. Davis NC, Evans EB, Cohen JR, Theile DE (1984) Staging of colorectal cancer. The Australian Clinico-Pathological Staging (ACPS) system compared with Dukes' system. Dis Colon Rectum 27: 707–713
4. Dukes CE, Bussey HJR (1958) The spread of rectal cancer and its effect on prognosis. Br J Cancer 12: 309–320
5. Hadfield GJ, Hobsley M, Morson BC (1985) The surgeon and the pathologist: an editorial introduction. In: Hadfield GJ, Hobsley M (eds) Pathology in surgical practice. Arnold, London

6. Jass JR, Love SB, Northover JMA (1987) A new prognostic classification of rectal cancer. Lancet i: 1303–1306
7. Jass JR, Morson BC (1987) Reporting colorectal cancer. J Clin Pathol 40: 1016–1023
8. Jensen J, Andersen J (1978) Lymph node identification in carcinoma of the colon and rectum. Acta Pathol Microbiol Scand Sect A 86: 205–209
9. Kyriakos M (1985) The President's cancer, the Dukes classification, and confusion (editorial). Arch Pathol Lab Med 109: 1063–1066
10. Morson BC, Dawson IMP (1979) Technical methods, chap. 48. In: Morson BC, Dawson IMP (eds) Gastrointestinal pathology, 2nd edn. Blackwell, Oxford, pp 781–790
11. Qizilbash A (1982) Pathologic studies in colorectal cancer. A guide to the surgical pathology examination of colorectal specimens and review of features of prognostic significance. Pathol Ann 17 (1): 1–46
12. Whitehead R (1979) Mucosal biopsy of the gastrointestinal tract, 2nd edn., Saunders, Philadelphia
13. Wolmark N, Fischer B, Wieand HS (1986) The prognostic value of the modifications of the Dukes'C class of colorectal cancer. An analysis of the NSABP clinical trials. Ann Surg 203: 115–122
14. Zinkin LD (1983) A critical review of the classifications and staging of colorectal cancer. Dis Colon Rectum 26: 37–43

6 Radiological Investigations

D. Mirescu and F. Sadry

Introduction

Because the anorectum can be easily examined digitally and endoscopically, it has long been believed that radiology has nothing to offer in its exploration. This opinion has been mostly maintained by the use of a single-contrast barium enema technique, known for its lack of sensitivity in the detection of many lesions. The advances in the technique of barium enema (double-contrast), the fast development of new imaging methods (ultrasonography, computerized tomography, nuclear magnetic resonance), and a better understanding of the physiology and physiopathology of the anorectum have contributed to making radiological investigations essential before any therapeutic procedure.

Normal Radiological Anatomy

Located within the true pelvis, the rectum has a curved shape which fits along the anterior concavity of the sacrum. It begins at the level of S3, ends 2.5 cm above the tip of the coccyx and measures approximately 13 cm in length. If continues as the anal canal which is 3.5–4 cm long [30].

The rectum is a fixed organ except for its upper third. This segment is more or less mobile depending on the inferior extension of the mesocolon [9]. The lower third of the rectum is totally extraperitoneal. Its posterior wall is separated from the sacrum by the presacral or retrorectal space which is situated between two fascial layers: Waldeyer's fascia posteriorly and the fascia propria anteriorly [9]. This space contains connective tissue, fat, the upper rectal vessels, and the presacral lymph nodes. It can be well visualized between S3 and S5 on a lateral view of the rectum. Its width, measured at the level of S5, depends on age and obesity, the accepted maximum being 1.5–2 cm [2].

With a double-contrast enema technique, where the mucosa and its folds are coated by a thin layer of barium, the rectal valves of Houston and the columns of Morgagni in the anal canal can be visualized. There are usually three valves of Houston, but the two on the left side are not always seen. The middle fold, which is seen more frequently, arises from the right side, is 4–5 mm thick, extends anteriorly, and delineates the inferior border of the peritoneal reflection. It has also been called the valve of Kohlrausch. The columns of Morgagni are longitudinal folds of the anal mucosa and consist of venous plexuses.

On condition that the examination is of good quality, any lesion inducing a change in the barium coating will be detected, be it mucosal, submucosal, or extraluminal. With computerized tomography, a third dimension has become available in radiology: the possibility of axial contiguous sections has lead to the visualization of the morphology of the rectum and of its relationship to the adjacent pelvic organs.

As the anatomy of the pelvis has been described in detail in the literature [1, 15], we shall point out only a few relevant facts:

- The rectum, but not its wall constituents, is opacified using contrast agents.
- The perirectal fascia is not normally seen.
- The pelvic muscles, fat planes, and spaces between adjacent organs (rectovesical, rectouterine, presacral and uterovesical spaces, and ischiorectal fossa) are well identified.
- Normal lymph nodes are not detected, and certain vascular structures will only be seen in a segmental fashion.

Imaging of Anorectal Disease

The radiological investigation of anorectal pathology offers two aspects: a morphological study of the area concerned as well as adjacent structures and a dynamic study of the anorectum.

Chest Radiograph

Even though it is a routine examination, a chest radiograph as a preliminary investigation of anorectal pathology may reveal interesting changes: enterococcal pneumonia, pulmonary metastasis, a possibility of hepatic metastatization when the right diaphragm is elevated can all lead to suspicion of a colorectal primary tumor. A previous mastectomy must suggest a malignant infiltration of the colon or rectum when the presenting symptoms are intestinal.

Plain Abdominal Film Series

Two projections are essential: an upright radiograph centered on the diaphragm and a supine anteroposterior view of the whole of the abdomen and pelvis. When the patient cannot stand, a left lateral decubitus with a horizontal beam is a suitable alternative to the upright projection.

Sometimes, the plain film can localize the point of intestinal obstruction. It will indicate perforation when free intraperitoneal air is visualized or a probable colo- or rectovesical fistula when there is air in the bladder.

When the clinical picture includes diarrhea and fever, an excessive colonic distension must lead to the diagnosis of toxic megacolon, a complication of parasitic or inflammatory colitis (Crohn's disease and ulcerative colitis).

Schistosomiasis [10] or rectal hemangiomas may be suspected when the plain film reveals amorphous or linear calcifications over the anorectal region, sometimes associated with calcifications of the wall of the bladder.

A prostatic or gynecological tumor compressing or infiltrating the rectum can first be seen as a mass, sometimes showing calcification with presenting symptoms of recent and unremitting constipation.

A careful study of the bony structure of the spine and pelvis can reveal a new pathology responsible for rectoanal symptoms through local compression or infiltration: bone metastasis, sacral chordomas, bacterial or tuberculous spondylitis, as well as known or unknown fractures may all be causes.

Barium Enema

Barium enema still remains one of the main methods of investigating endoluminal anorectal pathology.

Preparation and Contraindications

Except for emergency cases, a clean colon is the prerequisite to a reliable diagnosis. There are two ways of achieving this:

- Fast preparation consisting of the oral intake of 2–3 liters of a colonic lavage solution. It has proved ideal for colonoscopy [6] and is used prior to colonic surgery. Its main disadvantage is the persistence of fluid in the gut lumen, leading to mediocre barium coating.
- A classical method including a 3-day fiber-free diet, laxatives, and a cleansing enema the day before and a couple of hours before the examination. Some advocate a clear liquid diet, others [17] find no advantage in the fiber-free diet. Whatever the variations to this standard preparation, it has proved perfectly adequate for a diagnostic barium enema.

The major contraindications to barium enema are toxic megacolon, suspected perforation, recent biopsy, and myocardial infarction.

Single-Contrast Barium Enema

The single-contrast examination has the advantage of being relatively easy and quick to perform. It finds its main indication in the investigation of elderly and debilitated patients. Advanced colorectal carcinoma and diverticular disease are undoubtedly as well diagnosed as with the double-contrast technique, but small and superficial lesions will not be detected [21, 28], and the method is too basic for proper evaluation of inflammatory proctocolitis. It is justifiably argued that such patients will not benefit from the diagnosis of a 5-mm polyp [23].

Double-Contrast Barium Enema

Double-contrast barium enema has now been accepted as an invaluable advance in the detection of anorectal lesions [27, 28, 43]. The idea is to enable the detailed analysis of any perceptible pathological element by obtaining a uniform coating of the mucosa followed by air distension of the colorectal lumen (Fig. 6.1). The examination is simple to perform, provided that the radiologist has the skill and experience and that the patient participates.

The radiological features differ from that of the single-contrast technique [27, 28]. A correct study of the anorectum entails four conditions: a rectum empty of feces, sufficient air distension after complete evacuation of the rectal barium, the obtainment of early views to avoid overprojecting bowel loops, and radiographs taken without the rectal probe for a correct visualization of the lower rectum and anal canal (Fig. 6.2). The accuracy of diagnosis also depends on the type of projections employed, such as a lateral upright film, a supine and

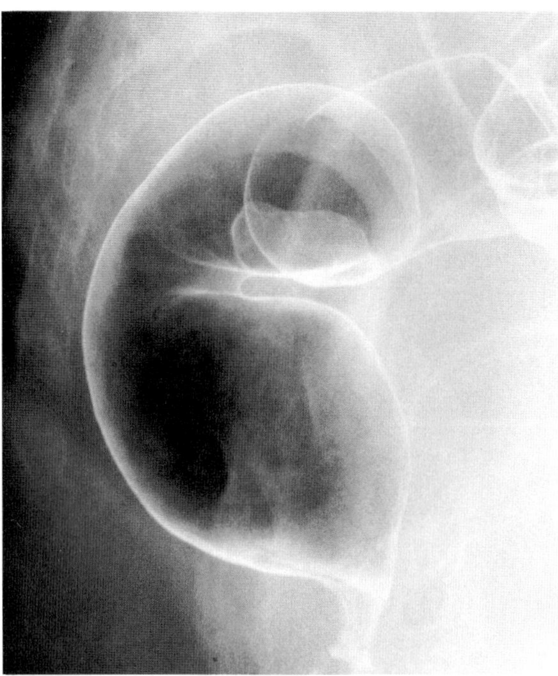

Fig. 6.1. Polypoid tumor of the upper rectum. Histological diagnosis: tubular adenoma

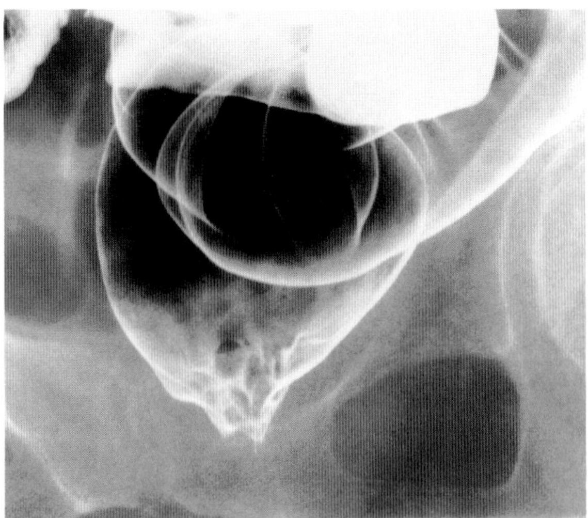

Fig. 6.2. Villous adenoma of the anorectal junction

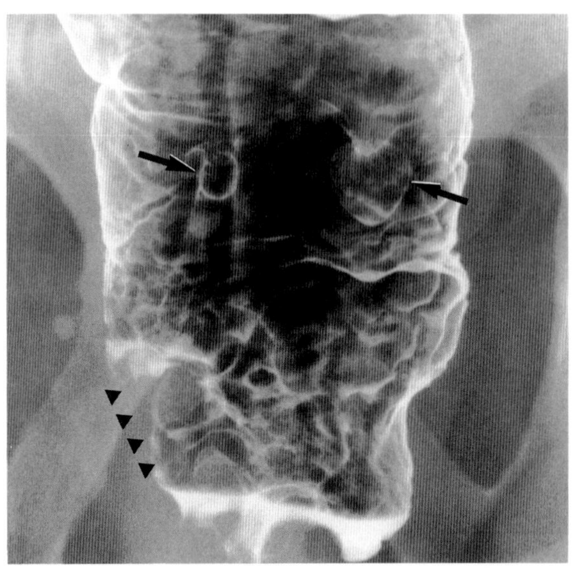

Fig. 6.3. Carcinoma of the lower rectum *(arrowheads)* and two "sentry" pedunculated polyps *(arrows)*

prone radiograph, with and without angling the beam, and possibly, a prone translateral view, not considered as important if the previous films provide satisfactory information.

Barium Enema Versus Endoscopy

The use of endoscopy and of barium enema in the investigation of colorectal pathology has lead to a debate regarding the accuracy in the literature. Both methods have false-positives and false-negatives, the rate depending on the type of study and the individual inclination of the authors [11, 21, 36]. Laufer [27], for example, finds that 15% of rectal cancers diagnosed on double-contrast barium enema are not discovered on digital or endoscopic examination. Hallmann [16], on the other hand, reports a rate of 50% of lesions missed on barium enema, but he does not distinguish the two techniques. Thoeni [43] reports an overall accuracy of 95% using double-contrast enema in detecting colorectal lesions compared to 84% with endoscopy. Both methods are complementary: their association accounts for a high degree of sensitivity (92.5% according to Brekkan.

The easy use of endoscopy, the direct visualization of a lesion that it offers and its immediate access to a diagnostic or therapeutic (polypectomy) procedure explain its obvious advantage in exploring the rectum. Nevertheless, barium enema also has benefits: it can overcome stenotic segments of bowel, allowing an overall exploration of the colon and, as a single procedure, the inventory and extension of a disease (synchronous tumors, polyposis coli, lymphoma, inflammatory colitis) (Figs. 6.3–6.5). Certain complications of Crohn's disease, such as fistulae and sinus tracts, can only be demonstrated on an enema (Fig. 6.6).

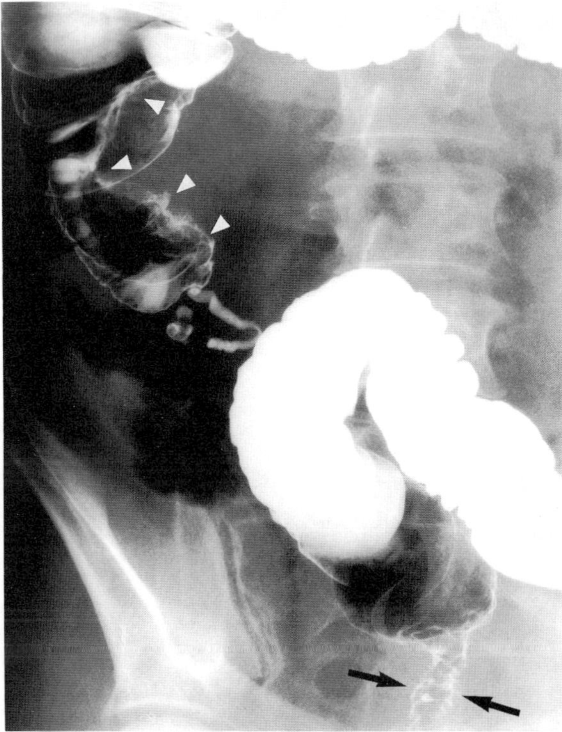

Fig. 6.4. Synchronous carcinomas: an infiltrating carcinoma of the rectum *(arrows)* and a polypoid carcinoma of the cecum *(arrowheads)*

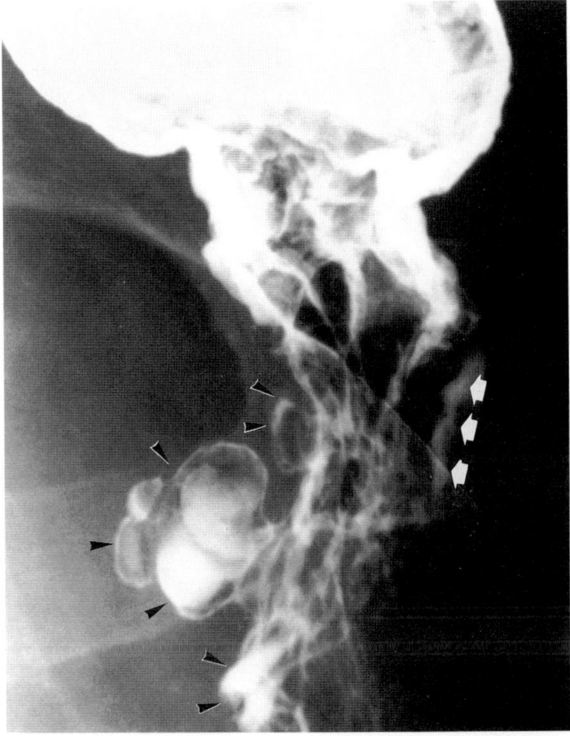

Fig. 6.6. Crohn's disease of the rectosigmoid colon: sinus tract *(arrows)* and pararectal and -anal abscesses *(arrowheads)*

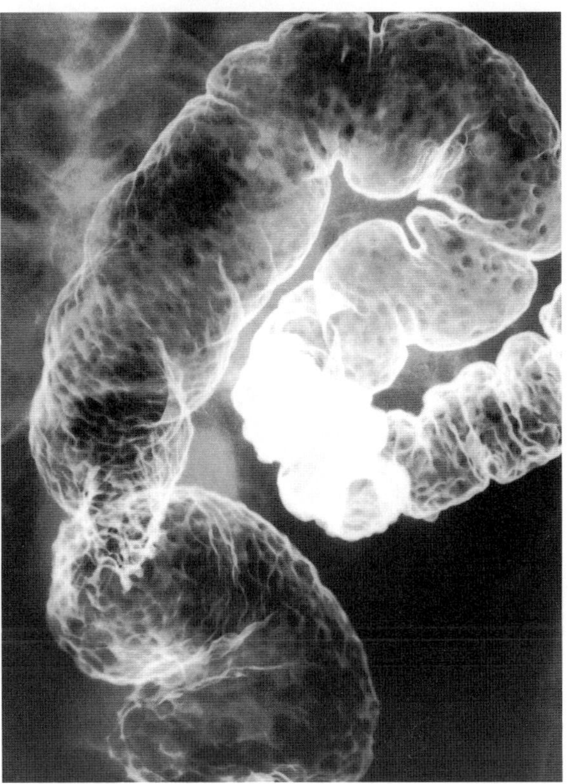

Neither Barium enema [12] nor endoscopy are free of complications, the most dangerous being perforation. A review of the literature brings out a rate of 1/2250–1/12000 examinations with a high mortality. The rectum is the most vulnerable site: a misplaced probe, especially if the rectal wall is weakened, and an excessive use of the inflatable contention balloon are the main causes.

Hydrosoluble Agents

The use of hydrosoluble agents is restricted to cases of suspected perforation and verification of recent anastomosis.

◁

Fig. 6.5. Diffuse secondary lymphoma: nodular type

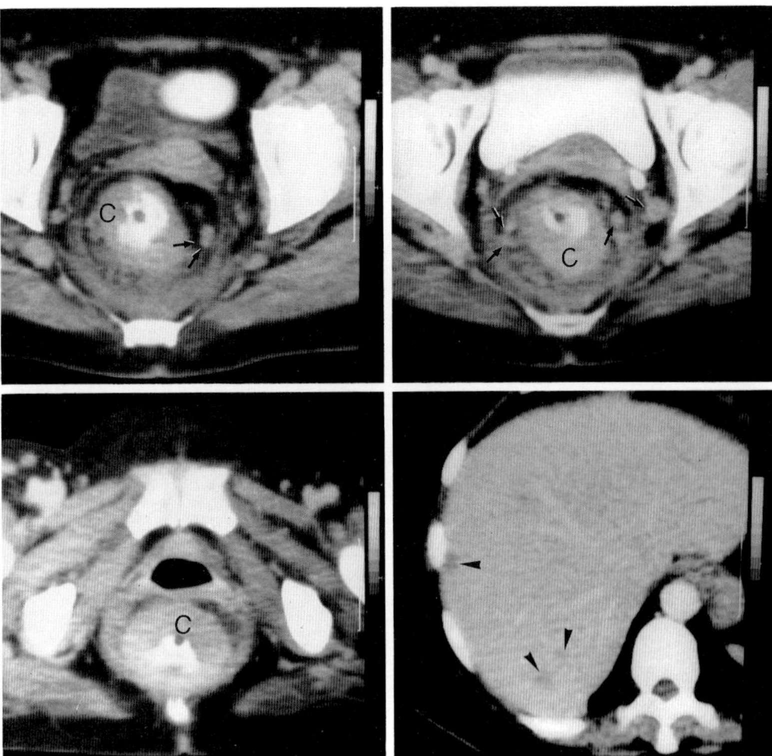

Fig. 6.7. Infiltrating rectal carcinoma *(C)* with invasion of perirectal fat and fascia. Enlarged lymph nodes *(arrows)*. Hepatic metastases *(arrowheads)*

Computerized Tomodensitometry

Computerized tomodensitometry (CT) has become an indispensable tool in the evaluation of the pathology of the anorectum: the axial sections provide direct visualization of the extraluminal environment. The major indications for a CT scan are:

- Pretherapeutic assessment of local and distant tumor spread (Fig. 6.7)
- Detection of primary or postoperative infectious processes (Fig. 6.8)
- Systematic investigation of local tumor recurrence, CT being the only nonaggressive approach, after abdominoperineal resection (Fig. 6.9)

CT remains a complementary method to endoscopy and barium enema. It must not be called on as an initial diagnostic measure [35, 42].

Several studies have established diagnostic criteria for malignant tumors on CT: a mass of more than 2 cm in the rectal wall; a thickened perirectal fascia; the invasion of adjacent organs; and the presence of local, regional, or distant lymph nodes of more than 1,5 cm [15, 35, 45] (Fig. 6.7 and 6.8 A, B). Using these elements, Moss [35] has proposed a ra-

diological staging of tumors that could serve as a guideline for therapeutic decisions [42].

Other authors have shown that CT cannot detect normal-sized pathological lymph nodes or distinguish lymph node enlargement of an inflammatory from a tumoral origin. Furthermore, it does not differentiate the fascial thickenings or assess transmural infiltration by tumor correctly [7, 13, 15, 44]. CT is the method of choice in the evaluation of advanced tumors with infiltration of adjacent organs. It is inefficient in the staging of early cancer [15].

The detection of locoregional recurrences after adominoperineal resection is the apanage of CT [34]. Even though reliable criteria for differentiating inflammatory masses from recurrence of tumor still do not exist, systematic checks at regular intervals can adjust the diagnosis (Fig. 6.9). An immediate postoperative examination is very helpful providing a base for future comparative studies. In most cases, a CT-guided biopsy will provide a definite answer [22, 24]. One pitfall must be avoided: nonopacified small bowel may present as a pelvic mass or collection.

CT also has an important part to play in the detection of some postoperative complications: the percutaneous guided drainage of a collection is useful

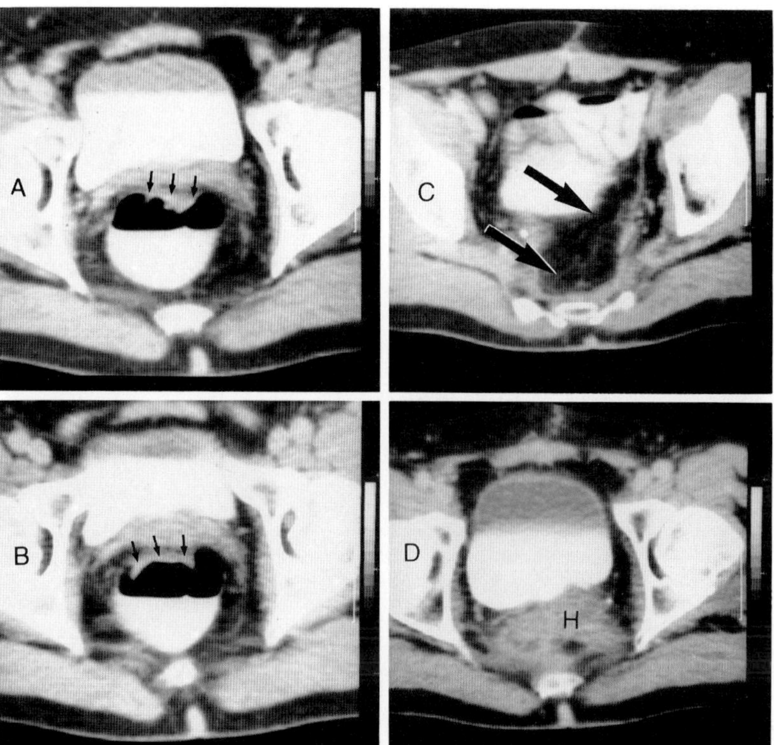

Fig. 6.8. *A, B* Polypoid carcinoma of the anterior wall of the rectum *(arrows)*. *C, D* Early investigation after abdominoperineal resection with omental transposition *(arrows)* and a hematoma in the resection bed *(H)*

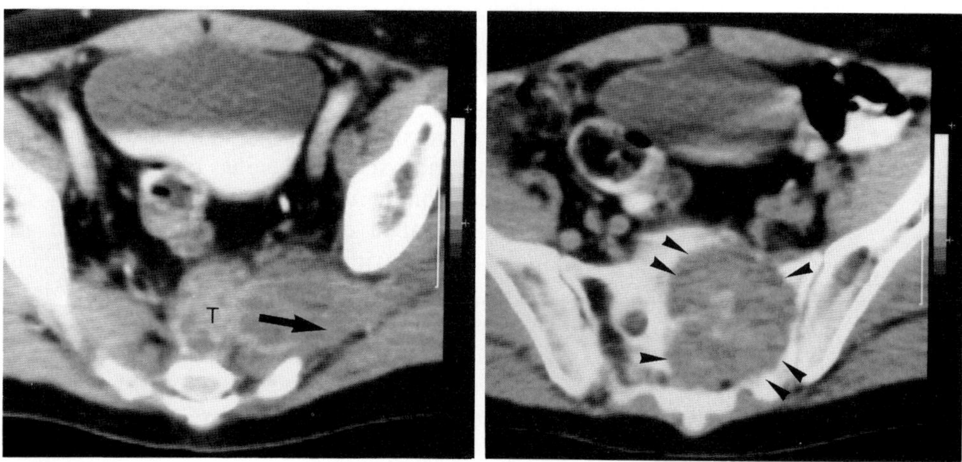

Fig. 6.9. Follow-up 3 years after an anterior resection of a rectal carcinoma: locoregional recurrence *(T)* with invasion of the left piriform muscle *(arrows)* and of the sacrum *(arrowheads)*

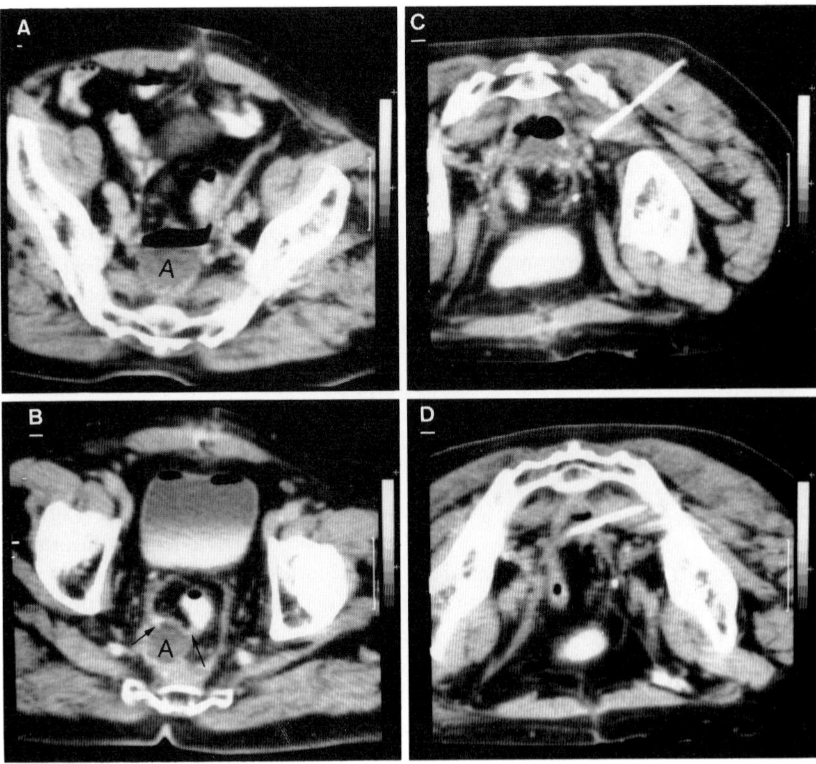

Fig. 6.10 A–D. Investigation 3 weeks after an anterior resection of a carcinoma of the lower rectum: *A, B* Anastomotic leak *(arrows)* and presacral abscess *(A). C, D* Transgluteal abscess drainage (prone)

in avoiding a second surgical procedure and its potential morbidity (Fig. 6.10).

Magnetic Resonance Imaging

The advantages of magnetic resonance imaging (MRI) over CT are the avoidance of ionizing radiation and iodine contrast agents, and the possibility of multiplanar imaging. MRI provides the best anatomic delineation. According to recent studies, MRI offers a similar, if not superior, accuracy to CT in the staging of rectal neoplasms, providing the examination is done after rectal air insufflation [5]. However, it is still not reliable in detecting the extension of parietal infiltration (stages I–II). The superiority of MRI is in being able to distinguish lymph nodes from tortuous vessels but, unfortunately, without histological specificity. There is controversy as to the possibility of differentiating between tumor recurrence and benign postsurgical reaction. There is hope that future technical progress will overcome these difficulties [41].

Ultrasonography

There are two totally different techniques, as outlined below.

Transabdominal Approach

Already widespread, the transabdominal approach is to be considered as a complementary method, remaining a quick, easy, and inexpensive method for the inventory of metastasis, hydronephrosis secondary to a pelvic mass, and for follow-up [19]. Ultrasound-guided aspiration biopsy is a rewarding and rarely complicated procedure.

Endorectal Approach

The endorectal approach, which is relatively new, is proving to be extremely valuable in the staging of rectal cancer as well as the detection of early recurrence, and it may prove to be reliable as a screening method [8, 25, 37]. Using a rotating probe of 7 MHz, five interfaces are seen, from the mucosa to the perirectal fat. The extension of a lesion can be evaluated according to the four stages determined by the Union Internationale Contre le Cancer (UICC), and this obiously determines the choice of surgery. In females with abdominoperineal resection, the vagina is used as an adequate alternative for follow-up.

Some problems still have to be overcome: the reliable diagnosis of pathological lymph nodes, the correct diagnosis of recurrence at the site of anastomosis, the need for narrower probes when there is relative stenosis, and the addition, now being tested, of a biopsy guide [40]. Nevertheless, endorectal ultrasonography has a sensitivity of 73% and a specificity of 72% as compared to 56% and 50% for CT [38].

Angiography

The indication of an angiographical examination for anorectal pathology is actually limited. It is used for the detection of a bleeding source not discovered by endoscopy or nuclear scanning, for the diagnosis of rectal vascular malformations or tumors, and for selectively placing a catheter for intra-arterial chemotherapy and embolization.

Fistulography

Fistulography is the only method available for the assessment of the course of a fistulous tract with a cutaneous outlet, be it perianal, perineal, or gluteal. The technique requires two precautions: the use of sterile iodinated contrast agents and the avoidance of fistula obstruction as any venous reflux may lead to septic shock.

Intravenous Urography

Today, intravenous urography has been replaced by CT with intravenous contrast injection when a preoperative assessment is necessary for rectal tumors of inflammatory lesions with perirectal infiltration. The aspect and topography of the bladder and ureters can always be viewed, when in doubt, by conventional abdominal films immediately after a CT examination.

Defecography

Included in the numerous means of investigation (digital, manometry, sphincter electromyography, endoscopy), defecography offers an excellent documentation of the morphology and dynamic aspects of the anorectum [2, 14, 26, 30, 33, 39]. Unremitting constipation, incomplete rectal emptying, incontinence, and anorectal pain can be the expression of a hypertonic puborectal sling, of an intussusception or prolapse, of a rectocele, or a descending perineum syndrome, all pathologies that a defecography can show [3].

The ideal set-up for defecography includes a tilting table, enabling the patient to be seated on a radiotransparent chamber pot, a radiocamera with a possible rate of one to two frames per second or a videotape. Without prior preparation, the colon is filled with a thick barium suspension. In the female, a tampon soaked in iodinated contrast medium is inserted in the vagina.

The first radiographs are taken with the patient in a lateral decubitus position, first lying down, then upright and sitting, for the exact anorectal morphology to be appreciated at rest and any incontinence, passive or on changing positions, to be detected.

Once seated on the chamber pot, profile views are taken by camera at a rate of one to two per second during straining and until complete emptying of the rectum. Complementary frames are particularly important in the dynamic evaluation of the pelvic floor and sphincteric muscles: these radiographs are taken during an effort of retention and a Valsalva maneuver.

Massive incontinence is the only source of failure of defecography.

The interpretation of this examination implies the understanding of certain radiological landmarks:

- The pubococcygeal line, representing the pelvic floor and its most important constituant the puborectal muscle, also called "puborectal sling" (Fig. 6.11).
- The anorectal junction, situated at a maximum of 2 cm from the pubococcygeal line (Fig. 6.11).
- The anorectal angle, formed by the intersection of a line tangent to the rectal inferior wall and a line drawing the anal axis. At rest it measures 90°–100° (Fig. 6.12). When above 135°, there is nearly always incontinence of mechanical origin.
- The defecation angle, or anorectal angle during defecation. It must be above 105°. An underlying pathology must be looked for when this angle does not reach at least 140°.

The most frequent pathologies encountered in the investigation of continence and defecation disorders are sometimes difficult to diagnose clinically or by endoscopy [14]:

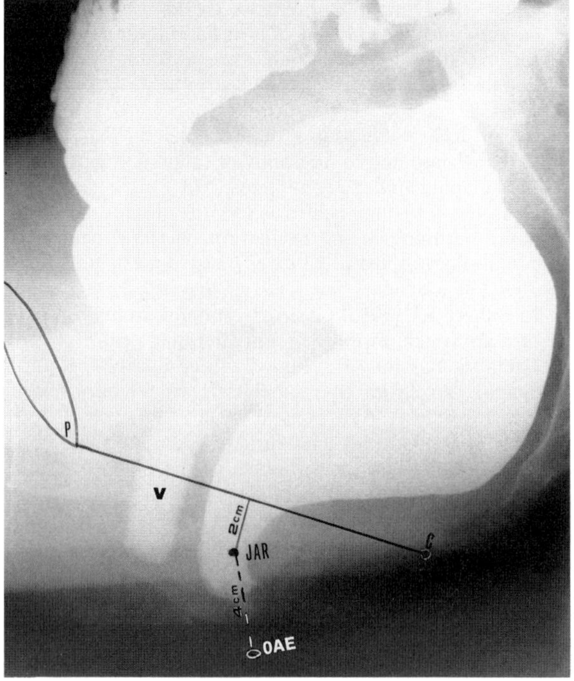

Fig. 6.11. Lateral view of the rectum at rest. *PC*, pubococcygeal line; *JAR*, anorectal junction; *OAE*, anal verge; *V*, vagina

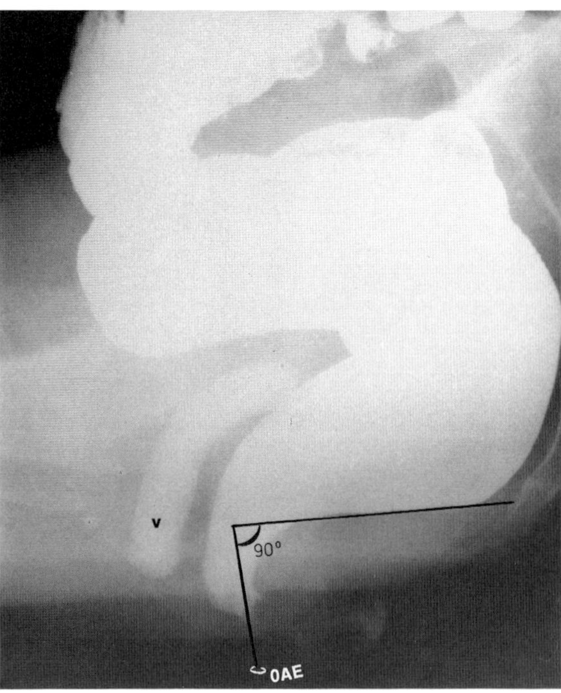

Fig. 6.12. Normal anorectal angle at rest. *V*, vagina

1. Intussusception: most frequently anteriorly situated, this is an invagination of the rectal mucosa in the lumen, generally occurring 6–8 cm above the anorectal junction. It progresses to a prolapse [18, 20] (Fig. 6.14).

2. Prolapse: described as incomplete when mucosal and complete when involving the rectal wall, it can remain situated in the rectum, reach the anal canal, or protrude through the anal verge (Fig. 6.13).

3. Rectocele, an anterior protrusion of the rectal wall, is variable in size, usually appears at the end of defecation, and often empties after the rectal ampulla. It is frequently a radiological finding as it is often hidden behind an intussusception or a prolapse.

4. The descending perineum syndrome is due to a general weakness of the pelvic floor often associated with other pathologies. Radiologically, one can find a detachment of the rectum from the concave anterior sacral border (mesorectum or Berman's mobile rectum theory), a lowering of the anorectal junction (of more than 2 cm); and sometimes an intussusception, a prolapse, and a rectocele (Fig. 6.14). Even though many of its constituents can be corrected by surgery, a des-

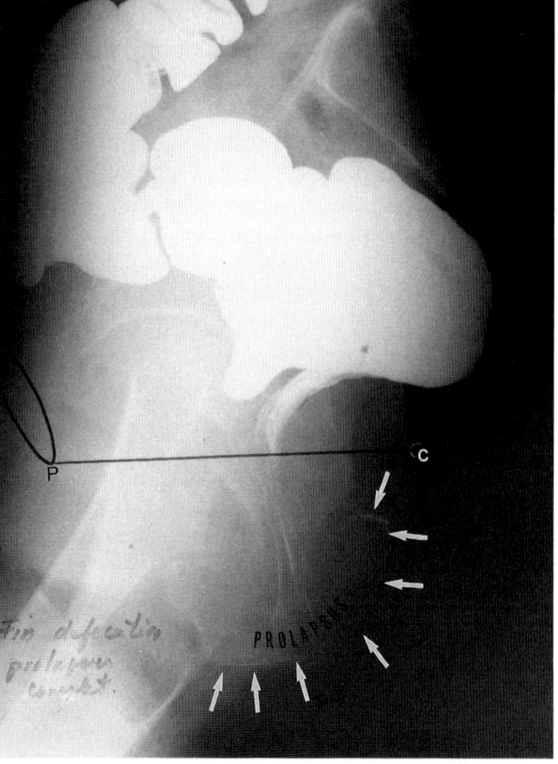

Fig. 6.13. Complete protruding prolapse. *PC*, pubococcygeal line

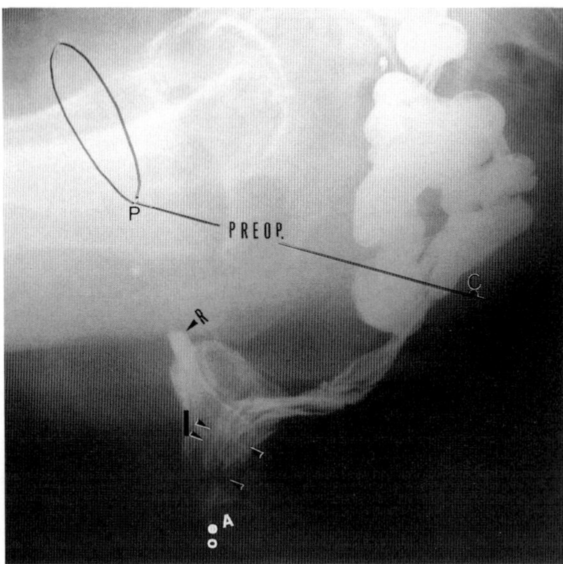

Fig. 6.14. Rectoanal intussusception and descending perineum syndrome. Preoperative view. *PC*, pubococcygeal line; *OA*, anal verge; *R*, rectocele; *vertical bar*, rectoanal intussusception

cent of the whole pelvic floor cannot be cured, as shown in postoperative studies.

5. The hypertonic puborectal sling, a curious pathology, may explain certain refractory constipations. The sling does not relax during straining. It is incriminated in the genesis of the solitary ulcer of the rectum [29].
6. The solitary ulcer of the rectum has a nonspecific radiological aspect [29]: it may present as a stenotic segment, as an ulcer niche or a polypoid nodule. The ultimate diagnosis is histological.

References

1. Balfe DM, Peterson RR, Lee JKT (1983) Normal abdominal anatomy. In: Computed body tomography. Raven, New York, pp 154–411
2. Bartram CI, Mahieu PHC (1985) Radiology of the pelvic floor. In: Coloproctology and the pelvic floor. Pathophysiology and management. Butterworth, London, pp 151–186
3. Berman IR, Manning DH, Dudley-Wright K (1985) Anatomic specificity in the diagnosis and treatment of internal rectal prolapse. Dis Colon Rectum 28: 816–826
4. Brekkan A, Kjartansson O, Tulinius H et al. (1983) Diagnostic sensitivity of X-ray examination of the large bowel in colorectal cancer. Gastrointest Radiol 8: 363–365
5. Butch RJ, Stark DD, Wittenberg J et al. (1986) Staging rectal cancer by MR and CT. AJR 146: 1155–1160
6. Chan CH, Diner WC, Fontenot E (1985) Randomized single-blind clinical trial of a rapid colonic lavage solution (Golytely®) VS standard preparation for barium enema and colonoscopy. Gastrointest Radiol 10: 378–382
7. Cohan RH, Silverman PM, Thompson WM et al. (1985) Computed tomography of epithelial neoplasms of the anal canal. AJR 145; 569–573
8. Dragsted J, Gammelgaard J (1983) Endoluminal ultrasonic scanning in the evaluation of rectal cancer: a preliminary report of 13 cases. Gastrointest, Radiol 8; 367–369
9. Eisenberg RL (1983) Gastrointestinal radiology. A pattern approach. Lippincott, Philadelphia, pp 779–791
10. Fataar S, Bassiony H, Hamed MS et al. (1984) Radiographic spectrum of rectocolonic calcification from schistosomiasis. AJR 141; 933–936
11. Fork F, Lindstrom C, Ekelund G (1983) Double contrast examination in carcinoma of the colon and rectum. Acta Radiol Diagn 24 (3): 177–188
12. Fox H, Legmann P, Levesque M (1985) Complications colorectales des explorations radiologiques. Ann Gastroenterol Hepatol 21: 377–381
13. Freeny PC, Marks WM, Ryan JA et al. (1986) Colorectal carcinoma evaluation with CT: preoperative staging and detection of postoperative recurrence. Radiology 158; 347–353
14. Fry R, Kodner I (1985) Anorectal disorders. Clin Symp 37 (6): 1–32
15. Grabbe E, Lierse W, Winkler R (1983) The perirectal fascia: morphology and use in staging of rectal carcinoma. Radiology 149: 241–246
16. Hallman JR, Howland WJ, Wolf BH (1986) Retrospective review of the sensitivity of barium enema examination in a community hospital setting. Ohio State Med J 2; 126–130
17. Hellstrom M, Brolin J (1987) Dietary fibers in the preparation of the bowel for diagnostic barium enema. Gastrointest Radiol 12: 76–78
18. Hoffman MJ, Kodner IJ, Fry RD (1984) Internal intussusception of the rectum. Diagnosis and surgical management. Dis Colon Rectum 27 (7): 435–441
19. Hollmann JP, Goebel N (1985) Computer tomographie (CT) und Sonographie (US) in der Rezidivdiagnostik kolorektraler Tumoren. ROFO 143 (6): 665–671
20. Johansson C, Ihre T, Ahlbäck SO (1985) Disturbances in the defecation mechanism with special reference to intussuspection of the rectum (internal procidentia). Dis Colon Rectum 28: 920–924
21. Kelvin F (1982) Radiologic approach to the detection of colorectal neoplasia. Radiol Clin North 20 (4): 743–759
22. Kelvin FM, Korobkin M, Heaston DK et al. (1983) The pelvis after surgery for rectal carcinoma: serial CT observations with emphasis on nonneoplastic features. AJR 141: 959–964
23. Kelvin FM (1987) Imaging the colon. Refresher course. RSNA, Chicago
24. Kindynis PH (1986) Etude TDM de l'évolution tumorale et non tumorale de la loge d'amputation rectale après amputation abdomino-périnéale. Thesisno 7047, University of Geneva
25. Konishi F, Muto T, Takahashi H et al. (1985) Transrectal ultrasonography for the assessment of invasion of rectal carcinoma. Dis Colon Rectum 28: 889–894

26. Kuijpers HC, Strijk SP (1984) Diagnosis of disturbances of continence and defecation. Dis Colon Rectum 27 (10): 658–662
27. Laufer J (1979) Double contrast gastrointestinal radiology with endoscopic correlation. Saunders, Philadelphia, pp 690–713
28. Laufer J (1983) Double contrast examination of the gastrointestinal tract in alimentary tract radiology, vol 1, 3rd edn. Mosby, St Louis, pp 148–191
29. Levine MS, Piccolello ML, Sollenberger LC et al. (1986) Solitary rectal ulcer syndrome: a radiologic diagnosis. Gastrointest, Radiol 11: 187–193
30. Lieberman DA (1984) Common anorectal disorders. Ann Intern Med 101: 837–846
31. Mahieu P, Pringot J, Bodart P (1984) Defecography: I. Description of a new procedure and results in normal patients. Gastrointest, Radiol, 9: 247–251
32. Mahieu P, Pringot J, Bodart P (1984) Defecography: II. Contribution to the diagnosis of defecation disorders. Gastrointest, Radiol, 9: 253–261
33. Marti MC, Mirescu D (1982) Utilité du défécogramme en proctologie. Ann Gastroenterol, Hepatol (Paris) 18: 379–384
34. McCarthy SM, Barnes D, Deveney K et al. (1985) Detection of recurrent rectosigmoid carcinoma: prospective evaluation of CT and clinical factors. AJR 144: 577–579
35. Moss AA (1982) Computed tomography in the staging of gastrointestinal carcinoma. Radiol Clin North 20 (4): 761–780
36. Ott DJ, Gelfand DW, Ramquist NA (1980) Causes of error in gastrointestinal radiology. Gastrointest Radiol 5: 99–105
37. Rifkin MD, Marks GJ (1985) Transrectal US as an adjunct in the diagnosis of rectal and extrarectal tumors. Radiology 157: 499–502
38. Rifkin MD, Wechsler RJ, Marks G (1987) Comparison of CT and endorectal US in staging rectal cancer. Radiology 165 [Suppl]: 174
39. Sadry F, Mirescu D, Marti M-C (1986) L'exploration radiologique des troubles de la défécation. In: Bessler W et al (eds) Neue Aspekte radiologischer Diagnostik und Therapie, Jahrbuch 1986. Huber, Bern, pp 8–91
40. Givel JC, Spinosa GP, Chapuis G (1988) Valeur de l'ultrasonographie endorectale pour la chirurgien.
41. Stark DD, Bradley WG (1988) Magnetic resonance imaging. Mosby, St Louis, pp 1130–1133
42. Thoeni RF, Moss AA, Schnyder P et al. (1981) Detection and staging of primary rectal and rectosigmoid cancer by computed tomography. Radiology 141: 135–138
43. Thoeni RF, Petras A (1982) Detection of rectal and rectosigmoid lesions by double-contrast barium enema examination and sigmoidoscopy. Accuracy of technique and efficacy of standard overhead views. Radiology 142: 59–62
44. Thompson WM, Halvorsen RA, Foster WL et al. (1986) Preoperative and postoperative CT staging of rectosigmoid carcinoma. AJR 146: 703–710
45. Zaunbauer W, Haertel M, Fuchs WA (1981) Computed tomography in carcinoma of the rectum. Gastrointest, Radiol 6: 79–84

7 Manometry and Electromyography

M.-C. Marti

Introduction

Several investigative methods are available to study the neuromuscular function of the pelvic floor and anal sphincters.

Manometry

Pressure is measured using three different devices:

- Small single or multiple balloons mounted on a catheter which is connected to pressure transducers in an air-free, waterfilled system
- Water-perfused open-tipped tubes
- Catheters in which microtransducer pressure gauges are mounted [2, 8, 19].

Pressure changes are converted into electrical impulses which are amplified and recorded on a computer system for further data work or are printed on moving paper. Furthermore, the system may also be connected to a television monitor and used for biofeedback training [4]. The system must be calibrated and the voltage on the amplifier adjusted to the expected pressure range.

Several contraindications exist in the use of some devices: an open perfused catheter can be blocked by feces; microtransducer pressure gauges are not useful in cases of incontinence with a dilated sphincter.

Anal Canal Pressure

The pressure within the anal canal can be measured at rest and during voluntary maximal contraction [2]. The resting pressure in the anal canal undergoes regular fluctuation: slow waves of 5–25 mm H_2O at a rate up 10–20/mn and ultraslow waves with 30–100 mm H_2O amplitude and a frequency of <3/mn are observed [10].

Using Arhan's two-balloon probe, it is possible to distinguish the pressure due to the internal sphincter in the upper anal canal from the pressure resulting from contraction of the external lower sphincter; 60%–80% of the resting pressure is due to the permanent contraction of the internal sphincter and the external sphincter. The voluntary contraction of the external sphincter and of the puborectalis muscle produces the maximal voluntary contraction pressure.

With simultaneous recording of the anal pressure and electromyography (EMG) of the external sphincter, the part of the resting tone which is due to the internal sphincter can be estimated by extrapolation as described by Schweiger [20].

Duration of Maximal Voluntary Contraction

The duration of the maximal voluntary contraction can be recorded. It usually ranges between 30 and 60 s. Owing to the fatiguability of the sphincters, the pressure may fall progressively.

Pressure Profile

The pressure profile of the anal canal can also be registered using a single-balloon probe or a Millar pressure gauge catheter [3, 14]:

1. The probe is withdrawn mechanically at a constant speed, allowing continuous registration of pressure.
2. The probe is withdrawn 0.5 or 1 cm at a time: at each point, the pressure at rest and during maximal voluntary contraction is registered.

Rectoanal Reflex

Distension of the rectum produces a reflex relaxation of the internal sphincter with a fall in the anal canal pressure in normal individuals [5]. This reflex is probably intramural as it is not necessarily suppressed by spinal anesthesia.

Viscoelasticity

Using the Arhan catheter with a large balloon mounted on its tip, it is possible to record anal pressure while the rectum is dilated [1]. After a baseline recording, increasing air volumes are injected into the balloon for 2–3 s. Usually with 20–50 ml of air, a sudden fall in the anal canal pressure occurs, followed by a spontaneous rise toward the baseline level within a few seconds. The volume of air necessary to produce the pressure drop is measured. If air is not withdrawn after injection and if the balloon is progressively dilated by repeated injections, the recovery of the anal pressure decreases, finally to zero, with each increment in the volume of the rectal balloon.

Manometry is useful in evaluating the function of the sphincters and the severity of incontinence [11]. Low voluntary squeeze pressures have a greater incidence of postoperative incontinence in cases of sphincter repair and rectal prolapse [9]. The absence of the anal inhibitory reflex is pathognomonic of Hirschsprung's disease and may be used to prove aganglionosis of the rectum. In cases of low anterior resection, the reflex is also suppressed; it reappears if sufficient nerve growth has occurred between the lower rectum and the anastomosed colonic segment [12].

Electromyography

EMG is an investigative technique which is employed, in particular, to evaluate disorders in which the nerve supply of muscles is damaged [7, 8, 10]. The electrical activity in muscle fibers is recorded using surface electrodes, concentric needle electrodes, and single-fiber EMG electrodes at rest, during voluntary contraction, and during stimulation of nerves.

EMG allows the recording and measurement of action potentials (amplitude, duration, number of phases, and firing rates) derived from motor units within a contracting muscle. With the use of single-fiber EMG, it is possible to record the activity of single muscle fibers. In proctology, EMG recordings allow functional muscle activity to be mapped and provides information on normal or deficient muscle innervation. Integrity of reflex activity can be tested during coughing, straining, and scratching of the anal skin.

In correlation with pressure recordings, EMG may help to distinguish insufficient functional activity due to myogenic lesions resulting from neurogenic or denervation damage [16]. EMG has proved that sphincter insufficiency and perineal descent may be the result of nerve stretching due to repeated straining, childbirth, and various types of neuropathy [8, 15, 16, 17]. Electrical stimulation – perineal, pudendal, or spinal – allows determination of nerve latency reaction and is useful in determining the level of motor conduction delay.

Volumetry

Using a water-filled balloon, it is possible to determine the minimal volume perceptible by the patient, the volume required to create a need to evacuate and the maximal tolerable volume before pain is induced [13]. If an air- or water-filled balloon connected to a pressure transducer is used, the rectal volume can be measured, values for rectal compliance (V/P) can be calculated, and accommodation properties of the rectum to the balloon distension can be evaluated. These data may be greatly altered in cases of constipation, rectal sclerosis due to inflammatory bowel diseases, and irradiation injuries. Tension of the rectal wall can be calculated from the pressure data by the Laplace law [1].

Sphincter Resistance

Henricksen [6] has developed a quantitative method for measuring sphincter resistance. A 2-cm diameter metal ball is inserted into the rectum. Using a dynamometer, the force necessary to withdraw the ball is measured at rest and during voluntary contraction.

Anal Sensation

Several quantitative experimental methods studied to measure anal and rectal sensitivity to electrical and thermal stimulation [18] are currently being.

References

1. Arhan P, Faverdin C, Persoz B, Devroede G, Dubois F, Dornic C, Pellerin D (1976) Relationship between viscoelastic properties of the rectum and anal pressure in man. J Appl Physiol 41: 677–682
2. Arhan P, Devroede G, Pellerin D (1979) Physiologie de la motricité de l'intestin terminal. Gastroenterol Clin Biol 3: 911–918

3. Blessing H (1984) The value of pullthrough manometry employing a microtransducer in anal emergencies. Coloproctology 6: 152–155
4. Denis P, Colin, Galmich JP, Muller JM, Hecketsweiler P, Merrien JF, Teniere P, Pasquis P (1983) Traitement de l'incontinence fécale de l'adulte. Gastroenterol Clin Biol 7: 857–863
5. Duthie HL, Bennett RC (1963) The relation of sensation in the anal canal to the functional anal sphincter: a possible factor in anal continence. Gut 4: 179–182
6. Henricksen FW, Huthouisen B (1972) Measurement of the anal sphincter through a simple method suitable for routine use. Scand J Gastroenterol 7: 555
7. Henry MM, Swash M (1978) Assessment of pelvic floor disorders and incontinence by electrophysiological recording of the anal reflex. Lancet 1: 1290–1291
8. Henry MM, Swash M (1985) Coloproctology and the pelvic floor. Butterworths, London
9. Keighley MRB, Fielding JWL (1983) Management of faecal incontinence and results of surgical treatment. Br J Surg 70: 463–468
10. Kerremans R (1969) Morphological and physiological aspects of anal continence and defecation. Arscid, Brussels
11. Kuypers JD (1982) Anal manometry: its applications and indications. Neth J Surg 34: 153–158
12. Lane RHS, Parks AG (1977) Function of the anal sphincters following coloanal anastomosis. Br J Surg 64: 596–599
13. Meunier P, Louis D, Jaubert de Beaujen M (1984) Physiologic investigation of primary chronic constipation in children: comparison with the barium enema study. Gastroenterology 87: 1351–1357
14. Nivatvongs S, Stern HS, Fryd DS (1981) The length of the anal canal. Dis Colon Rectum 24: 600–601
15. Parks AGP, McPartlin JG (1971) Late repair of injuries of the anal sphincter. Proc R Soc Med 64: 1–3
16. Parks AG, Swash M (1979) Denervation of the anal sphincter causing idiopathic anorectal incontinence. J R Coll Surg Edinb 24: 94–96
17. Parks AG, Swash M, Urich H (1977) Sphincter denervation in anorectal incontinence and rectal prolapse. Gut 18: 656–665
18. Roe AM, Bartolo DCC, Mortensen NJMcC (1986) New method for assessment of anal sensation in various anorectal disorders. Br J Surg 73: 310–312
19. Schuster MM, Hockman P, Hendrix TR, Mendeleff AI (1965) Simultaneous manometric recording of internal and external sphincter reflexes. Bull Johns Hopkins Hosp 116: 79–88
20. Schweiger M (1982) Funktionelle Analsphinkteruntersuchungen. Springer, Berlin Heidelberg New York

8 Positioning and Anesthesia for Anorectal Surgery

A. Forster and M.-C. Marti

Good operating conditions require proper placement of the patient on the operating table and adequate anesthesia. The aim of this chapter is to emphasize the principles that must be followed to obtain good operating conditions with optimal safety.

Positioning

Supine Position

For surgical procedures on the colon and for anterior resection of the rectum, the patient lies supine on the operating table [7]. In the case of very low anterior resection and if reanastomosis with the EEA stapler is planned, legs must be apart (Fig. 8.1) to give access to the anal canal.

Lithotomy Position for Abdominoperineal Excision

In the lithotomy a position roll must be placed below the sacrum and the patient must be drawn well down until the buttocks are beyond the end of the table. The legs are elevated with Lloyd Davies leg rests or leg supports. In abdominoperineal excision or pull-through procedures with one or two teams, flexion of the hips should be minimal to avoid any inguinal skin fold which would embarrass the abdominal surgeon. Furthermore, the operating table must be elevated with a 15%–20% head-down tilt (Trendelenburg) to give the surgeon good access to and vision of the perineum [7]. Surgeons operating simultaneously from the abdomen will stand on small steps to be in an optimal position (Fig. 8.2). To prevent the patient sliding headwards, shoulder rests are applied to the tip of the acromion. Both arms of the patient are fixed to the sides of the trunk. Optimal positioning of the patient should allow good and comfortable access to both the abdominal and perineal surgeons.

The instrument table is fixed over the head of the patient. A small instrument trolley is placed over the knees of the perineal surgeon.

A simplified lithotomy position is the best one for minor rectal operations (Fig. 8.3). In this case, the legs are elevated with leg supports and the hips are flexed at 90° or more. The patient must be drawn well down until the buttocks are beyond the end of the table.

Prone Jackknife Position

The prone jackknife position is preferred by many surgeons as it provides good surgical access and diminishes venous bleeding. To obtain these benefits, the abdomen and pelvis must be elevated with a roll placed exactly under the hips (Fig. 8.4). If the

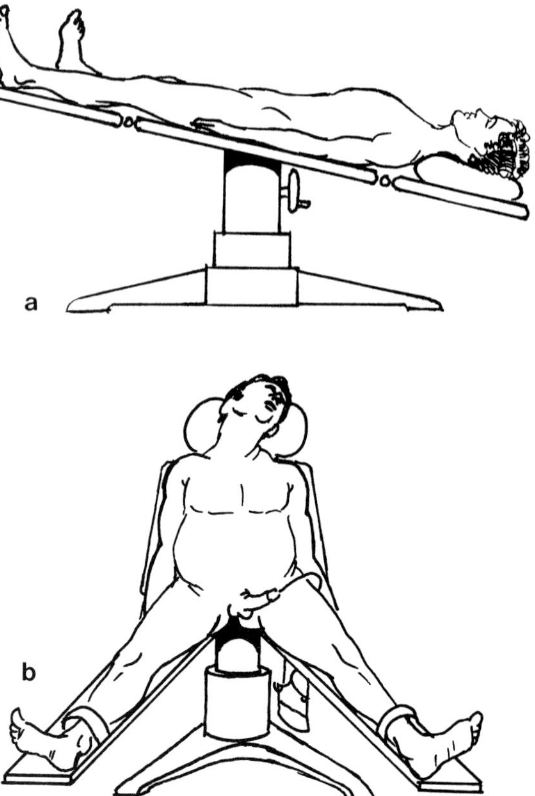

Fig. 8.1 a, b. Supine position

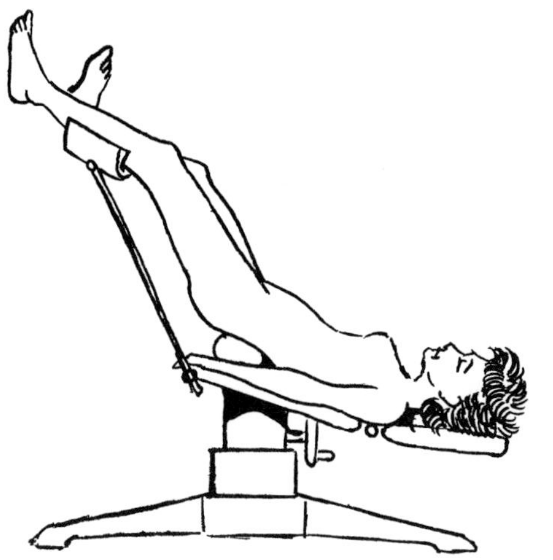

Fig. 8.2. Lithotomy position for abdominoperineal excision

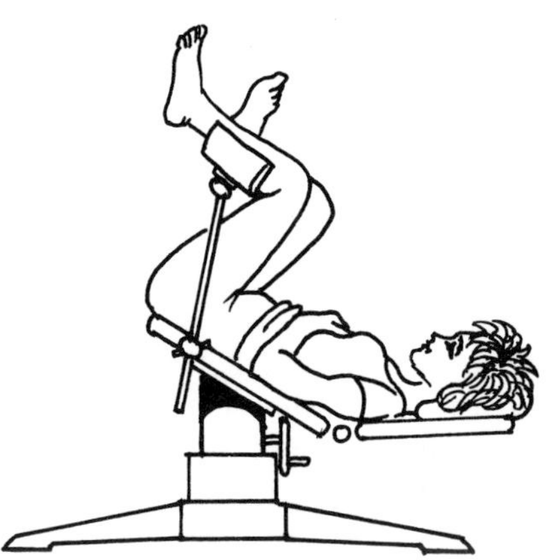

Fig. 8.3. Simplified lithotomy position for minor rectal operation

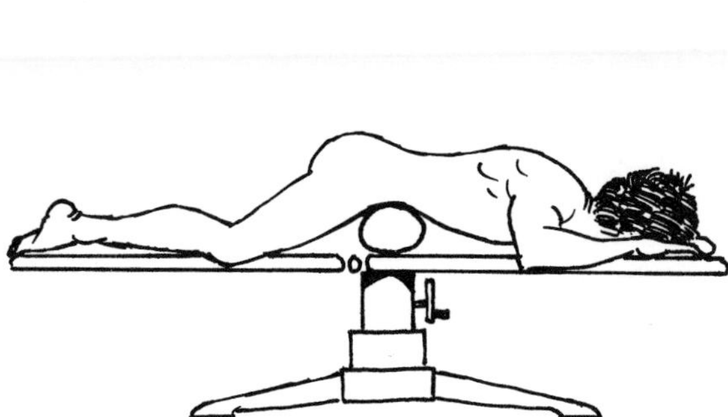

Fig. 8.4. Prone Jackknife position

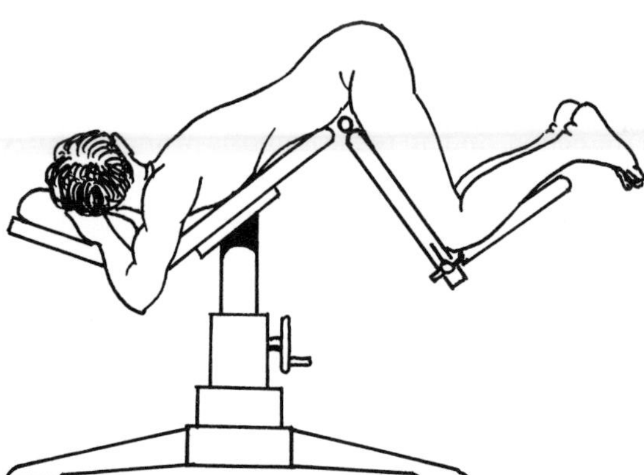

Fig. 8.5. Position on a proctological operating table

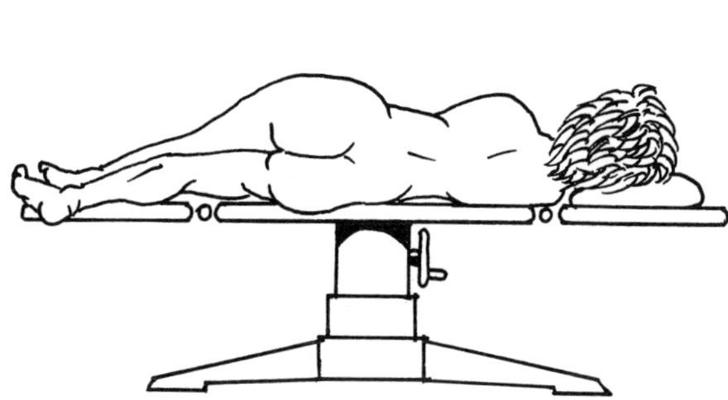

Fig. 8.6. Position for one-stage abdominosacral resection

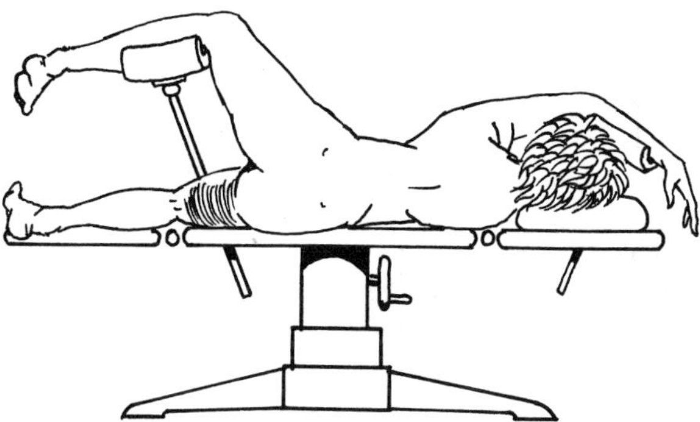

Fig. 8.7. Position for one-stage abdominosacral resection with elevated left leg

roll is placed higher, exposure will be less optimal, the vena cava inferior may be compressed resulting in increased surgical bleeding, and ventilation may be adversely affected [6, 7]. A special proctological operating table may be used (Fig. 8.5).

Position for One-Stage Abdominosacral Resection

In the case of midrectal carcinoma, Localio [10] favors an abdominosacral resection. To give simultaneous access to the rectum through the abdomen and through the sacrum, the patient is placed on the right side (Fig. 8.6). The left leg may be elevated (Fig. 8.7). Access to the sacrum is facilitated by raising the left buttock with some deep sutures.

Anesthesia

Efficacious anesthesia for proctology should fulfill at least five criteria [11]:

- Deep and lasting analgesia of the anal canal
- Blood-free operative field
- No side effects on the bladder
- Suppression of vagal reflex
- Easy use in outpatients

Several different types of technique can be used:
- Local anesthesia
- Local infiltration analgesia associated with sedative or light general anesthesia
- Locoregional or posterior perineal block
- Caudal anesthesia
- Epi- and peridural anesthesia
- General anesthesia

Local anesthesia, posterior perineal block, and caudal block give good operating conditions to perform nearly all proctological procedures. These methods do not require a long bed rest as compared to spinal block. They may be performed by the surgeon and may be used in outpatients [2, 8, 12, 17]. Careful patient selection is nevertheless necessary. The proctologist should be able to recognize and treat any cardiovascular and respiratory complication; adequate resuscitation equipment must be immediately accessible.

Advantages, disadvantages, and optimal indications in proctology are summarized in Table 8.1. Techniques requiring the presence of an anesthesist will not be discussed, but more details will be reported regarding techniques which can be performed by the surgeon him- or herself [2, 6, 8, 9, 11–13].

Locoregional Anesthesia

Choice of Local Anesthetic Agents

Local anesthetic agents may be classified [1, 16] according to their intrinsic potency compared to that of procaine, to the time needed until the onset of action, and to the duration of anesthesia (Table 8.2). All local anesthetic agents have a relaxant effect on the musculature of blood vessels resulting in vasodilatation. This effect is directly related to the potency of the drug: more potent and long-acting agents produce a greater and longer duration of vasodilatation.

Use of a Vasoconstrictor

Addition of a vasoconstricting [4, 16] agent into the local anesthetic solution contributes to constrict blood vessels, to reduce absorption, and hence to diminish the risk of systemic toxic reaction. Adrenaline and 8-ornithine vasopressin (POR 8) have been widely used at the following concentrations:

Adrenaline: 1:200000
8-Ornithine vasopressin: 1 unit in 4–10 ml

This results in:
- Reduced capillary bleeding
- Reduced reabsorption and risk of toxic effect
- Prolonged duration of analgesia

Caution is mandatory in cases of hypertension as well as coronary and cerebrovascular disease.

Use of Hyaluronidase

Hyaluronidase is a mucolytic enzyme which allows anesthetic solutions to spread into the tissue by inactivating the hyaluronic acid present in the interstitial space. It reduces swelling and increases absorption. Hyaluronidase is not toxic and rarely produces allergic reactions. Thanks to the increased diffusion of the anesthetic solution, a smaller volume may be used, but toxic reactions to the local anesthetic agent and to the vasoconstricting drug may be increased [3, 16]. Usually 150 units hyaluronidase are added to 50 ml solution.

Systemic Toxicity of Local Anesthetics

Surgeons should be well aware of toxic reactions due to local anesthetics and to vasoconstrictors; they must be able to manage and to treat them [1, 4–6, 16, 18]. Allergic reactions to local anesthetics

Table 8.1. Choice of anesthesia according to proctological procedures

	Technical problems	Complications and side effects	Advantages	Disadvantages and contraindications	Optimal indications in proctology
Local anesthesia	Easy to perform Does not need any premedication	Rare at the recommended dose Tissue deformation	Well tolerated by poor risk patients Dry operative field with vasoactive drugs Useful in outpatient surgery	Not acceptable to a number of patients Septic lesions	Sphincterotomies Anal and skin tags Excision
Posterior perineal block	Easy to perform after premedication	Depends on the drug used	Dry operative field No tissue deformity Partial relaxation of anal canal Useful in outpatient surgery	Contraindicated when area infected	Sphincterotomies Hemorrhoidectomies Cure of anal prolapse Anoplasties Thiersch wiring
Caudal block	Easy Does not need any premedication Failure if sacral hiatus not well located and in obese patient	Depends on the drug used Systemic reaction if inadvertent i v injection No tissue ischemia No hypotension	Excellent relaxation of anal canal and rectum No tissue deformity possible in outpatient Surgery with short-acting anesthetics	Contraindicated when area infected and in cases of pilonidal sinus	Fistulas Abscess Villous adenoma Sphincter repair
Rachi- and epidural block	Difficult in old patients Needs preoperative evaluation	No tissue ischemia Urinary retention Hypotension Spinal headache At least 1 day's hospitalization Postoperative nausea and vomiting	Excellent relaxation of anal canal and rectum	Contraindicated in cases of coagulopathy, when area of injection is infected, and in the case of neurological problems	Septic anal lesions
General anesthesia	Necessity of preoperative cardiovascular and pulmonary assessment Premedication necessary	Hospital stay may be necessary Requires intubation particularly in prone jackknife position Postoperative nausea and vomiting	Better accepted Excellent relaxation and analgesia	Poor-risk patients	Examination under anesthesia High pararectal and rectal lesions Extensive septic lesions

are rare and are usually limited to ester-linked agents, such as procaine and tetracaine, and not to amino-linked drugs like lidocaine and prilocaine. The majority of systemic reactions are due to inadvertent intravascular injection or to administration of an excessive dose. Toxic reactions can be classified, according to their severity, as light, medium, or severe (Table 8.3). Central nervous system excitation represents the earliest manifestation of toxicity. Respiratory and cardiovascular complications result from direct cardiac and vascular action due to overdosage or from indirect action by blockade of the autonomic nerve fibers. Bupivacaine causes the greatest cardiac toxicity [15].

Toxicity of Vasoactive Drugs

If vasoactive drugs have been injected with local anesthetics, side effects due to them should also be considered and recognized [16].

Table 8.2. Dosage and toxicity of local anesthesic agents

	Toxicity[a]	Analgesic power[a]	Maximal dosage		Onset of action (min)	Duration of action
			Without adrenaline (mg)	With adrenaline (mg)		
Procaine	1	1	500	1000	5–10	45–60 min
Tetracaine	10	10	100	20	10	60–90 min
Lidocaine	2	2	200	500	<2	60–120 min
Prilocaine	1,5	2	400	600	<2	60–120 min
Hostacaine	2	4	?	?	<2	60–120 min
Mepivacain	2	2	300	500	<2	60–120 min
Tolycaine			250	600	2–5	60–90 min
Bupivacaine	6	8	150	150	5–10	5–15 h

[a] In comparison to procaine.

Table 8.3. Signs and symptoms of local anesthetic toxicity

	Central nervous system effects	Cardiovascular effects
Light	Dizziness Lightheadedness Daze Tinnitus Tremor Agitation Disorientation	PR interval ↑ QRS duration ↑ Cardiac output ↓ Blood pressure ↓
Medium	Speach difficulties Confusion Vomiting Unconsciousness Muscle twitching Tremor of face and extremities	PR interval ↑↑ QRS duration ↑↑ Sinus bradycardia Hypotension
Severe	Coma Generalized convulsions Respiratory problems Respiratory arrest	Atrioventricular block Asystole

Table 8.4. Treatment of local anesthetic toxicity

Light	Oxygen administration Sedatives (benzodiazepine barbiturate)
Medium	Sedatives Clear airway if unconscious Respiratory assistance i. v. fluid
Severe	Sedatives Mask ventilation; if not successful: succinylcholine 1 mg/kg i. v. with eventual intubation i. v. fluid to restore volume Thiopental within 30 s to 1 min Adrenaline Cardiac massage if arrest Correction of the acidosis

Side Effects due to Vasoconstrictors

- Apprehension
- Excitation
- Sweating
- Tremor
- Palor
- Dizzines
- Hypertension
- Arrythmia
- Tachycardia

Treatment is different according to whether toxic reactions are due to local anesthetics or to vasoconstrictors, especially in the most severe forms (Table 8.4). Oxygen should be administered and sedatives injected in cases of arrythmia or tachycardia; i. v. lidocaine or β-blockers should be considered in cases of toxic reactions due to vasoconstrictors. Electric defibrillation may be necessary. To prevent severe complications some rules must be observed:

1. Complete resuscitation equipment (suction, mask and intubation set, O_2, resuscitative drugs) must always be available.
2. Maximal dosage of the local anesthetic drugs must not be exceeded.
3. Premedication is not reliable in preventing systemic toxic reactions.
4. Patients have to be observed carefully after completion of the injection.
5. Any complication should be correctly evaluated.
6. Any type of complication must be expected and, if necessary, treated.
7. Any type of complication or reaction should not be over- or undertreated.

Technique of Local Anesthesia

Local anesthesia is useful for many minor anorectal procedures not requiring muscular relaxation. Indications to local anesthesia are very restrictive [1, 2, 9]. Local injection is used to perform sphincterotomies in the treatment of fissures, to excise hypertrophic anal papillae and skin tags, to treat short fistulous tracts, and to treat perianal hematoma. Contraindications include local septic conditions, the patient's anxiety, the patient's insufficient compliance, and the prolonged time required for the procedure.

If necessary, the patient can be given premedication 30 min to 1 h before the procedure: 5–10 mg diazepam administered orally is very effective.

The skin is cleaned and disinfected with an antiseptic solution. The anesthetic solution is injected at first subdermally and then submucosally around the lesion to be treated with a continuous motion of the needle or frequent aspiration to prevent intravascular injection. Injection within the muscle may be avoided depending on the depth of the lesion. One should never inject near a septic lesion to avoid bacteremia.

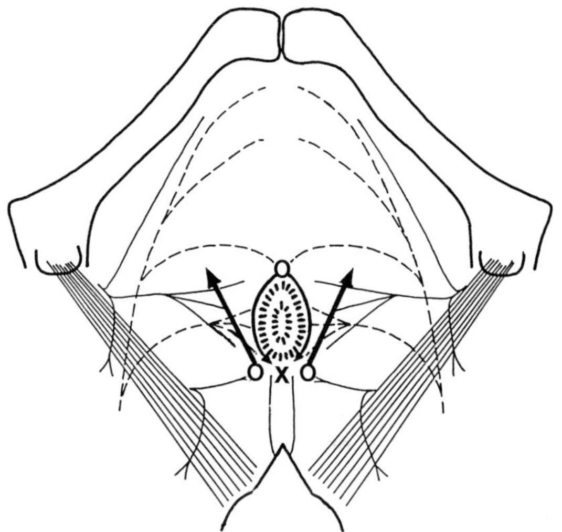

Fig. 8.8. Posterior perineal block

Posterior Perineal Block [11–13] (Fig. 8.8)

After subdermal infiltration at four sites, the anococcygeal ligament is deeply infiltrated with 5 ml 0.5% lidocaine; 10 ml solution is injected into both ischiorectal spaces when withdrawing the needle which is oriented at 45° cranially and 45° laterally. This allows anesthesia of the deep nerve endings. Through a skin puncture in front of the anus, 10 ml solution is then infiltrated subdermally on each side at the level of the rima ani to secure analgesia of the more superficial nerve endings. The total amount injected is 60 ml 0.5% lidocaine and 10–15 units 8-ornithine vasopressin.

This type of anesthesia is routinely used to perform hemorrhoidectomies. It allows a short hospital stay, a dry operative field, prolonged anesthesia with a low rate of bladder retention. An outpatient should not leave the hospital until he or she has completly recovered from the premedication and has passed urine.

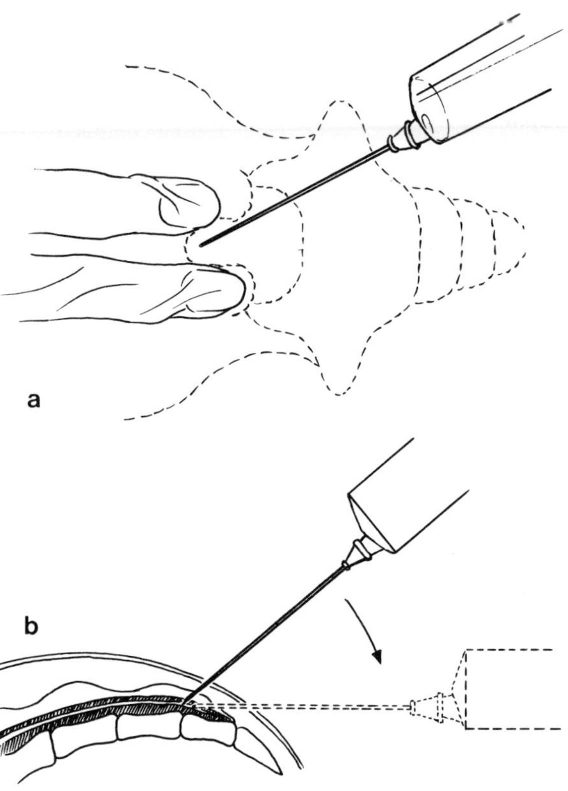

Fig. 8.9 a, b. Caudal block

Caudal Block (Fig. 8.9)

Caudal block is a type of epidural block [8, 11, 16]. With the patient in a prone jackknife position, 15–20 ml 2% lidocaine with epinephrine or 0.25% bupivacaine with epinephrine are injected into the sacral canal through the sacrococcygeal space after ensuring by suction that no blood or cerebrospinal fluid can be withdrawn. Immediately after injection, the patient is turned on the back and put in an anti-Trendelenburg position to ensure sacral distribution of the drug. This technique should not be used in patients with inadequate coagulation as in the case of hepatic insufficiency.

Unsatisfactory results and failures in the performance of caudal block occur in fewer than 5% of cases [11, 14, 16]. These are due to the failure to identify the sacral hiatus, to improper placement of the needle, or to a too narrow sacral hiatus not permitting insertion of a needle. Two complications may occur: unrecognized dural puncture which results in a so-called total spinal with profound hypotension, respiratory distress, and coma; too rapid an injection or injection within epidural veins may result in systemic toxicity.

A caudal block allows nearly all proctological surgical procedures, even septic ones. Local infiltration with vasoconstrictors may be useful in providing a dry field. Caudal block should not be performed in cases of infection in the area of intended puncture as, for example, in cases of pilonidal sinus or extensive infected fistulas.

Spinal Block

Spinal block provides excellent operative conditions with a much smaller dose of anesthetics. Contraindications, as for caudal block, are skin infection in the area of intended puncture, neurological diseases, and coagulopathy. Failures are less frequent than for caudal block [14, 16, 19]. Postspinal headache is the main disadvantage. We use spinal block in cases of extensive perianal septic lesions, for rectovaginal fistula, and in cases of failed or insufficient caudal block.

General Anesthesia

In long surgical procedures general anesthesia requires endotracheal intubation, but in most cases short procedures can be performed with a mask. We use general anesthesia in cases of contraindication to any other type of anesthesia. General anesthesia can be light when complemented by local anesthesia.

General anesthesia is used for some special proctological procedures when good relaxation is necessary, to treat an interspincteric abscess or an extensive abscess or fistula, and if the abdominal cavity is to be opened.

References

1. Auberger HG (1969) Praktische Lokalanästhesie, ein Kompendium. Thieme, Stuttgart
2. Barry BA (1985) Die Lokalanästhesie bei ambulanten Eingriffen. In: Kinoch HG, Hager TH, Frank WL (eds) Aktuelle Koloproktologie I. Nymphenburg, München, pp 73–78
3. Clery AP (1973) Local anaesthesia containing hyaluronidase and adrenaline for anorectal surgery: experiences with 576 operations. Proc R Soc Med 66: 680–681
4. Covino BG, Vasallo HG (1976) Local anesthetics, mechanisms of action and clinical use. Grune and Stratton, New York
5. De Jong RH (1978) Toxic effects of local anesthetics. JAMA 239: 1166–1168
6. Goldberg SM, Gordon PH, Nivatvongs S (1980) Essential of anorectal surgery. Lippincott, Philadelphia
7. Goligher J (1980) Surgery of the anus rectum and colon. Baillière Tindall, London
8. Knoch HG (1985) Bewährte Anästhesieverfahren in der ambulanten Proktologie. In: Kinoch HG, Hager TH, Frank WL (eds) Aktuelle Koloproktologie I. Nymphenburg, München, pp 68–72
9. Kratzer GL (1965) Local anesthesia in anorectal surgery. Dis Colon Rectum 8: 441–446
10. Localio SA, Baron B (1973) Abdomino-sacral resection and anastomosis for mid-rectal cancer. Ann Surg 178: 540–546
11. Marti MC, Froidevaux A, Rifat K (1977) Préparation pré-opératoire et choix de l'anesthésie en proctologie. Med Hyg 35: 2334–2338
12. Marti MC (1985) Chirurgie proctologique ambulatoire. Schweiz Rundsch Med Prax 74: 755–756
13. Marti MC (1981) Choix d'un type d'anesthésie en proctologie et intérêt des blocs périnéaux postérieurs. Ann Gastroenterol Hepatol (Paris) 17: 195–197
14. Massey Dawking CJ (1969) An analysis of the complications of extradural and caudal block. Anaesthesia 24: 554–561
15. Moore DC, Bridenbaugh LD, Thompson GE, Balfour RI, Horton WG (1978) Bupivacaine: a review of 11080 cases. Anesth Analg (Cleveland) 57: 42–53
16. Moore DC (1981) Regional block, 4th edn. Thomas, Springfield
17. Opperbecke HW (1982) Voraussetzungen und Grenzen ambulanten Operierens aus anästhesiologischer Sicht. Anaesthesiol Intensivmed 23: 186
18. Pittet JF (1987) Pharmacologie et toxicité des anesthésiques locaux. Schweiz Rundsch Med Prax 76: 865–871
19. Sadove MS, Levin MJ (1954) Neurological complications of spinal anesthesia. A statistical study of more than 10000 consecutive cases III. Med J (Engl Transl Lijec Vjesn) 105: 169–176

9 Hemorrhoids

M.-C. Marti

Hemorrhoidal disease is the most frequently observed anal pathology; 50%–90% of all individuals complain of hemorrhoids at least once in their lives. Fifty percent of all patients attending a proctological clinic present more or less severe symptoms due to hemorrhoids. This disease has been recognized and treated since antiquity [34, 78, 82].

Definition

Today hemorrhoids should be considered as a hypertrophy of the normal anal cushions lying in the upper part of the anal canal. Because of their apposition, these cushions are responsible for the precise closure of the anal canal [19, 99, 100]. They comprise a thick submucosa which contains blood vessels, smooth muscle, elastic and connective tissue. The vessels present a glomerular pattern; the blood supply comes from the mid- and inferior rectal arteries [105]. This concept is supported by the finding of bright red arterial bleeding at time of operation, by tissue oxymetric measures and thermoconductibility studies [107].

At the level of the dentate line, the submucosal space is divided into two parts by the ligament of Parks and the muscle of Treitz. This muscle is made up of smooth muscle originating from the longitudinal muscle of the rectum and crossing the internal sphincter. Its action is reinforced by muscle fibers of the internal sphincter. These muscular fibers end in the submucosa and prevent mucosal prolapse during defecation [52, 105, 106].

The position of the cushions is constant (Fig. 9.1): left lateral at 3 o'clock in the gynecological position; right posterior at 7 o'clock, and right anterior at 11 o'clock. Smaller cushions may be located in between. This configuration is constant with no relation to the branching of the superior rectal artery.

Pathophysiology

Internal hemorrhoids result from congestion and hypertrophy of the cushion located above the den-

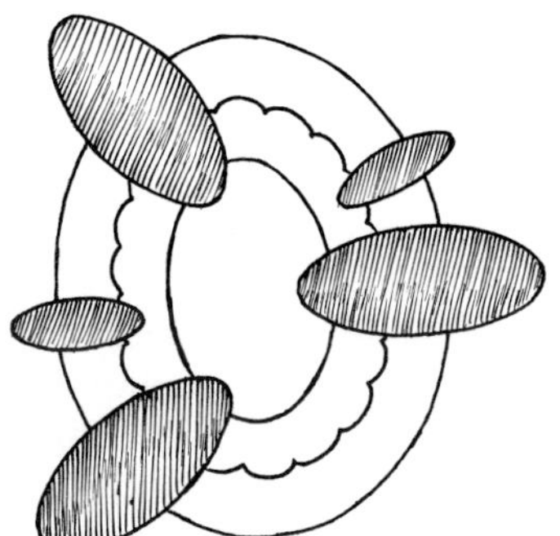

Fig. 9.1. Position of hemorrhoidal cushions

tate line, called the "corpus cavernosum recti" by Stelzner [99, 100]. As these vessels are connected with those located below the dentate line, so-called external hemorrhoids may develop [84]. Repeated episodes of venous congestion produce redundancy of the mucous membrane and perineal skin.

Hemorrhoids may be the result of several different mechanisms:

- Dysregulation of the arteriovenous shunt at the level of the glomerular formation
- Insufficient return of blood through the superior rectal veins resulting in a swelling of the cushions
- Increased intra-abdominal pressure with compression of the venous pedicle during straining in obstipation, during efforts to empty the bladder in cases of prostatic adenoma, and during pregnancy
- Prolonged sphincter hypertonicity diminishing return of blood through the transsphincteric shunts [40]

Chronic or repeated congestion results in a stretching of the ligament of Parks and hypertrophy followed by breaking of the muscle of Treitz. As the mucosa is no longer fixed to the muscular coat, an intermittent prolapse may appear followed by a permanent prolapse [34, 82, 83].

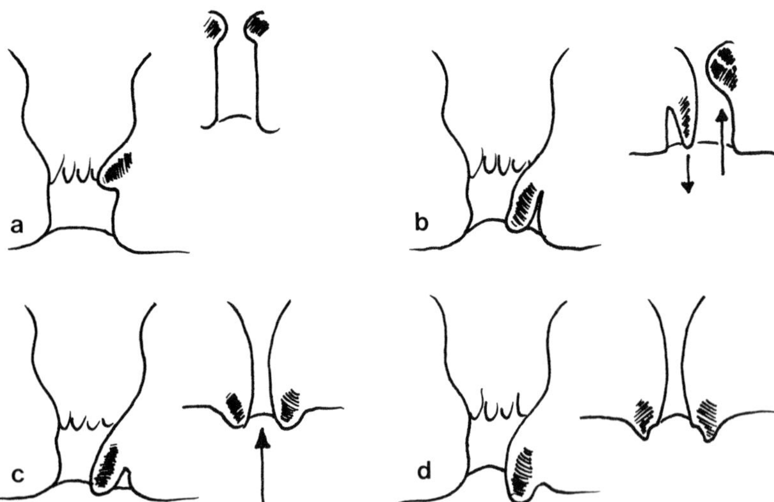

Fig. 9.2 a–d. Classification of hemorrhoids. *a* First degree; *b* second degree; *c* third degree; *d* fourth degree (see text for details)

Classification

Hemorrhoidal disease may be staged as follows (Fig. 9.2):

First-degree hemorrhoids, or simple hypertrophy of the corpus cavernosum recti, are said to be present when they bulge into the lumen of the anus, without prolapse. They can be observed only by proctoscopy. They may result in painless bleeding.

Second-degree hemorrhoids prolapse upon straining during bowel movements but reduce spontaneously. At this stage, the corpus cavernosum recti loses its properties of continence; patients complain of intermittent watery and mucosal exudate.

Third-degree hemorrhoids may lead to the prolapse becoming permanent, but it can be digitally replaced. The protruding cushions may become sclerotic with painful epidermal metaplasia. As prolapsed vessels are no longer under intra-anal pressure but under atmospheric pressure, surface venectasia may develop.

Fourth-degree hemorrhoids are those which can no longer be replaced digitally; they are irreducible, sclerotic, and frequently accompanied by skin tags.
The individual cushions may present at different stages in the same patient.

Etiology and Predisposing Factors

The incidence of hemorrhoids increases with age but lesions may be present at any age, even in childhood. Males seem to be affected twice as frequently as females. Different predisposing factors have been proposed [34, 43]: heredity, climate, age, sex, pregnancy, obstipation, abuse of laxatives, repeated enema, mucosal irritation, sedentary lifestyle, obesity, chronic use of suppositories, cirrhosis, and use of a pessary. No occupational group seems to be especially prone to hemorrhoids except military aircraft pilots submitted to high gravitational pressures [63].

Hemorrhoids are not cause by one individual mechanism but by the interaction of many factors. Among all the factors proposed, nutrition seems to play an important role. In epidemiological studies, Burkitt [21] has demonstrated that a highly refined, low-fiber, high-carbohydrate diet results in a significant increase of abdominal and intrarectal pressure resulting in the formation of small and hard stools which are therefore the main causes of constipation. On the other hand, a fiber-rich diet stimulates defecation and reduces the risk of hemorrhoidal congestion.

This hypothesis is not totally satisfactory and does not explain, for example, the occurrence of hemorrhoids in patients not suffering from obstipation or chronic diarrhea. Any increase of intra-abdominal or intraportal pressure does not necessarily result in a hypertrophy of the anal cushions [46]. A prostatic adenoma or an intrapelvic tumor may produce an increase of the intra-abdominal pressure, especially during micturation, but does not result in the development of hemorrhoids. A chronic respiratory insufficiency with chronic coughing results in an intra-abdominal pressure rise but does not seem to produce anal disease more frequently. According to these observations, factors other than mechanic and dietetic ones must be considered, e. g., vascular fragility and abnormal sensitivity to estrogens [90].

Symptoms

Several symptoms may be present in hemorrhoids, especially internal ones. Bleeding is the most common symptom. Bright red and painless bleeding occurs at the end of defecation. Bleeding may also be occult. Chronic iron deficiency anemia may occur as a result. Any other cause of bleeding must be excluded.

A prolapse develops during straining. In the case of second-degree hemorrhoids, reduction occurs spontaneously. In third-degree hemorrhoids, a prolapse can be replaced digitally. A prolapse predisposes to soreness, mucous and fecal leakage which induce pruritus, skin excoriation, and secondary mycotic infection.

A prolapse, if irreducible, may become strangulated and results in necrosis, secondary fistula, and gangrene. Pylephlebitis is a potential but rare complication.

Pain becomes a marked feature of the disease when thrombosis occurs, when a prolapse with severe edema develops, or when the prolapse becomes strangulated. Severe pain also suggests an associated anal fissure.

Examination

Correct examination is necessary to ensure the diagnosis, to evaluate the stage of the lesion and any complications, and to exclude other associated disease and coincidental lesions. General assessment is necessary as is local examination, proctoscopy, and even colonoscopy. Barium enema or panendoscopy must be performed in any patient with unusual clinical symptoms or if symptoms are more severe than those expected to result from the lesions observed.

When there is an unsuspected carcinoma in the upper rectum, cancer cells may implant on the scar tissue after hemorrhoidectomy and eventually lead to a need for abdominoperineal excision.

Nonsurgical Treatment

Various treatment modalities are available with the following goals:

- To correct dietetic factors in order to avoid straining during defecation and to stimulate regular production of bulky, large, and soft stools
- To diminish any swelling of the submucosa and corpus cavernosum recti
- To stimulate the venous return of blood through the reduction of sphincter spasms and intra-abdominal pressure
- To stimulate adhesion between mucosa and muscular coats
- To reconstruct normal anatomy and physiology of the anal canal
- To avoid scars, skin tags, and stenosis
- To treat any concomitant lesion

Not every patient with hemorrhoids will require active treatment. They will just learn from their physician that they do not have a tumor. Treatment should not be thrust on a patient who does not want it.

The hemorrhoids of pregnancy result mainly from a transient engorgement of the perianal venous plexus and do not need aggressive treatment. In the postpartum period, after reassessment, the need for treatment should be reevaluated.

Bowel Regulation

It is essential to regulate bowel movement in a patient with hemorrhoids. Both constipation and diarrhea should be avoided. The passage of hard stools results in congestion of the corpus cavernosum recti; diarrhea irritates the mucosa which becomes less resistant and predisposes to the development of hemorrhoids or to the aggravation of preexisting disease.

It is important to give the patient an adequate fluid intake and to increase the intake of bulk in the form of vegetable fiber or unprocessed cereal fiber like bran. A bulk-forming agent may be prescribed. Such a treatment should be followed indefinitely, even after surgical treatment, to avoid recurrences. Dietetic treatment seems more effective if the intra-anal pressure is raised [8].

Topical Treatment

To be useful, any topical treatment should be applied in the anal canal and not on the skin or into the rectum. Creams may be introduced using a smooth canula or a glove. Suppositories go too far into the rectum and therefore have no local efficacy. Their main action is to lubricate the anal canal and to produce soft stools.

All commercial preparations currently available are composed of antiseptic, anesthetic, anti-inflammatory, vasoactive, or antithrombotic drugs. Topical treatment may be useful in acute exacerbation of hemorrhoids at any stage but never helps in reducing a prolapse or changing the stage of the lesions.

As a histological study of 200 hemorrhoidectomy samples could not prove any signs of inflammation [31], the use of anti-inflammatory drugs is still debatable. It is therefore necessary to evaluate the side effects of any prolonged or abused application. Steroids, especially, may induce an atrophy of the anoderma and the skin, and favor mycotic infection and chronic eczematic changes.

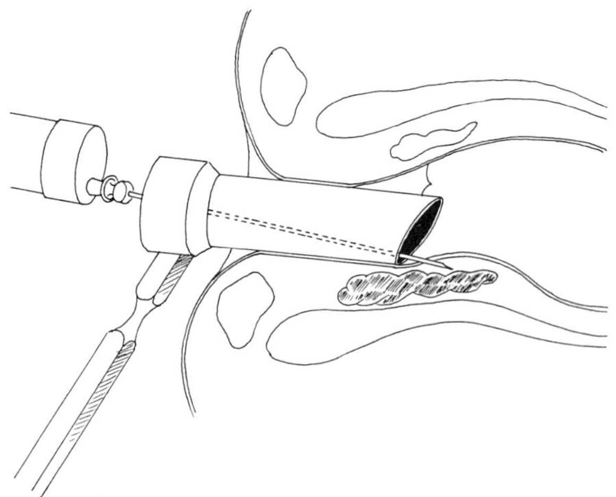

Fig. 9.3. Submucosal sclerosis

Sclerosing Injection Therapy

Sclerotherapy was developed in the United States during the second half of the nineteenth century by Blackwood and initially caused great controversy. It was introduced in Europe at the beginning of this century [13, 14, 69]. Two different procedures have been described.

Submucosal Sclerosis According to Bensaude

Submucosal sclerosis according to Bensaude [13] is the method most commonly used. The solution is inserted into the interstitial tissue of the submucosa (not into the veins) above the anal cushions, at the anorectal junction, and around the pedicles of the efferent vessels (Fig. 9.3). Injection produces a scarring in the submucous layer which will fix to the muscular layers, and retract and atrophy the cushions preventing further prolapse. The most commonly used solution is 5% phenol in almond or arachide oil with some drops of menthol to remove the unpleasant odor of the solution. It is nontoxic and harmless [36]. The injection of 2–5 ml in a single area produces good interstitial fibrosis without necrosis. As the viscosity of the solution is very high, the 10-cm 20-gauge straight needle used should be pushed firmly onto the nozzle of the syringe; a Luer-lock Gabriel needle fixed on a special syringe is useful and prevents undesiderable unlocking.

The proctoscope is inserted and the obturator withdrawn to allow exact identification of the anorectal ring by sliding the proctoscope up and down within the anal canal. Feces are cleaned off or pushed back with some cotton swabs. The mucosa is not disinfected. The needle is passed through the anuscope and inserted through the mucosa into the submucosa just above the anal cushions. The three cushions at 3, 7, and 11 o'clock are injected in one session. Some cotton swabs are left inside the anal canal to press the mucosa against the muscular layers. The injection should be done slowly and does not require undue force; a light swelling must be produced with the vessels becoming visible. If painful, the injection should be stopped since the needle has been placed in an incorrect position. Replacement and injection can be immediately performed in the correct way. Instead of phenol solution, some authors use a small amount (0.5–1 ml) of quinine and urea or iodides. The low pH of quinine solution may induce more severe necrosis.

After injection, the patient is asked to avoid movement for 24 h if possible. He or she is checked again 3–4 weeks later; injection can be completed if necessary but previous sites of sclerosis should be avoided. Subsequent injection with smaller doses can be given if symptoms reappear. The larger the hemorrhoids, the shorter the duration of remission.

Complications as a result of sclerotherapy are rare and result mainly from an incorrect technique [113]. Injections which are too superficial may produce necrosis and rectal ulceration resulting in pain, bleeding, and delayed healing. Too deep an injection may be damaging, especially after injection of the right anterior hemorrhoid in the male resulting in hematuria by direct trauma to the urinary tract and prostate. Extrarectal injection can result in stricture by scarring [87]. Abscess and fistula in ano may occur. Oleogranuloma is rare but very severe.

Intravenous injection results in an oil embolus. Jaundice has been reported due to injection directly into the inferior hemorrhoidal veins [112].

The cure rate in the treatment of first- and second-degree hemorrhoids is in the order of 75%. In 1934 Kilbourne [51] reviewed 25000 cases and estimated that recurrence took place in at least 15% of cases within 3 years.

Sclerosis According to Blond

Blond [15] described a technique of sclerosis with direct injection into the submucosa of the cushion. Using a proctoscope with a lateral window and a special needle, 0.2 ml 20% quinine solution is injected into the submucosa at two to three different levels of each cushion. Only one cushion should be treated at each session. Stein [96, 97] used this technique with success, even in the treatment of prolapsed third-degree hemorrhoids.

Complications [97] are more frequent with this technique than with Bensaude's procedure. Injection of too large an amount of solution may result in necrosis and bleeding. Allergic reaction is possible. Rectosigmoidal necrosis has been described after accidental injection within hemorrhoidal vessels [97].

Sclerosis is contraindicated during pregnancy, when there are coagulation problems, inflammatory bowel disease, and septic anal lesions.

Infrared Coagulation

Photocoagulation of the mucosa and submucosa with infrared light was introduced in the treatment of hemorrhoids by Neiger [76, 77] (Fig. 9.4). Photocoagulation produces thermal necrosis followed by ulceration which heals by cicatrization within 2–3 weeks. The scar fixes the mucosa to the underlying tissue and so prevents prolapse. Infrared coagulation has a hemostatic effect which is superior to the usual methods of sclerosis.

Photocoagulation is performed through an anuscope. Three to four areas of mucosa, at 2, 4, 8, and 10 o'clock, just above the internal cushions and usually above the inner anal ring are coagulated in one session. Two sessions are usually sufficient to coagulate also at 3, 6, 9, and 12 o'clock. The tip of the infrared photocoagulator, coated with a polymer to prevent tissue adherence, is applied for 1–1.5 s to ensure sufficient effect. The complete procedure can be performed by one surgeon without an assistant.

Infrared coagulation is a simple, fast, and effective method, with fewer complications and side effects than sclerosis by injection or rubber band ligation [5, 54, 55, 103]. Postoperative pain and secondary bleeding are rare, resulting in less time off work than after rubber band ligation. Cure at 12 months can be achieved in 75% of first- and second-degree hemorrhoids. Fifteen percent of all patients experience a recurrence of their symptoms within 3 years. Treatment may then be repeated.

Rubber Band Ligation

Already in the Middle Ages, hemorrhoids were treated by ligation. The procedure was very painful as skin, anoderm, and mucosa were strangulated to-

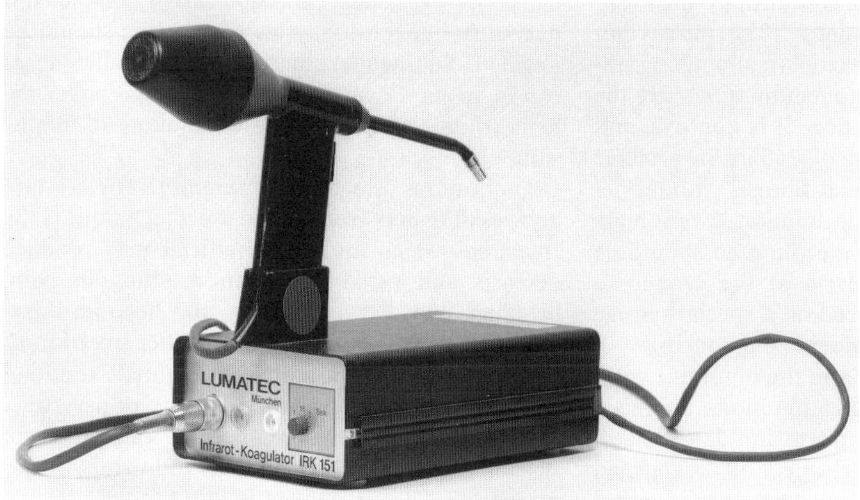

Fig. 9.4. Infrared coagulator

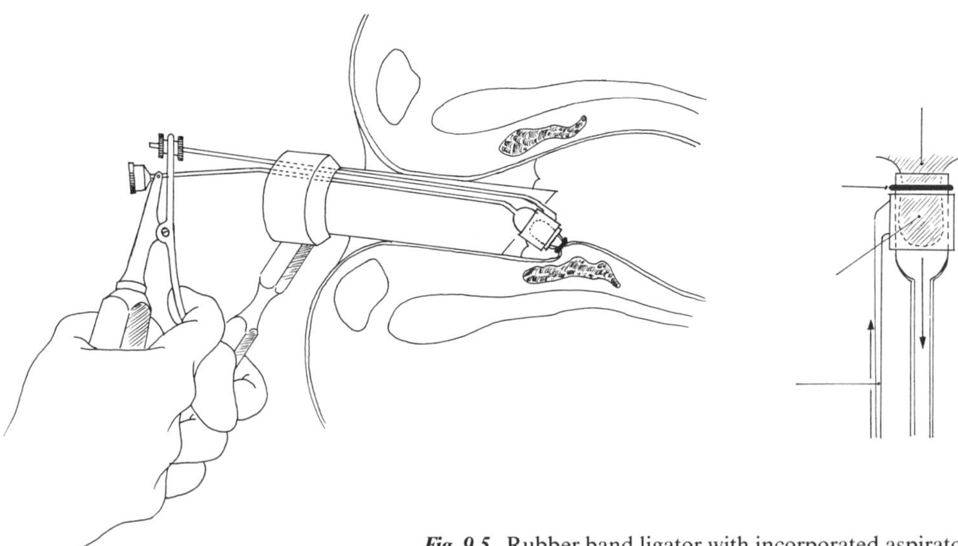

Fig. 9.5. Rubber band ligator with incorporated aspirator

gether. In China and New Caledonia, prolapse of the rectum was treated by strangulating the prolapsed gut with the help of two tubes of bamboo fitted one inside the other and slotted. Special instruments for ligation of internal hemorrhoids have been devised. Barron [11] improved the procedure by ligating only the mucosa and submucosa with a rubber band. This method is now universally accepted as the treatment of choice for second-degree hemorrhoids with normal or almost normal perianal skin. Third- and fourth-degree hemorrhoids with venous engorgement are best treated by surgery; nevertheless, good palliation in the form of symptomatic relief can be obtained by ligation.

The instrument designed by Barron comprises two drums which can be moved, one inside the other, by using a handle fitted with a trigger device. Two rubber bands are loaded on the inner drum by means of a cone. Special forceps are inserted through the inner drum and grasp the internal hemorrhoids. Using the trigger, the outer drum pushes the rubber bands onto the base of the internal hemorrhoids.

Soulard [94] replaced the forceps by incorporating an aspirator into the inner drum (Fig. 9.5). This instrument may be used by one person and does not require an assistant to hold the proctoscope. The diameter of the inner drum is usually 8–10 mm; larger instruments with a diameter of 14 mm have been also designed [75].

The procedure can be performed as an outpatient or office procedure. It does not usually need anesthesia or preparation except routine endoscopic examination.

The instrument is inserted onto the most redundant part of the rectal mucosa at the anorectal junction immediately above the internal hemorrhoid. The mucosa is sucked to determine the size of tissue to be strangulated and to ensure that it is painless. Application which is too low, near the dentate line, or too deep, grasping underlying musculature, would induce severe pain.

As a rubber band may break when rolling on the applicator, two bands should always be applied; immediate breakage of one is still possible and would result in incomplete constriction; breakage occurring before scarring would produce bleeding.

The procedure is described as painless in most patients. Nevertheless, many complain of more or less severe discomfort and a sensation of fullness and false bowel movement [3, 73]. This sensation may persist for several days. The patient should be aware of this fact and adequate analgesic should be prescribed. A local anesthetic (1–2 ml) may then be injected at the base of the strangulated hemorrhoid below the rubber band [104]. If the pain is very severe, the bands should be removed with scissors.

To produce a speed'er sloughing down of the strangulated tissue, it may be deep frozen by cryosurgery [61, 85, 87, 88]. Strangulated tissue sloughs in 7–14 days leaving a limited area of inflammation resulting in a small scar. This scar fixes the mucosa to the deeper lyers and prevents prolapse. A small trace of blood will occur during the sloughing. Occasionally, bleeding may be more severe and may require new banding of the bleeding point or the application of infrared coagulator or electrocoagulation 7–14 days after the original banding. A repeat sigmoidoscopy should always be performed when there is bleeding.

Table 9.1. Results after rubber band ligation

Reference	Patients	Follow-up	Healed (%)	Improved (%)	No effect (%)
Alexander-Williams and Crapp 1975 [3]	200		46 by single ligature		
Bartizal and Slosberg 1977 [12]	670	1–12 months	95.7		4.3
Groves et al. 1971 [38]	156	4–40 months	66	25	9
Soullard and Contou 1979 [94]	1074	1–10 years	69	21	10
Steinberg et al. 1975 [98]	125	4.8 years	89	10	1

Only one or two areas should be banded at a time to prevent severe discomfort. Three bands in one session would result not only in frequent pain, but also in a large area of ulceration with subsequent risk of stenosis. Further treatment can be performed after healing, 3–6 weeks after the first banding.

Banding may precipitate acute thrombosis. In the case of external hemorrhoidal thrombosis alone, simple excision may be performed; a hemorrhoidectomy may be required in acute internal and external hemorrhoidal thrombosis with prolapse.

Good symptomatic relief can be obtained with rubber band ligation. Results appear to last a long time (Table 9.1). Repeated application may be performed. Surgery is still possible later on if there is recurrence and seems to result in more permanent relief.

External hemorrhoids are not treated by rubber band ligation but may be partially reduced in size. Cosmetic results are not as good as those obtained by surgery. Skin tags may persist and, if unpleasant, should be excised under local anesthesia.

Manual Dilatation of the Anus

Lord [58–60] described a treatment for the cure of third-degree hemorrhoids by anal stretching. He proposed that hemorrhoids were caused by bands of constriction around the lower rectum and anal canal, such as the pecten bands described by Miles [72]. The pecten bands have never been satisfactorily demonstrated. The narrowing due to these bands would interfere with normal defecation, increase the anorectal pressure, and cause venous congestion of the cushions. Obstruction leads to straining and causes engorgement of the venous plexus which results in further obstruction, thus producing a vicious circle favoring bleeding and prolapse. This vicious circle should be broken by anal stretching.

The procedure is performed as an outpatient procedure. Under general anesthesia, in the lateral position, the constricting bands are identified and disrupted by increasing digital dilatation. Up to eight fingers are inserted into the left and right lateral areas of the anus. The sphincter and the overlying anoderm must not be damaged, particularly at the anterior and posterior midline which are the weakest zones. A foam sponge is inserted in the anus for 1 h to avoid hematoma. The patient must insert a specially designed plastic dilatator daily for 2–3 weeks and then weekly for at least 6 months. Taylor [102] has designed an inflatable dilatator to carry out Lord's procedure in a standardized way.

Any degree or stage of hemorrhoidal disease is said to be suitable for anal dilatation, even prolapsed and thrombosed hemorrhoids [102]. However, the procedure should be performed in a very cautious way in men and in elderly patients. Lord described a low incidence of complications, particularly of incontinence: there is transient and minor incontinence but no permanent lesions. In contrast, several authors have reported more or less severe cases of postoperative incontinence due to sphincter damage, particularly flatus incontinence. Records of anal pressure show a significant reduction of resting anal pressure after dilatation in comparison to preoperative values [6, 25, 39, 53]. A prolapse remains unchanged or may even get worse after treatment: mucosal prolapse occurs in 20% of cases within 2 weeks [59].

Results 6 months and 1 year after dilatation, with a success rate of 84%, compare favorably with 98% after hemorrhoidectomy [6]. Dilatation seems to be as effective as surgery in curing bleeding and pain but does not affect a prolapse [23, 41]. In 66 patients MacInthyre [62] observed 43.6% skin tags and prolapse, 21.8% flatus incontinence, and 3.6% partial fecal incontinence.

Partial Internal Sphincterotomy

Partial internal sphincterotomy (see Chap. 10) is now recognized as the treatment of choice for anal fissures due to hypertonicity of the internal sphincter [1, 44]. Whether such a dysfunction accounts for the occurrence of hemorrhoids is still controversial. Partial sphincterotomy has been advocated to overcome such an abnormality. Internal sphincterotomy allows precise division of the internal sphincter and does not result in any lesion of the external sphincter as can be the case after anal dilatation. Best results are obtained if the procedure is performed under general anesthesia and if the sphincter is visualized as opposed to a blind lateral submucosal sphincterotomy [4, 7].

This procedure is without effect on external hemorrhoids, prolapse and skin tags all of which may require further treatment. Incontinence of varying degrees may result in as many as 25% of patients. If a hyperactive sphincter is evident and if anal fissure is present, partial internal sphincterotomy should be considered at least as part of the treatment. Arabi [7] did not find any advantages of internal sphincterotomy over rubber band ligation in the treatment of first- and second-degree hemorrhoids. Sphincterotomy is a simple technique but still has not gained general acceptance.

Cryosurgery

Lewis [56, 57] was the first to introduce cryosurgery in the treatment of hemorrhoids. Tissue destruction by freezing is an effective method of dealing with certain dermatological conditions. To destroy tissue, the temperature should be rapidly lowered to at least below $-60°-150°C$. Immediate anesthesia is produced at low temperatures. If a sufficiently temperature is not achieved, deep freezing will not occur, and severe pain is induced. The amount of tissue destroyed depends on the vascularity of the tissue and its heat capacity, of the temperature of the cryoprobe, and the duration of the application [81].

Cryodestruction of hemorrhoids can be performed as an outpatient procedure. The cryoprobe is introduced through the anuscope and placed on the cushion; through rapid lowering of the temperature an ice ball is formed which delineates the tissue which will slough. The three cushions are destroyed in one session; of necessity, the mucosa and anoderm between the hemorrhoids should be preserved to avoid strictures [26, 35, 81].

The procedure takes 10-15 min, is usually painless, although uncomfortable, and can be performed as an outpatient procedure [49]. Local anesthesia may be required; sedation or prescription of analgesic is necessary. The main disadvantage of cryosurgery is that it results in profuse watery discharge which starts within 3 h and may last for 4 weeks [26, 35]. This requires the patient to wear anal pads for 2-3 weeks.

Complete healing is achieved in 4-6 weeks. Secondary bleeding occurs in 3% of patients. Large skin tags may result and have to be treated by secondary surgical excision.

Very different and even disappointing results have been reported. Successes range from 45% to 88% of patients treated [16, 35, 85, 112]. Of the patients treated by Goligher [35] 70% had satisfactory results. Smith et al. [95] compared surgical hemorrhoidectomy and cryodestruction in the same patients. Hemorrhoidectomy is more painful than cryosurgery 2 days after the operation; later on cryosurgery results in longer-lasting pain. A total of 75% of the patients preferred surgery to cryotherapy.

Cryosurgery has been associated with several other procedures, particularily with rubber band ligation. The cryoprobe may be applied to the banded hemorrhoid for 3 min twice within 15 min, and the rubber band should then be removed. Freezing after banding allows more exact delineation of the cryodestruction [85, 99]. This combination speeds up the whole process but at the expense of turning a very simple office procedure into an unnecessarily complex and cumbersome one.

Proctotherm

The application of an endoanal plug, heated to $30°-41°C$, for 15 min twice daily relieves pain and bleeding due to hemorrhoids. The rationale for this treatment has not been clearly established [18]. Heat and local compression of the cushions may produce relaxation of the internal sphincter which results in better venous drainage and regression of the hemorrhoidal congestion. Short-term results are very interesting but long-term results are not yet available. Such a treatment takes time: 15-20 min two or three times per day for at least 1 month.

Zeroid

The endoanal application of a plastic cannula containing a solution of glycol cooled to $10°-15°C$ diminishes the congestion of the anal cushions [91].

The application should be performed for 3–5 min several times a day. This treatment modifies the vascular pattern within the cushions. The application results in immediate relief of pruritus, pain, and anal congestion. Long-term results are still not available. This treatment should not be applied during menstruation and in cases of prostatitis or cystitis.

Surgical Treatment

Principals and Preoperative Evaluation

Several surgical procedures for destroying hemorrhoids have been described:

- Excision of the anal canal mucosa according to Whitehead [111]
- Submucosal stripping of the hemorrhoidal plexus as proposed by Eisenhammer [27]
- Open excision as described by Milligan et al. [71]
- Semi-open or semi-closed excision with suture of the mucosa [29, 89]
- Closed hemorrhoidectomy with complete suture of the wounds as described by Parks [83]

Hemorrhoidectomy is unpopular and nowadays has an unjustifiably bad reputation due mainly to fear of pain, incomplete or delayed healing, anal stenosis, skin tags, mucous prolapse, urinary retention, and more or less severe incontinence. Today's techniques should prevent all of these complications [19, 22].

Each patient undergoing hemorrhoidectomy must be submitted to sigmoidoscopy, or at least rectoscopy, to exclude additional pathology, inflammatory bowel disease, and rectosigmoidal polyps or cancer. In patients beyond the age of 50 years and if symptoms suggest additional pathology or are not absolutely related to anuscopy findings, a barium enema or colonoscopy is indicated.

Crohn's disease is a contraindication to hemorrhoidectomy. Portal hypertension, leukemia, lymphomas, spontaneous or medically induced bleeding diathesis, severe renal insufficiency treated by dialysis are absolute contraindications to hemorrhoidectomy.

No special preoperative measures or restrictions on diet are required. Shaving is unnecessary and should be avoided. Limited shaving can be done after anesthesia in the theater if necessary. No laxative or enema should be prescribed. Mucilage or bran should be taken for as long as possible before the operation to stimulate regular bowel movement.

The patient is anesthetized and placed in the lithotomy position. A semi-prone or jackknife position is recommended by several authors. We usually use a posterior perianal block [64]. In the case of general anesthesia, a local anesthetic with vasopressin or adrenaline (lidocaine 0.5% or 1% or, better, carboesthesine with long-acting effect) is injected locally; this allows the anesthesist to proceed with light anesthesia and avoids pain when the patient recovers consciousness. The administration of intravenous fluid should be restricted to less than 100 ml to avoid postoperative bladder retention.

The perineum is washed and swabbed with an antiseptic solution. The surgeon and his or her assistant are seated in front of the perineum. An instrument nurse is not necessary. The surgeon should examine the patient once again to exclude any other concomitant lesion.

Ligation and Excision

It is not necessary to stretch the anal sphincters or to use a bivalve retractor like Parks's retractor or an operative scope like Fansler's scope. Artery forceps are placed on the perianal skin opposite each of the, usually, three anal cushions. They are placed in the left lateral position at 5 o'clock, right posterior at 7 o'clock, and right anterior at 11 o'clock. Gentle traction on the forceps allows better examination of the internal hemorrhoids. To ensure preservation of sufficiently large bridges of anoderm after dissection, their limits are determined by small longitudinal incisions.

Dissection is then started on the perianal skin outside the rima ani (Fig. 9.6). The largest hemorrhoid is excised first. With curved scissors, an eliptical incision is made to join the previous longitudinal incision at the anal verge. The flap created in this way is elevated and drawn toward the anus to expose the lower edge of the sphincter. Dissection is continued down to the internal sphincter and all external hemorrhoidal tissue is excised. The fibers of the muscle of Treitz should be observed and cut. When there is exaggerated traction of the flap, there is a risk of cutting within the internal sphincter.

As soon as the muscle of Treitz at the level of the dentate line is cut, the flap can be mobilized better. Dissection is then continued in the well-defined submucosal plane. The longitudinal incisions are extended on both sides of the hemorrhoids, within the anus to the upper part of the anal canal or the tip of the anal cushions. A ligature of absorbable 00 synthetic suture material transfixed the upper level

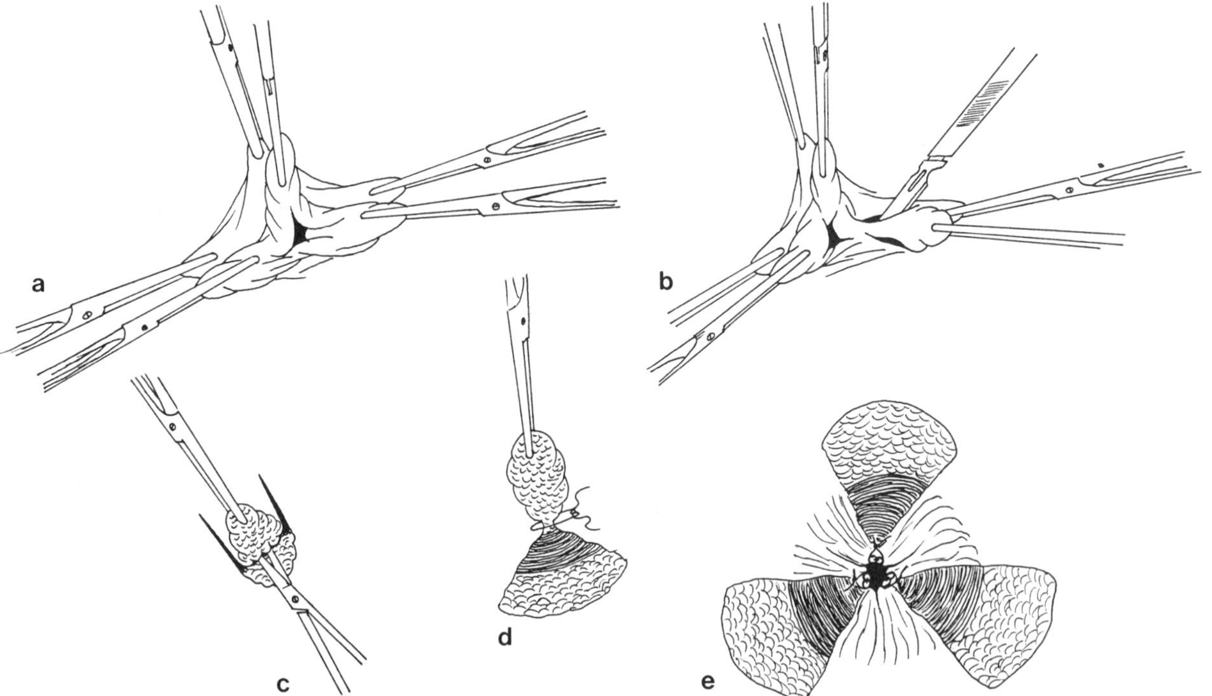

Fig. 9.6 a–e. Ligation and excision of hemorrhoids. *a* Traction on the three anal cushions with forceps; *b* limits of skin bridges are determined by small incisions; *c* dissection; *d* ligation; *e* end result

of the dissection and is tied tightly. The hemorrhoid is excised. Forceps are placed on the suture until the end of the procedure. Traction on the suture will permit better control of any bleeding vessel.

The two other hemorrhoids are dissected and excised in the same way. Any hemorrhoidal tissue which is left is excised. Vessels below the anoderm usually stop bleeding spontaneously, but electrocoagulation may be required. Any skin tags should be excised to leave only flat wounds. Accessory hemorrhoids may be present between the three main primary hemorrhoids. They can be excised by separate longitudinal incision or by undermining the mucocutaneous bridges [9]. If too much skin is excised, there is a significant risk of anal stricture.

We usually complete the procedure with a partial internal sphincterotomy at the level of the left posterior excision. A nonadherent dressing is inserted into the anal canal. We usually use a latex glove with a generous amount of anesthetic cream. The glove ensures pressure on the skin bridges and may be easily withdrawn the day after surgery. All excised tissue must be sent to the pathologist for histopathological examination. Unsuspected malig-

nancy or inflammatory lesions may be diagnosed.

The wounds can be closed with a continuous suture line of catgut 000 or another absorbable material, or an atraumatic needle [89]. Some prefer interrupted sutures. The suture will bite the internal sphincter, creating a longitudinal scar which will prevent further prolapse and improve hemostasis. With suturing there is a great risk of skin tags and anal stenosis [110].

If a skin bridge, especially the posterior one, prolapses, further treatment in the form of an anodermoplasty may be necessary (Fig. 9.7). Two traction stitches are placed 1–2 mm above the dentate line, one on either side. The mucosa is cut transversely between the two stitches located laterally. The anodermal flap is mobilized and undermined until it is fully stretched. The mucosa above the incision is resected as far as necessary to allow the anodermal flap to lie flat without tension and without prolapse. The transverse incision is closed by separate stitches of absorbable 00 or 000 suture material.

If a posterior fissure is present, the treatment policy should not be changed: a hemorrhoidectomy with

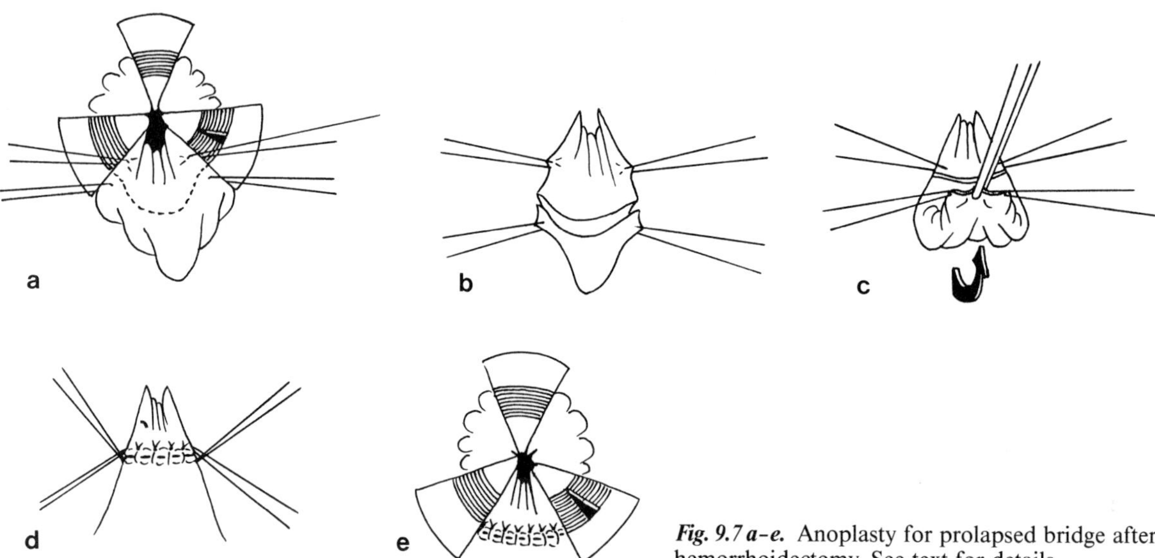

Fig. 9.7 a–e. Anoplasty for prolapsed bridge after hemorrhoidectomy. See text for details

sphincterotomy should be performed. The edges of the fissure and the skin tags, if present, are excised. Instead of a single posterior anodermal bridge two smaller ones will be left.

Semiopen, Semiclosed, and Closed Hemorrhoidectomy

Many operative procedures have been described which have the aim of leaving minimal scarring of the anal canal. After excision of all hemorrhoidal tissue and redundant mucosa, after ligation of vascular pedicles, the wounds are partially or totally closed. This should allow healing of wounds, reduce drainage and soiling, diminish postoperative discomfort, and simplify postoperative care resulting in a reduced hospital stay.

Semiopen Technique. In the semiopen technique (Fig. 9.8), after excision has been completed, the two edges of each wound are sutured to the sphinc-

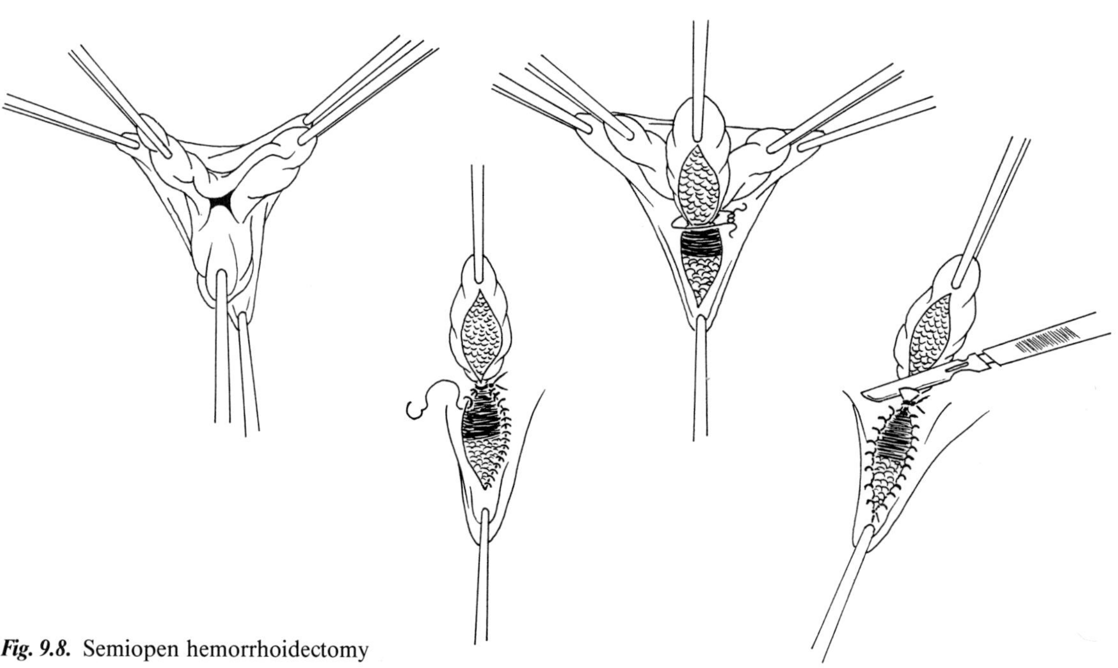

Fig. 9.8. Semiopen hemorrhoidectomy

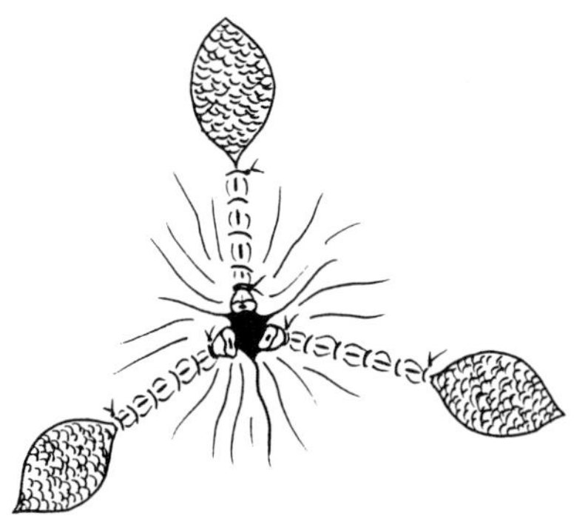

Fig. 9.9. Semiclosed hemorrhoidectomy

ter and subcutaneous fatty tissue starting from the upper part of the wound to the lower, external part (Fig. 9.8).

Semiclosed Technique. In the semiclosed technique (Fig. 9.9) the mucous membrane is closed as far as the dentate line, but the external wound is left open [88].

Closed Hemorrhoidectomy. In closed hemorrhoidectomy (Fig. 9.10), after excision and ligation, the an-

oderm and mucosa are elevated and redundant tissue excised only as much as necessary. The wound is closed, starting from the apex, with a running suture of absorbable suture material. The mucous membrane is sutured down to the internal sphincter to prevent further prolapse [19, 20]. It is essential that the wounds be closed without tension to prevent postoperative stenosis.

Submucosal Hemorrhoidectomy

Parks described a technique for submucosal hemorrhoidectomy [82, 83]: after infiltration of the submucosa with saline and adrenaline, a specially designed speculum is inserted. The skin over the lower extremity of the hemorrhoid is grasped with artery forceps. An incision is made around the forceps and the two limbs joined at the mucocutaneous junction or just above the dentate line (Fig. 9.11). From this point the mucosa is incised longitudinally up to the anorectal junction. The two flaps are raised by submucosal dissection. All hemorrhoidal tissue is excised at the level of the internal sphincter by cutting the adherence between submu-

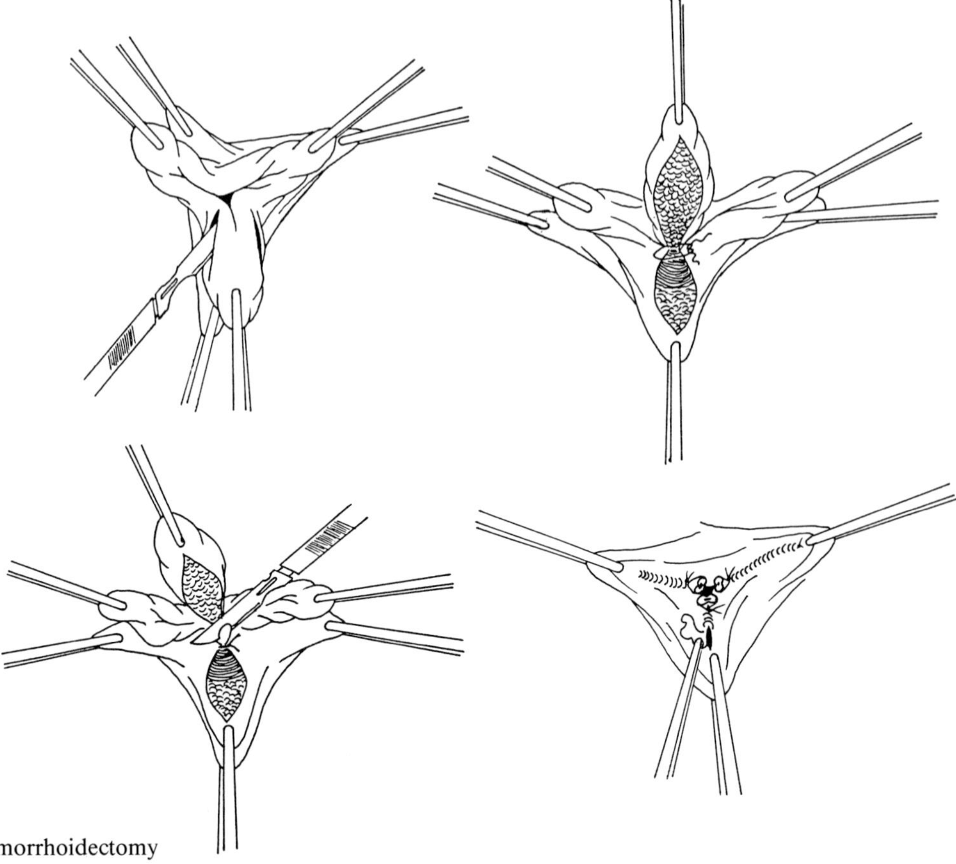

Fig. 9.10. Closed hemorrhoidectomy

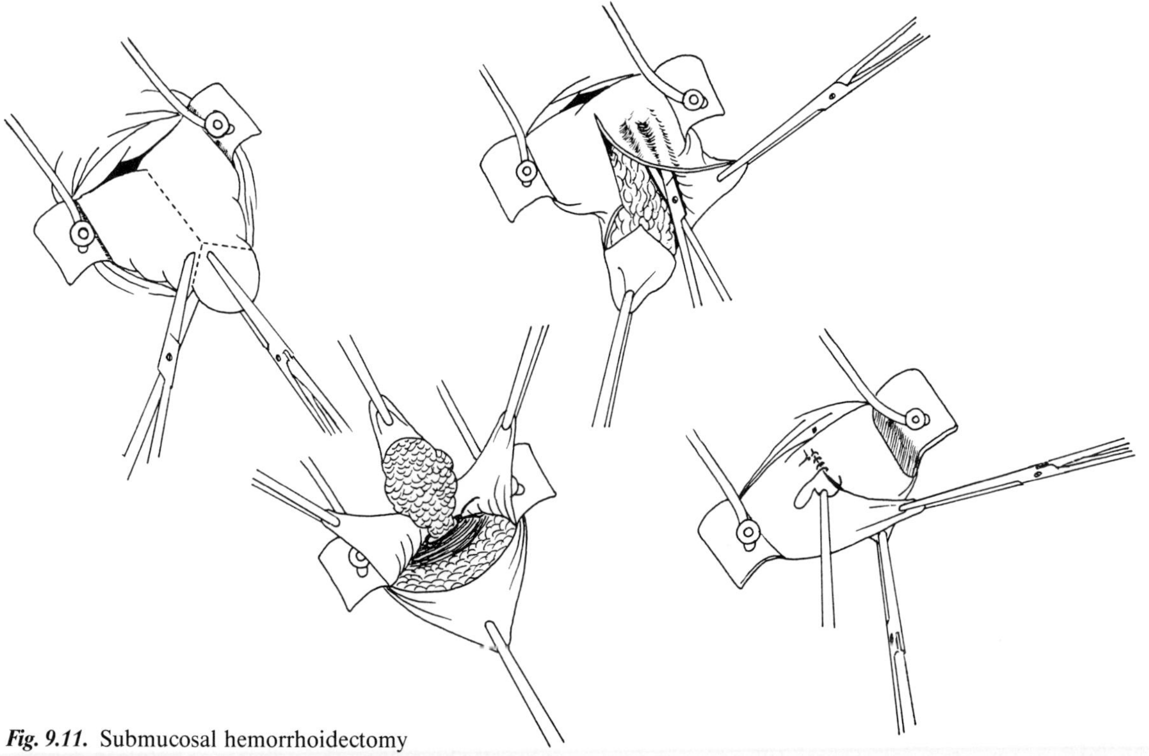

Fig. 9.11. Submucosal hemorrhoidectomy

cosa and muscle. The pedicle is transfixed and ligated by absorbable 0 or 00 suture material, and the hemorrhoidal tissue excised. All three hemorrhoidal areas are dissected.

The speculum is inserted again, and hemostasis is completed by electrodiathermy or coagulation. The mucosa is reconstructed. The mucocutaneous junction is first reconstructed with separate stitches and fixed to the internal sphincter to prevent prolapse. The upper part of the mucosal wound is then closed by separate stitches. If necessary, excess mucosa should be resected. The skin wounds are left unsutured but may be approximated.

Postoperative Care

Patients require analgesic drugs for 24–48 h if there is any pain. No routine prescription is recommended. The analgesic compound can be injected or taken orally. There is less pain if the surgical procedure was performed under locoregional anesthesia rather than under general anesthesia. No restriction is placed on diet. The first bowel movement takes place 24–48 h after surgery. If it does not occur, a laxative and paraffin oil may be prescribed. A sitz bath with a mild antiseptic solution or vegetable extracts such as extr. chamomillae

fluid is recommended three to four times a day and should be performed after each bowel movement to ensure clean wounds. It may be useful to apply an anesthetic ointment during the day and a small amount of wound cream during the night. The wounds are protected by light pads which help to alleviate any soreness. The wounds heal spontaneously by granulation and retraction within 3–4 weeks when left open and within 2 weeks when closed. The risk of stenosis is reduced if bowel actions are regular therefore obviating the need for repeated digital examination or application of an anal dilatator [30, 34].

Some discomfort is felt for 7–10 days and then rapid improvement is achieved, especially if wounds are kept clean [20, 110]. After the first bowel movement, if no bleeding occurs, the patient can leave hospital. In our experience, the patient can leave hospital on the 2nd or 3rd postoperative day. He or she should be warned about the possibility of secondary hemorrhage which may occur within 2 weeks in less then 1% of cases. Any severe bleeding at home leads to emergency readmission to hospital. The patient should be checked by the surgeon once a week until total healing is achieved.

Complications of Operative Treatment

Hemorrhoidectomy is not a minor procedure as it may end in major tragedy if not correctly performed. Complications are few: early and secondary bleeding, infection, fistula, fissure, healing delay, stenosis, skin tags, incontinence, urinary retention, fecal impaction. Buls [20] analyzed 500 consecutive hemorrhoidectomies and noted the complications listed in Table 9.2.

Hemorrhage

Hemorrhage may occur early or late. Early bleeding, on the day of operation, occurs from skin wounds or from an incompletely ligated pedicle. Any bleeding vessel should be visualized by anuscopy and ligated, coagulated, or pressed. Blood replacement may be necessary if there is severe bleeding. If the bleeding point cannot be identified, compression might be necessary and should be performed by a large-sized Foley bladder catheter placed in the rectum and submitted to gentle traction in the same way as a Stengstaken-Blackmoor sond for esophageal bleeding.

If secondary bleeding occurs after the patient has left hospital, immediate readmission is mandatory. The bleeding presumably comes from sloughing and lysis of the ligated internal hemorrhoids. With the use of absorbable synthetic material instead of catgut, the complication is far less frequent. Treatment requires reexamination under anesthesia and oversewing of the bleeding area.

Infection

Infection is very rare, even in closed hemorrhoidectomy [34]. Perianal and ischiorectal abscesses can occur during the convalescent period and probably result from activation of an overlooked fistulous tract. Injection of adrenaline solutions have been criticized. No evidence that they may induce or promote infection has been obtained. Even thrombosed and gangrenous hemorrhoids can and must be removed. The fear of pylephlebitis is no longer actual.

Pain

Postoperative pain is more or less present in every patient. It is mainly a discomfort due to the inci-

Table 9.2. Complications of operative treatment (in %)

Abscess	0.0
Fistula	0.4
Anal fissure	0.2
Anal stenosis	1.0
Incontinence	0.4
Skin tags	6.0
Fecal impaction	0.4
Thrombosed external hemorrhoid	0.2
Urinary retention	10.0

sional wounds which lasts for 2–3 days. The pain is exacerbated by the first two to three bowel movements. Topical ointments with an anesthetic like cinchocaine are very useful but may induce allergic reactions. Spasms may occur especially if internal sphincterotomy or anal stretch have not been performed. They may be aggravated by the administration of morphine. If they occur later on, after 1 week for example, they are mainly produced by fecal impaction and may be relieved by a simple enema and laxatives. There seem to be no significant differences in the severity of postoperative pain among the various type of hemorrhoidectomies. According to Parks [83], submucosal hemorrhoidectomy has been advocated to reduce postoperative pain.

Stenosis

Anal stenosis can be prevented by careful surgery. Stenosis can occur at the anal verge, on the dentate line, or above. Stenosis at the anal verge mainly results from excessive removal of anal skin and anoderm leaving bridges which are too small. With contraction of the wounds the anus contracts. The scarring is accompanied by fissure due to tears induced by bowel action. Digital or instrumental dilatation is unsuccessful. Secondary surgical correction is necessary.

Stenosis on the dentate line may occur after a closed hemorrhoidectomy. Stenosis above the dentate line is the result of a too generous ligation of the hemorrhoidal pedicle. This can be easily prevented by careful dissection or by several smaller ligations of the mucosa instead of only one. This type of stenosis requires repeated dilatation but can be also treated surgically (see Chap. 24).

patients with than in patients without portal hypertension [46, 101] or alcoholic liver disease. Hemorrhoidectomy is still possible but should not be performed before correction of any coagulopathy. Closed hemorrhoidectomy with careful hemostasis is preferable to open procedures.

Leukemia and Lymphoma

Patients with leukemia, lymphoma, Hodgkin's disease, and other causes of immunosuppression may present with hemorrhoidal disease. If not treated, there is a great risk of septic complication, necrosis, and gangrene [33]. Operation results in poor wound healing and even abscess with sepsis. Surgery should be undertaken only after correction of blood coagulation and after prophylactic antibiotic treatment. If complete healing cannot be achieved, the remaining wound may nevertheless be easier to manage and will be more comfortable for the patient than bleeding, discharging, and painful prolapsing hemorrhoids. Leukemia or lymphomatous infiltration should not be excised surgically but treated by irradiation.

Intestinal Bypass for Obesity

Hemorrhoids and even prolapse may develop in association with diarrhea in patients who have undergone an intestinal bypass operation for obesity. Rubber band ligation may be useful for early stages of the disease. Hemorrhoidectomy should be reserved for third-degree lesions. Control of the diarrhea by drugs is necessary.

Management

There are many conservative and surgical ways to treat hemorrhoids. No one method is suitable for all degrees of hemorrhoids. The proctologist must select the most appropriate method not only for each patient but also for each cushion in the same patient [17, 65, 66]. Our rationale is summarized in Table 9.3. Dietetic measures should be prescribed in every case. First-degree hemorrhoids can be treated by topical methods, infrared coagulation, and sclerosis. Small second-degree hemorrhoids can be treated by sclerosis and infrared coagulation, but best results are achieved by rubber band ligation. Large second-, third- and fourth-degree hemorrhoids should be operated. The choice of procedure depends on the experience of the operator. The most didactic procedure with constant results is the open hemorrhoidectomy as described by Milligan et al. [71]. Under special circumstances and with skill, closed or semiclosed hemorrhoidectomy can be performed but may result in prolapse and anal stenosis. Cryosurgery should not be used any more. The efficacity of the proctotherm procedure has still to proved.

Results

Many reports of trials that compare different types of treatment are now available (Table 9.4). Results must be assessed not just for 3 or 6 months after treatment but for at least 1 year, as we know that among the different clinical manifestations of hemorrhoids, bleeding may disappear spontaneously in up to 60% of patients followed up over a long period [48]. As mentioned by Nicholls [79], symptomatic improvement noted after a few months falls by 15%–30% when the patients are seen at 1 year.

Results vary considerably for a given treatment. Injection, infrared coagulation, and rubber band ligation are equally effective for bleeding hemorrhoids, but rubber band ligation is more effective for a prolapse. Dilatation and sphincterotomy are useless for prolapses. Hemorrhoidectomy gives better results particularly in third-degree hemorrhoids.

Table 9.3 see p. 73

Table 9.4. Hemorrhoids: choice of treatment

	First degree	Second degree	Third degree	Fourth degree
Systemic treatment	?	?	?	?
Topical treatment with or without steroids	+	±	Useful in case of inflammation	
Sclerotherapy	+	±	−	−
Infrared coagulation	+	±	−	−
			Hemostatic effect may be useful	
Proctotherm	+	+	−	−
Zeroid	+	+	−	−
Cryosurgery	+	±	?	?
Rubber band ligation	0	+	±	−
Sphincterotomy	+	−	−	−
Hemorrhoidectomy	0	+	+	+

?, Controversial; 0, no indication; −, useless; ±, inconstant efficacity; +, best indication.

Table 9.3. Results of randomized clinical trials on treatment of hemorrhoids

Reference	Follow-up (months)	Symptom	No. of asymptomatic patients/No. of patients followed						
			Injection	RBL	MDA	IR	C	LS	H
Keighley et al. 1979 [50]	12	Not specified	–	16/35	11/37	–	4/36	6/34	–
Cheng et al. 1981 [24]	12	Bleeding	14/21	15/20	19/22	–	–	–	18/19
		Prolapse	4/9	10/10	5/8	–	–	–	11/11
Sim et al. 1981 [93]	12	Bleeding	14/24	15/22	–	–	–	–	–
		Prolapse	0/7	5/7	–	–	–	–	–
Greca et al. 1981 [37]	12	Not specified	13/33	15/28	–	–	–	–	–
Murie et al. 1982 [74]	42	Bleeding	–	27/38	–	–	–	–	32/38
		Prolapse	–	17/25	–	–	–	–	27/29
O'Callaghan et al. 1982 [80]	48	Not specified	–	–	–	–	65/89	–	64/88
Leicester et al. 1983 [55]	12	Bleeding	17/35	–	–	20/38	–	–	–
		Prolapse	–	12/34	–	17/43	–	–	–
Templeton et al. 1983 [103]	3–12	Not specified	–	33/62	–	34/60	–	–	–
Ambrose et al. 1983 [5]	12	First degree	–	6/17	–	8/22	–	–	–
		Second degree	–	20/62	–	26/68	–	–	–

RBL, rubber band ligation; MDA, maximal dilatation of the anus; IR, infrared coagulation; C, cryotherapy; LS, lateral sphincterotomy; H, hemorrhoidectomy.

References

1. Abcarian H (1975) Lateral internal sphincterotomy. Surg Clin North Am 55: 143
2. Acklany TH (1961) The treatment of prolapsed gangrenous hemorrhoids. Aust NZ J Surg 30: 201
3. Alexander-Williams J, Crapp AR (1975) Conservative management of hemorrhoids. Clin Gastroenterol 4: 595–600
4. Allgöwer N (1975) Conservative management of hemorrhoids, part III: partial internal sphincterotomy. Clin Gastroenterol 4: 608–618
5. Ambrose NS, Hares MM, Alexander-Williams J, Keighley MRB (1983) Prospective randomised comparison of photocoagulation and rubber band ligation in treatment of hemorrhoids. Br Med J [Clin Res] 1: 1389–1391
6. Anscombe AR, Hancock BD, Humphreys WV (1974) A clinical trial of the treatment of hemorrhoids by operation and the Lord procedure. Lancet ii: 250–253
7. Arabi Y, Alexander-Williams J, Keighley MRB (1977) Anal pressures in hemorrhoids and anal fissure. Am J Surg 134: 608
8. Arabi Y, Marcuria T, Buchmann P, Alexander-Williams J, Keighley MRB (1987) Trial of high fiber diet or local treatment for patients with hemorrhoids. Gut 19: 1987
9. Arnous J, Parnaud E, Denis J (1971) Une hémorroïdectomie de sécurité. Presse Med 79: 87–90
10. Barrlos G, Khubuchandani M (1979) Urgent hemorrhoidectomy for hemorrhoidal thrombosis. Dis Colon Rectum 22: 159
11. Barron J (1963) Office ligation of internal hemorrhoids. Am J Surg 105: 573
12. Bartizal J, Slosberg PA (1977) An alternative to hemorrhoidectomy. Arch Surg 112: 534–536
13. Bensaude A (1967) Les hémorroïdes et affections courantes de la région anale. Maloine, Paris
14. Blanchard CE (1928) Textbook of ambulant proctology. Medical Success Press, Youngstown, OH, p 134
15. Blond K, Hoff H (1936) Das Hämorrhoidalleiden. Denticke, Leipzig
16. Brulé J (1981) La cryothérapie des hémorroïdes. Rev Proctol 2: 85–93
17. Buchmann P, Mineruini S, Keighley MRB, Alexander-Williams J (1979) Individuell differenzierte Behandlung von Hämorrhoiden. Schweiz Rundsch Med Prax 68: 1600–1604
18. Buchmann P, Hodel T (1980) Proctotherm, ein neues Prinzip der Hämorrhoidentherapie. Praxis 49: 1836–1838
19. Buchmann P (1988) Lehrbuch der Proktologie, 2nd edn. Huber, Bern
20. Buls JG, Goldberg SM (1978) Modern management of hemorrhoids. Surg Clin North Am 58: 469–478
21. Burkitt DP (1972) Varicose veins, DVT and hemorrhoids; epidemiology and suggested aetiology. Br Med J 2: 556–561
22. Bennett RC, Friedman MHW, Goligher J-C (1963) Late results of hemorrhoidectomy by ligation and excision. Br Med J 2: 216–219
23. Chant ADB, May A, Wilken BJ (1972) Hemorrhoidectomy versus manual dilatation of the anus. Lancet ii: 398–399
24. Cheng FCY, Shum DWP, Ong GB (1981) The treatment of second degree hemorrhoids by injection, rubber band ligation, MDA and hemorrhoidectomy – a prospective clinical trial. Aust NZ J Surg 51: 458–462
25. Creve U, Hubens A (1979) The effect of Lord's procedure on anal pressure. Dis Colon Rectum 22: 483–485

26. Detrano SJ (1973) Cryosurgical hemorrhoidectomy. Surgery 3: 118
27. Eisenhammer S (1974) Internal anal sphincterotomy plus free dilatation versus anal stretch procedure for hemorrhoids. Dis Colon Rectum 17: 493–522
28. Fallet P, Marti M-C (1982) Complications urinaires et choix de l'anesthésie lors d'hémorroïdectomies. Rev Proct 2: 101–110
29. Ferguson JA, Heaton JR (1959) Closed haemorrhoidectomy. Dis Colon Rectum 2: 176–179
30. Gabriel WB (1939) Treatment of hemorrhoids. Br M J 2: 1266
31. Gass OC, Adams J (1950) Hemorrhoids. Etiology and pathology. Am J Surg 79: 40–43
32. Ganchrow MJ, Bowman HE, Clark JF (1971) Thrombosed hemorrhoids. Dis Colon Rectum 14: 331–340
33. Goldberg SM, Gordon PH, Novatvongs S (1980) Essential of anorectal surgery. Lippincott, Philadelphia
34. Goligher JC (1975) Surgery of the anus, rectum and colon, 3rd edn. Ballière Tuidall, London
35. Goligher JC (1976) Cryosurgery for hemorrhoids. Dis Colon Rectum 19: 213–218
36. Graham-Stewart CW (1962) Injection treatment of hemorrhoids. Br Med J 1: 213
37. Greca F, Hares MM, Nevah E, Williams JA, Keighley MRB (1981) A randomised trial to compare rubber band ligation with phenol injection of hemorrhoids. Br J Surg 68: 250–252
38. Groves AR, Evans JCW, Alexander-Williams J (1971) Management of internal hemorrhoids by rubber band ligation. Br J Surg 58: 923–924
39. Hancock BD, Smith K (1975) The internal sphincter and Lord's procedure for hemorrhoids. Br J Surg 62: 833–836
40. Hancock BD (1977) Internal sphincter and the nature of hemorrhoids. Gut 18: 651–655
41. Hancock BD (1982) How do surgeons treat hemorrhoids? A study with special reference to Lord's procedure. Ann R Coll Surg Eng 64: 397–400
42. Hansen JB, Jorgensen SJ (1975) Radical emergency operation for prolapsed and strangulated hemorrhoids. Acta Chir Scand 141: 810–812
43. Hansen HH (1977) Neue Aspekte zur Pathogenese und Therapie des Hämorrhoidalleidens. Dtsch Med Wochenschr 102: 1244
44. Hochnli R, Allgöwer M (1968) Weitere Erfahrungen mit der Spaltung des sphinkter internus nach Eisenhammer bei Analfissuren, Fisteln und Hämorrhoiden. Helv Chir Acta 35: 266–273
45. Howard PM, Pingree JH (1968) Immediate radical surgery for hemorrhoidal disease with acute extensive thrombosis. Am J Surg 116: 777–778
46. Jacobs DM, Bubrick MP, Onstad GR, Hitchcock CR (1980) The relationship of hemorrhoids to portal hypertension. Dis Colon Rectum 23: 567–569
47. Jeffery PJ, Ritchie JL, Parks AG (1977) Treatment of hemorrhoids in patients with inflammation bowel disease. Lancet i: 1084
48. Jones CB, Schofield PF (1974) A comparative study of the methods of treatment for hemorrhoids. Proc R Soc Med 67: 51–53
49. Kaufman HD (1976) Outpatient treatment of hemorrhoids by cryotherapy. Br J Surg 63: 462–463
50. Keighley MRB, Alexander-Williams J, Buchmann P et al. (1979) Prospective trials of minor surgical procedures and high fiber diet for hemorrhoids. Br Med J 2: 967–969
51. Kilbourne J (1934) Internal haemorrhoids: comparative value of treatment by operative and by injection methods: a survey of 62910 cases. Ann Surg 99: 600–608
52. Kohlrausch O (1854) Zur Anatomie und Physiologie der Beckenorgane. S Hirzel, Leipzig, pp 9–10
53. Lane RH, Casula G, Parks AG (1976) Anal pressure before and after hemorrhoidectomy. Br J Surg 63: 158
54. Leicester RJ, Nicholls RJ, Mann CV (1981) Infrared coagulations. A new treatment for hemorrhoids. Dis Colon Rectum 24: 602–605
55. Leicester RJ, Nicholls RJ, Mann CV (1983) Vergleichende Studie über Infrarot-Koagulation und konventionelle Methoden in der Hämorrhoiden-Therapie. Proktology 3: 313–315
56. Lewis MI (1972) Cryosurgical hemorrhoidectomy: a follow-up report. Dis Colon Rectum 15: 128–134
57. Lewis MI (1973) Cryohemorrhoidectomy. Dis Colon Rectum 15: 171
58. Lord PH (1968) A new regime for the treatment of hemorrhoids. Proc R Soc Med 61: 935–936
59. Lord PH (1969) A day-case procedure for the case of third-degree hemorrhoids. Br J Surg 56: 747–749
60. Lord PH (1972) A new approach to hemorrhoids. Prog Surg 10: 109–124
61. Lurz KH, Götner E (1978) Kombinierte Gummibandligatur und Kryochirurgie von Hämorrhoiden. Med Klin 73: 1392–1395
62. Macintyre IMC, Balfour TW (1972) Results of the Lord non-operative treatment for hemorrhoids. Lancet 1: 1094–1095
63. Mahlberg FA (1980) Hämorrhoidenentwicklung bei Piloten durch 6. Belastung. Phlebol Proktol 9: 36–40
64. Marti M-C (1976) Anesthésie locale en proctologie. Nouv Presse Med 5: 2075
65. Marti M-C (1982) La maladie hémorroïdaire et son traitement. Rev Med Suisse Romande 102: 359–368
66. Marti M-C (1983) Quand faut-il opérer des hémorroïdes. Med Hyg 41: 3010–3014
67. Marti M-C, Rochat CH (1983) Faut-il opérer en urgence les prolapsus hémorroïdaires thrombosés? Med Hyg 41: 2280–2281
68. Marti M-C, Rochat CH (1985) Affections proctologiques et grossesse. Schweiz Rundsch Med Prax 74: 615–618
69. Martin CF (1904) The injection treatment of internal hemorrhoids. Am J Med 8: 365
70. Mazier WP (1973) Emergency hemorrhoidectomy. A worthwhile procedure. Dis Colon Rectum 16: 200–205
71. Milligan ETC, Morgan CM, Jones LE, Officer R (1937) Surgical anatomy of the anal canal and the operative treatment of hemorrhoids. Lancet ii: 1119
72. Miles E (1919) Observations upon internal piles. Surg Gynecol Obstet 29: 497–506
73. Muller CA (1980) Innere Hämorrhoidektomie mittels Gummibandligatur. Colo-Proctology 5: 317–319
74. Murse JA, Sim AJW, Mackenzie I (1982) Rubber band ligation versus hemorrhoidectomy for prolapsing hemorrhoids. A long term prospective clinical trial. Br J Surg 69: 536–538

75. Neiger A (1977) Experience acquise avec le strangler appareil à ligaturer. Ann Gastroentérol hépatol (Paris) 13: 997–998
76. Neiger A, Moritz K, Kiefhaber P (1977) Hämorrhoiden-Verödungsbehandlung durch Infrarotkoagulation. (Fortschritte der gastroenterologischen Endoskopie, vol 6.) Witzstrock, Baden-Baden, pp 102–106
77. Neiger A (1981) Treatment of bleeding hemorrhoids with infrared coagulation. Proktology 3: 310
78. Nesselrod JP (1964) Clinical proctology, 3rd edn. Saunders, Philadelphia, p 76
79. Nicholls J, Glass R (1985) Coloproctology. Springer, Berlin Heidelberg New York
80. O'Callaghan JD, Matheson TS, Hall R (1982) In patient treatment of prolapsing piles. Cryosurgery versus Milligan Morgan hemorrhoidectomy. Br J Surg 69: 157–159
81. Oh C (1975) Role of cryosurgery in management of anorectal disease. Dis Colon Rectum 18: 289–291
82. Parks AG (1956) The surgical treatment of hemorrhoids. Br J Surg 43: 337–351
83. Parks AG (1965) Hemorrhoidectomy. Surg Clin North Am 45: 1305
84. Parnaud E, Guntz M, Bernard A, Chom J (1976) Anatomie normale macroscopique et microscopique du réseau vasculaire hémorroïdal. Arch Fr Mal Appar Dig 65: 501–514
85. Parnaud E, Brulé J, Bidart JM (1980) Traitement ambulatoire des hémorroïdes par congélation contrôlée. Gastroenterol Clin Biol 4: 875–880
86. Raynham WH (1970) Strangulated prolapsed hemorrhoids. S Afr J Surg (S Afr Tydskr Chir) 8: 29–34
87. Rosser C (1931) Chemical rectal stricture. JAMA 96: 1762
88. Rudd WH (1977) Hemorrhoidectomy. How I do it: ligation with and without cryosurgery in 3000 cases. Dis Colon Rectum 20: 186–188
89. Ruiz-Moreno F (1977) Hemorrhoidectomy. How I do it: semiclosed technique. Dis Colon Rectum 20: 177
90. Saint-Pierre A, Palayodan A (1974) Anus et oestroprogestatifs de synthèse. Rapport de la 2ème réunion annuelle de la Société Nationale Française de Proctologie, Toulouse
91. Saint-Pierre A (1980) Fünf Jahre Erfahrungen mit dem Zeroid-Stab. Proctology 2: 119–120
92. Schottler JL, Balcos EG, Goldberg SM (1973) Postpartum hemorrhoidectomy. Dis Colon Rectum 16: 395
93. Sim AJW, Murie JA, Mackensie I (1981) Comparison of rubber band ligation and sclerosant injection for 1st and 2nd degree hemorrhoids. A prospective clinical trial. Acta Chir Scand 147: 717–720
94. Soullard J, Contou JF (1979) La ligature élastique. Nouv Presse Med 8: 1681–1682
95. Smith LE, Goodyear JJ, Fouty WJ (1979) Operative hemorrhoidectomy versus cryo destruction. Dis Colon Rectum 22: 10–16
96. Stein E (1982) Praktische Erfahrungen mit der Sklerotherapie. Colo Proctology 3: 144–149
97. Stein E (1986) Proktologie. Springer, Berlin Heidelberg New York
98. Steinberg D, Liegois H, Alexander-Williams J (1975) Long term review of the results of rubber band ligation of hemorrhoids. Br J Surg 62: 144–146
99. Stelzner F, Staubesand J, Machleidt H (1962) Das Corpus cavernosum recti – die Grundlage der inneren Hämorrhoiden. Langenbecks Arch Klin Chir 299: 302–312
100. Stelzner F (1963) Die Hämorrhoiden und andere Krankheiten des Corpus cavernosum recti und des Analkanals. Dtsch Med Wochenschr 88: 689–696
101. Taylor FW (1954) Portal hypertension and its dependence on external pressure. Ann Surg 140: 652
102. Taylor TV (1976) An instrumental method of performing Lord's procedure for hemorrhoids. Br J Surg 63: 460–461
103. Templeton JL, Spence RAJ, Kennedy TL et al. (1983) Comparison of infrared coagulation and rubber band ligation for first and second degree hemorrhoids: a randomised prospective clinical trial. Br Med J 286: 1387–1389
104. Tchirkow G, Haas PA, Fox TA (1982) Injection of a local anesthetic solution into hemorrhoidal bundels following rubber band ligation. Dis Colon Rectum 25: 62–63
105. Thomson WHF (1975) The nature of hemorrhoids. Br J Surg 62: 542–552
106. Thomson WHF (1982) The real nature of "perianal haematoma". Lancet ii: 467
107. Thulesins O, Gjöres JE (1973) Arteriovenous anastomoses in the anal region with reference to the pathogenesis and treatment of hemorrhoids. Acta Chir Scand 139: 476–478
108. Tinckler LF, Baratham G (1964) Immediate hemorrhoidectomy for prolapsed piles. Lancet ii: 1145–1146
109. Treitz F (1853) Über einen neuen Muskel am Duodenum des Menschen, über elastische Sehnen, und einige andere anatomische Verhältnisse. Viertel Jahrschrift Prag Heilkunde (Prager) I: 113–144
110. Watts JM, Bennett RC, Duthie HL, Goligher JC (1964) Healing and pain after different forms of hemorrhoidectomy. Br J Surg 51: 88
111. Whitehead W (1887) Three hundred consecutive cases of hemorrhoids cured by excision. Br Med J 1: 449
112. Wilson MC, Schofield P (1976) Cryosurgical hemorrhoidectomy. Br J Surg 63: 497
113. Wright AD (1950) Complications of rectal injections. Proc R Soc Med 43: 263
114. Zollinger RM, Howe CT (1968) The small and large intestine. In: Davis L (ed) Christophers textbook of surgery, 9th edn, vol 2. Saunders, Philadelphia, p 731

10 Anal Fissure

M.-C. Marti

Definition

An anal fissure is a painful linearly or eliptically shaped ulceration situated in the lower part of the anal canal extending from the dentate line more or less to the anal verge. This lesion is very common and results in severe pain.

Pathogenesis and Physiopathology (Fig. 10.1)

In the acute phase, the fissure is shallow and the edge ill-defined. The floor is constituted by the subcutaneous fibers of the longitudinal ligament [11, 12]. This lesion may heal spontaneously or with topical treatment.

When there is delayed healing, the lesion may become chronic. The lower part is swollen and a so-called sentinel pile develops. Through chronic inflammation and infection, this pile undergoes fibrosis resulting in the formation of a skin tag. At any stage, a suppuration may occur extending into the surrounding tissues [35]. Acute infection due to fecal retention may result in a subcutaneous abscess followed by fistulization and extension under the fissure edges. The sinus is usually short, not exceeding 2 cm in length. At the proximal end, at the level of the anal valve, swelling and fibrosis may produce a pseudopolypoid, hypertrophied anal papilla.

Different ethiopathogenic mechanisms have been proposed.

Mechanical Etiology

There is no doubt that a fissure is a tear of the anoderm due to the passage of hard stools [8]. During straining, modification of the anorectal angle and the position of the sphincters are responsible for the occurrence of the greatest number of traumatic lesions on the posterior midline, especially in men. In women, a weak zone situated between the vulva, vagina and the fibrous center of the perineum is responsible for the frequent anterior fissures. This concept provides a good explanation for acute fissures and for their location.

Epithelial Theory

Histological studies of the anoderm in cases of fissure reveal a parakeratosis with loss of epithelial elasticity [3]. Such a parakeratosis may be due, maintained, or aggravated by the use of irritating laxatives, chronic diarrhea of any etiology, or alkaline feces and results in inflammation and loss of elasticity. These factors explain why a fissure never develops above the dentate line where the mucosa is more mobile. They are responsible for the trend to chronicity of acute fissures and for their delayed healing. These modifications are aggravated by topical steroids which are responsible for epithelial atrophy.

Scars due to previous surgery, delivery and childbirth injuries also diminish epithelial elasticity and sphincter stretch during straining

Vascular Theory

Fissures are frequently associated with hemorrhoids. Impairment of blood supply in the anterior and posterior midline could result in the formation of a varicose ulcer with perhaps, thrombosis. This concept is attractive but does not explain the occurrence of fissures in patients without hemorrhoids [4].

Infectious Theory

According to the infectious theory [50], a fissure could result from infections of an anal crypt. As anal glands are more frequently located in the posterior part of the anal canal, their infection could explain the occurrence of posterior fissures. Chronic inflammation would result in fibrosis and loss of elasticity. In our opinion, fissure and cryptitis could coexist, but infection produces a true ulcer and not a fissure. For example, syphilis and tuberculosis result in more or less extended ulceration with a totally different aspect from that of a chronic fissure.

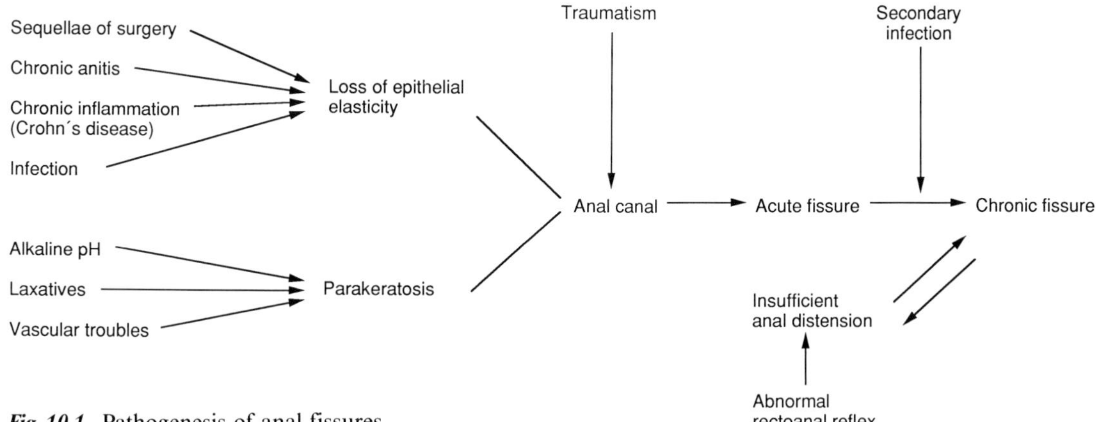

Fig. 10.1. Pathogenesis of anal fissures

Neuromuscular Theory

Arabi [2] demonstrated a high maximal pressure in patients with anal fissure, even if resting pressure was no different from that noticed in patients without a fissure [10, 23, 24]. Kuypers [32] also observed an increased anal resting pressure. Northmann and Schuster [44] have demonstrated that patients with a fissure may have an abnormal "overshoot contraction" of the internal sphincter after rectal distension instead of a normal reflex relaxation. This phenomenon accounts for the sphincter spasm, the acute pain during defecation, and delayed healing. These changes may represent a primary abnormality or may be due to the fissure as this abnormal reflex disappears after healing of the fissure.

A fissure is not the result of a single mechanism (Fig. 10.1) but of an interaction of several factors. As Arnous and Denis [3] said: "A fissure may occur in one second but the conditions necessary for its formation need several years."

Epidemiology

Fissures are encountered in both sexes, in young and middle-aged adults, as well as in children and in the elderly. The site of the fissure differs. In 80% of cases they are located in the midline posteriorly, in 10% anteriorly, and in 5%–10% laterally. In 4% of cases, fissures are simultaneously present in the anterior and posterior midline. Anterior fissures are found nearly exclusively in women [9, 18, 20, 38, 39, 50].

Symptoms and Signs

The main symptom of an anal fissure is an acute pain occurring during or just after defecation. The pain diminishes and disappears over several hours and reoccurs at the next bowel action. The pain may be prolonged, remaining for hours. It has been described as a burning, shooting, aching, tearing sensation. It is located on the anal verge but radiates into the lower back or down to the legs. As bright red bleeding in small amounts is frequently noticed, patients complain of hemorrhoids.

Constipation is a frequent symptom and may be responsible for the occurrence of a tear, but the pain due to the fissure is such a distressing symptom that it may induce severe fecal retention with encopresis. Furthermore, it may result in disturbances in micturation; dysuria, retention, or frequency.

The diagnosis may be established by history alone. It is necessary to rule out by history and physical examination any associated disease such as inflammatory bowel disease, anal carcinoma, venereal infection. Inspection alone is sufficient to confirm the diagnosis. The buttocks should be separated gently to see the fissure. When there is a chronic lesion, a sentinel pile, fibrotic edges, and, occasionally, a fistulous tract may be observed.

When there is severe pain and anal spasm, it may be useful to apply a topical anesthetic prior to examination. Palpation will confirm the anal spasm. Digital examination to exclude other lesions may be impossible or incomplete at the initial examination and should be postponed. Instrumental examination should also be avoided as it would cause unnecessary pain. An acute fissure that fails to heal with adequate treatment should be biopsied to exclude Crohn's disease, anal carcinoma, or implanted adenocarcinoma.

Differential Diagnosis

History alone is enough to exclude most conditions presenting with anal pain. Careful differentiation is necessary.

Perianal Suppuration

Among the different degrees of perianal suppuration, the intersphincteric abscess may mimic a fissure and can only be confirmed by digital examination under general anesthesia.

Pruritus Ani

In the case of pruritus ani, multiple superficial linear skin "cracks" which never extend up to the dentate line are observed with signs of chronic irritation but without anal spasms. Pruritus can occur when there is an anal fissure due to discharge and insufficient local hygiene.

Ulcerative Colitis

Fissures are encountered in 7% of colitis patients. They are multiple, broad, inflamed, and located away from the midline. Exact diagnosis is obtained by endoscopy.

Crohn's Disease

In anal Crohn's disease, the anal lesion is much greater than when there is an idiopathic fissure. The ulceration is extensive and is associated with edema, overhanging edges, and large skin tags. The lesion may be painless. Biopsy will confirm the diagnosis.

Squamous Cell Carcinoma of the Anus

A squamous cell carcinoma of the anus or an extensive adenocarcinoma of the rectum may involve the anoderm and produce severe pain during defecation. At the time of presentation, the lesions are usually at an advanced stage. Digital examination reveals induration of the lateral edges and base. Histological examination is necessary to make a correct diagnosis.

Syphilis

The primary lesion of syphilis may be found at the anal verge. The chancre resembles an ordinary fissure but frequently appears as symmetrical lesions on both sides of the anal canal. The surface of the lesion is covered by a serous discharge. The body is indurated. Inguinal lymph nodes are almost always enlarged. Other venereal conditions, such as condyloma acuminatum, may occur simultaneously. As a rule, the lesions are painful, but not necessarily so. Diagnosis will be confirmed at this stage by dark-field microscopy and later by an appropriate serological examination.

Tuberculosis

Tuberculous lesions may be difficult to differentiate from Crohn's disease. They are distinguished by large irregular ulceration with eroded edges. They are associated with pulmonary tuberculosis. Biopsy and guinea pig inoculation should be carried out. After chemotherapy they should be treated conservatively like idiopathic fissures.

Hematological Conditions

Leukemic lesions are indurated and may be infected. They produce severe anal pain. They occur at any stage of the disease but especially during exacerbation. Abscesses should be drained.

Conservative Treatment

The aim of treating an acute or chronic anal fissure is to break the vicious circle of hard stools, pain, and reflex spasm. In the main this can be done using simple measures: regular bowel action with stool softeners and bulkforming foods like bran to avoid obstipation and laxative abuse, and warm baths to help in relieving anal spasm. Anesthetic ointment inside the anal canal may be successful, but prolonged application can lead to allergic skin reactions and dermatitis. Anal dilators lubricated with an anesthetic jelly and inserted just before defecation was already proposed by Gabriel in 1929 [14, 15]. This kind of treatment may be successful but is very painful [33]. The dilator does not seem to contribute to the success of conservative treatment [22, 40]. Injection of a long-acting anesthetic below the fissure is effective for only a few hours. It results in temporary incontinence due to paralysis of the external sphincter. Injection of a sclerosing agent such as a 5% solution of quinine urea has been proposed by some authors [2, 4]. These injections, which are very popular in France, relieve pain but are without effect on wound healing. They induce a great number of complications: abscesses, fistulas, oleogranuloma. Despite the popularity of these measures, there is probably no longer any place for this type of treatment.

Anal Dilatation Under Anesthesia

In 1838 Recamier [47] proposed sphincter stretching for anal fissure. The manual dilatation of the anus or forceful stretching of the anal sphincter with four [19], five [7], or even eight fingers [34] has been performed. The effect is to produce a temporary paralysis of the internal and external sphincter lasting several days or even a week. This results in more or less severe long-lasting incontinence.

Dilatation is performed under general anesthesia but does not require a hospital stay. There is no anal wound and early return to work is possible.

Relief of pain is very good in 80%-90% of cases [51]. The disadvantages of this method are persistence or recurrence of the fissure in 20% of cases, imperfect sphincter control in 12%-23% [7, 13, 51], and acute thrombosed hemorrhoids. Controlled trials to compare anal dilatation with lateral sphincterotomy give controversial results [13, 36].

Surgical Treatment

Various surgical procedures have been proposed for the treatment of acute or chronic fissures.

Classical Excision (Fig. 10.2)

Gabriel [15] popularized the excision of the fissure with a broad triangle of skin. He also stretched the anal canal and cut the lower part of internal sphincter. This procedure results in major discomfort for the patient, delayed wound healing, bleeding, abscess, stenosis, failure to heal, recurrence, or incontinence of varying degree. Hughes [30] applied an immediate split-thickness skin graft to stimulate

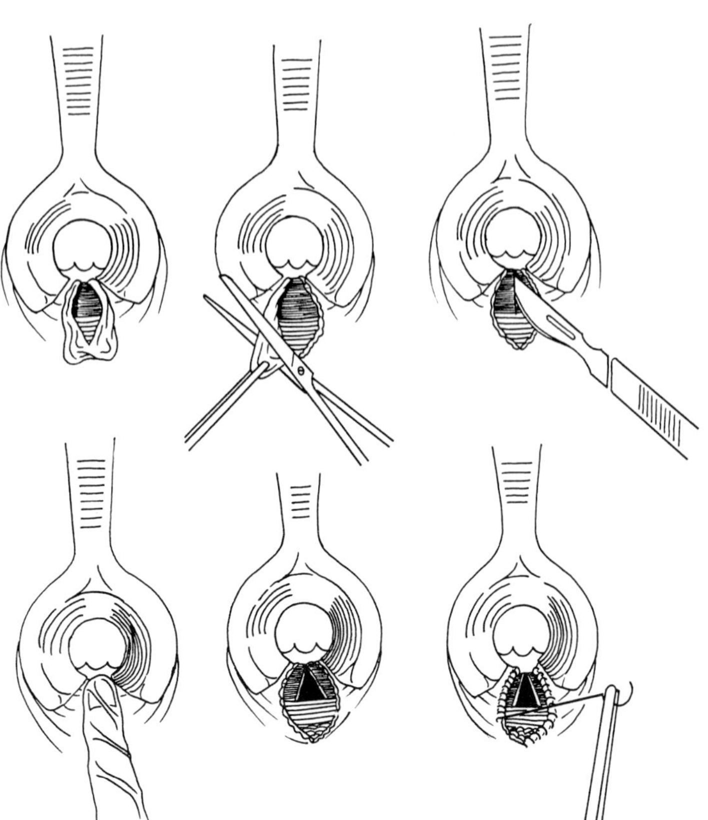

Fig. 10.2. Excision of the fissure, partial sphincterotomy, and hemostatic suture of the edges of the wound

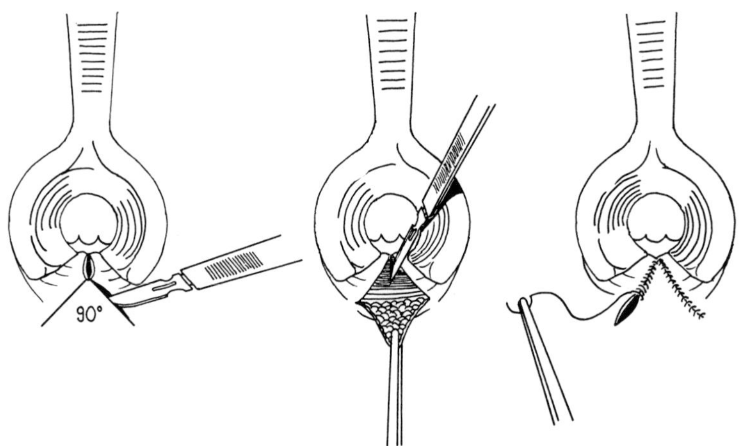

Fig. 10.3. V–Y anoplasty after fissure excision and sphincteroplasty

healing. The patient submitted to this treatment should stay in hospital for about 1 week, and bowel action should be confined.

Y-V Anoplasty (Fig. 10.3)

Samson and Stewart [49] reported wide experience with a Y-V anoplasty. A large-based skin flap is mobilized after excision of the fissure up to the dentate line and partial internal sphincterotomy. The flap is stiched with a continuous suture. The healing is first without leaving a scar or a deformity. The procedure needs considerable dissection, a prolonged operating time and it is more complicated than seems necessary. It is impracticable when there is an associated fistula, infection, or irritated skin.

Sphincterotomy

Posterior midline sphincterotomy was already being practiced in the last century by Boyer [6] and Goodsall [21]. Miles [41] treated anal fissures by what he called a "pectenotomy" but which was in fact, as shown in retrospect by Eisenhammer [11, 12] a sphincterotomy of the lower part of the internal sphincter.

Open Sphincterotomy

The original method consisted of a division of the lower half of the internal sphincter in the posterior midline through the fissure. Any anal and skin tags are excised. This procedure relieves pain but leaves a wound which heals very slowly taking about 4–8 weeks and results in keyhole deformity. Such a deformity is accompanied by imperfect continence,

lack of control of flatus or even occasionally feces, fecal soiling. Eisenhammer [11] suggested that these complications could be reduced by lateral sphincterotomy. Parks [45] recommended lateral sphincterotomy (Fig. 10.4). He performed a 1-cm long incision along the lower edge of the internal sphincter after anal stretching with the retractor. After exposure of the internal sphincter, the intersphincteric space is dissected and the internal sphincter is separated from the mucosa and from the external sphincter up to the dentate line. The internal sphincter is cut longitudinally under eye control. Bleeding is stopped by diathermy and digital pressure. The wound is closed by interrupted stitches. Lateral sphincterotomy results in fewer complications than posterior sphincterotomy, faster healing and fewer recurrences [26, 28].

An open lateral internal sphincterotomy can also be performed through a longitudinal incision (Fig. 10.5). The wound is closed with a running absorbable suture such as 3–0 chromic catgut. The fissure itself is not treated, but sentinel piles, anal tags, and prolapsing hemorrhoids may be removed.

Open sphincterotomy, especially a lateral one, may require general anesthesia because of the sphincter stretching. Results are no different if the procedure is performed under local or general anesthesia [16, 31]. Tissue may be infiltrated with a solution of lignocaine and a vasoconstrictor (adrenaline or 8-ornithine vasopressin) to diminish the bleeding and to reduce the amount of drugs needed for the general anesthesia.

Subcutaneous Sphincterotomy

Internal subcutaneous sphincterotomy (Fig. 10.6) has been described by Notaras [43]. It is a more simple and expeditious procedure than open

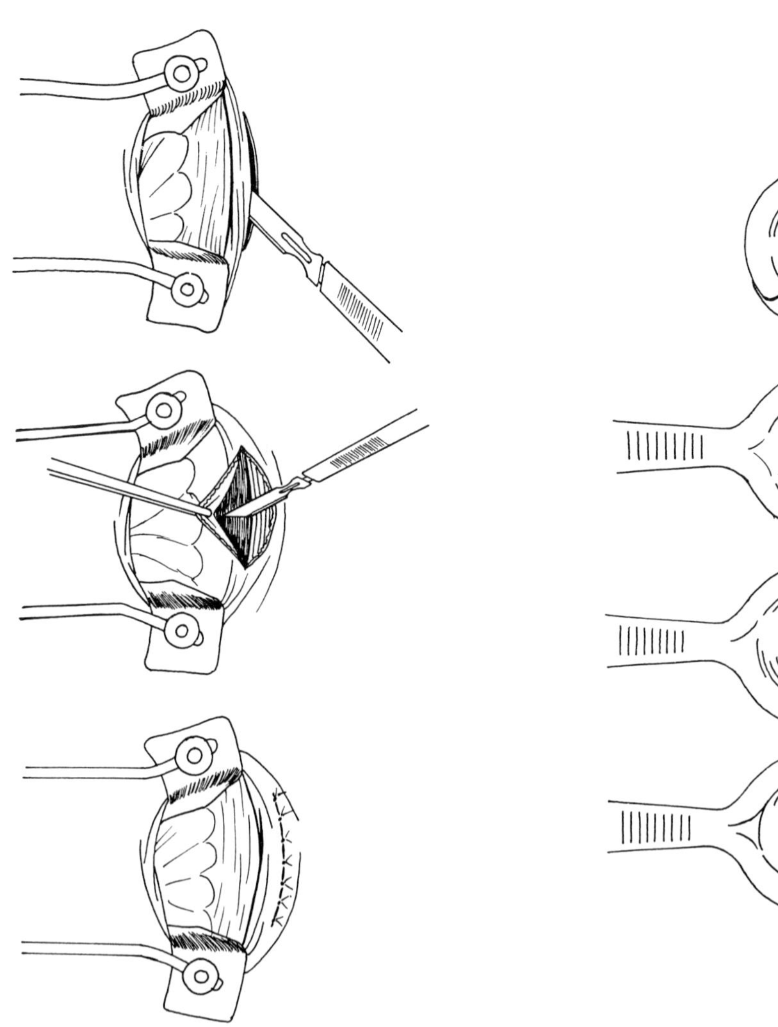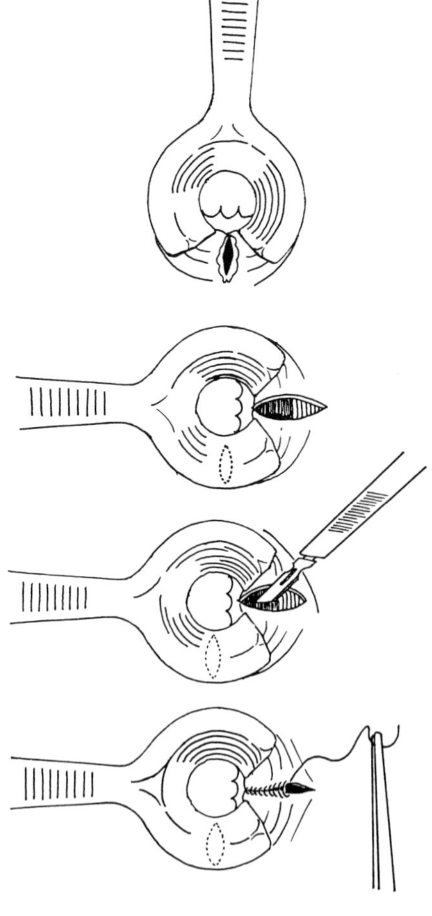

Fig. 10.4. Lateral sphincterotomy through a 1-cm lateral incision

Fig. 10.5. Open lateral sphincterotomy through a longitudinal incision

Table 10.1. Lateral internal sphincterotomy

Author	Year	Ref.	Patients (n)	Impaired control		Fecal soiling (%)	Untreated or recurrence (%)
				Flatus (%)	Feces (%)		
Hardy & Cuthbertson	1969	[25]	17	29	6–12	4	18
Hawley	1969	[26]	24	?	0	0	0
Hoffmann	1970	[28]	99	6	1	7	3
Notaras	1971	[43]	82	2	1	6	~10
Millar	1971	[42]	99	2	1	1	0
Gemsenjaeger	1972	[17]	30	0	0	0	0
Fischer	1976	[19]	32	0	0	6	3
Ray	1974	[46]	21	?	?	?	0
Marti	1976	[37]	30	3.3	0	0	0
Abcarian	1977	[1]	125	0–30	0	0	1.5
Rudd	1975	[48]	200	0	0	0	0.5
Herzog	1979	[27]	33	?	0	9	3
Collopy	1979	[7]	86	17.4	11	18	53

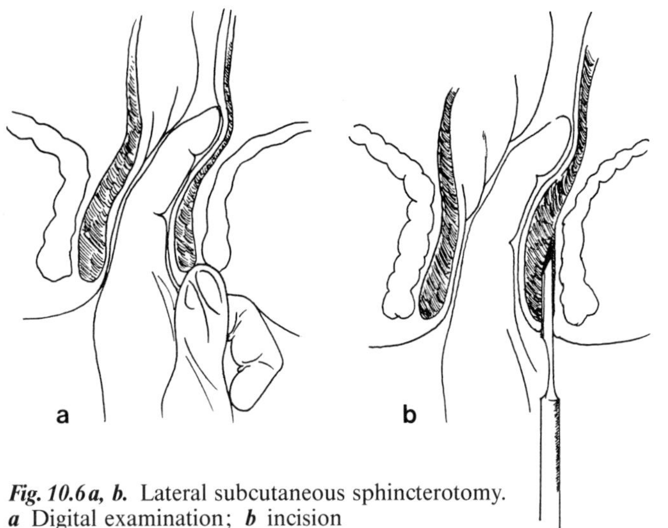

Fig. 10.6 a, b. Lateral subcutaneous sphincterotomy.
a Digital examination; *b* incision

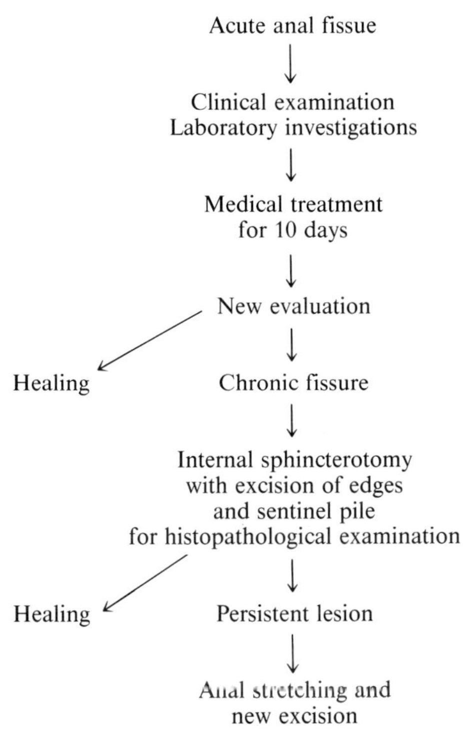

Fig. 10.7. Treatment policy for anal fissures

sphincterotomy. It cannot be used for training purposes nor is it a suitable procedure for the occasional surgeon. It is best performed in the lithotomy position. It can be performed as an outpatient procedure [37, 48]. After digital examination, the intersphincteric groove is palpated. Lignocaine (2–5 ml) with 8-ornithine vasopressin or adrenaline is infiltrated. A narrow-bladed scalpel is inserted through the skin, flat side adjacent to the muscle, and advanced submucosally, or preferably in the intersphincteric space, to the level of the dentate line. The sharp edge is then turned toward the internal sphincter and the sphincterotomy is performed. As soon as the sphincter is cut, a "give" will result. Digital pressure will stop any bleeding. Again, any associated lesion will be excised. This sphincterotomy leaves virtually no wound or one which is less than 5 mm long. This wound heals in a few days. Both subcutaneous and open sphincterotomy result in a significant reduction of anal canal pressure [5].

Postoperative Care

The need for postoperative care is reduced after sphincterotomy. Sitz baths, correct anal cleaning, wound liniment, and dry dressings are prescribed for 1 week. Formation of large soft stools should be stimulated by bran or stool softeners.
Complications are few. They are less frequent with subcutaneous blind sphincterotomy than after an open one and include ecchymoses, bleeding, abscess, fistula, prolapse, and minor incontinence. Experience and careful technique reduce the complication rate, especially after closed sphincterotomy.

In comparison to fissurectomy and posterior midline sphincterotomy, lateral sphincterotomy gives better results, reduces the length of the hospital stay, relieves pain faster, and ensures faster healing [1, 27, 29].

Results of Sphincterotomy

Results of internal sphincterotomy are very good. They are summarized in Table 10.1. Pain disappears by the first bowel movement in about 90% of cases. Healing of the fissure nevertheless takes 2–4 weeks. Our treatment policy is summarized in Fig. 10.7.

References

1. Abcarian H (1980) Surgical correction of chronic anal fissure: results of lateral internal sphincterotomy vs fissurectomymidline sphincterotomy. Dis Colon Rectum 23: 31–36
2. Arabi Y, Alexander-Williams J, Keighley MRB (1977) Anal pressures in hemorrhoids and anal fissure. Am J Surg 134: 608–610
3. Arnous J, Denis J (1969) Les bases anatomiques et pathogéniques du traitement des fissures anales. Revue du Praticien 19: 1811–1818
4. Bensaude A (1972) La fissure anale. Rev Prat 22: 1779

5. Boulos PB, Araujo JO (1984) Adequate internal sphincterotomy for chronic anal fissure: subcutaneous or open technique? Br J Surg 71: 360–362

6. Boyer A (1818) Remarques et observations sur quelques maladies de l'anus. Journal complémentaire du dictionnaire des sciences médicales 2: 24

7. Collopy B, Ryan P (1979) Comparison of lateral subcutaneous sphincterotomy with anal dilatation in the treatment of fissure in ano. Med J Aust 2: 461–495

8. Crapp AR, Alexander-Williams J (1975) Fissure-in-ano and anal sclerosis. Clin Gastroenterol 4: 619–628

9. Duhamel J, Hueber D (1978) Nouvelles études statistiques portant sur 500 cas de fissures anales. Ann Gastroenterol Hepatol (Paris) 14: 35–39

10. Duthie HL, Bennett RC (1964) Anal sphincter pressure in fissure-in-ano. Surg Gynecol Obstet 118: 19–21

11. Eisenhammer S (1951) The surgical correction of chronic internal anal (sphincteric) contracture. S Afr Med J 25: 2486–2489

12. Eisenhammer S (1959) The evaluation of the internal anal sphincterotomy operation with special reference to anal fissure. Surg Gynecol Obstet 109: 583–590

13. Fischer M, Thermann M, Trobisch M, Sturm R, Hamelmann H (1976) Die Behandlung der primär-chronischen Analfissur durch Dehnung des Analkanals oder Sphincterotomie. Langenbecks Arch Chir 343: 35–44

14. Gabriel WB (1929) Treatment of pruritus ani and anal fissures; the use of anaesthetic solutions in oil. Br Med J 1: 1070–1072

15. Gabriel WB (1948) Principles and practice of rectal surgery, 4th edn. Lewis, London

16. Gatehouse D, Arabi Y, Keighley MRB, Alexander-Williams J (1978) Lateral subcutaneous sphincterotomy-local or general anaesthesia. Proc R Soc Med 71: 29–30

17. Gemsenjaeger E (1972) Die Sklerose des Sphincter ani internus. Schweiz Med Wochenschr 102: 336–339

18. Goldberg S, Gordon P, Nivatvongs S (1980) Essentials of anorectal surgery. Lippincott, Philadelphia

19. Goligher J.-C. (1965) An evaluation of internal sphincterotomy and simple sphincter-stretching in the treatment of fissure-in-ano. Surg Clin North Am 45: 1299–1304

20. Goligher J.-C. (1980) Surgery of the anus, rectum and colon, 4th edn. Baillière Tindall London

21. Goodsall DH (1892) Fissure, non-syphilitic and syphilitic of the rectum and anus. St Bartholome's Hosp Reports 28: 205–210

22. Gough MJ, Lewis A (1983) The conservative treatment of fissure-in-ano. Br J Surg 70: 175–176

23. Graham-Stewart CW (1962) The etiology and treatment of fissure-in-ano. Int Abstr Surg 115: 511

24. Hancock BD (1977) The internal sphincter and anal fissure. Br J Surg 64: 92–95

25. Hardy KJ, Cuthbertson AM (1969) Lateral sphincterotomy – an appraisal with special reference to sequelae. Aust NZ J Surg 39: 91–92

26. Hawley PR (1969) The treatment of chronic fissure-in-ano. Br J Surg 56: 916–918

27. Herzog U, Gemsenjaeger E (1980) Fissura ani. Schweiz Rundsch Med 47: 1734–1743

28. Hoffmann DC, Goligher JC (1970) Lateral subcutaneous internal sphincterotomy in treatment of anal fissure. Br Med J III: 673–675

29. HSU TC, MacKeigan JM (1984) Surgical treatment of chronic anal fissure. A retrospective study of 1753 cases. Dis Colon Rectum 27: 475–478

30. Hughes ESR (1953) Anal fissure. Br Med J 2: 803–805

31. Keighley MRB, Greca F, Nevah E, Hares M, Alexander-Williams J (1981) Treatment of anal fissure by lateral subcutaneous sphincterotomy should be under general anesthesia. Br J Surg 68: 400–401

32. Kuypers HC (1983) Is there really sphincter spasm in anal fissure. Dis Colon Rectum 26: 493–494

33. Lock MR, Thomson JPS (1977) Fissure-in-ano: the initial management and prognosis. Br J Surg 64: 355–358

34. Lord PH (1972) A new approach to haemorrhoids. Progress in Surgery 10: 109–124

35. Magee HR, Thompson HR (1966) Internal anal sphincterotomy as an outpatient operation. Gut 7: 190–193

36. Marby M, Alexander-Williams J, Buchmann P, Arabi Y, Kappas A, Menervini S, Gatehouse D, Keighley MRB (1979) A randomized controlled trial to compare anal dilatation with lateral subcutaneous sphincterotomy for anal fissure. Dis Colon Rectum 22: 308–311

37. Marti M.-C. (1976) Les fissures anales. Praxis 65: 1398–1403

38. Marti M.-C. (1979) Les fissures anales. Méd Hyg 37: 285–288

39. Mazier WP (1972) An evaluation of the surgical treatment of anal fissures. Dis Colon Rectum 15: 222–227

40. McDonald P, Driscoll AM, Nicholls RJ (1983) The anal dilator in the conservative management of acute anal fissures. Br J Surg 70: 25–26

41. Miles WE (1944) Rectal surgery – a practical guide to the modern surgical treatment of rectal diseases. Cassell, London

42. Millar DM (1971) Subcutaneous lateral internal anal sphincterotomy for anal fissure. Br J Surg 58: 737–739

43. Notaras MJ (1971) The treatment of anal fissure by lateral subcutaneous internal sphincterotomy - a technique and results. Br J Surg 58: 96–100

44. Northmann BJ, Schuster MM (1974) Internal anal sphincter derangement with anal fissures. Gastroenterology 67: 216–220

45. Parks AG (1967) The mangement of fissure-in-ano. Br J Hosp Med 1: 737–738

46. Ray JE, Penfold JCB, Gathright JB, Roberson SH (1974) Lateral subcutaneous internal anal sphincterotomy for anal fissure. Dis Colon Rectum 17: 139–144

47. Recamier JCA (1838) Extension, massage et percussion cadencée dans le traitement des contractures musculaires. Revue Méd française et étrangère 1: 74–89

48. Rudd WWH (1975) Lateral subcutaneous internal sphincterotomy for chronic anal fissure: an outpatient procedure. Dis Colon Rectum 18: 319–323

49. Samson RB, Williams RC, Stewart RC (1970) Sliding skin grafts in the treatment of anal fissures. Dis Colon Rectum 13: 372–375

50. Soullard J (1975) Proctologie. Masson, Paris

51. Watts J MCK, Bennett RC, Goligher JC (1964) Stretching of anal sphincters in the treatment of fissure-in-ano. Br Med J 2: 342–343

11 Anorectal Abscesses and Fistulas

M.-C. Marti

Introduction

Anorectal abscesses and fistulas are among the most frequently observed anorectal lesions. As anorectal abscesses frequently result in more or less complex and extensive fistulous tracts, the two pathologies should be regarded as the same condition. Abscesses and fistulas are two phases of the same disease: a fistulous abscess [9]. However, for practical and therapeutical reasons, they should be considered separately.

Abscesses

Etiology

Perianal septic lesions may be the result of several etiologies. They may be due to skin lesions like hidradenitis suppurativa, localized pyoderma, or infection of a sebaceous adenoma. They may follow perianal trauma: injections as, for example, in sclerotherapy of hemorrhoids; surgical wounds; impaction of ingested fish or rabbit bones; or introduction of sharp foreign bodies into the anal canal. An anal fissure with a skin tag may also be complicated by an abscess. However, most commonly, a perianal abscess has a cryptoglandular origin [14].

The anal glands, described in 1844 by Hermann and Desfosses [19], are located in the intersphincteric space and empty through a duct crossing the internal sphincter into the base of an anal crypt at the level of the pectineal line (Fig. 11.1).

Not all crypts contain anal glands, and two glands may open into one crypt. The higher-density of anal glands are in the posterior half of the anus. Cystic formation may be present. Stasis, increased back pressure due to occlusion of a duct and secondary to fecal material, foreign bodies, or trauma result in stasis and secondary infection with abscess formation in the intersphincteric space. The isolation of gut-specific organisms such as colonic aerobes and *Bacteroides fragilis* in the culture of pus tends to confirm the cryptoglandular origin of anal fistulas [11, 16].

Spread of Infection

Infection may spread and seek the path of least resistance (Fig. 11.2). It may extend downward into the intersphincteric space resulting in a perianal abscess, upward inside the longitudinal muscle layer within the gut wall causing an intermuscular abscess, or upward outside the gut wall resulting in a supralevator abscess. It may spread across the external sphincter at any level resulting in an ischiorectal abscess which may also extend upward or downward. Furthermore, circumferential spread is possible at any level within the intersphincteric space, the ischiorectal space, or the supralevator

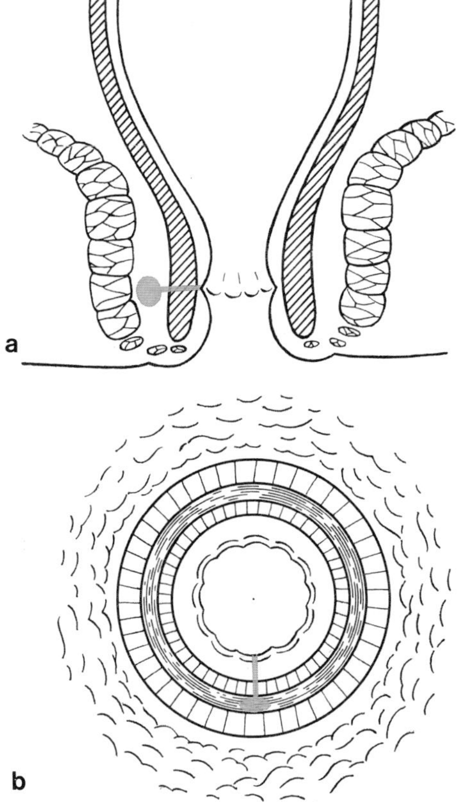

Fig. 11.1 a, b. Position of intersphincteric anal gland on frontal (*a*) and horizontal (*b*) section

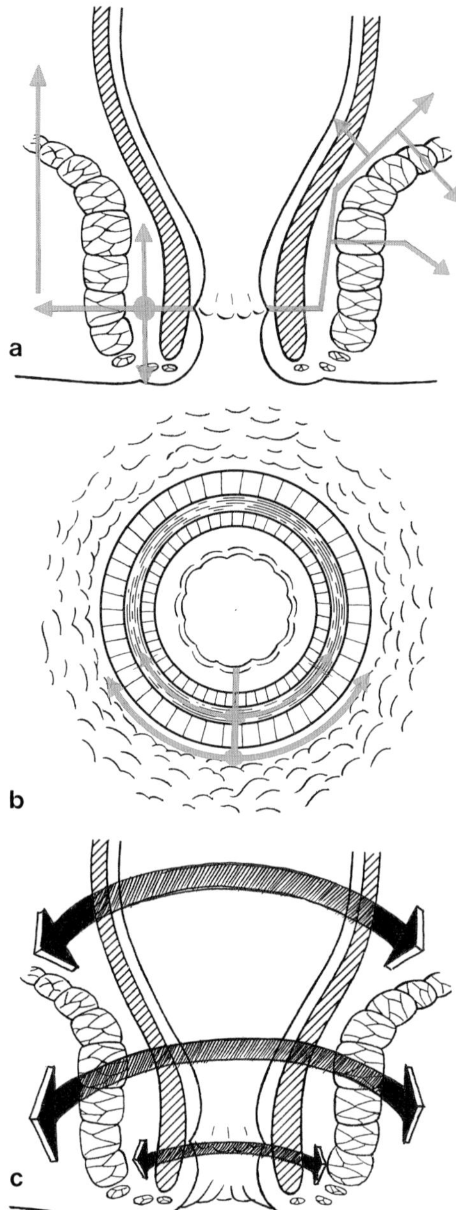

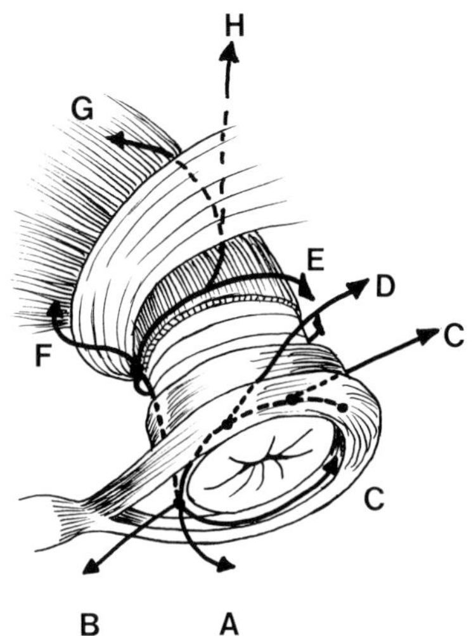

Fig. 11.3. Various extensions of anal abscesses: *A,* intersphincteric; *B,* para-anal; *C,* horseshoe, superficial; *D,* horseshoe superficial; *E,* horseshoe, deep; *F,* ischiorectal; *G,* pelvirectal; *H,* supralevator

Fig. 11.2a–c. Possible ways of extension of an anal abscess downward, upward, and along the various planes and fatty spaces of the perineum

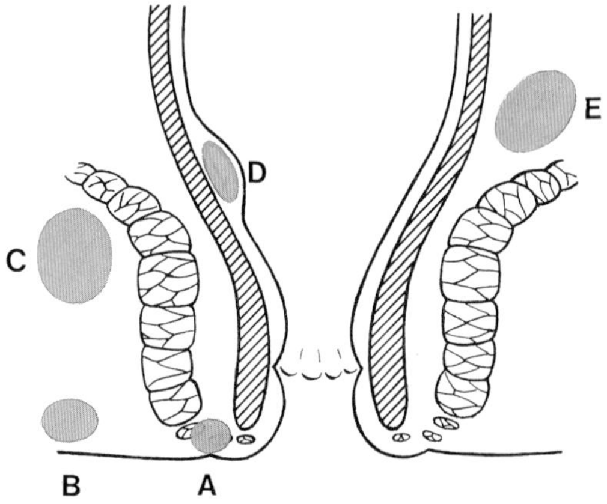

Fig. 11.4. Classification of anal abscesses: *A,* perianal; *B,* perineal; *C,* ischiorectal; *D,* submucosal; *E,* pelvirectal

space. It may extend from one ischiorectal fossa to the controlateral one via the intersphincteric space of Courtney or deep postanal space (Fig. 11.3) [17] resulting in a so-called horseshoe abscess.

A pelvirectal abscess resulting from a cryptoglandular infection extending above the levator ani in close contact with the rectal wall and below the peritoneum is rare; a pelvirectal abscess originates more frequently in pelvic pathology.

The location of anorectal abscesses may be classi-

fied according to Fig. 11.4. The incidence of the various sites of anorectal abscesses (Table 11.1) differs among the published series for several reasons: classification and patient recruitment are different from one institution to another. Anal abscesses may be complicated by extensive perineal gangrene due to streptococci, *Pseudomonas aeruginosa,* mixed aerobic and anaerobic infections, and purely clostridial germs [5, 33, 43, 44]. Fournier's disease is an uncommon form of gangrene involving the scrotum

Table 11.1. Frequency of various types of anorectal abscesses

	Ellis 1953 [10] (%)	Goldberg et al. 1980 [13] (%)	Abcarian 1989 [1] (%)
Perianal	54.5	26	44.6
Intersphincteric		16	22.9
Ischiorectal	39	54	22.4
Supralevator		4	6.2
Submucosal, high intramuscular	0		3.9
Atypical	6.5		

and the perineum (see Chap. 31): this necrotizing infection requiring extensive skin excision may be secondary to an anal abscess or fistulous abscess [7, 12, 42]. Tetanus as a complication of anorectal surgery and anal abscess has also been reported [31]. Delay in treatment, inadequate examination and initial drainage may result in extensive infection with a fatal outcome [4, 28].

Signs, Symptoms and Diagnosis

The main symptoms of an abscess are discomfort, perianal pain, and swelling. The symptoms develop more or less rapidly within hours or days. They are aggravated by sitting, walking, and defecation. Minor anal bleeding and discharge of a small amount of pus may occur if the abscess opens into the anal canal. An obvious cause for the pain is usually detected; swelling, tenderness, and induration at palpation, asymmetry of the buttocks, redness, superficial cellulitis, or even gangrenous skin. Inguinal lymph nodes may be enlarged. Systemic symptoms like fever, chills, malaise, and tachycardia occur more frequently with high abscesses than with more superficial ones. In the most severe cases, patients may be hospitalized for severe fever of unknown origin or acute urinary retention. Only a careful rectal examination reveals the development of a high anorectal abscess.

Bidigital examination allows an appreciation of an induration in the deep postanal space and in the ischio- and/or pelvirectal spaces. A small intersphincteric abscess may be very painful and could be confused with an acute anal fissure. Examination under general anesthesia may be required to allow palpation of a small nodule, no bigger than a grain of rice, within the intersphincteric space, at the level of the dentate line [35]. An anorectal examination with sigmoidoscopy must be performed at some stage for three main reasons:

- To identify the anal crypt responsible for the infection.
- To determine the presence of underlying septic or inflammatory proctitis.
- To look for a perforated anorectal cancer.

In men, an abscess situated anterior to the anus should be distinguished from a periurethral abscess and, in women, from infections of Bartholin's glands.

An internal fistulous opening can be identified on careful examination in about 30%–40% of patients undergoing drainage of an abscess [30, 40]. It may be missed at the time of the initial drainage of the abscess as the tissues are distorted and inflamed by the septic conditions and may also not be recognized as a result of spontaneous closure [9]. One-third of patients have a history of anorectal abscess which had ruptured spontaneously, had been drained surgically, or had undergone spontaneous remission [41].

Treatment of Anorectal Suppuration

To treat anorectal abscesses, some guidelines must be followed:

- Spontaneous healing and complete resolution without suppuration of perianal cellulitis is very rare and should not be expected.
- Broad-spectrum antibiotics without drainage delay the need for surgery and create more complex lesions.
- Microbiological investigations must be performed to confirm or rule out the presence of a fistulous tract and to obtain evidence of venereal anal disease.
- Incision should not be delayed.
- Incision should allow optimal drainage without pocketing.
- A fistulous tract must be looked for carefully and may be recognized in 30%–40% of abscesses. A lay-open or one-stage operation should only be performed by a skilled and well-trained surgeon.

Surgical Treatment of Perianal Abscesses

A perianal abscess can almost always be drained under local anesthesia in the office. The skin must be shaved and prepared with antiseptics; 2 ml 0.5% lidocaine with a vasoconstrictor are injected into the skin at the level of the most tender point. The incision must be radial and long enough to allow free drainage (Fig. 11.5). A diamond-shaped skin

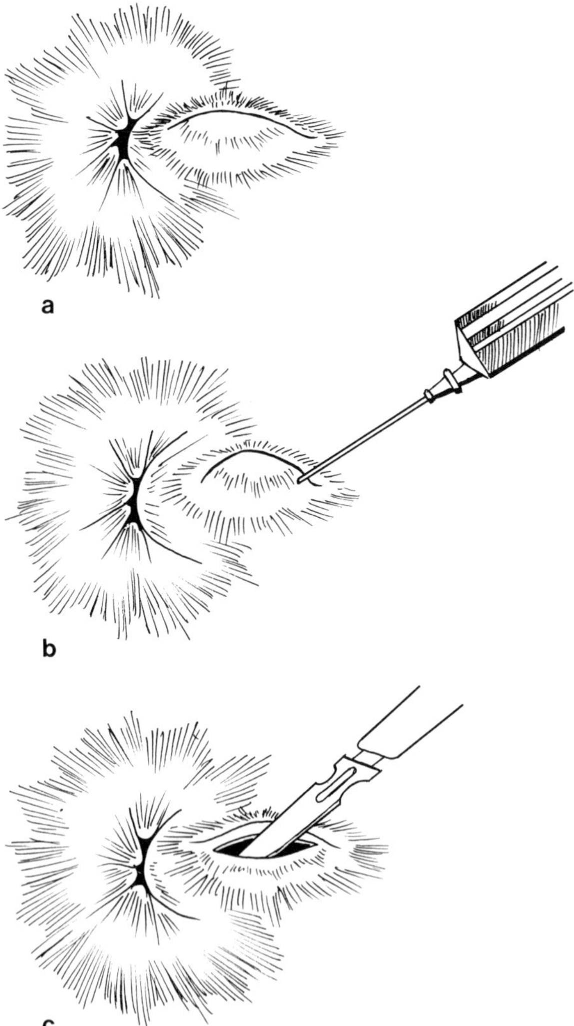

Fig. 11.5 a–c. Incision and drainage of an anal abscess

Fig. 11.6 a–c. Treatment of an intersphincteric abscess: excision of a flap of anoderm, division of the internal sphincter and curettage of the intersphincteric space. If a fistulous tract is identified, curettage may be performed ▽

flap may be excised to prevent early closure with recurrence of the abscess. Packing to control bleeding should be reduced to a minimum as it would interfere with drainage.

Surgical Treatment of Intersphincteric Abscesses

Locoregional or general anesthesia is required to allow examination and adequate exposure. Incision starts at the level of the intersphincteric groove, just beyond the lower edge of the internal sphincter (Fig. 11.6). The anoderm is incised, or a strip of it is excised up to the level of the dentate line. The internal sphincter fibers are divided from the lower end up to the level of the highest cavity. The intersphincteric space is cleaned, and curettage is performed to remove any trace of the infected anal gland.

Surgical Treatment of Ischiorectal Abscesses and Pelvirectal Abscesses

These lesions are too deep to be treated under local anesthesia; caudal, locoregional, or general anesthesia is required. After proctoscopy to identify the anal crypt involved in the process, a radial incision is made in the perianal tissue and continued into the ischiorectal space. If bidigital examination confirms extension into the pelvirectal space, the levator muscle fibers are separated to allow drainage of the highest septic cavities (Fig. 11.7). A rubber tube drain or a Penrose drain is inserted and fixed to the skin with a stitch. After gentle curettage, the wounds are loosely packed with a mesh dressing for 24–48 h. A second stage will be required to treat the trans-sphincteric fistulous tract.

A pelvic abscess extending from the anal canal should never be drained into the rectum as it would

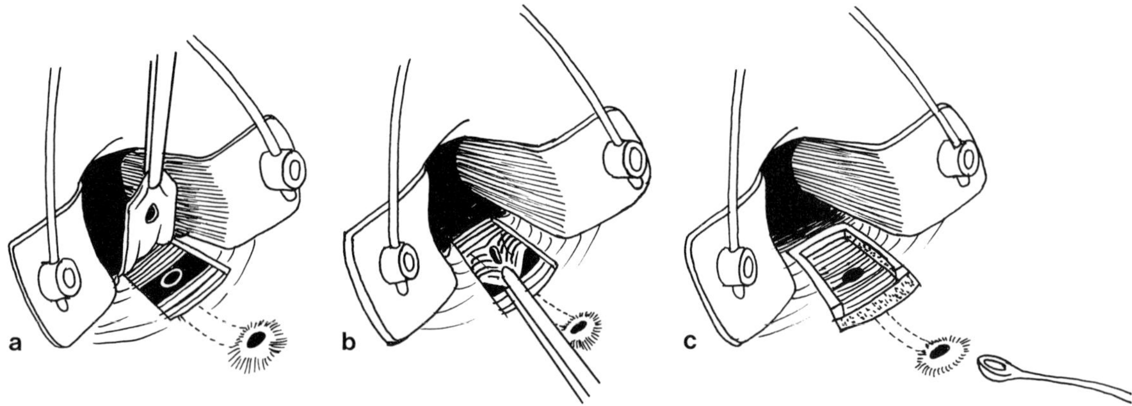

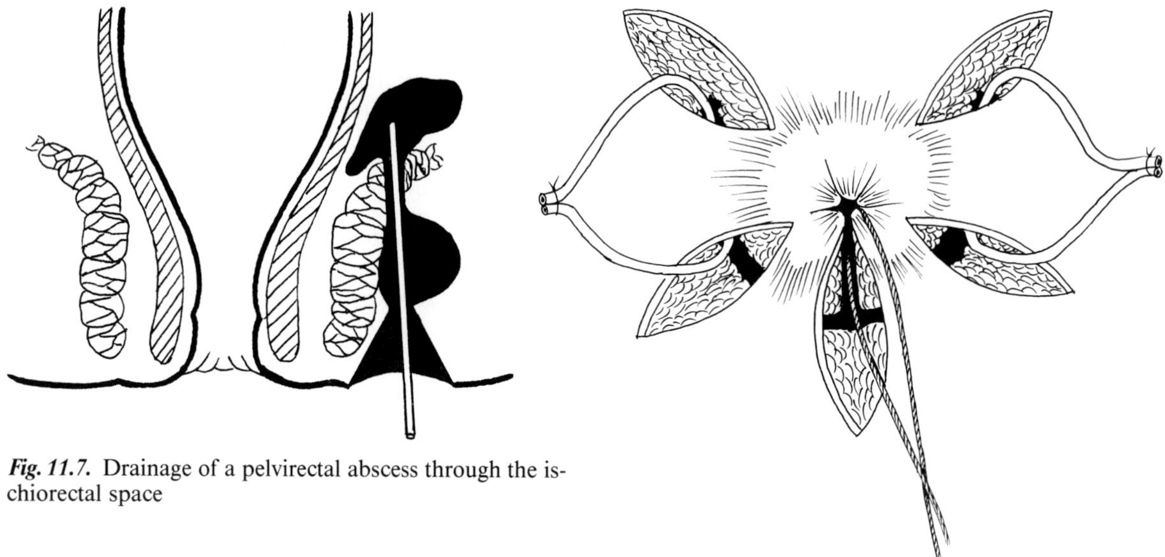

Fig. 11.7. Drainage of a pelvirectal abscess through the ischiorectal space

Fig. 11.8. Horseshoe abscess. The postanal space is opened. A seton drainage is placed through the posterior tract. Lateral and anterior extensions of the abscess are drained through several radial incisions

result in an extrasphincteric fistula which is a much more complex problem to treat. If the pelvic abscess is caused by a pelvic disease such as complicated diverticulitis, Crohn's disease, or appendicitis, it should be drained through the abdominal wall or, as a Douglas abscess, through the rectal lumen.

Surgical Treatment of Postanal Abscesses and Horseshoe Abscesses

A deep postanal abscess should be drained by a posterior radial incision on the midline. The primary opening is usually located in a crypt in the posterior midline. It is easy to identify as pus can be seen draining from it. A probe is inserted into the tract and passed into the deep postanal space. The radial incision is performed with the tip of the probe. The postanal space is opened to allow free drainage of the pus-filled space (Fig. 11.8). The fistulous tract should not be submitted to immediate fistulotomy in order to prevent excessive sphincter damage. A seton drainage is placed to allow easy identification of the tract at a later stage and to allow better drainage.

In the case of a horseshoe abscess, the lateral and anterior extensions of the abscess are drained by one or more separate radial incisions on each side. Curettage is performed in the lateral limbs of the abscess which are then drained and packed separately.

Primary Suture Under Systemic Antibiotic Cover

Some superficial abscesses may be treated not by the classic incision and drainage method but by incision, curettage, and primary suture under the cover of broad-spectrum and high-dosage systemic antibiotherapy [10, 22, 45, 48] (Fig. 11.9). Intravenous antibiotherapy should begin before anesthesia. Bacteriologic samples are cultured. All granulation tissue and fibrous linings of the abscess should be removed to leave a clean, well-bleeding cavity with a good supply of antibiotics. Deep vertical mattress sutures of monofilament, nonabsorbable material are placed to close the whole cavity. Antibiotics are given for 5–10 days; the choice of drug is adapted to the results of the bacteriologic cultures. Sutures are removed on the 5th or 7th day. In the case of recurrence or extension of the septic lesions, sutures must be removed earlier.

This treatment allows outpatient treatment and eliminates the need for frequent painful changes of dressing. Unfortunately, however, it results in at least a 15% recurrence rate (as the cryptoglandular origin of the lesion is not adequately treated) and a 7% rate of secondary fistulous tracts. It is therefore no longer to be recommended.

Are Antibiotics Necessary?

As antibiotics do not remove the cause of anorectal infection, they have very little place in the management of anorectal abscesses. They are useful in cases of extensive cellulitis to prevent bacteriologic dissemination due to the surgical procedure. They

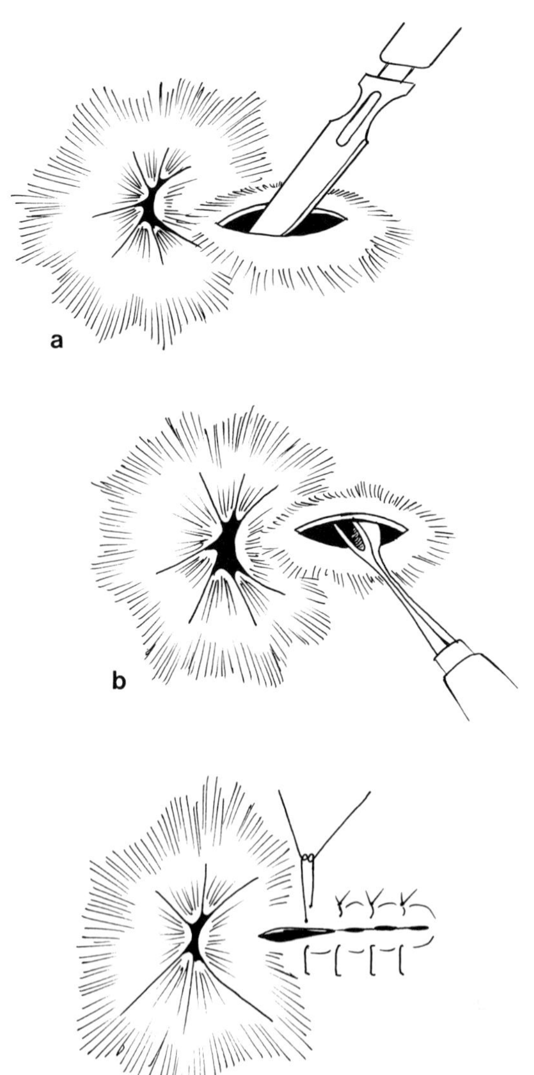

Fig. 11.9a–c. Mattress suture of an abscess. After incision, curettage, and excision of granulomatous and fibrous tissue, the cavity is closed with a deep mattress suture of nonabsorbable monofilament material which encircles all the excision

must be given if the patient is diabetic, immunodepressed, suffering from valvular lesions of the heart, or wearing prosthetic material.

One- or Two-Stage Operation; Value of Seton Drainage

The primary opening in a crypt may be identified when treating an acute abscess. A one-stage or a two-stage operation may be considered. A one-stage operation is possible in the case of an intersphincteric abscess or a low trans-sphincteric fistu-

lous tract. The lay-open technique should only be performed if it results in minimal sphincteric division. In every other instance, a two-stage operation should be planned. The abscess is incised and drained as previously described, and the fistulous tract should be drained using a seton drainage [39].

Nonabsorbable monofilament sutures are placed from the incision of the abscess along the tract to the primary crypt or in the opposite direction. Three or four 3-0 nylon or polyester sutures are placed and tied separately and loosely without tension, as the extremities of a single heavy suture may be painful as a result of the perineal skin being damaged and as the knots of several stitches tied together may become too loose early.

The seton will allow drainage and promote fibrosis around the fistulous tract. At a second stage, traction on the seton drainage is useful to evaluate the thickness of the spared anal muscle and to select the treatment modality according to the amount of sphincter involved: fistulotomy, fistulectomy, rerouting, or sliding flap advancement.

Postoperative Care After Abscess Drainage

The wounds are dressed with dry gauze, and not with gauze impregnated with petroleum jelly, to prevent small collections of remaining pus and to facilitate further changes of dressing. The patient should have a bath or a shower after each bowel action and clean the wound at least three times a day. After a short hospital stay, the wound must be supervised weekly until complete healing occurs. A possible initially unrecognized fistulous tract must be looked for carefully after 2–3 weeks. A second-stage operation can be planned as soon as sufficient wound healing has been achieved, usually after 3–6 weeks.

Anal Fistula

Etiology

Only 10% of anal fistulas are due to a specific etiology (Table 11.2); 90% of cases have a cryptoglandular origin [1]. A previous history of abscesses may not be recorded in nearly one-third of the patients; in these cases, discharge is the first indication of trouble [37, 41]. In a study of 562 consecutive fistulous abscesses (unpublished data), 190 fistulous tracts were evident at first examination; 101 were discovered at the second stage. In 143 cases of a fis-

Table 11.2. Etiology of anorectal fistulas

Nonspecific (90%)
  Cryptoglandular origin

Specific (10%)
  Anorectal disease
    Fissure in ano
    Hemorrhoidectomy
    Sclerotherapy of hemorrhoids
  Inflammatory bowel disease
    Crohn's disease
    Ulcerative colitis
  Infections
    Tuberculosis
    Actinomycosis
    Lymphogranuloma venereum
    Bursitis ischiadica
  Malignancy
    Anal carcinoma
    Low rectal carcinoma
    Blood dyscrasia
    Postirradiation
  Trauma
    Penetrating injuries
    Episiotomy
    Surgery of the prostata
    Ingested foreign bodies
    Impalement
    Injuries due to enema

tulous tract, no abscesses were recorded; 209 abscesses were incised and no fistulous tract was evident at the first stage or later over a period of 5 years.

A specific etiology of anal fistulas must be recognized as early as possible to avoid the risk of inadequate treatment. Particularly in cases of Crohn's disease, more or less extensive lesions may be recognized in the distal colon. One-third of those initially free from intestinal Crohn's disease will develop the disease within 5 years (see Chap. 13).

Signs and Symptoms

Anorectal fistula causes chronic purulent, fecal or serosanguine discharge with skin irritation. Intermittent swelling, pain, and even fever are due to fecal stasis in the tract; spontaneous rupture and drainage will result on improvement. More frequently, in the absence of acute suppuration, a fistula is seen as a draining sinus in the perineal area. A long history may result in the formation of several lateral secondary openings with a "watering-can" appearance.

Examination

If there is no abscess, palpation is painless, and the examining physician can appreciate a cord-like indurated structure stretching more or less radially from the draining sinus toward the anal canal. If the fistulous tract is in a high localization, perineal palpation near the external sphincter is insufficient. Bidigital examination is then useful to appreciate the fibrous tract crossing the external sphincter and to palpate a retraction at the level of an anal crypt. A primary opening should be identified if this has not already been done when draining an abscess.

Goodsall's rule is still very useful [15] (Fig. 11.10). Fistulas opening in front of an imaginary line dividing the anus transversely have a direct course to the anus, while those with an external opening behind this line have a curved course and usually reach the anal canal in the midline. Anterior openings, located more than 3 cm from the anal verge, also have a posterior curved course.

Identification of the fistulous tract is best performed with a curved blunt-tipped probe introduced through the secondary opening. It is a very painful procedure which traumatizes the tract and may create a false passage into the anal canal. Such an examination therefore requires anesthesia. The primary opening, at the depth of an anal crypt, can be identified according to Goodsall's rule by use of a blunt crypt hook.

Injection of air into the secondary opening helps in the identification of the primary opening and, to

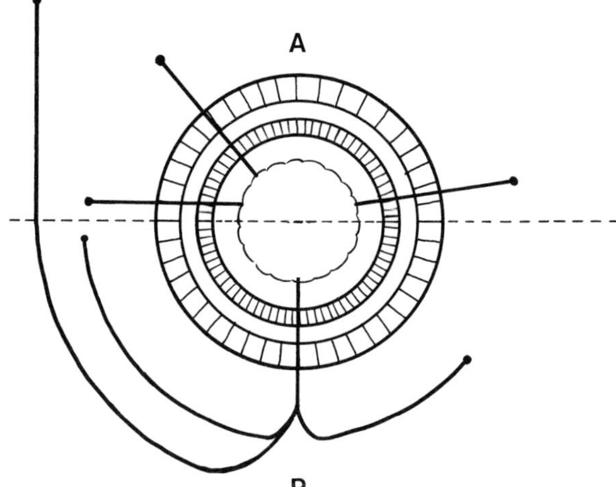

Fig. 11.10. Goodsall's rule: anterior (A) fistulous tracts are linear, whereas posterior (P) tracts are curved. Anterior secondary openings located more than 3 cm from the anal margin communicate through a curved tract with a posteriorly located anal gland

some extent, distends the fistulous tract. The passage of air into the anal lumen is confirmed by digital perception of air bubbles or by anuscopy. Air is far more useful than the injection of a dye solution as it does not stain the various structures. As this examination is painless, unlike the use of metallic probes, it can be performed without anesthesia.

Fistulography is useful to identify the various tracts in cases of complicated and/or recurrent fistulas. Radiographs in the supine and lateral decubitus positions should be obtained with a probe in the anal canal. Recently, CT combined with fistulography and endoanal ultrasonography have been used for complex cases with involvement of adjacent organs.

Classification

A fistulous tract of cryptoglandular origin crosses the sphincters or extends in the same way as abscesses [46]: upward, downward, and around the anal canal along the various spaces, resulting in

Table 11.3. Parks' classification of fistula in ano [36]

1. Intersphincteric
   a, Simple low tract
   b, High blind tract
   c, High tract with rectal opening
   d, Rectal opening without a perineal opening
   e, Extrarectal extension
   f, Secondary to pelvic disease

2. Trans-sphincteric
   a, Uncomplicated
   b, High blind tract

3. Suprasphincteric
   a, Uncomplicated
   b, High blind tract

4. Extrasphincteric
   a, Secondary to anal fistula
   b, Secondary to trauma
   c, Secondary to anorectal disease
   d, Secondary to pelvic inflammation

more complex lesions. The various tracts must be recognized so that they can be optimally treated. Various classifications of anal fistulas have been described. The most useful is that of Parks et al. [36]. This classification has optimal correlations with the anatomical structures and helps in the planning of surgical treatment (Table 11.3, Fig. 11.11). Intersphincteric and trans-sphincteric fistulas are more frequent than extrasphincteric and complex ones (Table 11.4).

Surgical Treatment of Anal Fistula

Anal fistulas do not heal spontaneously without surgery. As anal fistulas are the result of an infection of the anal glands, in 90% of cases the "infecting source" – i.e., the anal gland and duct – must be removed to allow healing of the tract. A precise definition of the anatomy of the fistula should be obtained before treatment. Surgery must achieve the following goals:

- Deroofing or excision of the intersphincteric abscess.
- Laying open of the primary tract.
- Drainage of any secondary tracts.
- Minimal or even no division of the external sphincter to prevent incontinence.
- Safe healing with minimal scarring.

Although the lay-open technique is the most widely accepted method to cure superficial or low anal fistulas, several techniques have been recently used to treat high and complex fistulas. The treatment policy must therefore be adapted to the anatomical and operative conditions.

One-Stage Fistulotomy and Fistulectomy

Fistulotomy involves the deroofing or the laying open of a fistulous tract along a probe. Fistulectomy means excision of all the fistulous tract, granu-

Table 11.4. Frequency of various anal fistulas

	Parks et al. 1976 [36] (%)	Marks and Ritchie 1977 [27] (%)	Arnous et al. 1972 [2] (%)
Superficial		16	
Intersphincteric	45	54	61.1
Trans-sphincteric	30	21	19.1
Suprasphincteric	20	3	5.5
Extrasphincteric	5	3	
Multiple and complex		3	14.2

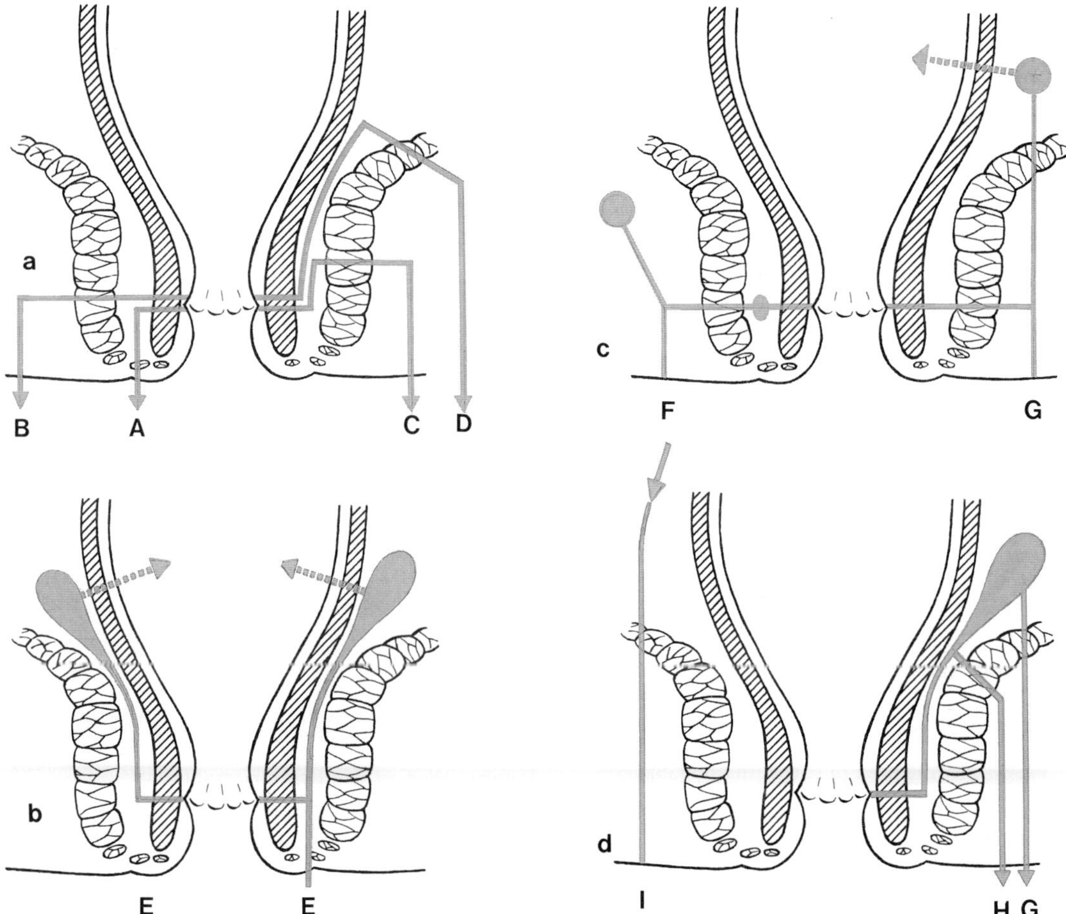

Fig. 11.11 a–d. Classification of anal fistulas according Parks [36]: *A*, intersphincteric fistula; *B*, low trans-sphincteric fistula; *C*, high trans-sphincteric fistula; *D*, suprasphincteric fistula, *E*, intersphincteric fistula with high tract extension and possible rectal opening; *F*, trans-sphincteric fistula with high blind tract; *G*, extrasphincteric fistula secondary to anal fistula; *H*, suprasphincteric fistula; *I*, extrasphincteric fistula

lation, and dense fibrous tissue. Fistulectomy creates larger wounds and a greater separation of the ends of the sphincter resulting in a longer healing time and increased risk of incontinence.

Fistulectomy and fistulotomy are easy to perform in cases of perineal, intersphincteric, and low trans-sphincteric fistulas. If the fistulous tract crosses the external sphincter, a lay-open technique or fistulotomy results in some sphincter damage depending on the amount of sphincter which is divided.

Healing by Second Intention

After excision or incision of a fistulous tract, with more or less extensive excision of the skin, and after removing the intersphincteric anal gland, the wound is left open for healing by second intention (Fig. 11.12). Wounds are irrigated or washed several times a day and dressed by a nurse during the hospital stay or by the patient him- or herself.

Primary Suture

Primary suture of wounds resulting from fistulectomy (Fig. 8.12) is unsound for several reasons: a contaminated hematoma may develop and lead to infection and recurrence of a fistula; exploration of any secondary or deep tract may be difficult; if skin is excised, the suture will be under tension with a risk of becoming loose.

After excision of the internal opening, partial suture at the level of the pectineal line and anoderm may nevertheless achieve hemostasis, speed up healing time, and prevent an anal key-hole deformity. The outer part of the excision is left open to ensure drainage.

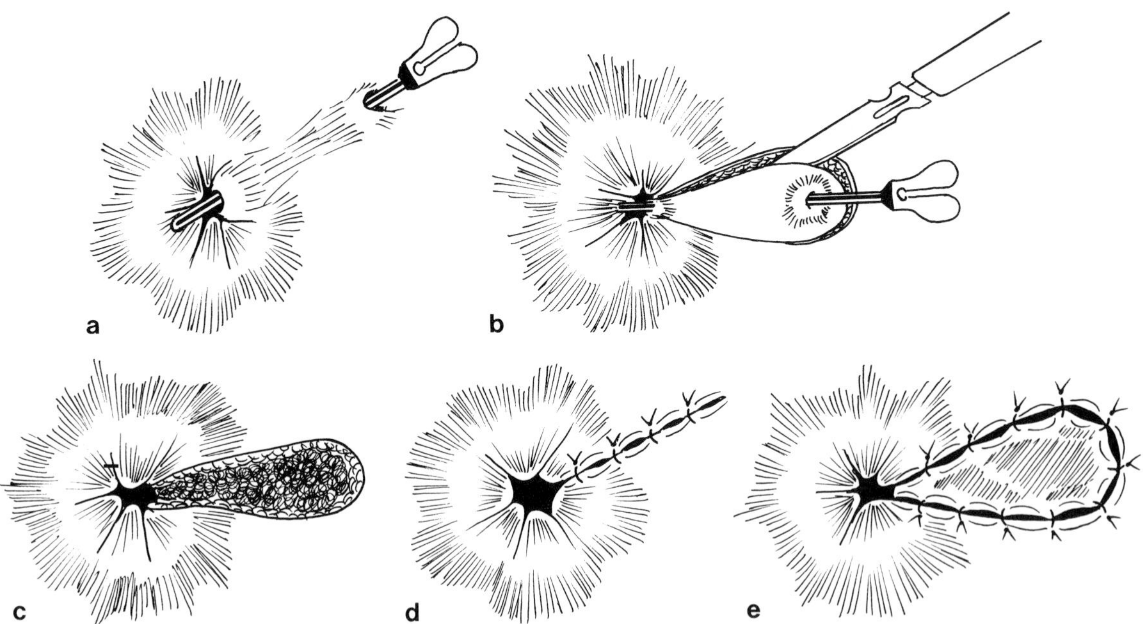

Fig. 11.12a–e. Management of fistulectomy wounds: excision may be left open for healing by second intention (*c*); partially or totally closed (*d*); and skin grafted (*e*)

Skin Graft

Primary or delayed skin graft, as a free graft of thin "split-thickness" skin, has been advocated for fistulectomy wounds (Fig. 8.12). Wound healing is speeded up even if the graft is only partially successful. If the skin graft sloughs, no harm has been done. The wound can then be left open or regrafted. A skin graft has the disavantage of preventing wound retraction and it therefore leaves a persistent deformity.

Two-Stage Fistulectomy

For trans-sphincteric fistula, in a low or a high localization, and for suprasphincteric fistula, a two-stage procedure must be usually planned. In the first stage, the original abscess is exposed within the intersphincteric space as previously described (see p. 87). The relationship of the primary tract to the external sphincter and the puborectalis muscle must be determined. If the tract is low and if a sufficient amount of external sphincter is left above, a fistulotomy may be performed in the same session; the fistulous tract may be curetted or cored out. This tract may close spontaneously, but recurrences are frequent.

If there are doubts about the amount of sphincter left, the external tract outside the sphincter and within the ischiorectal space is excised widely to al-low good drainage (Fig. 11.13). The external sphincter is denuded for 1–2 cm. A seton drainage of rubber or nylon is passed through the tract across the external sphincter and tied loosely. No bridge of skin should be left between the anal excision and the ischiorectal incision. The wounds are drained and dressed.

The amount of functioning muscle enclosed by the seton is estimated later when the patient is conscious. The seton drainage allows healing of the external wound with fibrous tissue bridging the external sphincter outside the fistulous tract. When complete healing of the external wound is achieved – from several weeks to 6 months later – the muscle may be divided if necessary, preventing sphincter edges from retracting and minimizing the risk of postoperative incontinence [34]. The rubber band seton drainage may also be tied progressively every 2–3 weeks to cut the external sphincter and puborectalis sling slowly [2].

Rerouting the Tract for a High Fistula

Several treatments have been developed to minimize the risk of sphincter damage while treating a high-level fistula. The rerouting of the tract, as described by Mann and Clifton [26], is a staged procedure in which the extrasphincteric part of the tract is moved inward to a site where it can be laid open without any sacrifice of sphincter muscle

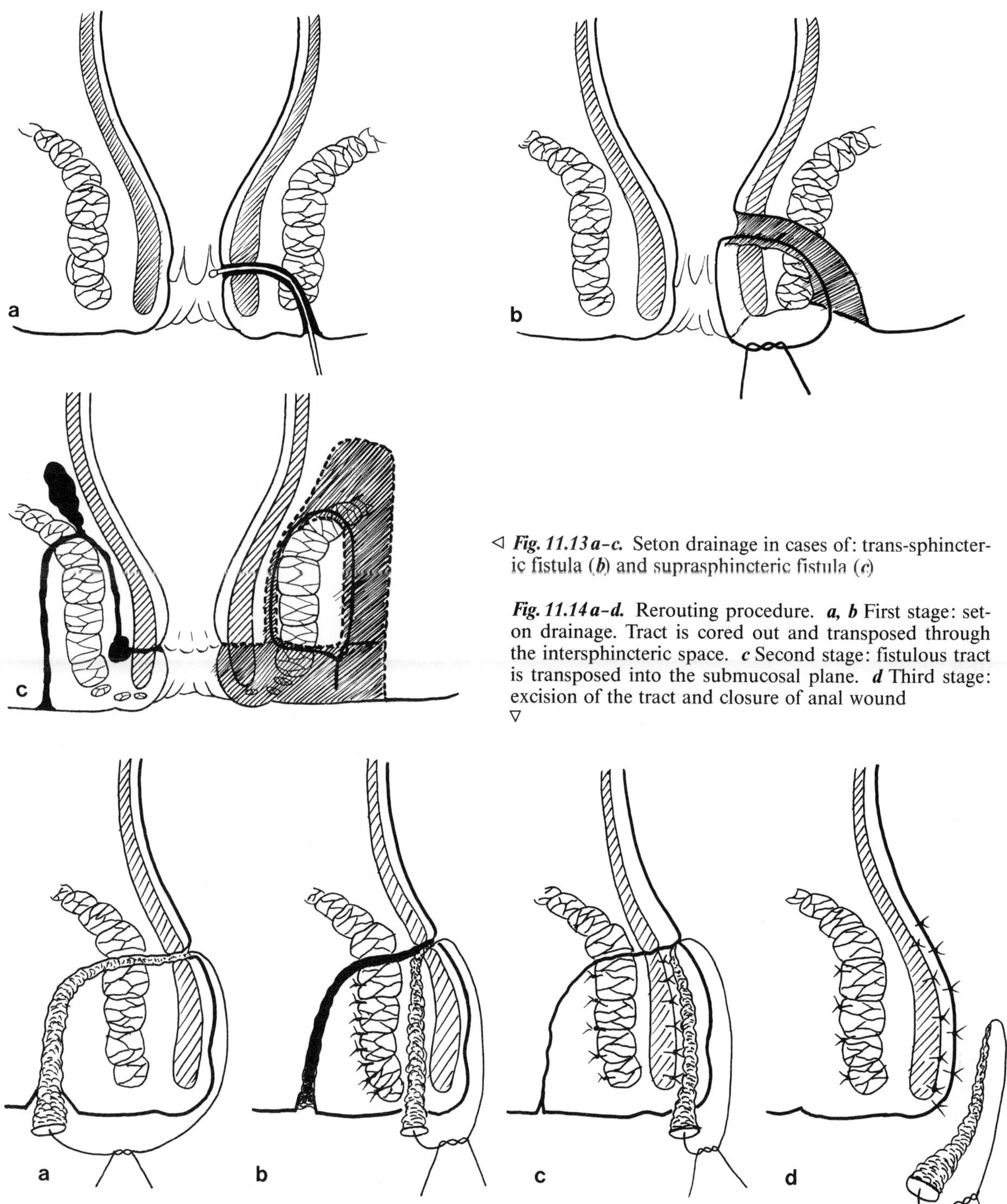

◁ **Fig. 11.13 a–c.** Seton drainage in cases of: trans-sphincteric fistula (*b*) and suprasphincteric fistula (*c*)

Fig. 11.14 a–d. Rerouting procedure. *a, b* First stage: seton drainage. Tract is cored out and transposed through the intersphincteric space. *c* Second stage: fistulous tract is transposed into the submucosal plane. *d* Third stage: excision of the tract and closure of anal wound
▽

(Fig. 11.14). This technique can only be used for a chronic well-established fistula and not for acute cases with abscess.

In the first stage, a nylon seton is passed through the tract and tied loosely. The skin around the external opening is incised sufficiently to allow exposure of the external sphincter and puborectalis muscle. The fistulous tract is cored out up to the point where it crosses the external sphincter. The intersphincteric space is dissected up to the same level. The external tract is passed through or above the external sphincter and brought down into the intersphincteric space. The gap in the external sphincter is closed. The external wound is left open; it heals rapidly.

The second stage is undertaken 4–6 weeks later when the external wound has closed. The fistulous tract is transposed into the submucous plane by division and immediate repair of the internal sphincter. As the connection between the external and internal sphincter has not been destroyed, the external sphincter acts as a splint for the divided internal sphincter and prevents deformity of the muscles and anal canal. A third stage may be necessary to excise the tract and close the mucosal and anodermal lining of the anal canal. The first and second stages may be combined.

This technique of treating a high fistula has been used in only a small number of cases. Two or three stages are necessary. The external muscle must be partially divided and resutured. Nevertheless, the healing time is shorter, and results ought to be better than after two-stage fistulectomy.

Sliding Flap Advancement

Instead of two-stage fistulotomy and rerouting, some authors core out all the fistulous tract from the external to the internal opening (Fig. 11.15) [21, 32, 47]. The intersphincteric space is curetted. The gap through the external and internal sphincters is closed by separate stitches of absorbable material starting from the anal lumen. The mucosa and anoderm, depending on the level of the tract, are excised around the internal opening. A flap of mucosa is undermined, with a base which is twice the width of the apex, and sutured to the lower edge of the mucosa. The suture line must lie distal to the previous muscle closure. The external wound is left open.

This technique preserves a greater amount of sphincter than any other, it minimizes scar formation, avoids anatomic deformity, and does not require any intestinal diversion. The technique is used for chronic fistula; it can also be performed as the second stage after incision and drainage of a fistulous abscess with a seton. In some selected cases of localized and small ischiorectal abscesses, we have used it as the first and therefore the only stage.

Technique for Intramural or Intermuscular Fistula

Intramural or intermuscular fistula may extend from the pectineal line high up into the rectum. If the tract below the anorectal ring is adequately opened and destroyed, the remaining tract above the ring will close spontaneously. If an abscess is present, a seton drainage may be applied for some days or weeks before the tract is opened. If the intramural abscess constitutes a diverticular extension of trans-sphincteric fistula, it must be opened at the first stage of a two-stage fistulectomy [6].

Extrasphincteric Fistula

This fistula can have a cryptoglandular origin but occurs more frequently as a result of Crohn's disease and as a complication of probing too deeply and surgical drainage of an abscess. In the case of Crohn's disease, a permanent seton should be kept in place for several months to prevent the formation of an abscess and to promote the growth of an epithelial lining. If the patient does not respond to this treatment nor to metronidazole, proctectomy must be considered (see Chap. 13). If the extrasphincteric fistula has a traumatic origin, a sliding flap advancement, as previously described or a low anterior resection with coloanal anastomosis must be considered.

Horseshoe Fistula

Horseshoe fistula is one of the most difficult conditions that a surgeon must face [18, 46]. The primary fistulous opening is usually in a posterior midline crypt. If not previously drained by a seton, the primary tract is deroofed through a sagittal incision at the tip of the coccyx. The posterior anal space is opened. The Y-shaped portion of the tract in the postanal space, below the anococcygeal raphe, is excised. The remaining trans-sphincteric tract is drained with a seton (Fig. 11.8). The secondary openings are excised through radial incisions. The tracts are excised or curetted but not deroofed in order to prevent large scars. As soon as the lateral wounds have closed, the primary tract may be excised or cored out as previously described.

Postoperative Care After Fistulectomy

At the end of an operation for fistula, the wounds are kept apart with a light gauze dressing soaked in antiseptic. Oily dressings are best avoided. Baths or wound irrigations are recommended three to four times daily. The wound must be kept clean.

Weekly inspection should be carried out by the surgeon. Pocketing and early bridging of the wounds must be avoided. Silver nitrate may be applied to prevent overgranulation. Sphincter function must

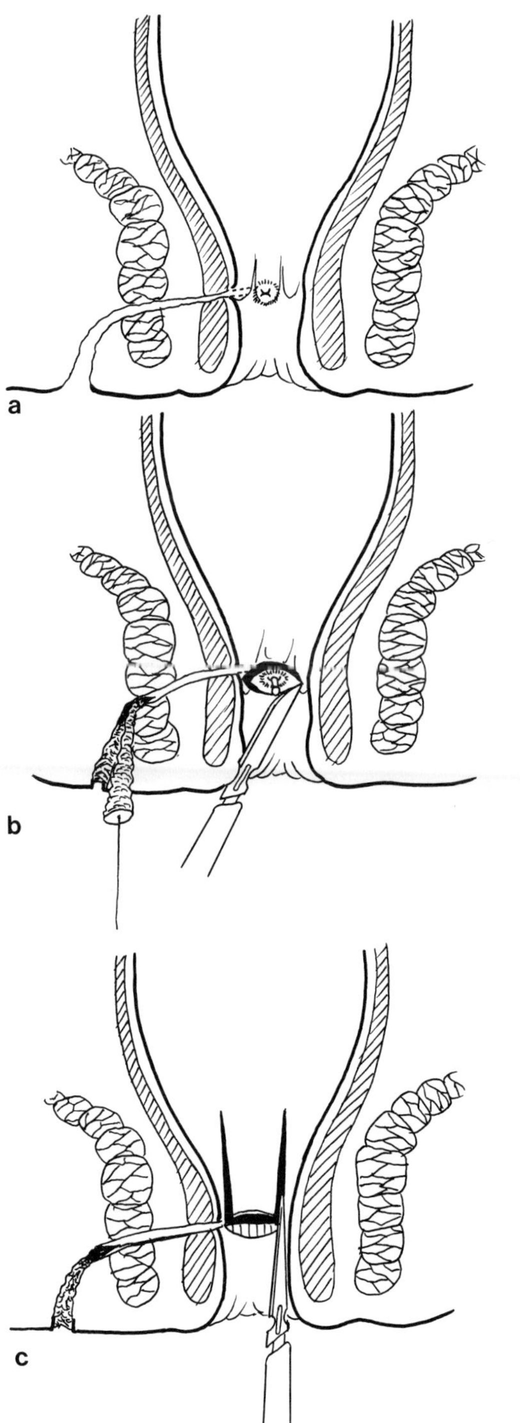

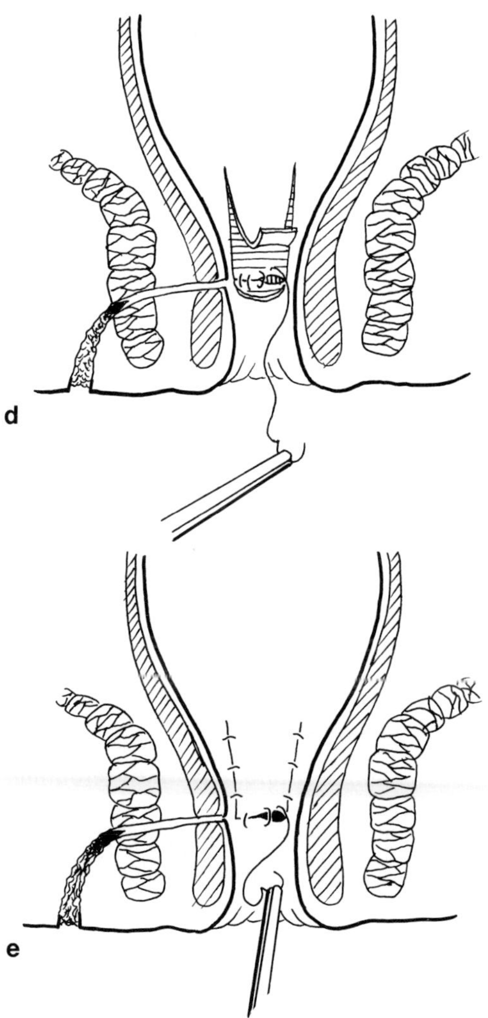

Fig. 11.15 a–e. Sliding flap. *a, b* Coring out of all the fistulous tract and anal gland. *c* Mobilization of a mucosal flap. *d* Closure of muscular gap. *e* Suture of the mucosa

be evaluated soon after surgery, especially if a seton drainage is in place. Bowel action should not be delayed. Bulky laxatives must be given to allow passage of stools without straining and to reduce pain.

Results and Complications After Treatment of Anal Fistula

Satisfactory results may be achieved in the treatment of anal fistula. Results depend on the type of fistula. The healing time varies from 6 weeks for the low type to 16 weeks or more for the complex variety. Fistula surgery should be reserved for experienced surgeons in order to reduce, as much as possible, the high incidence of recurrence. Three main postoperative complications may occur after treatment of an anal fistula: recurrence, incontinence, and rectal prolapse. The incidence of these complications is listed in Table 11.5

Table 11.5. Results and complications after surgical treatment of fistula in ano

	Patients (n)	Recurrence (%)	Incontinence (%)
Bennett 1962 [3]	108	2	36
Hill 1967 [20]	626	1	4
Kubchandani 1984 [23]	137	5.8	
Lilins 1968 [25]	150	5.5	13.5
Marks and Ritchie 1977 [27]	793		17–31
Mazier 1971 [29]	1000	3.9	0.01
McElwain et al. 1975 [30]	1000	3.6	7.0–3.2
Parks and Stitz 1976 [34]	400	9	
Pearl et al. 1986 [38]	1732	1.8	

Recurrence

Recurrence of anal fistula in cases of cryptoglandular origin is due essentially to the failure to remove the right anal gland. The internal opening may not be found and part of the tract may be buried under the granulation tissue. A recurrence rate of around 10% is observed. It is also difficult to assess the adequacy of the initial management from reports in the literature. If a fistula has been adequately treated and still recurs, the possibility of Crohn's disease must be considered.

Incontinence

Partial early postoperative incontinence is frequent after surgery of any fistulous tract and is the result of inflammation, tissue deformity, pain, and the dressing. If the sphincter has been divided, the initial weakness regresses, and continence has proved to be adequate within 2–3 weeks. As many as one-third of the patients have some permanent disturbance in anal continence, varying from loss of flatus control to severe fecal incontinence. To prevent incontinence, there must be a sufficient space of time between the two operative sessions in a two-stage procedure. Division of the sphincter muscle must be kept to a minimum. In cases of trans-sphincteric fistula, a sliding flap is preferable to long and high fistulotomies. If sphincter division results in persistent incontinence, sphincter repair must be considered.

Prolapse of the Rectum

Mucosal prolapse frequently occurs after sphincter division below the anorectal ring. The hypertrophic mucosa tends to obliterate the postoperative deformity. This prolapse is usually asymptomatic and should not be excised. If the anorectal ring has been divided, rectal prolapse with incontinence may occur. An abdominal rectopexy with suture of the levator ani must be considered.

Carcinoma

The occasional development of a carcinoma in a fistulous tract has been reported. The tumor is situated in the perianal and perirectal tissues and is of the mucoid adenocarcinoma type [8]. Furthermore, free viable cancer cells from an upper rectal tumor may be grafted on the granulation surface of a perianal fistula [24].

References

1. Abcarian H (1989) Anorectal fistulae. Postgrad Adv Colorectal Surg 1-X: 1–6
2. Arnous J, Parnaud E, Denis J (1972) Quelques réflexions sur les abcès et les fistules à l'anus. Rev Prat 22: 1793–1814
3. Bennett RC (1962) A review of the results of orthodox treatment for anal fissure. Proc R Soc Med 55: 756–757
4. Bevans DW, Westbrook KC, Thomson BW, Carldwell FT (1973) Perirectal abscess: a potentially fatal illness. Am J Surg 126: 765–768
5. Bubrick MP, Hitchcock CR (1979) Necrotizing anorectal and perineal infections. Surgery 86: 655–662
6. Denis J, Ganansia R, Arnous-Dubois N, du Puy-Montbrun T, Lemarchand N (1983) Les abcès intra-muraux du rectum. Presse Med 12: 1285–1289
7. Di Falco G, Guccione C, D'Annibale A, et al. (1986) Fournier's gangrene following a perianal abscess. Dis Colon Rectum 29: 582–585
8. Dukes CE, Galvin C (1956) Colloid carcinoma arising within fistulae in the anorectal region. Ann R Coll Surg Engl 18: 246–261
9. Eisenhammer S (1966) The anorectal fistulous abscess and fistula. Dis Colon Rectum 9: 91–106
10. Ellis M (1953) The new treatment of ischiorectal abscesses. Univ Leeds Med J 2: 84
11. Eykyn SJ, Grace RH (1986) The relevance of microbiology in the management of anorectal sepsis. Ann R Coll Surg Engl 68: 237–239
12. Fournier AJ (1883) Gangrène foudroyante de la verge. Sem Med 3: 345–348
13. Goldberg S, Gordon PP, Nivatvongs S (1980) Essentials of anorectal surgery. Lippincott, Philadelphia
14. Goligher J-C, Ellis A, Pissidis AG (1967) A critique of anal glandular infection in the aetiology and treatment of idiopathic anorectal abscess and fistulas. Br J Surg 54: 977–983

15. Goodsall DH, Miles WE (1900) Diseases of the anus and rectum. Longmans Green, London, pp 92–173
16. Grace RH, Harper IA, Thompson RG (1982) Anorectal sepsis: microbiology in relation to fistula in ano. Br J Surg 69: 401–403
17. Hamilton CH (1975) Anorectal problems. The deep postanal space. Surgical significance in horseshoe fistula and abscess. Dis Colon Rectum 18: 642–645
18. Hanley PH (1965) Conservative surgical correction of horseshoe abscess and fistula. Dis Colon Rectum 8: 364–368
19. Hermann G, Desfosses L (1880) Sur la muqueuse de la région cloacale du rectum. C R Séances Acad Sci 90: 1301–1304
20. Hill JR (1967) Fistulas and fistulous abscesses in the anorectal region: personal experience in management. Dis Colon Rectum 10: 421–434
21. Jones IT, Fazio VW, Jagelman DG (1987) The use of transanal rectal advancement flaps in the management of fistulas involving the anorectum. Dis Colon Rectum 30: 919–923
22. Jones NAG, Wilson DH (1976) The treatment of acute abscesses by incision, curettage and primary suture under antibiotic cover. Br J Surg 63: 499–501
23. Khubchandani M (1984) Comparison of results of treatment of fistula in ano. J R Soc Med 77: 369–371
24. Killingback M, Wilson E, Hughes ESR (1965) Anal metastases from carcinoma of the rectum and colon. Aust NZ J Surg 34: 178–187
25. Lilius HG (1968) Fistula in ano: an investigation of human foetal anal ducts and intramuscular glands and a clinical study of 150 patients. Acta Chir Scand [Suppl] 383: 88
26. Mann CV, Clifton MA (1985) Rerouting of the track for the treatment of high anal and anorectal fistulae. Br J Surg 72: 134–137
27. Marks CG, Ritchie JK (1977) Anal fistulae at St. Mark's Hospital. Br J Surg 64: 84–91
28. Marks G, Chase WV, Mervie TB (1973) The fatal potential of fistula in ano with abscess. Dis Colon Rectum 16: 224–230
29. Mazier WP (1971) The treatment and care of anal fistulas. A study of 1000 patients. Dis Colon Rectum 14: 134–144
30. McElwain JW, McLean MD, Alexander RM, et al. (1975) Experience with primary fistulectomy for anorectal abscess: a report of 1000 cases. Dis Colon Rectum 18: 646–649
31. Myers KJ, Heppell J, Bode WE, Culp CE, Thurber DL, van Scoy RE (1984) Tetanus after anorectal abscess. Mayo Clin Proc 59: 429–430
32. Oh C (1983) Management of high recurrent anal fistula. Surgery 93: 330–332
33. Oh C, Lee C, Jacobson J (1982) Necrotizing fasciitis of the perineum. Surgery 91: 49–51
34. Parks AG, Stitz RW (1976) The treatment of high fistula in ano. Dis Colon Rectum 19: 487–499
35. Parks AG, Thomson JPS (1973) Intersphincteric abscess. Br Med J 2: 537–539
36. Parks AG, Gordon PH, Hardcastle JD (1976) A classification of fistula in ano. Br J Surg 63: 1–12
37. Paul M. Fernando M (1957) Fistula in ano. Med Press 238: 557–562
38. Pearl RK, Nelson RL, Orsay CT, Abcarian H (1986) Anorectal abscess: the importance of early surgical exploration. Scientific exhibit, American College of Surgeons Clinical Congress. New Orleans LA, October 1986
39. Ramanujam P, Prasad ML, Abcarian H (1983) The role of seton in fistulotomy of the anus. Surg Gynecol Obstet 57: 419–422
40. Ramanujam P, Prasad ML, Abcarian H, Tan AB (1984) Perianal abscesses and fistulas. A study of 1023 patients. Dis Colon Rectum 27: 593–597
41. Read DR, Abcarian H (1979) A prospective survey of 474 patients with anorectal abscess. Dis Colon Rectum 22: 566–568
42. Riegles-Nielsen P, Hessefeldt-Nielsen B, Bang-Jensen E, Jacobsen E (1984) Fournier's gangrene: 5 patients treated with hyperbaric oxygen. J Urol 132: 918–920
43. Rosenberg PH, Shuck JM, Tempest BD, Redd WP (1978) Diagnosis and therapy of necrotizing soft tissue infections of the perineum. Ann Surg 187: 430–434
44. Slim K, Ben Slimene T, Largueche S, Bard K, Guiga M, Mzabi R (1988) Les gangrènes périnéales secondaires aux abcès de la marge anale. J Chir 125: 270–275
45. Stegwart MPM; Laing MR, Krukowski ZH (1985) Treatment of acute abscesses by incision, curettage and primary suture without antibiotics: a controlled clinical trial. Br J Surg 72: 66–67
46. Stelzner F (1981) Die anorektalen Fisteln, 3rd edn. Springer, Berlin Heidelberg New York
47. Wedell J, Meier zu Eissen P, Banzhaf G, Kleine L (1987) Sliding flap advancement for the treatment of high level fistulae. Br J Surg 74: 390–391
48. Wilson DH (1964) The late results of anorectal abscess treated by incision, curettage and primary suture under antibiotic cover. Br J Surg 51: 828

12 Pilonidal Sinus

A. Froidevaux

Definition

Pilonidal sinus is caused by an epidermal invagination allowing hairs to be drawn in and to form a foreign body granuloma. Pilonidal sinus is a chronic inflammatory lesion. It is mainly located between the buttocks but may also be observed in the interdigital webs, the umbilicus, the axilla, the scalp, the perineum, the anus, and amputation stumps.

Pathogenesis

Since 1847 various theories have been put forward to explain the pathogenesis of pilonidal sinus [2, 3, 4, 8]:

Congenital Origin Theory. Embryonal remnants (sexual glands, spina bifida scars, neural rests) may be reactivated at puberty.

Acquired Origin Theory. Because of the muscular movements of the buttocks, hairs are drawn into the cutaneous lining of the natal cleft where they react as foreign bodies.

Mixed Congenital and Acquired Etiology Theory. According to our histopathological observations [4, 10], only a mixed theory can account for the pathogenesis. Histological sections across the primary pit show surface epithelium invagination (congenital component) through which hairs have entered, developing into a foreign body granuloma which will be secondarily infected (acquired component). The secondary openings are nothing more than discharge channels. No epithelium can be found within the excised pilonidal sinus. The hairs found in the sinus are free. They may be too long to originate from the vicinity of the sinus; they may have penetrated after becoming detached from the head, for example.

Clinical Findings

The epidemiology is well known: there is a clear male predominancy in hairy, Mediterranean-type patients aged between 20 and 29 [4, 10]. Clinically there is a characteristically long evolution before treatment: more than 1 year in one-third of cases. The natural history of pilonidal sinus is characterized by relapses and remissions of abscesses, discharges, and swelling (Fig. 12.1). Discharge is noted in 67% of cases, swelling in 52%, pain in 35%, and fever in 1%. The patient suffering from pilonidal sinus will complain of a swelling in the natal cleft or buttocks, which develops within a few days. There may be spontaneous discharge, or the lesion may require surgical drainage. Once the lesion has been drained, a chronic pilonidal sinus is formed. On examination we have found [4, 10] (Fig. 12.2):

- One or more primary pits in the natal cleft
- Secondary tracts with lateral openings

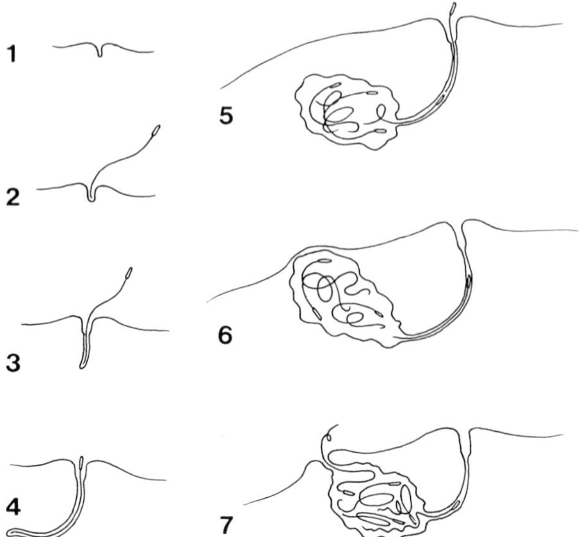

Fig. 12.1. Natural evolution and formation of pilonidal sinus. *1,* Small pit in the natal cleft; *2, 3* and *4,* penetration of hair; *5,* formation of a pilonidal sinus due to the penetration of many hairs; *6* and *7,* inflammatory reaction and fistulisation to the skin with formation of a secondary tract

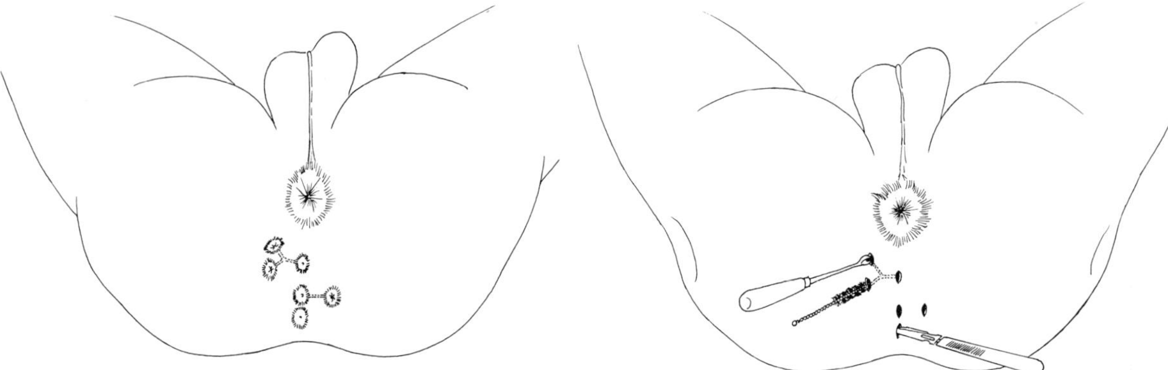

Fig. 12.2. Clinical aspects of a pilonidal sinus. Primary pits are within the natal cleft. Secondary openings are located laterally

Fig. 12.3. Surgical treatment of pilonidal sinus: excision of primary pits. Coring out of the various tracts, brushing to remove hairs, and curettage

Streptococci and *Staphylococci albi* may be found on bacteriological examination [10]. Pilonidal sinus should be distinguished from anal fistulas, hidrosadenitis suppurativa, simple furoncle, and scratching lesions complicated by an abscess.

Conservative Treatment

Various conservative treatment methods have been used with minimal success: topical or systematic anti-inflammatory drugs, antibiotics, or injection of 80% phenol solution within the sinus. Knowledge of the pathogenesis allows one to understand why conservative treatment that does not suppress the causal agent is useless.

Surgical Treatment

Surgical treatment aims at solving three problems definitively (Fig. 12.3) [8, 10]:

- Congenital epidermic invagination by excision
- Hairs entering into the invagination by careful and frequent shaving
- Wound superinfection by an open technique and frequent washing

The various procedures described can be divided into four groups: those in which the whole lesion is widely excised and left open, those in which the wound is partially or totally closed after excision, and the Lord-Millar procedure.

Open Techniques [1, 5, 9, 12]

Incision. Incision is the immediate treatment of a painful abscess but is not a curative procedure. The recurrence rate following incision is about 93%. A second curative procedure should be performed within 6–8 weeks after drainage of an abscess.

Marsupialization. After opening any incision of the various tracts, the wound edges are sutured. Removal of hairs and curetage of granulation tissue should facilitate healing. The recurrence rate is 5%–20%.

Excision. Without shaving, excision of a pilonidal sinus enables a cure in 70% of cases.

Half-Open Technique

The half-open procedure consists in a plain excision followed by a part suture. This technique allows a small opening for drainage, and at the same time the part suture enhances the recovery time. The recurrence rate ranges from 0% to 50% [1, 12].

Closed Technique

Following complete excision of the lesion, the wounds are closed either vertically, transversely, obliquely, or by using a Z or W skin plasty to reduce tissue tension [5, 6, 12]. Recurrence occurs in 4%–8%.

Lord-Millar Technique

The Lord-Millar procedure [7, 10, 11] is performed on a patient lying in ventral decubitus with the buttocks pulled apart with adhesive tape straps. Local anesthesia is performed.

- The primary and secondary openings are enlarged by circumcision: small circular strips of skin, less than 1 cm in diameter and centered on the primary pit, are excised. When there are several primary pits, each of them must be treated in the same way.
- All fibrotic tissue enclosing hair is dissected.
- Secondary subcutaneous tracts are cleaned, curated, and brushed using small electric razor brushes or pipet-cleaning brushes.
- Hemostasis may be necessary.
- No skin closure is required.

The same procedure is used in cases of an acute abscess. Identification of the primary pit may be difficult because of tissue swelling. Curetage may result in bacteremia. Administration of prophylactic broad-spectrum antibiotics is therefore required.

Postoperative Care. Hemostatic gauze may be applied for 24 h especially if the patient is treated on an outpatient basis. To keep the wound clean, the patient is asked to use a shower two to three times a day, directing the spray onto the wound; sitz baths are not sufficient. The wound should be dried using a hair-dryer. Dry dressings or, better, hygienic pads to avoid adhesive tape are applied. To prevent penetration of hairs into the wound, the skin edges should be shaved weekly by the surgeon him/herself. A magnifying glass may be useful to remove all the hairs growing near the wound. After the wound has healed, usually within 3-4 weeks, the patient has to apply an epilatory cream once a week for 3 months.

Results of the Lord-Millar Procedure. This procedure is so simple that it can be performed with local anesthesia on an outpatient basis in almost all cases. Postoperative pain is much reduced. The healing time does not exceed 3-4 weeks, resulting in a short time off work. The recurrence rate is low, with an average of 3% in our experience.

Complications

Recurrences occur in 1%-48% of cases according to the treatment technique used. The highest rate occurs after immediate closure. The lowest rate is observed after the Lord-Millar procedure. Recurrence occurs within 6 months of the primary treatment. Superinfection: this complication mainly occurs after closed techniques and requires re-opening of the incision which results in a prolonged healing time.

References

1. Abramson DJ (1977) Excision and delayed closure of pilonidal sinuses. Surg Gynecol Obstet 144: 205-207
2. Bascom J (1980) Pilonidal disease: origin from follicles of hairs and results of follicle removal as treatment. Surgery 87: 567-572
3. Bascom J (1983) Pilonidal disease: long-term results of follicle removal Dis Colon Rectum 26: 800-807
4. Froidevaux A (1976) Kystes sacro-coccygiens, étude de 422 cas. Lyon Chir 72: 408-412
5. Hodgson WJB (1981) A comparative study between Z-plasty and incision and drainage or excision with marsupialization for pilonidal sinuses. Surg Gynecol Obstet 153: 842-844
6. Karydakis GE (1975) Pilonidal sinus. Communication to the Congress of the Royal Society of Proctology. London 1975
7. Lord PH (1965) Pilonidal sinus: a simple treatment. Br J Surg 52: 298-300
8. Lord PH (1975) Etiology of pilonidal sinus. Dis Colon Rectum 18: 661-664
9. Marks J (1985) Pilonidal sinus excision - healing by open granulation. Br J Surg 72: 637-640
10. Marti MC (1977) Les sinus pilonidaux sacro-coccygiens. Lyon Chir 73: 33-37
11. Marti MC (1987) Traitement ambulatoire des kystes sacro-coccygiens. Présentation au Congrès français de chirurgie
12. Sood SC (1975) Results of various operations for sacrococcygeal pilonidal disease. Plast Reconstr Surg 56: 559-566

13 Anorectal Crohn's Disease

P. Buchmann

Definition

Anorectal Crohn's disease includes lesions of the perianal skin, the inner lining of the anal canal and lower rectum as well as pathological formations originating from these regions related to Crohn's disease.

Etiology

Despite the amount of research that has been done in recent years to identify the cause of Crohn's disease, the precise etiology is still unknown [18]. Interesting hypotheses have been formulated on the basis of immunological disorders [10]. The suggestion that Crohn's disease mainly affects part of the bowel where there are aggregations of lymphoid tissue [19] and narrowing of the bowel [12] may explain the predominance of lesions in the anal area. In the future we might learn more from the research into the human immunodeficiency virus (HIV), as this infection creates a similar impairment of wound healing as observed after fistulectomy in Crohn's disease.

Classification

The clinical feature of anorectal lesions in patients suffering from Crohn's disease are listed in Table 13.1. However, not all the pathology seen in these patients is to be contributed to inflammatory bowel disease, especially when it is quiescent. Therefore incidental lesions can be found as in any otherwise healthy subject. Erosions frequently occur during periods of diarrhea (Fig. 13.1). These superficial epithelial defects turn from excoriations to large macerations, especially during periods of acute proctitis (Fig. 13.2). Pruritus in ano is then replaced by a continuous pain. With increasing age, skin tags become more common as perianal alterations. However, lymphedematous swelling of these skin tags is almost diagnostic for Crohn's disease, especially when coupled with inflammation in the anal canal and lower rectum (Fig. 13.3).

Abscess formation is frequently observed in Crohn's disease, but symptoms are less striking compared with intestinally healthy patients. This carries the danger that the patient and even the physician accept some anal pain as a normal symptom of the disease leading to delay in surgery. Destruction of the tissue might progress, requiring a diverting enterostomy to overcome the suppuration.

The typical Crohn's fissure in ano is painless, broadly based and with no preference for location in the outer anal canal. With careful examination and a good light source, these lesions may be the most frequently found lesions beside skin tags. Nevertheless, there are occasionally typically pain-

Table 13.1. Classification of anorectal lesions

Localization	Related to Crohn's disease	Incidental
Skin lesions		Erosion
	Maceration/ulceration	
	Edematous skin tags	Skin tags
		Abscess
Anal canal lesion	Painless fissure	Painful fissure
	Ulcer	
	Stenosis with induration	Hemorrhoids
Fistulas		Low (from dentate line)
	High (rectum to skin)	
	Rectovaginal	Anovaginal

ful fissures in the posterior, or less frequently anterior, position as in the healthy population.

Deep ulcerations causing a great deal of pain can occasionally be found higher up in the anal canal. These might give rise to a high fistula. These ulcerations and fistulas sometimes heal leaving behind a stenosis with induration. This narrowing of the anal canal often inhibits penetration of the rectum even with the little finger (Fig. 13.4).

Contrary to claims quoted in earlier publications, hemorrhoids are not seen more frequently in Crohn's disease. In our series we found hemorrhoids to be extremely rare, which could be explained by the fact that a thickened mucous mem-

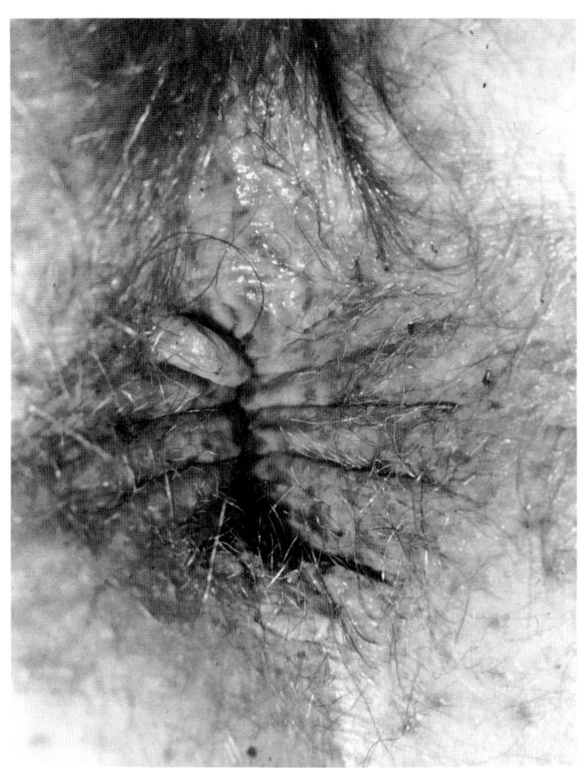

◁

Fig. 13.1. Erosions of the perianal skin. All dark dots near the anal margin represent superficial ulcers

Fig. 13.2 *(below left).* Maceration of the perianal skin. Near the anus the wet inflamed skin is red and very painful. Anteriorly there is a small swollen skin tag

Fig. 13.3 *(below right).* Large edematous skin tags at 5 and 7 o'clock in lithotomy position

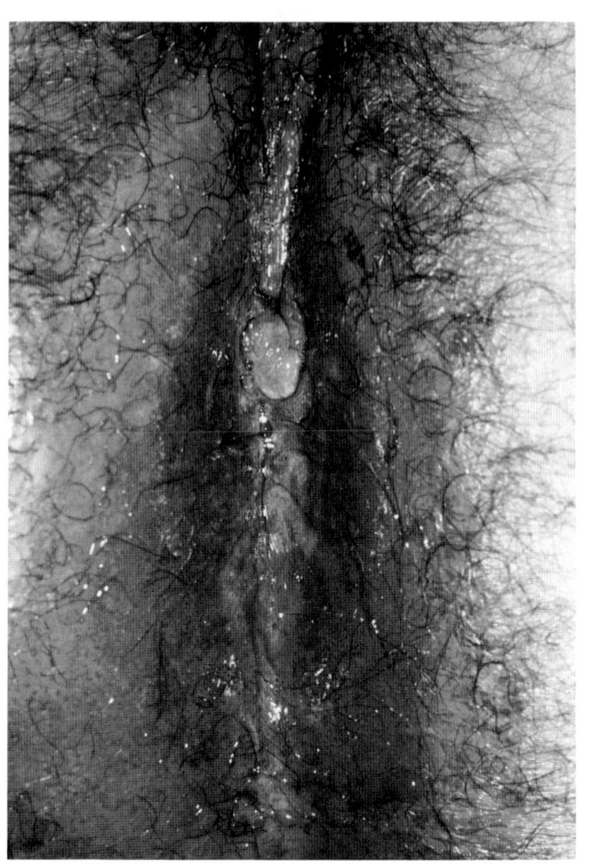

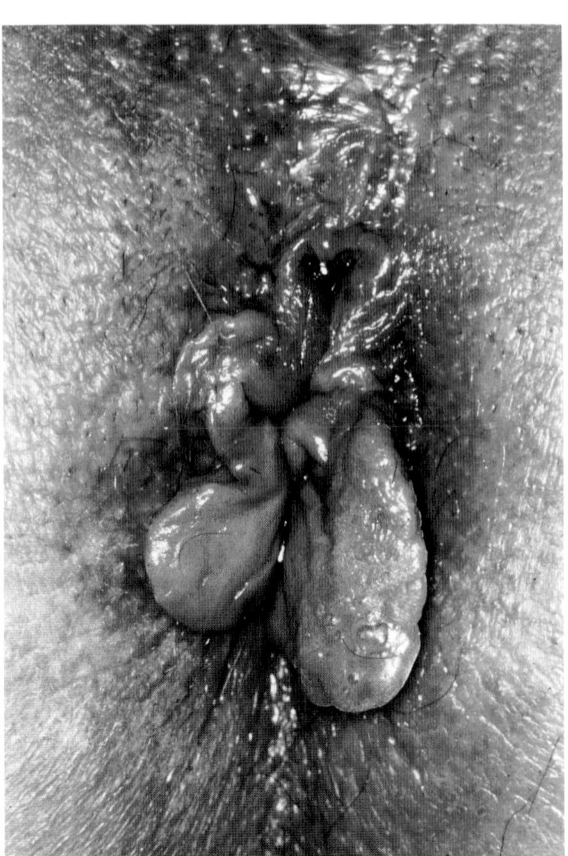

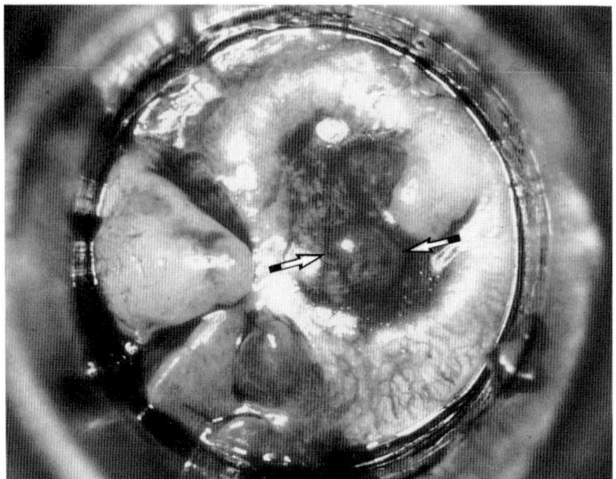

Fig. 13.4. Hypertrophic anal papillae are seen through the anoscope at 7 and 9 o'clock. The anal canal is severely stenosed in the upper part, with an opening of about one fifth of the diameter of the anoscope *(arrows)*

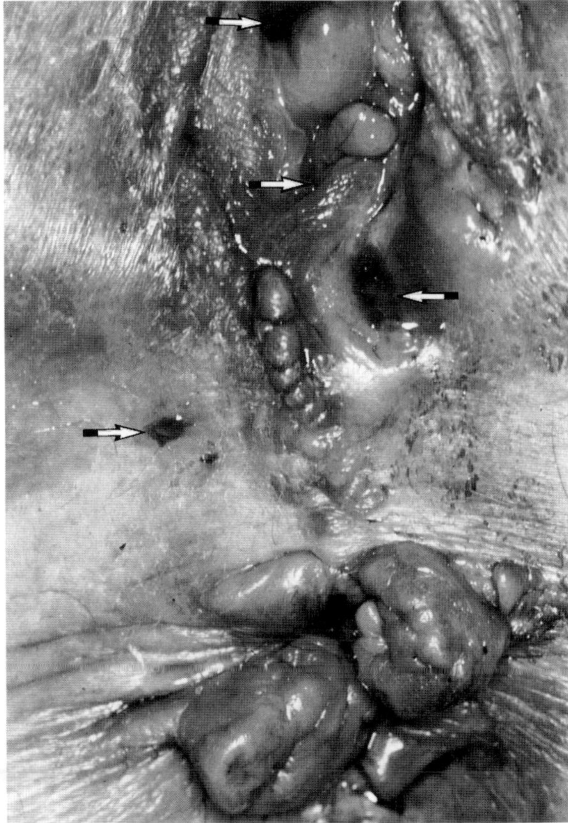

▷

Fig. 13.5. Multiple fistula openings at the perineum and introitus vaginae with severe edema of the skin tags *(arrows)*

brane does not allow the hemorrhoid vascular plexus to swell [4].

It is important to distinguish between two forms of fistulas. The first runs from the dentate line to the perianal skin and probably has the same etiology (infection of the proctodeal glands) as is thought to be the case in patients without Crohn's disease. Most fistulas are of this low type [17]. Secondly a fistula from the anal canal to the introitus vaginae sometimes develops (anovaginal) (Fig. 13.5). High fistulas usually run an extrasphincteric course and originate in a rectal ulcer caused by proctitis. This type of fistula can open outside the anus or vagina (rectovaginal fistula).

Epidemiology

The frequency of anorectal lesions in Crohn's disease varies between 60% and 80% in the literature if patients are examined with a special interest in these alterations [9, 16]. Figures below this frequency are suspect, as they are taken either from retrospective analysis or superficial exploration. However, in children anorectal manifestation is mostly related to active intestinal disease. Perianal lesions sometimes preceding gastrointestinal inflammation by months or even years.

It is common knowledge that Crohn's disease should be considered when recurrent fistulas are observed, especially in a population where tuberculosis is more or less under control. The frequency of fistulas varies between 25% and 45%, including rectovaginal fistulas and abscesses [5, 13]. The discussion whether there is an increased risk of perianal suppuration in ulcerative colitis is still open to debate. Figures of up to 19% are to be found in the literature [13]. However, we believe, in agreement with others, that many of these patients will have a definite diagnosis of Crohn's disease in the future, as ulcerative colitis is confined to the mucous membrane and therefore the pathophysiological background explaining an increased risk of developing fistulas is missing.

Differential Diagnosis

Differentiation can be done in two ways: (a) whether it is Crohn's disease or whether there is any other illness to be taken into account: (b) in patients with Crohn's disease, whether the anorectal manifestations are caused by the disease or whether they are just incidental lesions (Table 13.1). The first differentiation has to be made under the comparatively rare circumstances where the existence of Crohn's disease has not yet been identified. Abscess and fistula formation due to tuberculosis are often related to an active organ tuberculosis and there is either direct contamination or manifestation in the form of a descending abscess from the retroperitoneum. The diagnosis can be easily established by microbiological cultures. Microbiological tests and reactions allow confirmation of a chancroid (ulcus molle), an infection caused by *Hemophilus ducreyi* with painful ulcerations and suppurating abscesses. Direct immunofluorescence leads to the demonstration of chlamydiae causing rectal strictures and abscesses as well as fistula formation.

The differentiation of Crohn's disease and tuberculosis from an actinomycosis can be difficult. This rare condition often progresses to strictures from which biopsies help the diagnosis.

Fistulas from gonorrhea never have access to the anus but always to the urethra. The only proctological manifestation of infection with *Neisseria gonorrhoeae*, an anoproctitis, is usually seen in individuals practicing anal intercourse.

A dermoid located perianally, a teratoma, or a chordoma may fistulate or, in the case of a dermoid, even form an abscess, especially when excision was incomplete. Pathological diagnosis has to be made from a specimen.

Acute leukemia is often followed by a perianal abscess and fistulation. The incidence increases during periods of granulocytopenia induced either by the disease or the therapy. Adequate hematological tests make differentiation easy.

Superficial skin lesions are usually nonspecific when caused by a period of diarrhea, incompetence of the anal sphincter, or deformation of the anal canal. However, in more extended lesions or in delayed wound healing, tuberculosis and herpes simplex infection have to be excluded. The latter infection is especially frequent in patients with positive HIV serology.

Patients from the Mediteranian area and Japan may present with Behçet's disease, a symptom of which is painful aphthous ulceration. The etiology is thought to be immune vasculitis which can be demonstrated by immunohistological tests [21].

Primary syphilitic ulceration or anal fissure can be localized allround the anus as in Crohn's disease. However, these are usually painful. If untreated they develop into deep indurated ulcers which have the appearance of a necrotic carcinoma. Diagnosis is made by the demonstration of *Treponema pallidum* in darf-field microscopy of a sample of serous exudate taken from the base of this lesion. As already mentioned, all these diagnostic steps are unnecessary if Crohn's disease has already been confirmed.

The risk of confusing Crohn's disease with cancer is small. Anal carcinoma can take the form of a swollen skin tag with a cartilaginous consistency on digital examination. If there is any suspicion of malignancy or the carcinoma is to be classified, a biopsy is mandatory. In very rare cases carcinoma can arise in a long-standing Crohn's fistula (see "Natural History").

If Crohn's disease has already been diagnosed, the differentiation has only to be made between "related to" and "incidental." If there are no changes in therapy as a result of this classification, it is only of academic interest. Skin tags in Crohn's disease are lymphedematous, corrugated perianal skin folds which slacken as soon as active inflammation disappears. When they cause hygiene problems after defecation, resection should be considered. However, it is a good idea to wait until active intestinal inflammation has resolved, then it is of no importance whether these skin tags are due to Crohn's disease or not. Erosions of perianal skin and abscesses have to be treated in the same manner whether or not they are specific, but this decision has more importance in hemorrhoids, fistulas, and fissures. Although internal hemorrhoids are common in the average patient, they are fortunately rare in Crohn's disease because active treatment often gives rise to complications (see below). Fistulas originating from the dentate line may be treated as unspecific fistulas in quiescent disease. However, they should always be considered to be Crohn's fistulas when they arise higher up in the gastrointestinal tract.

Diagnostic Procedure

The diagnosis of Crohn's disease is sometimes not very easy to confirm. Several facts, including the natural history of the disease, symptoms, radiological or endoscopic features, and histological findings must be considered together. One more aspect in this puzzle is the presence of the typical perianal lesions described above (Table 13.1). Therefore, if diagnosis is still uncertain, histological examination of all resected skin specimens should be made.

However, in a patient with an established diagnosis, special pathology is not necessary.

In connection with anorectal manifestations, the distribution and activity of intestinal Crohn's disease is of interest,especially if surgical intervention is planned. The physical signs should not be overlooked. Pain, diarrhea, sporadic bleeding, and reduced general health indicate that perianal disease might be of secondary interest, except when an abscess has to be opened. Diagnostic procedures consist of either X-ray examination using barium meal for the upper intestine or a double-contrast enema for colitis. Alternatively, for the exploration of the esophagus, stomach, duodenum, colon, and terminal ileum the endoscope should be used. In quiescent intestinal disease, a careful digital examination and anoscopy conclude the necessary explorations. Preoperative fistulography prevents an intraoperative surprise. It is particularly important to mark the anal canal with a probe, and the fistula opening and anal margin with a small piece of lead to be able to interprete the X-ray correctly.

Treatment

Four possibilities exist to deal with anorectal Crohn's disease:

- Wait and observe the natural course of the lesion
- Treatment of the concomitant intestinal manifestation
- Conservative treatment concentrated on the perianal disease
- Minor or extended local surgery

These four alternatives have to be considered carefully because in each individual patient the optimal combination is necessary for the best treatment. Hughes and Jones [12] strongly advocate a classification of perianal lesions in Crohn's disease into three categories:

- Primary lesions which are strongly related to the pathological processes in the gastrointestinal tract: anal fissures, ulcerated edematous skin tags, and cavitating ulcers (in the anal canal).
- Secondary lesions which follow the primary, such as subcutaneous fistula, skin tags, anal strictures, deep perianal abscess/fistula, are responsible for most of the morbidity.
- Incidential lesions are unrelated to the inflammatory bowel disease and occasionally occur in patients with Crohn's disease: hemorrhoids, perianal abscess/fistula, skin tags, cryptitis.

Hughes et al. [12] stress that there is no way to treat primary lesions locally, however, that secondary lesions might be dealt with successfully by local surgery.

Natural History

The most frequent anal lesions in Crohn's disease are fistulas and fissures in ano, and their natural history has been studied more carefully. Because an abscess is almost the same as in patients without inflammatory bowel disease, the minimal pain experienced often delays the patient's consultation with a physician, and he or she may unfortunately be tempted to play down the complaint. It is not infrequent that in the end a huge suppuration in both buttocks is present while the patient still tolerates the situation.

A fistula may be the result of a deroofed abscess or it can occur spontaneously. Apart from a fistula in an otherwise healthy person, an asymptomatic fistula or one with only few symptoms should often be left alone. These findings are based on a 10-year follow-up study of a series of 61 patients of whom 21 presented with a fistula [5]. A spontaneous cure was observed in eight, and in six healing was achieved after deroofing of the fistulous tract. In one cases the operative treatment failed, while five patients developed a new fistula within the 10-year interval [5]. There is small risk of developing a malignant process in perianal fistulas, as reported in a few cases [4]. The common feature in these cases is the presence of a fistula for more than 10 years with a marked change in the symptoms – there is increased tenderness or the discharge is suddenly stained with blood. Compared with the frequency of 25%–45% anal fistulas in anorectal Crohn's disease, malignant changes can be judged as a very rare complication.

A fissure in ano is even less symptomatic and frequently overlooked. However, during a careful proctological examination fissures can be detected in about 70% of patients with Crohn's disease. After a 10-year interval healing was observed in 17 of 54 patients with Crohn's fissure [5], 27 had progressed to an induration of the anal canal or stenosis without an active fissure. Only ten patients presented wit an active fissure after 10 years.

Treatment of Intestinal Inflammation

Some anorectal manifestations of Crohn's disease seem to be closely related to the degree of intestinal inflammation. However, only skin tags show a statistically significant relationship which correlates with albumin and osoromucoid serum concentration indicating activity of the enteritis [9]. In addition, increased proctitis is followed by a reduced rectal capacity [6], and the importance of quiescent intestinal disease for successful anal surgery is stressed in many publications (see "Surgery" below). In this respect, a conservative therapy with 5-aminosalicylate, steroids, and, in severe inflammation, bedrest and parenteral nutrition creates optimal conditions for healing of anorectal lesions.

However, resolution of perianal Crohn's disease has only been noted after proximal resection of a diseased bowel if this is curative and no recurrence occurs [23]. Proctectomy for anorectal lesions is indicated only in about 4%–5% of all proctectomies in Crohn's disease [4, 11]. A loop ileostomy or colostomy with the same indication is thought to be a temporary solution, but unfortunately reclosure is rarely possible [8].

Medical Treatment

The early results with metronidazole were remarkable [2]; The drug (20 mg/kg bodyweight) was administrated over a period from 3 months to over 1 year. However, with an increased follow-up time recurrences occurred in two-thirds of the patients after medication was discontinued [3]. In half of the patients paraesthesia developed on average after 6½ months. This side effect was dose related and disappeared only sometime after the intake of metronidazole was reduced or discontinued. Unfortunately in many of these cases this step was followed by an increase of symptoms. This is why metronidazole is no longer the wonder drug it was first thought to be in Crohn's disease.

Similar results have been published with 6-mercaptopurine [15]. In a double-blind randomized series, 1.5 mg/kg bodyweight (rounded off to the nearest 50 mg) was given. Complete blood and platelet counts were performed until both were stabel. The Dose was adjusted to maintain the white blood count at 5000 (not below 4500) and the platelet count at not below 100000. Nausea was common in the initial stage of treatment. During periods with fever, rash, upper respiratory infection, or other intercurrent diseases, drug therapy was interrupted.

At 1 year, 72% of the patients treated with 6-mercaptopurine had improved compared with 14% in the placebo group. These results seem to be excellent but are unique in the literature. Metronidazole and 6-mercaptopurine can both occasionally be tried in cases of complex anorectal fistula, but one has to be aware of the side effects and risks associated with their use.

Currently no other conservative treatment is known with a specific local effect. However, 5-aminosalicylate (e. g. sulphasalzine) and/or corticosteroids have been proved beneficial in active ileocolitis or Crohn's colitis and therefore may help in lesions related to intestinal manifestations (fissure in ano, ulcerated edematous skin tags, and cavitating ulcers). In fistulas drug therapy has no effect, and the choice is either surgery or spontaneous healing.

Surgery

For a long time the majority of surgeons emphasized the fact that surgical treatment in anorectal Crohn's disease should play a minor role and that surgery should be concentrated on the drainage of pus collection. This statement is still valid although under certain circumstances the treatment may be more aggressive. It is always good advice for the inexperienced to do as little as needed to relieve pain and leave the more sophisticated therapy to the specialized surgeon in order to avoid postoperative incontinence which in most cases necessitates a definitve stoma. Surgery for anorectal lesions never exacerbates underlying Crohn's disease [22].

The general assumption is that a good postoperative result is obtainable when intestinal disease is quiescent, especially in the absence of active proctitis. Therefore one should wait and have the enteritis under control before anorectal manifestations are dealt with. The only exception is the acute suppuration already mentioned where a simple deroofing of the abscess cavity gives immediate relief of the symptoms. In a stable almost healthy condition of the patient, skin tags, fistulas (including rectovaginal fistula) and strictures can be operated upon following the techniques used in patients without any inflammatory bowel disease.

Abscesses

Anal or perirectal pain is either caused by pus under tension or a deep lesion in the skin or anal ca-

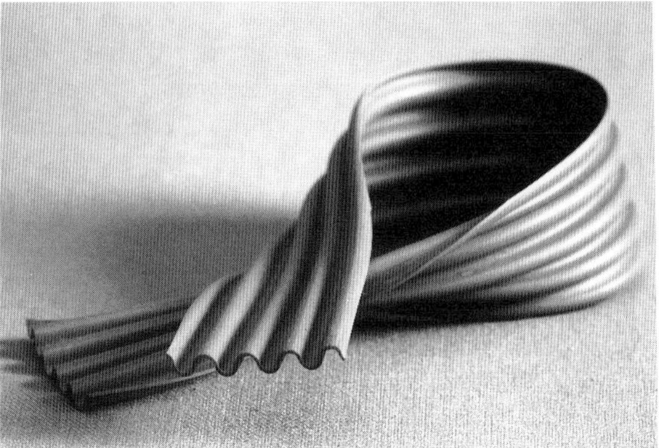

Fig. 13.6. Rubber drain used for extended abscess formations

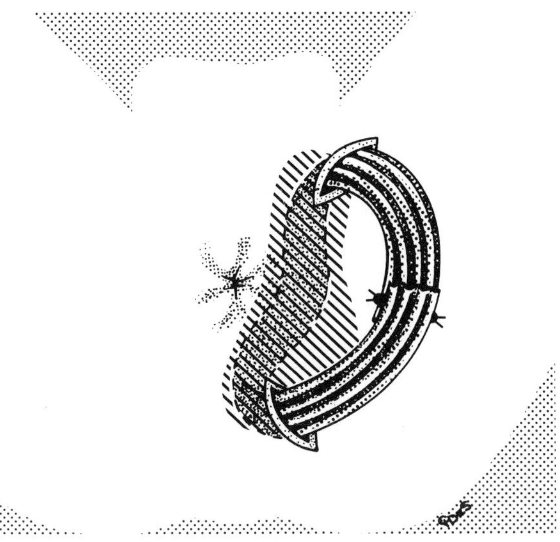

Fig. 13.7. A large abscess is drained by two incisions and a rubber drain, as shown in Fig. 13.6 (the *hatched area* demonstrates the extension of the abscess)

nal. The last two conditions mentioned are related to acute proctitis and in the main, have to be treated conservatively. The perianal abscess, however, needs to be opened. We prefer a very simple technique as in patients without Crohn's disease:

The patient is put into the lithotomy position, usually under general anesthesia. At the point where the abscess seems to be closest to the skin, a round skin fragment about 2 cm in diameter is excised (deroofing). After pus has escaped, a digital exploration of the cavity is performed, the exploration for fistula must be avoided. If the cavity is very much extended, one or two more incisions are made at the extremity of the lesion. Sometimes exploration with forceps simplifies the determination of the extent of the abscess. A corrugated rubber drain (Fig. 13.6) is pulled through the incisions (Fig. 13.7). With the help of a disposable female catheter, irrigations are easy along this drain. It should be replaced with a female catheter when the cavity has decreased and the walls lie on the drain. If the primary fistula tract has closed spontaneously, healing without excessive skin damage is possible. More often a fistula is left behind, possibly with one or two side tracts situated immediately under the skin. Should these fistulas be asymptomatic, they may be left untreated or the fistula operation can be performed in a second step with a much smaller wound (see below).

A horseshoe abscess can be dealt with in the same way. However, if the suppuration continues, caused mostly by a large opening in the rectum leading to a constant loss of bowel contents into the abscess cavity, a diverting colostomy or ileostomy has to be established. The severity of the condition is mirrored by the fact that, in order to control perianal abscesses and fistulas, only two out of ten stomata made could be closed [8].

Fistulas

There is disagreement about the role of surgery in the treatment of anal fistulas. Some authors follow a conservative protocol and operate only when the fistulas cause pain or a lot of discharge [4, 23]. Others advocate laying open all fistulas originating from the dentate line [17]. A possibly prolonged healing time has to be taken into account when deciding whether an operation should be done or not [1]. In addition, the tendency to spontaneous closure of a fistula is obvious (see "Natural History"). On the other hand, in quiescent intestinal disease, laying open a simple transphincteric or subcutaneous fistula carries little risk. The recommendation, therefore, is to operate if the patient is inconvenienced by the fistula and if moderate or severe proctitis is absent. The surgical procedure follows the guidelines for any uncomplicated fistula (see Chap. 11). In patients with proctitis and pain as a result of the fistula, fistulography usually demonstrates a stenosis in the fistular tract together with a prestenotic cavity. There is an alternative procedure to fistulotomy if the fistula originates from the rectum, is very complex, or the bowel inflammation is too active for radical surgery. In order to release the pus and help the fistula to become smooth walled and obstruction free a resection of the tissue distal to the stenosis is performed as indicated in

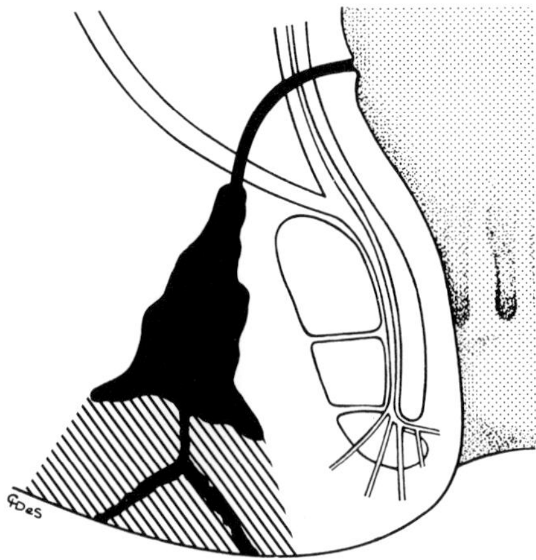

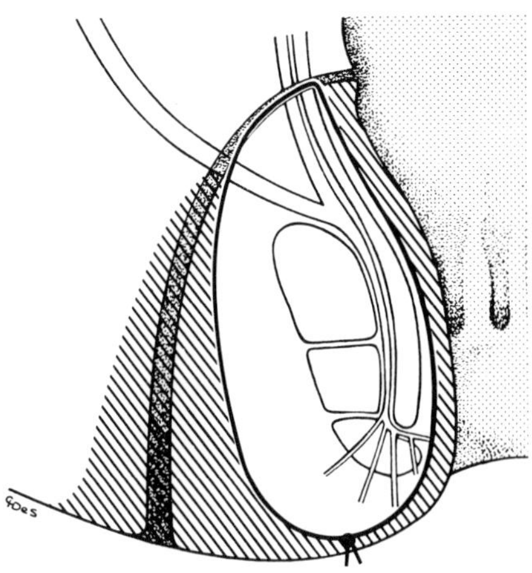

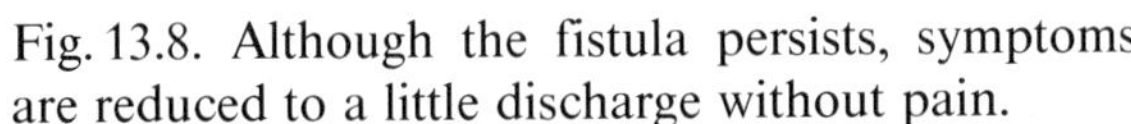

Fig. 13.8. An extrasphincteric fistula is very painful due to the abscess caused by stenoses in the fistular tract. Palliative therapy is by excision of the *hatched area* leading to an asymptomatic fistula

Fig. 13.9. An extrasphincteric fistula is treated by excision of the infralevatoric portion of the tract, the mucous membrane, and skin layer from the inner opening to the external wound *(hatched area)*. A seton (monofilament synthetic suture) is knotted tightly avoiding any traction

Fig. 13.8. Although the fistula persists, symptoms are reduced to a little discharge without pain.

Another possibility, especially in extrasphincteric fistula without proctitis, is the use of a seton. The mucous membrane is taken off in a small strip from the internal opening of the fistula down to the anal margin, and the external part is excised up to the levator ani muscle. A nonabsorbable monofilament thread is brought through the fistula into the rectum and out agian transanally. It is tightly knotted externally so that the thread lies on the muscle but does not cause traction (Fig. 13.9). The mucous membrane will grow over the thread and thus close the inner opening of the fistula. As soon as epithelialization is complete and the thread is pulled out, healing of the external wound occurs spontaneously.

As already mentioned under "Abscesses," the construction of a diverting colostomy or ileostomy is the ultimate solution. Nevertheless, it might be indicated in a complex fistular system with multiple inner openings, troublesome pain, and discharge. The site of the stoma has to be chosen very carefully so as not to use an actively inflammed part of the bowel. A loop ileostomy should be constructed if there is any suspicion of the presence of colitis. Before closure of the stoma, anal continence should be checked by filling the distal limb of the loop with semisolid material.

Rectovaginal fistulas never close spontaneously because the epithelia of the bowel and the vagina come into contact preventing a spontaneous cure. Depending on the position and size of the connec-

tion, symptoms range from a litte suppuration to a huge discharge of stool or air through the vagina. In addition, the consistency of the stool plays an important role as liquid or semisolid stools may cause disabling incontinence through the vagina, whereas in the same patients symptoms are quite tolerable with a formed stool. Last but not least, the attitudes of the patient and her partner to this problem are of great importance. Women with a large rectovaginal fistula may have normal intercourse and even normal deliveries without any complications. On the other hand, girls are often so embarrassed that they do not dare to form a close relationship with a man because they are afraid of rejection. Beside the regulation of the defecation with constipating drugs, important support comes from repeated talks with the patient to help her deal with the problem. Surgical correction is only possible if intestinal disease is absolutely quiescent. A diverting colostomy is not mandatory, and the technique depends on the site and extent of the fistula. Surgical techniques are no different from the closure of a rectovaginal fistula in patients without inflammatory bowel disease (see Chap. 16).

Stricture

Symptoms from anal strictures are often suprisingly minimal especially when the motion is semisolid. An anal stretch in the manner of a Lord's procedure or even only with four fingers is dangerous and leads to incontinence. The best therapy comprises gentle dilatation with a dilator, initially under anesthesia, and then bougienage twice or three times daily with the aim of keeping the anal canal open to accomodate the index or at least the small finger. Bougienage has to be continued for some months with decreasing frequency, and the intensity needed has to be judged by regular consultation.

Incontinence

The symptoms of incontinence have to be differentiated from discharge caused by a fistula or from the vagina. Etiologically one can distinguish three groups:

- Diarrhea
- Urgency
- An impaired function of the pelvic floor and sphincter muscles

Diarrhea alone rarely causes incontinence but, in addition to some induration in the anal canal or impairment in sphincter function, the patient might be unable to control motions. With constipating drugs continence can often be regained. Urgency (the need to go to the toilet as soon as the urge of defecation is signalized) may give rise, in its severe from, to uncontrolled evacuation. In a study of 39 patients with Crohn's disease and 20 normal controls, no correlation between urgency and the following parameters was found: basal anal sphincter pressure, squeeze pressure, rectal capacity, and the degree of proctitis on sigmoidoscopy. However, it was found that in some patients with Crohn's colitis, colectomy and ileorectal anastomosis were able to prevent urgency, even when associated with incontinence [7]. Reduced rectal capacity, inversely related to the degree of proctitis, is not a major reason for incontinence as has been shown in a study on the relationship of proctitis and rectal capacity [6]. Surgical intervention can be considered in cases of descending perineum syndrome and sphincter-related incontinence. The same conditions as already mentioned for the closure of a rectovaginal fistula have to be applied for any local reconstructive surgery of the anus. In absolutely quiescent disease a sphincter repair to correct an, in most instances iatrogenic, sphincter lesion can give good results, the technique is described in Chap. 20. In some patients postanal repair to lift the pelvic floor in the case of an incidental descending perineum has been performed successfully. Should the procedure fail, the condition of the patient might be worse than before the operation. Therefore a careful preoperative evaluation is mandatory. Unfortunately, in many cases only a diverting stoma is of help because the anal canal is destroyed by ulceration and induration, and local surgery does not give satisfactory results.

Skin Tags

Swollen skin tags indicating active Crohn's disease of the lower rectum and anal canal are not suitable for surgery. However, if in quiescent disease these skin folds interfere with hygiene in this region, a local excision can be performed, preferably with a primary closure of the wound by a continuous catgut suture.

Hemorrhoids

A complete review of the possible treatments for hemorrhoids is given in Chap. 9. With regard to Crohn's disease, we have to remember that in active proctitis the alteration of the mucous membrane gives rise to rectal bleeding and thickening of the wall. With stiffness of the upper anal canal, swelling of the hemorrhoidal cushions is prevented. If the active inflammation is located more proximally, incidental symptomatic hemorrhoids are possible. However, it seems to be a rare condition.

The therapy of symptomatic hemorrhoids should be concentrated on conservative treatment avoiding everything which could cause ulceration (for example, rubber band ligation or injection treatment). It has been demonstrated that, especially after hemorrhoidectomy, fistulas frequently occur which can only be dealt with by proctectomy [14].

References

1. Baker WNW, Milton GJ (1974) Mangement of fistulae in Crohn's disease. Proc R Soc Med 67: 58
2. Bernstein LH, Frank NS, Brandt LJ, Boley SJ (1980) Healing of perianal Crohn's diseases with metronidazole. Gastroenterology 79: 357–365
3. Brandt LJ, Bernstein LH, Boley SJ, Frank NS (1982) Metronidazole therapy for perineal Crohn's diseases: a follow-up study. Gastroenterology 82: 383–387
4. Buchmann P, Alexander-Williams J (1980) Classification of perianal Crohn's diseases. Clin Gastroenterol 9: 323–330
5. Buchmann P, Keighley MRB, Allan RN, Thompson H, Alexander-Williams J (1980) Natural history of perianal Crohn's diseases. Ten year follow-up: a plea for conservatism. Am J Surg 140: 642–644
6. Buchmann P, Mogg GAG, Alexander-Williams J, Allan RN, Keighley MRB (1980) Relationship of proctitis and rectal capacity in Crohn's disease. Gut 21: 137–140

7. Buchmann P, Kolb E, Alexander-Williams J (1981) Pathogenesis of urgency in defaecation in Crohn's disease. Digestion 22: 310–316

8. Buchmann P, Weterman IT (1981) Der perianale Morbus Crohn. Colo-Proctology 3: 77–81

9. Fielding JF (1972) Perianal lesions in Crohn's disease. J R Coll Surg Edinb 17: 32–37

10. Hanauer SB, Kraft SC (1983) Immunology of Crohn's disease. In: Allan RN, Keighley MRB, Alexander-Williams J, Hawkins C (eds) Inflammatory bowel diseases. Churchill Livingstone, Edinburgh, pp 356–371

11. Homan WP, Tang C, Thorgjarnarson B (1976) Anal lesions complicating Crohn's disease. Arch Surg 11: 1333–1335

12. Hughes LE, Jones KRG (1983) Peri-anal lesions in Crohn's disease. In: Allan RN, Keighley MRB, Alexander-Williams J, Hawkins C (eds) Inflammatory bowel diseases. Churchill Livingstone, Edinburgh, pp 321–331

13. Jaeger K, Stelzner F (1980) Colitis ulcerosa und Enteritis granulomatosa. Das Schicksal von 494 Kranken nach 2–22 Jahren. Dtsch Med Wochenschr 105: 49–54

14. Jeffrey PJ, Ritchie JK, Parks AG (1977) Treatment of hemorrhoids in patients with inflammatory bowel disease. Lancet i: 1084–1085

15. Korelitz BK (1981) Successful treatment of Crohn's disease with an immunosuppressive drug (6-Mercaptopurine). In: Peña AS, Weterman IT, Booth CC, Strober W (eds) Recent advances in Crohn's disease. Martinus Nijhoff, The Hague, pp 478–485

16. Lennard-Jones JC, Ritchie JK, Zohrab WJ (1976) Proctocolitis and Crohn's disease of the colon. A comparison of the clinical course. Gut 17: 477–482

17. Marks CG, Ritchie JK, Lockhart-Mummery HE (1981) Analfistulas in Crohn's disease. Br J Surg 68: 525–527

18. Mayberry JF, Rhodes J (1984) Epidemiological aspects of Crohn's disease: a review of the literature. Gut 25: 886–899

19. Parks AG, Morson BC (1962) The pathogenesis of fistulae in ano. Proc R Soc Med 55: 751–754

20. Puntis J, McNeish AS, Allan RN (1984) Long term prognosis of Crohn's disease with onset in childhood and adolescence. Gut 25: 329–336

21. Rufli T (1988) Dermatologie des Anus und der Perianalregion. In: Buchmann P (ed) Lehrbuch der Proktologie, 2nd edn. Huber, Bern, pp 119–159

22. Sohn N, Korelitz BK, Weinstein MA (1980) Anorectal Crohn's disease: definitive surgery for fistulas and recurrent abscesses. Am J Surg 139: 394–397

23. Wolff BG, Culp CE, Beart RW, Ilstrup DM, Ready RL (1985) Anorectal Crohn's disease. A long-term perspective. Dis Colon Rectum 28: 709–711

14 Ulcerative Colitis

H. Wehrli and A. Akovbiantz

Definition

Ulcerative colitis is a usually chronic inflammatory disease of the colon of largely unknown etiology [48, 60]. It was first described by Samual Wilkes of London in 1859 [19]. Ulcerative colitis, unlike Crohn's disease, is generally limited to the mucosa and submucosa of the colon [96] except in cases where the disease takes an acute, fulminating, toxic course. Inflammation of the terminal ileum ("backwash ileitis") is seen only when the disease process involves the entire colon. Ulcerative colitis begins distally and may spread proximally and continuously throughout the large bowel. The rectum is involved in 98% of cases [88]. The disease may have its onset at any age but most commonly appears in the 2nd–4th decades [21]. Childhood onset of ulcerative colitis, seen in 25% of cases [20], implies a very poor prognosis [96].

Symptoms

The cardinal symptoms of chronic ulcerative colitis are rectal bleeding and diarrhea. The latter may be profuse, consisting of up to 20 or 30 mucoid bloody stools per day [21, 48, 96, 100]. Systemic disease symptoms are frequently combined with abdominal pain. Systemic complications of ulcerative colitis involving the eye (episcleritis, uveitis), oral mucosa (aphthosis), skin (erythema nodosum, pyoderma), liver (pericholangitis, fatty liver, cirrhosis, etc.), joints (sacroiliitis, arthritis of the knee or ankle, ankylosing spondylitis), kidney (urolithiasis), and growth disturbances in juveniles are observed in up to 50% of cases [16, 20, 48, 53, 66, 96, 100] (Table 14.1). The acute, fulminating form of ulcerative colitis (toxic megacolon) is a very severe, often life-threatening condition that requires immediate, intensive medical care and may necessitate urgent surgical intervention (see "Chronic Active Colitis" and "Acute Complications" below).

Table 14.1. Symptoms of ulcerative colitis (Data from [16, 34, 48, 53, 63, 66, 91, 100])

Mild, subacute-chronic course

Cardinal symptoms:		Bloody mucoid diarrhea
Systemic symptoms:		Weakness, fatigue (anemia), fever, weight loss, abdominal pain.
	Children:	growth retardation, malabsorption (vitamin B_{12}, fat)
Extraintestinal manifestations	Skin:	Erythema nodosum (1.7%–10%) Pyoderma gangrenosum (rare)
	Mouth:	Aphthous stomatitis (common)
	Eyes:	Episcleritis Uveitis Conjunctivitis } 1.1%–12%
	liver:	Fatty liver 40%–55% Pericholangitis 30% Cirrhosis 2%–5% Sclerosing cholangitis 1% Bile duct carcinoma 1%
	Joints:	Arthritis 5%–12% Sacroileitis 18% Ankylosing spondylitis 2.1%–6%
	Kidneys:	Nephrolithiasis 2%–6%

Acute fulminating course (toxic megacolon)

Cardiopulmonary:	Tachycardia, tachypnea, hypotension, shock
Abdomen:	Distension, pneumoperitoneum, peritonitis (may be absent in patients on steroids), bloody diarrhea
Kidneys:	Oliguria or anuria
Sepsis:	Febrile state, chills
Sensory changes:	Confusion, apathy

Etiology and Pathogenesis

The etiology of ulcerative colitis remains poorly understood even after a century of experience with the disease [16, 34, 48, 84, 96, 100]. A great many theories on etiology have been advanced, but it does not appear that bacterial or viral agents (dysenteric bacteria, diplococci, rotaviruses, etc.) [12, 16, 72], food allergies [48, 100], mucolytic enzymes [44, 48,

100], or psychosomatic factors [48, 100] can be held solely accountable for the disease. Genetic factors appear to be significant in many cases. A familial incidence with a 10%–29.4% likelihood of acquiring the disease [16, 56, 60, 96] has been described, and the disease has appeared concurrently in monozygotic twins [62]. The incidence of ulcerative colitis is highest in the Jewish and white population of Europe and the United States, but its possible mode of inheritance remains unclear [48, 56]. Ulcerative colitis is rare among blacks, Indians, Asians, and Latin Americans [34].

It is likely that immunopathologic discoveries will contribute most to elucidating the etiology of ulcerative colitis, and it appears that the pathogenesis of the disease is multifactorial [80].

Classification of Ulcerative Colitis

Ulcerative colitis can be classified by the extent (severity) of disease or by its clinical course (Table 14.2).

Table 14.2. Classification of ulcerative colitis

Extent of disease:	Proctitis, proctosigmoiditis
	Left-sided colitis
	Pancolitis
Clinical course:	Single attack
	Chronic active disease
	Chronic recurring disease
	Acute fulminating disease

Extent of Disease

Proctitis and Proctosigmoiditis

The rectum is almost always involved in ulcerative colitis, with solitary rectal involvement representing a mild form with favorable prognosis [85]. The stool contains blood and mucus, but severe diarrhea is rare. In 5%–15% of cases the inflammation spreads proximally to involve the colon. Once the colon is affected, the colitis remains confined to the rectosigmoid in only 10%–40% of patients [48].

Left-Sided Colitis

Left-sided colitis is a common pattern in which the disease process is distal to the splenic flexure [47]. However, any attack can incite proximal extension to the transverse colon [48].

Pancolitis

Pancolitis is the most extensive and severe form of ulcerative colitis. Not infrequently the disease has an acute, fulminating onset or produces initial symptoms in childhood [48]. Patients with pancolitis have frequent, usually bloody stools as their predominant symptom [47].

Clinical Course

The onset of ulcerative colitis may be insidious or acute and fulminating. The cardinal symptom is always a mucoid bloody stool or diarrhea.

Single Attack

A single attack of ulcerative colitis followed by complete recovery is unusual (4%–10% [16, 88]). Retrospective analysis shows that most of these cases represent a bacterial dysentery (salmonella, shigella, campylobacter, yersinia) rather than true ulcerative colitis [59].

Chronic Active Colitis

Of the patients with ulcerative colitis, 5%–15% have a chronically active form which is as uncommon as the single attack [16]. Remissions are not achieved with conservative therapy. All grades of severity can occur, but the complication rate (fibrosis, stricture, cancer risk) is significantly higher than in the chronic recurring form, as is the mortality (25% versus 14% [42]) and the rate of operative treatment (82.8% versus 28.2% [42]).

Chronic Recurring Colitis

Chronic recurring ulcerative colitis is the most common form of the disease, accounting for 60%–75% of cases according to Truelove [96]. Mild acute flareups last for several weeks and are followed by periods of remission [48]. Severe attacks with toxemia and anemia may culminate in a complete or partial remission with persistent rectoscopic findings or may convert to an acute, fulminating form.

Acute Fulminating Colitis

Acute fulminating ulcerative colitis is the most severe form of the disease and is frequently life threatening. It is associated with a septic-toxic state and profuse, bloody diarrhea. It affects 5%–15% of colitis patients [2, 86] and is more prevalent in younger individuals [67]. It may represent an initial manifestation, an exacerbation, or a recurrence of the disease.

Usually the entire colon is involved. Complications such as toxic dilatation (50%) or perforation (30%) are frequent [48]. Mortality is high (5.3%–60% [2, 16, 48, 67]) but has declined significantly in recent years as a result of emergency colectomy and intensive medical care.

Epidemiology

Ulcerative colitis has a worldwide distribution although its prevalence and incidence vary greatly [96]. In contrast to Crohn's disease, the incidence of ulcerative colitis appears to have fallen slightly in recent years [27]. Highest case numbers are reported in the United States, Canada, Great Britain, and northern Europe, where the incidence ranges from 5 to 15 per 100000 population per year, and the prevalence from 40 to 225 per 100000 [16, 56, 92]. All age groups are affected, although the peak incidence is between 20 and 40 years [48, 92]. Reports on sex distribution vary [16, 48, 60, 92]. Familial and racial aspects of epidemiology are discussed under "Etiology and Pathogenesis".

Differential Diagnosis

The differential diagnosis of ulcerative colitis can be difficult, especially when dealing with a mild, initial attack [35, 93] where there may be no endoscopic evidence of colonic ulceration.

Even with histologic evaluation, 10%–15% of ulcerative colitides fall initially into the "nonclassifiable" category [28]. It is helpful for the clinician to differentiate between predominantly hemorrhagic and predominantly nonhemorrhagic forms of colitis [35]. This classification is employed in Table 14.3, which lists the diseases under each heading that should be considered for patients with suspected ulcerative colitis. Often the course is helpful in making a diagnosis, since infective and drug-induced colitides tend to clear rapidly. Early rectoscopy is justified in doubtful cases. Therapeutically, it is important to consider amebiasis, Crohn's disease, pseudomembranous enterocolitis, and venereal proctologic diseases to avoid the consequences of inappropriate therapy [35].

Table 14.3. Differential diagnosis of ulcerative colitis. (Data from [16, 28, 35, 93, 96])

Predominantly hemorrhagic forms

Infectious colitides:	Salmonellosis, shigellosis, campylobacter colitis, amebiasis, schistosomiasis, gonorrhea
Iatrogenic colitides:	Laxatives, salicylate suppositories, pseudomembranous enterocolitis, radiation colitis, colitis in a defunctionalized colon segment

Ischemic colitis
Pneumatosis cystoides intestinalis
Familial colonic polyposis
Diverticulotic bleeding
Hemorrhoids

Predominantly nonhemorrhagic forms
Crohn's disease
Irritable colon
Tuberculosis
Yersiniosis
Simple rectal ulcer
Actinomycosis
Venereal diseases (lymphogranuloma venereum, herpex simplex type II, syphilis, chlamydia)

Diagnosis of Ulcerative Colitis

The mainstay in the diagnosis of ulcerative colitis is proctosigmoidoscopy with the histologic examination of biopsy specimens. This will establish whether mild, moderate, or severe disease is present. A precise histologic diagnosis is assured only if multiple (six to eight) biopsy specimens of sufficient size are taken from various sites [70, 83]. The grading of dysplasia [71] by the pathologist at this stage often plays a critical role in selecting cases for surgical treatment [40]. Colonoscopy is an important means of follow-up and surveillance for carcinoma [65], but it is not always necessary for the diagnosis of ulcerative colitis since the rectosigmoid is almost always involved [16, 83, 96].

The clinical examination is of major importance for determining the patient's general condition, evaluating abdominal pain, and identifying any extraintestinal manifestations of the disease. Laboratory studies complete the diagnostic workup (Table 14.4). Microbiologic stool examinations are helpful for excluding bacterial dysentery [96]. Radiographic examination is of limited importance in patients with ulcerative colitis. The plain abdominal film can exclude toxic megacolon in cases that take a fulminating course [16, 48]. The double-contrast colon examination provides information about the severity and extent of the disease but is contraindi-

Table 14.4. Diagnosis of ulcerative colitis

Necessary	Desirable	Unnecessary
Proctosigmoidos-copy	Colonoscopy	Colon double-contrast enema
Biopsy (histology)		
Clinical examination	Abdomen plain film	
Blood examination (ESR, Hb, Lc, Quick's test, Tc, glucose, urea, creatinine, protein, liver values)	Bacteriologic stool examination	Anal manometry
		Selective mesenteric angiography

ESR, erythocyte sedimentation rate; Hb, hemoglobin; Lc, leukocytes; Tc, thrombocytes.

cated in acute fulminating cases. The colon contrast study is inferior to colonoscopy as a surveillance method for the early detection of dysplasia and carcinoma [16]. Anal manometry is occasionally useful as a final preoperative study, especially when an ileoanal anastomosis is proposed [8].

Pathoanatomic Features of Ulcerative Colitis

The lesions of ulcerative colitis are generally confined to the colonic mucosa [9] so that the colon, when viewed externally, appears grossly normal [96]. Transmural changes are seen only in toxic megacolon with crypt abscesses leading to disruption of the muscular layer and serosa [16]. The edematous, granulated, hypoglandular mucosa bleeds easily and forms ulcers. In the late phase the mucosa consists entirely of pseudopolypoid mucosal islands, and segmental strictures appear. Lieberkühn's crypts become obstructed with feces and mucus, leading to abscess formation. Histologically there is eosinophilic infiltration and hypervascularization of the mucosa with increased lymphocytes and plasma cells in the lamina propria. Carcinomatous change is frequently multifocal and occurs less frequently in the polypous mucosa than in the atrophic mucosa. Mucus-producing and undifferentiated tumors are the most common forms and at one time accounted for the dismal prognosis of carcinoma in colitis [16, 43, 69, 78]. Today this is no longer necessarily true owing to improvements in follow-up care [33].

Medical Treatment of Ulcerative Colitis

Principles

Except in patients with severe acute complications (toxic megacolon, perforation, severe hemorrhage), the primary treatment of ulcerative colitis is medical, and success rates are high. However, the risk of cancer increases with the duration of the disease to 7.5%–12.6% after 20 years and 11%–41.8% after 25 years [50, 61, 89]. Risk of future cancer is the major reason why 50% of patients with ulcerative colitis will require surgical treatment at some point in the course of their disease [88].

Available Therapies

Acute attacks are treated with corticosteroids, salazosulfapyridine, or more recently with 5-aminosalicylic acid (5-ASA). The latter two drugs are continued as maintenance therapy once remission has been achieved (Table 14.5).

Corticosteroids

Corticosteroids are administered systemically, topically (by enema), or by both routes. The initial dose is 40–60 mg prednisone daily, given in a single oral dose to reduce steroid side effects [16]. This regimen is continued for 4–6 weeks, depending on clinical response, while reducing the dose to 10–20 mg per day. Most patients show clinical improvement within 7–10 days [96]. Steroids should not be used as prophylaxis against recurrence [26]. Steroids do not increase rates of postoperative morbidity or mortality [3]. In 1956 Truelove introduced topical steroid application into the treatment of distal ulcerative

Table 14.5. Medical treatment of ulcerative colitis

Course		Mild	Severe
Corticoste-roids:	Prednisone	40–60 mg/day	60–100 mg/day
	Betamethasone (enema)	5 mg/day	5 mg/day
Salazosulfapyridine		2–4 g/day	6–8 g/day
		(0.75 g/day for maintenance)	
5-Aminosalicylic acid		1.5 g/day	1.5 g/day
		(0.75 g/day for maintenance)	
Azathioprine		2.5 mg/kg per day	

colitis [48]. Use of the appropriate topical steroid (betamethasone phosphate [6]) can induce remission in 75% of patients with virtually no endocrine side effects [6, 51].

Salazosulfapyridine

Salazosulfapyridine is less effective than steroids in treating acute attacks of colitis, but the combination of both is very beneficial [16, 96]. The daily dose in acute attacks is 2–4 g per day [16, 26, 48], with larger doses causing side effects such as nausea, allergic response, leukopenia, and anemia [26]. As these side effects are referrable to the sulfapyridine component of the drug, the active component, 5-ASA, has been isolated and administered orally as well as topically [36]. 5-ASA causes markedly fewer side effects and is as effective as salazosulfapyridine when given orally or by enema [36]. Several preliminary studies demonstrate the efficacy of 5-ASA even in patients who do not benefit from conventional therapy [13, 25, 36]. The oral dose is 3×0.5 g daily for 6–24 weeks [36, 54]. The recommended rectal dose ranges from 0.7 to 4 g per day [54].

The agents of choice for long-term maintenance therapy are salazosulfapyridine (2–3 g/day [16, 26, 48, 96]) and 5-ASA (3×0.25 g/day [13, 54]). Views differ regarding the duration of the prophylaxis, with reports ranging from 1 year to lifelong maintenance of remission [26]. The remission rate is 50%–87% [13, 36, 54].

Azathioprine

Several immunosuppressive drugs, most notably azathioprine, have been employed in the treatment of ulcerative colitis. Their efficacy is controversial [48], their side effects are severe (bone marrow depression, sepsis), and their use is justified only after all other therapeutic modalities have failed [16, 48, 96]. Even surgical treatment should be considered before azathioprine is tried [26]. Azathioprine is not indicated for the maintenance of remission [16].

Miscellaneous Therapies

The antiasthmatic compound *disodium cromoglycate* is frequently recommended, but its efficacy in the treatment of ulcerative colitis remains to be proved [16, 96]. *Metronidazol* has been used unsuccessfully in combination with steroids [17]. *Dietary measures* other than the elimination of milk are of no significant benefit [48]. The value of *parenteral nutrition* in ulcerative colitis is a subject of consider-

able dispute [18, 48, 55, 58]. It does not appear to alter the prognosis of the disease. Of course, there is a very strong rationale for instituting intravenous electrolyte and protein replacement in patients who are severely ill.

Medical Treatment in Pregnancy

The medical treatment of pregnant patients with ulcerative colitis may be continued with salazosulfapyridine and corticosteroids [64, 96]. The slightly increased rate of fetal complications is referrable to the colitis itself and not to the medical therapy. Azathioprine is absolutely contraindicated. It should be added that salazosulfapyridine has been found to cause reversible infertility in males [64].

Surgical Treatment of Ulcerative Colitis

The importance of surgery in the treatment of ulcerative colitis is underscored by the fact that colectomy offers patients a definitive cure.

Indications for Surgery

From the surgeon's standpoint there are three overriding indications for the surgical management of ulcerative colitis (Table 14.6):

1. The presence of a major acute complication
2. Lack of response to medical treatment
3. The prevention of colonic cancer

Table 14.6. Indications for surgical treatment of ulcerative colitis

Acute complications (massive hemorrhage, perforation, refractory fulminating colitis, toxic megacolon)
Lack of response to medical therapy with significant discomfort or debilitation
Prevention of future cancer

Consistently good surgical results can be achieved only if high-risk emergency operations are avoided. This requires close cooperation among the internist, endoscopist, surgeon, and pathologist [21, 90, 96].

Acute Complications

Approximately 15% of all patients with ulcerative colitis develop a major complication in the course of their illness constituting a surgical emergency [2].

Hemorrhage, Perforation. From 4.8% to 16% of all emergency operations are performed for massive hemorrhage [2, 37, 60], and 1%–11% for perforation [2, 31, 60]. The procedure of choice for most of these cases is subtotal colectomy with ileostomy, or proctocolectomy [2, 60, 98].

Toxic Megacolon. With a mortality of 20%–60% [37, 60, 67], toxic megacolon is the most dreaded acute complication of ulcerative colitis. It may represent the initial manifestation of the disease. Fortunately, the incidence of toxic megacolon has been declining in recent years [98]. Determining the optimal timing for surgical intervention remains a difficult problem.

Because remission is achieved in 30% of cases with conservative therapy, surgery may be deferred initially, although one must be careful about overlooking a colon perforation in the critically ill patient who is receiving steroids. Severe electrolyte disturbances and metabolic derangements are poor prognostic signs [15]. Absolute indications for surgery in toxic megacolon are listed in Table 14.7.

We reject the Turnbull procedure of loop ileostomy with multiple colostomies [97] for this condition, as it leaves the septic, toxic organ in place (Fig. 14.1). We prefer a subtotal colectomy and end ileostomy, favoring a sigmoid loop fistula over Hartmann's technique of stump closure both for therapeutic (rectal stump irrigation) and prophylactic reasons (stump leak with fistula formation). The rectal stump may be removed later, or in rare cases it may be used to reestablish continuity. Generally we feel that a proctocolectomy is too extensive an operation as concerning the severity of the patient's condition and the urgency of the situation.

Lack of Response to Medical Treatment

Failure of conservative therapy with a debilitating course (intolerance of medication, frequent recurrences despite prophylaxis, local strictures, hemorrhagic anemia) or systemic complications (skin, eye, liver, see "Definition"), the presence of pancolitis or disease of more than 10 years' duration, as well as growth disturbances in children are considered indications for the surgical eradication of disease [21, 26, 39, 48, 61, 96, 98]. Surgery is also indicated in cases where a severe, acute exacerbation cannot be medically controlled within a period of 1–2 weeks [26].

Various surgical options are available (see "Surgical Options" below). Total proctocolectomy with end ileostomy, until recently cited as the standard oper-

Table 14.7. Absolute indications for surgical treatment of toxic megacolon

Free perforation
Confined or impending perforation
Deteriorating clinical status
Lack of response to medical treatment for 2–4 days
Recurrence of toxic megacolon

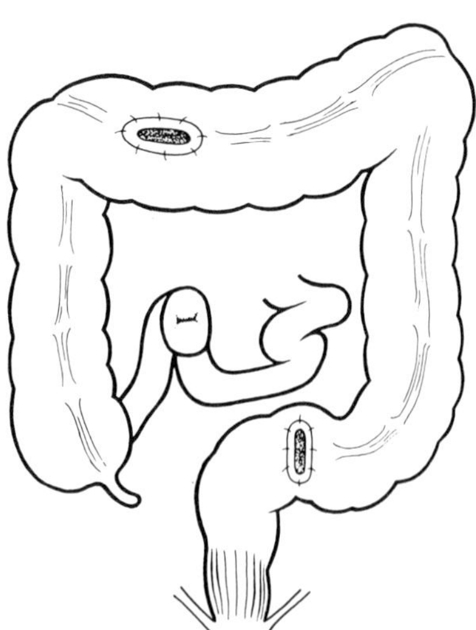

Fig. 14.1. Turnbull operation with multiple enterostomies [48]

ation for ulcerative colitis, has today been abandoned at many centers in favor of a more differentiated approach [1]. While total proctocolectomy can indeed cure the patient, it necessitates the construction of a permanent stoma, which is a major disadvantage when one considers the youth of many ulcerative colitis patients. Some 25% of proctocolectomy patients have been found to experience significant emotional and maintenance-related problems with their stomas [22, 88, 94]. Thus, the preservation of fecal continence is a highly desirable goal [29] and one that can be accomplished through any of several techniques (Table 14.8).

Table 14.8. Continence-saving operations in patients with ulcerative colitis

Ileorectostomy (Aylett)
Total colectomy with mucosal proctectomy and ileoanal anastomosis (Ravitch, Sabiston)
Total colectomy with mucosal proctectomy and ileoanal anastomosis with a fecal reservoir (Parks, Fonkalsrud, Utsonomiya, etc.)
Continent ileostomy (Kock)

Prevention of Colorectal Cancer

The controversial risk of cancer in ulcerative colitis is the main indication for surgical intervention. Of all colitis patients, 20% undergo prophylactic proctocolectomy during the first 10 years of their disease [50]. Factors that influence the risk of carcinoma in ulcerative colitis are listed in Table 14.9 [40, 43, 48–50, 52, 60, 71, 96]. Of patients who develop ulcerative colitis during childhood, 40% die within 20 years [48]. If the colitis remains confined to the rectosigmoid, the cumulative risk of cancer is no higher than in the normal population [49]. However, analysis of site distribution indicates that 50% of all carcinomas in colitis affect the rectum and sigmoid colon [39, 83, 89]. Multifocal carcinomas are observed in 13.5% of cases [40]. Chronic active disease without significant remission and a severe first attack increase the risk of carcinoma [52].

Data on the cumulative risk of cancer are summarized in Table 14.10. While the data on cancer risk vary greatly, it is apparent that the risk of developing cancer is increased by a factor of 10–20 compared with healthy individuals. These figures emphasize the need to maintain regular follow-up for an indefinite period to ensure early cancer detection in the colitis patient (Fig. 14.2). Similar follow-up is necessary following a surgical procedure, such as ileorectostomy, which leaves behind residual rectal mucosa (see "Ileorectostomy" below).

Table 14.9. Risk factors for carcinoma in ulcerative colitis

Childhood onset of disease
Disease present for more than 10 years
Extension of colitis
Repeated demonstration of low-grade epithelial dysplasia
Demonstration of high-grade epithelial dysplasia
Chronic active disease
Severe first attack

Table 14.10. Cumulative risk of cancer in patients with ulcerative colitis

Years after onset of symptoms	10–15 (%)	20–25 (%)	35–40 (%)
Mir-Nadjlessi et al. 1986 [65]	0.8	11.9	28.1
Kieninger in: Gaisberg and Töpfer 1984 [26]	5	42	–
Lennard-Jones 1986 [49]	1.7	7.1	24
De Domball in: Herfarth 1983 [39]	5.0	22	45
Truelove 1984 [96]	1.6	4.5	–
Kewenter et al. 1978 [43]	–	34	–
Morson 1983 [70]	3	24	–

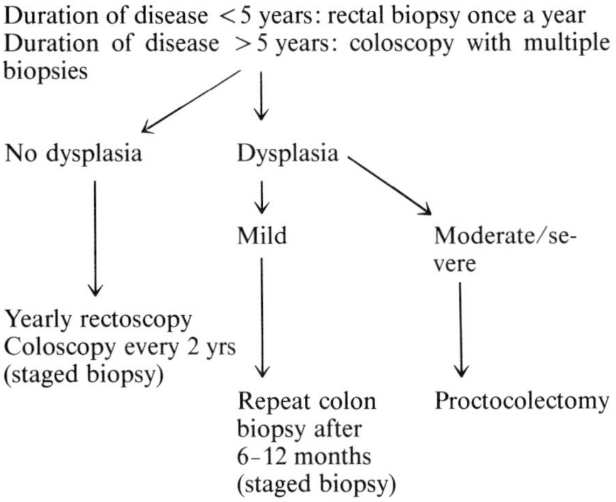

Duration of disease <5 years: rectal biopsy once a year
Duration of disease >5 years: coloscopy with multiple biopsies

No dysplasia — Dysplasia

Dysplasia → Mild — Moderate/severe

No dysplasia → Yearly rectoscopy / Coloscopy every 2 yrs (staged biopsy)

Mild → Repeat colon biopsy after 6–12 months (staged biopsy)

Moderate/severe → Proctocolectomy

Fig. 14.2. Carcinoma surveillance in ulcerative colitis. (Data from [39, 49, 61, 79, 89])

Disregarding Duke's classification, 5-year survival rates of between 18% and 54% are reported in the literature for colitis patients who develop carcinoma [29, 60]. These rates are significantly lower than for carcinoma in patients without colitis.

Surgical Options

Proctocolectomy With Ileostomy

Proctocolectomy with end ileostomy is still considered by some to be the standard operation for the definitive cure of ulcerative colitis [1]. Significant proctitis with bleeding, a shrunken rectum with stricturing, and rare perianal fistulas would contraindicate preservation of the rectum [61]. Proctocolectomy is generally performed as a one-stage elective procedure [88] with an early mortality of 2%–6% [40, 88, 89]. The two-stage emergency procedure (for toxic megacolon) is described in "Acute Complications" above.

Technique. With the patient standing, sitting, or supine, the ileostomy site is identified and marked on the right lower quadrant on the eve of the operation. The patient is placed on the operating table in the Lloyd-Davis position [48], and a bladder catheter is inserted. The abdomen is entered through a lower midline laparotomy, whereupon the ascending, transverse, and descending colon segments are mobilized, and the greater omentum is resected. If the latter shows inflammatory change, the mesocolon is skeletonized close to the colon wall. Dissection and mobilization of the rectum are performed

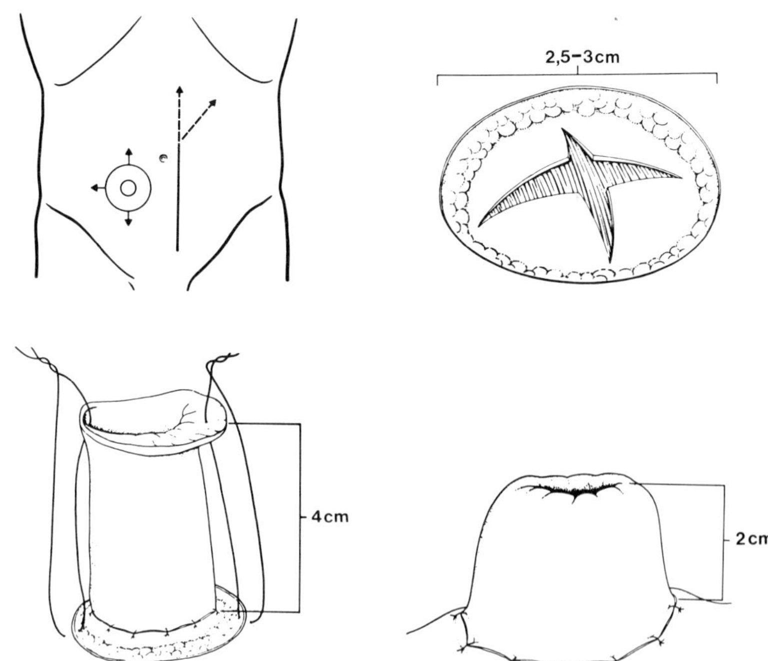

Fig. 14.3. End ileostomy [48]

close to the colon in males to avoid sexual dysfunction. A spindle-shaped incison is made around the anus from the perineal aspect, the anorectum is mobilized, and the specimen is removed. A soft drain is placed into the perineal cavity, and gentamycin-impregnated beads are inserted. The peritoneum of the pelvic floor and the defect in the ileal mesentery are closed.

A skin disc (2–3 cm) is excised over the proposed stoma site in the right lower quadrant, a cruciate incision is made in the anterior rectus layer, a longitudinal incision in the posterior layer and peritoneum, and the terminal ileum is exteriorized. The 5- to 6-cm long stump of ileum is sutured to the peritoneum and to the anterior rectus sheath with Dexon threads. The ileostomy is everted by the Brooke technique to produce a 2- to 3-cm long spout, which is secured with mucocutaneous Dexon sutures (Fig. 14.3).

Complications. The rate of complications following proctocolectomy is 18.8%–37% [10]. Disturbances of perineal wound healing are very common (25%–100%). Intra-abdominal septic and thromboembolitic [10] complications are rare. On the other hand, early or late bowel obstruction is described in 6%–21% of cases. Stoma problems are reported in 6.7%–24% [14, 39, 68] and mostly involve stricture and recession (6%–10% [68]). Revisional surgery is required in 12%–24% of ileostomy complications [14], which is why we cannot overstate the impor-

tance of a carefully constructed ileostomy that is easy for the patient to maintain. Sexual dysfunction develops in 6% of 20- to 30-year-olds and in 31% of patients over 60 [68]. Bauer [7] reports a 3% incidence of male impotence, with 1.3% of his female patients reporting dyspareunia. Female fertility is not impaired, nor is pregnancy affected [96].

Continent Ileostomy

Kock is recognized as the first surgeon able to preserve fecal continence by the construction of an ileal pouch [45]. In this procedure the distal segment of ileum is intussuscepted to create a valve mechanism which prevents leakage of bowel contents and makes it unnecessary for the patient to wear an external bag. The patient empties the ileal pouch with a catheter.

Technique. The continent ileostomy is generally an elective procedure, i.e., is performed in a second operation following proctocolectomy. The distal 5 cm of the terminal ileum are used for the stoma, the next 8–10 cm for the valve, and the proximal 30 cm for the pouch. The mesenteric peritoneum and fat in the proposed nipple area are resected, and a 2-cm opening is made in the transilluminated mesentery close to the ileal wall (Fig. 14.4). An incision is made along the antimesenteric side of the 30-cm ileal loop, and both limbs are sewn together in U-shaped fashion with a single row of continu-

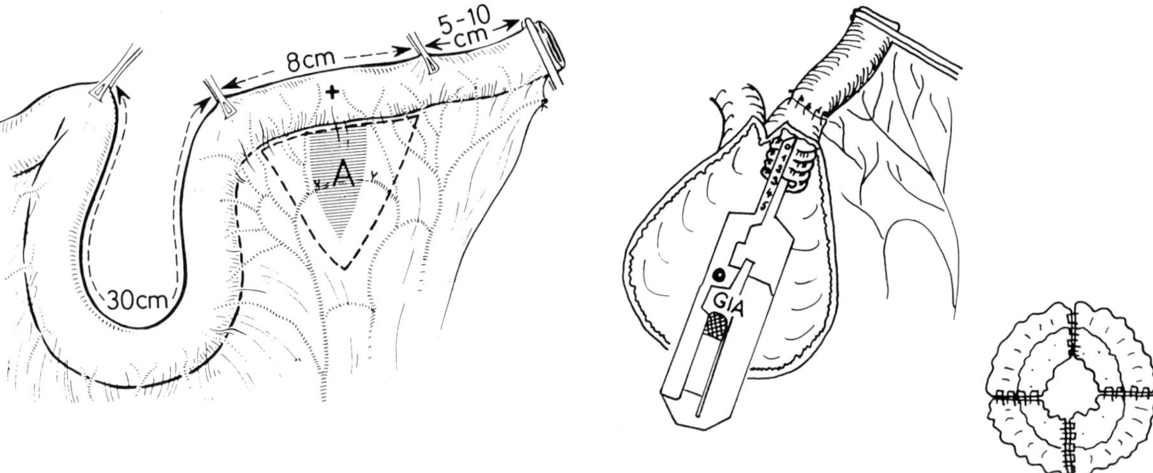

Fig. 14.4. Continent ileostomy of Kock [48] *A*, resected mesentery

Fig. 14.7. Fixation of the nipple valve with four rows of GIA staples

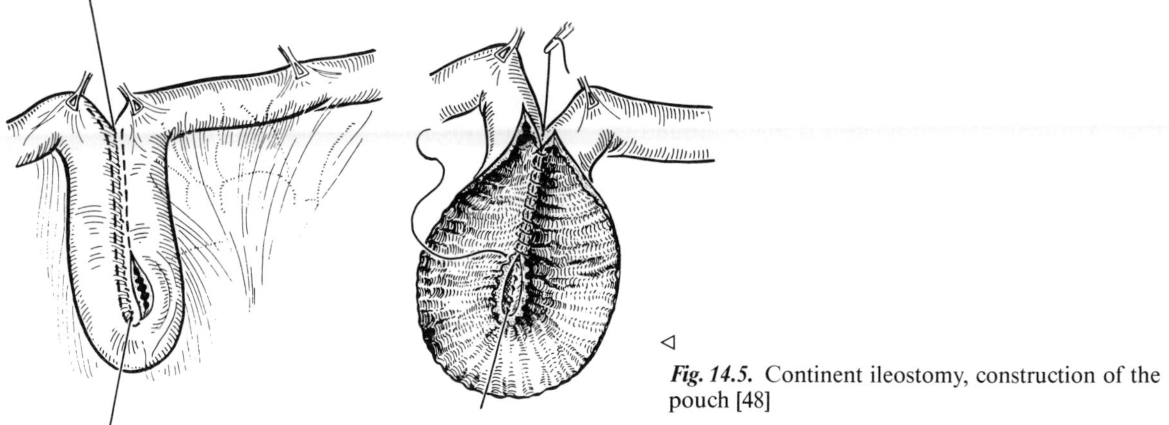

Fig. 14.5. Continent ileostomy, construction of the pouch [48]

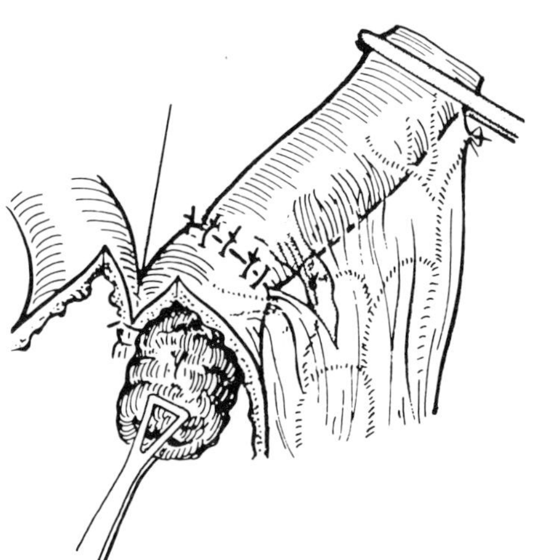

Fig. 14.6. Continent ileostomy, construction of the nipple valve [48]

ous 4/0 Dexon sutures (Fig. 14.5). The distal part of the ileum is intussuscepted into the more proximal bowel to create a 5-cm long nipple valve (Fig. 14.6), and the intussusception is secured with four rows of GIA staples (Fig. 14.7). The TA-55 staples may also be used. The nipple is fixed near its base with 4/0 Dexon. The open flap of bowel is turned upward and closed by continuous suture to create a pouch (Fig. 14.8). The ends of the reservoir are placed between the mesenteric layers so that the initially posterior part of the pouch is positioned anteriorly. The proximal limb of the ileum is clamped off, and air is insufflated through a tube. If the pouch and valve are properly constructed, there should be no escape of air. Next, the distal ileum is pulled through a finger-wide canal in the rectus muscle in the right lower quadrant, the pouch is sutured to the rectus muscle and parietal peritoneum, and the stoma is

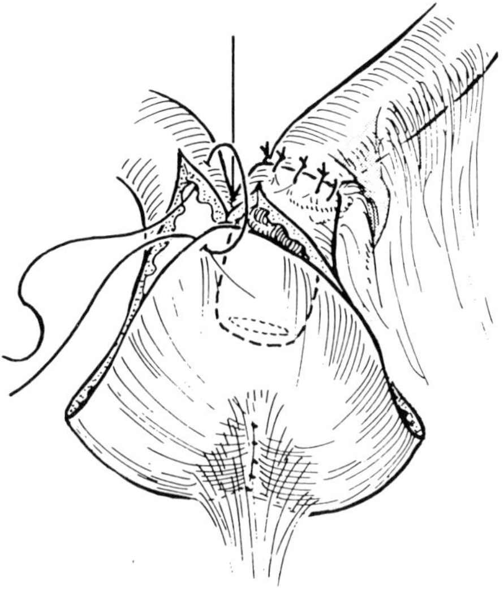

Fig. 14.8. Continent ileostomy, closed pouch

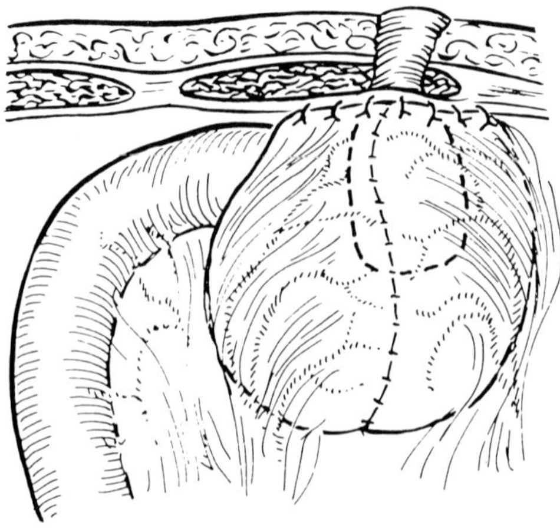

Fig. 14.9. Continent ileostomy, fixation of the pouch to the abdominal wall [48]

sutured to the skin; it should protrude no more than 1 cm above the skin surface [46] (Fig. 14.9).

Postoperative Care. Parenteral nutrition is maintained for 4–5 days and continuous pouch drainage for 2 weeks (a catheter fixed to the skin drains the base of the pouch and is flushed several times daily with 10–20 ml NaCl to confirm patency). After 2 weeks the catheter is clamped off hourly, and at 4 weeks the catheter is removed. The patient is instructed to empty the pouch two or three times daily and irrigate it with water as required [46].

Complications. Potential complications are listed in Table 14.11. By modifying the technique (GIA sta-

Table 14.11. Complications of the continent ileostomy. (Data from [1, 46])

Early complications:	Necrosis of pouch or nipple valve, anastomotic leak
	Perforation of pouch by catheter
	Bowel obstruction
Later complications:	Nipple valve displacement (partial or complete)
	Fistula formation in nipple valve
	Fistula formation between pouch and skin
	Inflammation of the pouch
	Volvulus of the pouch
	Catheter perforation of the pouch

pler, aspirating the pouch for 2–4 weeks, see above), Kock was able to lower the early complication rate from 23% to 8% and the mortality from 4.3% to 0%. These results are not always achieved by other authors. Potential late complications include nipple valve slippage (0.7%–5%), fistulas (10%), strictures (8%), and inflammation of the pouch (pouchitis, 17%) [46]. The rate of nipple valve slippage has fallen markedly since 1982 owing to use of the GIA or TA-55 staplers, as has the incidence of fistulas, most of which resulted from the use of nonabsorbable suture material. Strictures can usually be corrected under local anesthesia. Pouchitis is treated with metronidazole or salazosulfapyridine [46].

Results. Of patients undergoing the Kock operation, 97% are continent. The initially high revision rate of 54% has been reduced to 10% [20]. The most satisfying results are achieved by experienced surgeons in well-informed, younger, intelligent, psychologically stable patients who are in remission [1]. The continent ileostomy is contraindicated in patients with Crohn's disease and in insulin-dependent diabetics.

Ileorectostomy

Ileorectostomy advocated most strongly by Aylett and colleagues [5], is somewhat illogical in that the diseased rectum is left behind. The percentage of patients who are candiates for this procedure ranges from 10% to 90% in the literature [11, 40, 60]. Contraindications include severe proctitis, perianal fistulas, rectal stenosis or fibrosis, mucosal dysplasia, and extraintestinal manifestations of ulcerative colitis [1]. The patient must be willing to submit to follow-up rectoscopic examinations on a 6- or 12-monthly basis [48, 61]. The advantage of the ileorectal anastomosis is the short convalescence and preservation of sexual and bladder function [40]. Favorable functional results are reported in 20%–90% of cases [29, 60].

Technique. The patient retains approximately 12–15 cm of the rectum [29, 30]. The single-layer anastomosis is constructed in end-to-end or end-to-side fashion. Some authors [29] recommend a protective ileostomy for 2–3 weeks to provide a period of defunctioning [29, 48].

Complications. The foremost complication is a poor functional result with incontinence or diarrhea (more than eight stools per day). Good results are described in 50%–90% of cases. The perioperative mortality is 0%–13.3% [1, 22, 29, 32, 38, 60]. The incidence of cancer in the rectal stump reportedly ranges from 4.4% to 6% [5, 29, 32, 60]. Secondary excision of the rectum is necessary in 3.8%–46% of patients [1, 4]. On balance, one should be cautious about recommending this procedure today in view of the availability of other options.

Ileoanostomy (With or Without a Pouch)

A desire to preserve continence in patients with ulcerative colitis has led to the increasing use of colectomy with mucosal proctectomy and ileoanal pull-through, with or without a fecal reservoir and temporary protective ileostomy. This technically demanding operation is described in detail in Chap. 15 [1, 22–24, 30, 41, 48, 57, 73–77, 81, 82, 87, 94, 95, 99, 101].

References

1. Akovbiantz A (1981) Kontinenzerhaltende Operationen bei der Colitis ulcerosa. Helv Chir Acta 48: 789–796
2. Albrechtsen D, Bergau A, Nygaard K, Gjone E, Flatmack A (1981) Urgent surgery for ulcerative colitis: early colectomy in 132 patients. World J Surg 5: 607–615
3. Allsop JR, Lee E (1978) Factors which influenced postoperative complications in patients with ulcerative colitis or Crohn's disease of the colon on corticosteroids. Gut 19: 729–734
4. Athanasiadis S, Kuhlgatz CH, Girona J (1984) Zur Wertigkeit der ileorektalen Anastomose bei der Behandlung der Colitis ulcerosa. Zbl Chirurgie 109: 1179–1206
5. Baker W, Aylett SO, Glass RE, Ritchie JK (1978) Cancer of the rectum following colectomy and ileorectal anastomosis for ulcerative colitis. Br J Surg 65: 862–868
6. Bansky G, Bühler H, Stamm B, Häcki WH, Buchmann P, Müller J (1987) Treatment of distal ulcerative colitis with betamethasone enemas: high therapeutic efficacy without endocrine side effects. Dis Colon Rectum 30: 288–292
7. Bauer J, Gelernt IM, Salky B, Kreel I (1983) Sexual dysfunction following proctocolectomy for benign disease of the colon and rectum. Ann Surg 197: 363–367
8. Becker JM, Hillard HE, Mann FA, Kestenberg A, Nelson JA (1985) Functional assessment after colectomy, mucosal proctectomy and endorectal ileoanal pull-through. World J Surg 9: 598–605
9. Becker V (1982) Pathologische Anatomie entzündlicher Darmerkrankungen. Colo-proctology 4: 347–350
10. Berry AR, de Campos R, Lee ECG (1986) Perineal and pelvic morbidity following perimuscular excision of the rectum for inflammatory bowel disease. Br J Surg 73: 675–677
11. Buchmann P (1983) Colitis ulcerosa und Colonpolypose: Die Erhaltung des Rectums. Helv Chir Acta 509: 587–591
12. Burnham W, Lennard-Jones J, Stanford JL, Bird RG (1978) Mycobacteria as a possible cause of inflammatory bowel disease. Lancet 2: 693–696
13. Campbell DES (1986) Therapie der Colitis ulcerosa auf der Basis von 5-Amino-Salicylsäure. Schwerpunkt Med 9: 12–20
14. Carlstedt A, Fasth S, Hultén L, Nordgreen S, Palselius I (1987) Long-term ileostomy complications in patients with ulcerative colitis and Crohn's disease. Int J Colorect Dis: 22–25
15. Caprilli R, Vernia P, Colaneri O, Frieri G (1980) Risk factors in toxic megacolon. Dig Dis Sci 25: 817–822
16. Cello JP (1983) Ulcerative colitis. In: Sleisenger M, Fordtran J (eds) Gastrointestinal disease, 3rd edn. Saunders, Philadelphia
17. Chapman RW, Selby WS, Jewell DP (1986) Controlled trial of intravenous metronidazole as an adjunct to corticosteroids in severe ulcerative colitis. Gut 27: 1210–1212
18. Clark M (1986) Role of nitrition in inflammatory bowel disease: an overview. Gut 27: 72–75
19. Coran AG (1985) New surgical approaches to ulcerative colitis in children and adults. World J Surg 9: 203–213
20. Dick W (1986) Chronisch-entzündliche Darmerkrankungen. Der informierte Arzt 20: 8–12
21. Dölle W, Herfarth C (1979) Diagnose und Therapie chronisch-entzündlicher Darmerkrankungen. Med Welt 30/29: 1120–1124
22. Dozois RR, de Calan L (1985) Rectocolite ulcérohémorragique: alternatives chirurgicales à l'iléostomie conventionnelle de Brooke. Gastroenterol Clin Biol 9: 687–689
23. Feinberg S, McLeod RS, Cohen Z (1987) Complications of loop ileostomy. Am J Surg 153: 102–107
24. Fonkalsrud EW (1981) Endorectal ileal pullthrough with lateral ileal reservoir for benign colorectal disease. Ann Surg 194: 761–766
25. Friedmann LS, Richter JM, Kirkham SE, DeMonaco HJ, May RJ (1986) 5-Aminosalicylic acid enemas in refractory distal ulcerative colitis: a randomized controlled trial. Am J Gastroenterol 81: 412–418

26. Gaisberg U, Töpfer HU (1984) Medikamentöse Therapie der Colitis ulcerosa und des M. Crohn. In: Gaisberger U (ed) Colitis ulcerosa - M. Crohn: II. Fortbildungsveranstaltung, Bad Cannstatt 1984. Fak Foundation eV, Habsburgerstr. 81, D-7800 Freiburg i. Br.
27. Gilat T (1983) Incidence of inflammatory bowel disease: going up or down? Gastroenterology 85: 194-203
28. Gloor F (1981) Die nicht klassifizierbaren ulzerösen Kolitiden. Schweiz Med Wochenschr 111: 779-783
29. Goligher JC (1981) Current efforts to retain continence in the surgery of ulcerative colitis. Schweiz Med Wochenschr 111: 784-789
30. Goligher JC (1981) Eversion technique for distal mucosal proctectomy in ulcerative colitis: a preliminary report. Br J Surg 71: 26-28
31. Greenstein AJ, Barth JA, Sachar DB, Aufses AH (1986) Free colonic perforation without dilatation in ulcerative colitis. Am J Surg 152: 272-275
32. Grundfest SF, Fazio V, Weiss RA, Jagelmann D, Lavery I, Weakley FL, Turnbull RB (1981) The risk of cancer following colectomy and ileorectal anastomosis for extensive mucosal ulcerative colitis. Ann Surg 193: 9-14
33. Gyde SN, Prior P, Thompson H, Waterhouse JAH, Allan RN (1984) Survival of patients with colorectal cancer complicating ulcerative colitis. Gut 25: 228-231
34. Haferkamp O (1981) M. Crohn und Colitis ulcerosa - Standortbestimmung: pathologisch-anatomische Aspekte. Chirurg 52: 737-743
35. Halter F (1981) Differentialdiagnose der Colitis ulcerosa. Schweiz Med Wochenschr 111: 773-778
36. Hartmann F (1986) 5-Aminosalicylsäure: Neue Therapiemöglichkeit bei chronisch entzündlicher Darmerkrankung? Leber Magen Darm 16: 20-27
37. Hassler H, Grossmann S, Fischer L, Oesch A (1984) Colitis ulcerosa: Die notfallmäßige Operation beim toxischen Megacolon mit Perforation. Helv Chir Acta 51: 47-50
38. Hawley PR (1985) Ileorectal anastomosis. Br J Surg 72 [Suppl]: 75-82
39. Herfarth C (1983) Chronisch-entzündliche Darmerkrankungen - Indikation zur Operation. Z Gastroenterol 21: 27-34
40. Herfarth C, Otto HF (1987) Carcinom-praeventive Operationsindikationen bei entzündlichen Darmerkrankungen. Chirurg 58: 221-227
41. Herfarth C, Stern J (1986) Die kontinenzerhaltende Proktocolectomie. Chirurg 57: 263-270
42. Jalan K (1970) An experience of ulcerative colitis. II. Short term outcome, III. Long term outcome. Gastroenterology 59: 589-609
43. Kewenter J, Hultén L, Ahlman H (1978) Cancer risk in extensive colitis. Ann Surg 188: 824-828
44. Kim YS, Byrd JC (1984) Ulcerative colitis: a specific mucin defect? Gastroenterology 87: 1193-1195
45. Kock N (1977) Ileostomy. Curr Probl Surg 14: 18-47
46. Kock N, Myrvold HE, Nilsson LO, Philipson BM (1985) Achtzehn Jahre Erfahrung mit der kontinenten Ileostomie. Chirurg 56: 299-304
47. Kommerell B (1981) Colitis ulcerosa und M. Crohn. Der informierte Arzt 15: 34-40
48. Kremer K, Rumpf P, Ehms H, Strohmeyer G (1981) Colitis ulcerosa. In: Allgöwer M, Siewert JR, Blum AL (eds) Chirurgische Gastroenterologie. Springer, Berlin Heidelberg New York
49. Lennard-Jones JE (1986) Compliance, cost and common sense limit cancer control in colitis. Gut 27: 1403-1407
50. Lennard-Jones JE (1985) Cancer risk in ulcerative colitis: surveillance or surgery. Br J Surg 72: 84-86
51. Lennard-Jones JE (1983) Toward optimal use of corticosteroids in ulcerative colitis and Crohn's disease. Gut 24: 177-181
52. Lockart-Mummery HE (1968) Diffuse conditions of the large bowel which are premalignant. Br J Surg 55: 737
53. Lupinetti M, Mehigan D, Cameron JL (1980) Hepatobiliary complications of ulcerative colitis. Ann J Surg 139: 113-118
54. Maier K, Gaisberg U (1986) Klinische Erfahrungen mit der rectalen und oralen Applikation mit 5-Aminosalicylsäure. In: Ewe K (ed) Therapie chronisch-entzündlicher Darmerkrankungen. Schattauer, Stuttgart
55. Matuchansky C (1986) Parenteral nutrition in inflammatory bowel disease. Gut 27: 81-84
56. Mayberry JF (1985) Some aspects of the epidemiology of ulcerative colitis. Gut 26: 968-974
57. McCafferty MH, Fazio V (1985) Ileoanale Anastomose bei Colitis ulcerosa. Chirurg 56: 293-298
58. McIntyre PB, Lennard-Jones JE, Powell-Tuck J, Wood SR, Zerebours E, Hecketsweiler P, Colin R, Galmiche J-P (1986) Controlled trial of bowel rest in the treatment of severe acute colitis. Gut 27: 481-485
59. Mee AS, Shield AS, Burke M (1985) Campylobacter colitis: differentiation from acute inflammatory bowel disease. J R Soc Med 78: 217-223
60. Meister R, Schmidt R (1986) Chirurgische Therapie der Colitis ulcerosa. Colo-proctology 1: 15-23
61. Merkle P (1983) Colitis ulcerosa. Münch Med Wochenschr 125: 255-258
62. Meyer J (1973) Ulcerative colitis. In: Sleisenger M, Fordtran J (eds) Gastrointestinal disease. Saunders, Philadelphia, pp 1296-1349
63. Miller B (1978) Chronisch-entzündliche Darmerkrankungen: Colitis ulcerosa und M. Crohn. In: Bock E et al. (eds) Klinik der Gegenwart, vol 10. Urban and Schwarzenberger, München, pp 442a-E 460
64. Miller JP (1986) Inflammatory bowel disease in pregnancy: a review. J R Soc Med 79: 221-225
65. Mir-Nadjlessi SH, Farmer RG, Easley KA, Beck GJ (1986) Colorectal and extracolonic malignancy in ulcerative colitis. Cancer 58: 1569
66. Mock DM (1986) Growth retardation in chronic inflammatory bowel disease. Gastroenterology 91: 1019-1023
67. Morel P, Alexander-Williams J, Hawker PC, Allan RN, Dykes PW (1986) Management of acute colitis in inflammatory bowel disease. World J Surg 10: 814-819
68. Morowitz D, Kirsner JB (1981) Ileostomy in ulcerative colitis. Ann J Surg 141: 370-375
69. Morson BC (1968) Pathology of ulcerative colitis. Baillière Tindall and Cassell, London
70. Morson BC (1983) Kolorektale Biopsie bei entzündlichen Darmerkrankungen. Leber Magen Darm 13: 261-269

71. Mottet NK (1971) Histopathologic spectrum of regional enteritis and ulcerative colitis. Saunders, Philadelphia, Major problems in pathology, vol 2
72. Muto T, Kamiya J, Sawada T, Kubota Y, Morioka Y, Chida T, Okamura N, Nakaya R (1985) Die Beziehung zwischen Bacteroides und Colitis ulcerosa. Colonproctology 2: 73–74
73. Nasmyth DG, Johnston D, Godwin PGR, Dixon MF, Williams NS, Smith A (1986) Factors influencing bowel function after ileal pouch-anal anastomosis. Br J Surg 73: 469–473
74. Neal DE, Johnston D, Williams NS (1982) Rectal, bladder and sexual function after mucosal proctectomy with and without a pelvic reservoir for colitis and polyposis. Br J Surg 69: 599–604
75. Nicholls RJ, Pezim ME (1985) Restorative proctocolectomy with ileal reservoir for ulcerative colitis and familial adenomatous polyposis: a comparison of three reservoir designs. Br J Surg 72: 470–474
76. Nicholls JR, Moskowitz RL, Shepherd NA (1985) Restorative proctocolectomy with ileal reservoir. Br J Surg 72: 76–79
77. Nicholls J, Pescatori M, Motson RW, Pezim ME (1984) Restorative proctocolectomy with a three-loop ileal reservoir for ulcerative colitis and familial adenomatous polyposis. Ann Surg 199: 383–388
78. Nostrant TT (1987) Histopathology differentiates acute self-limited colitis from ulcerative colitis. Gastroenterology 92: 318–328
79. Nugent FW, Haggitt RC, Colcher H, Kutteruf GC (1979) Malignant potential of chronic ulcerative colitis. Gastroenterology 76: 1
80. Otto HF (1981) Immunpathologische und ultrastrukturelle Aspekte der Colitis ulcerosa. Schweiz Med Wochenschr 111: 768–773
81. Parks AG (1982) Die Rekonstruktion des Anus naturalis mittels Reservoir. Chirurg 53: 611–615
82. Pemberton JH, Beart RW, Hepell J, Dozois R, Telander RL (1982) Endorectal ileoanal anastomosis. Surg Gynecol Obstet 155: 417–424
83. Riddell RH, Morson BC (1979) Value of sigmoidoscopy and biopsy in detection of carcinoma and premalignant change in ulcerative colitis. Gut 1: 575–580
84. Riemann JF (1982) Aetiologische Aspekte von M. Crohn und Colitis ulcerosa. In: Gall FP, Groitl H (eds) Entzündliche Erkrankungen des Dünn- und Dickdarmes. Perimed, Erlangen
85. Ritchie J, Lennard-Jones J (1978) Clinical outcome of the first ten years of ulcerative colitis and proctitis. Lancet 2: 1140–1143
86. Roth JLA (1969) Ulcerative colitis. In: Bockus HL (ed) Gastroenterology. Saunders, Philadelphia, pp 645–749
87. Rothenberger DA, Vemevlen FD, Christenson CE, Balcos EG, Nemer FD, Goldberg S, Belliveau P, Nivatrongs S, Schottler JL, Kennedy HL, Fang DI (1983) Restorative proctocolectomy with ileal reservoir and ileoanal anastomosis. Am J Surg 145: 82–88
88. Säuberli H, Akovbiantz A, Hahnloser P (1982) Die chirurgische Behandlung der Colitis ulcerosa – Verbesserung der Lebensqualität durch kontinente Ileostomie? Extracta Gastroenterologica 11: 177–197
89. Säuberli H (1986) Colitis ulcerosa und M. Crohn – chirurgische Aspekte. Schweiz Rundschau Med (Praxis) 75: 283–289
90. Schofield PF, Manson JM (1986) Indications for and results of operation in inflammatory bowel disease. J R Soc Med 79: 593–595
91. Sigel A, Bötticher R, Supala K (1977) Urologische Komplikationen chronisch-entzündlicher Darmerkrankungen. Chirurg 48: 262–266
92. Stonnington CM, Phillips SF, Melton LJ, Zinsmeister AR (1987) Chronic ulcerative colitis: incidence and prevalence in a community. Gut 28: 402–409
93. Surawicz CM (1987) Diagnosing colitis: biopsy is best. Gastroenterology 92: 538–540
94. Taylor BM, Beart RW (1983) Straight ileoanal anastomosis versus ileal pouch-anal anastomosis after colectomy and mucosal proctectomy. Arch Surg 118: 696–701
95. Taylor BM, Beart RW, Dozois RR, Cranley B, Kelly KA, Phillips SF (1983) A clinico-physiological comparison of ileal pouch-anal and straight ileoanal anastomosis. Ann Surg 198: 462–468
96. Truelove SC (1984) Ulcerative colitis. Update postgraduate centre series. Update, London
97. Turnbull RB (1970) Choice of operation for the toxic megacolon phase of nonspecific ulcerative colitis. Surg Clin N Am 50: 1151–1169
98. Van Heerden J, McIlrath DC, Adson MA (1978) The surgical aspects of chronic mucosal inflammatory bowel disease. Ann Surg 187: 536–541
99. Utsonomiya MD, Iwama T, Imajo M, Matsudo S, Sawai S, Yaegashi K, Hirayama R (1980) Total colectomy, mucosal proctectomy and ileoanal anastomosis. Dis Colon Rectum 23: 459–466
100. Watkinson G (1973) Colitis ulcerosa. In: Demling L et al. (eds) Klinische Gastroenterologie. Thieme, Stuttgart
101. Williams WS, Johnston D (1985) The current status of mucosal proctectomy and ileo-anal anastomosis in the surgical treatment of ulcerative colitis and adenomatous polyposis. Br J Surg 72: 159–168

15 Ileoanal Anastomosis

A. Rohner

Introduction

An understandable repugnance to the idea of permanent ileostomy may influence the future of suffered from ulcerative colitis or familial polyposis coli in different ways. First, it tends to induce both the patients and their physicians to defer operation for as long as possible, accepting the risk of the serious complications inherent in these two conditions. At the same time, it orients surgeons towards a policy of rectal conservation by ileorectal anastomosis, with attendant persistence of unhealthy rectal mucosa, which in ulcerative colitis may finally lead to secondary proctectomy, and in polyposis may be the starting point of malignant change.

Although the incidence of malignancy is evaluated differently in different series, its unquestioned possibility calls for repeated endoscopy and fulguration, procedures which are physically and psychologically unwelcome. It was natural, therefore, that surgeons should seek a solution that would be intermediate between, on the one hand, proctocolectomy with permanent ileostomy bringing security at the price of disability, and, on the other hand, ileorectal anastomosis (IAA) providing comfort linked with potential risk. IAA, an old concept restored to favor in recent years, preserves anorectal function but, by removing potential disease-bearing mucosa, it rules out both the occurrence of malignancy and the recurrence of inflammatory disease.

History

Attempts to establish ileoanal continuity were made by Lisfranc in 1826 [41], Kraske in 1885 [39], and Nissen in 1933 [52], but the absence of sustained interest testified to their lack of success. The concept was taken up under experimental conditions by Ravitch and Sabiston in 1947 [60] and by Valiente and Bacon in 1955 [80], and later applied with increasing frequency in human subjects by workers such as Waugh and Turner [82], Black and Walls [7], and Bacon [1]. Its use by Soave [69] for the management of Hirschsprung's disease helped to make it better known. The fluctuations in its popularity were outlined by Pemberton et al. in 1982 [58]: out of 41 patients who had an IAA before 1960, acceptable continence was obtained in only 54%. From 1960 to 1976 attempts were relatively few but more successful, and 77% of the 45 patients reported, among whom were those of Safaie-Shirazi and Soper [65], had continence compatible with normal life. The number of operations performed rose again between 1977 and 1981 [42, 57, 76], and in 91% of 123 patients who had an IAA constructed during those years continence was satisfactory. IAA was commented on favorably by Fonkalsrud and Ament in 1978 [22] after a trial in five patients. Reporting on 50 patients who underwent the procedure between 1978 and 1981 on account of ulcerative colitis or familial polyposis, Beart et al. [2] concluded that it is "a viable alternative" to permanent ileostomy.

The idea of inserting an ileal reservoir to replace the excised rectal ampulla radically transformed the functional efficacy of IAA. The feasibility in humans of the ileal neorectum devised in animals by Valiente and Bacon in 1955 [80] was demonstrated by Kock in 1969 [36], when he constructed a continent cutaneous ileostomy, an essential element of which was an ileal reservoir or pouch made up of several juxtaposed segments of intestine opening into each other. In 1978 Parks and Nicholls [55], adapting Kock's invention, produced the first IAA with a reservoir, the three-loop (S) reservoir of Parks. There followed the two-loop side-to-end (J) reservoir described by Utsunomiya et al. in 1980 [78] and the two-loop isoperistaltic side-to-side (H) reservoir of Fonkalsrud [18, 19].

The encouraging results obtained by these pioneers stimulated interest in the procedure. The improvement in function brought about by placing an ileal storage reservoir proximal to the IAA was analyzed and sanctioned experimentally by Cranley and McKelvey [13], Schraut and Block [67], and Schraut et al. [68], and confirmed clinically in humans by Neal et al. [47] and Taylor et al. [74]. The four-loop (W) reservoir was introduced by Nicholls and Pezim in 1985 [50]. At a symposium reported by Williams in 1986 [84], 839 operations performed between 1976 and 1985 were reviewed. French experience with the procedure has been reported by Parc et al. [53].

In this short account we shall describe the various techniques that have been tried, discuss their respective advantages, disadvantages, indications, and contraindications, and attempt to evaluate them in terms of their functional results.

Operative Techniques

General

Thorough antibiotic bowel preparation and the perioperative administration of systemic antibiotics are necessary. The intermediate gynecological position used at St. Mark's Hospital, London for two-team rectal excision is the most suitable. The abdomen is opened through a left paramedian incision (setting aside and sparing the rectus abdominis muscle) which confers greater resistance in the long term than does incision in the midline. The operation is performed in two stages when it is elective, in three stages when colectomy is urgent. There is evidence that the three-stage technique has the lesser risk of pelvic sepsis. Williams [84] found major sepsis in 26% of his cases with the two-stage method, but in only 6% when a three-stage procedure was employed.

The mesenteric dissection during total abdominal colectomy can be done very close to the colon in ulcerative colitis and in familial polyposis in the absence of malignancy, but malignant change in one or several colonic polyps calls for wide mesenteric exeresis as in the presence of cancer. The greater omentum is usually removed. Its retention, recommended by some surgeons, does not seem to preclude the postoperative occlusion that often follows total colectomy.

Below the rectosigmoid junction the procedure differs from conventional colorectal exeresis. The plane of dissection must be kept close to the rectal wall to avoid damaging the pelvic autonomic nerves and consequent risk of urogenital complications. Hemostasis has to be meticulous and conducted in direct contact with individual rectal vessels. Also, to avoid nerve trauma, the pelvic vessels are spared electrocoagulation. No attempt should be made to raise the rectum by mobilizing it posteriorly in the plane normally used in rectal surgery, or at least not further than the level at which it will be transsected.

The three principal stages of the operation – rectal transsection, rectal mucosectomy, and construction of the ileal reservoir – will now be considered, with special attention to the variations that have been proposed by different workers. Finally, mention will be made of temporary protective ileostomy, which is generally necessary.

Transsection of the Rectum

In the technique initially described by Parks and Nicholls [55] and Parks et al. [56], the rectum was transsected "at or just below the peritoneal reflection" at the bottom of the rectovesical or rectovaginal pouch. Most surgeons today, however, prefer to transsect at a lower level than this, namely, 4–5 cm above the pectinate (dentate) line.

Parks believed that retention of a long rectal muscle cuff had the potential advantage of favoring fecal continence and perhaps also of protecting an anastomosis that is difficult to construct and is often dehiscent. The disadvantage of the long cuff – like other surgeons, Rothenberger et al. [62], for example, the author used it in his own early experience of this operation [61] – is that it prolongs the operating time required for rectal mucosectomy, making this latter procedure more difficult to perform and less certain in its outcome. The short cuff method allows the rectal stump to be closed through the abdominal approach and the rectal mucosa to be removed by the transanal route [14–16], thus reducing the critical surface and thereby minimizing the risk of septic complications. Surgeons who have changed from the long to the short rectal cuff have found that the shorter cuff gives a lower incidence of cuff abscesses [15, 21, 25, 79]. In the series of Utsunomiya et al. [79] this incidence fell from 33.3% to nil.

Local infection, even temporary, impairs the functional results, sometimes disastrously. By causing cicatricial retraction, for example, sepsis may impede expansion of the ileal neorectum. That sacrifice of the large part of the rectal muscle tube has no adverse effect on continence has been reported in several series [3, 14, 74], one of which [14] comprised 369 cases.

Dozois' [14] suggested closure of the rectum by a TA automatic stapler has proved difficult when the pelvis is narrow, especially in women. It can be replaced by interrupted sutures taking in all layers of the rectal wall.

A possible relation between length of rectal muscle cuff and urogenital sequelae is discussed under "Urogenital Sequelae."

Rectal Mucosectomy

The rectal mucosectomy stage of the operation, which has to be carried out with minute attention to detail, probably has most influence on the quality of the result of IAA. How far caudally the rectal mucosa should be stripped has been subject of debate. In the early days of the procedure, the practice was to retain some 2 cm of mucosa *above* the pectinate line, in the belief that this would promote good function and, in particular, preserve the ability to distinguish liquid feces from flatus. Later experience, however, has shown that retention of mucosa above the pectinate line has no functional utility [3, 14]. It may even be dangerous. Cancer has arisen near the pectinate line in patients with familial polyposis in whom mucosa had been left behind [78], and recurrence of rectal polyps in residual mucosa has been reported [28, 85]. In the two patients of Wolfstein et al. [85], polyposis recurred in the rectal segment 3 and 7 years after IAA for familial polyposis coli, and these investigators related the recurrence to the preservation of a 1-cm strip of mucosa above the pectinate line. To determine whether rectal mucosa does in fact regenerate after rectal mucosectomy and IAA, Heppell et al. [30] examined specimens of the IAA in eight patients who had required neorectal excision. They were able to identify islets of rectal mucosa and anal glands in two patients only, a finding which, they insisted, should be interpreted with caution.

Mucosectomy (Fig. 15.1) is technically the most difficult part of the ileoanal anastomotic procedure, so much so that surgeons regard the presence of severe rectal scarring or deep rectal ulcers as sufficient reason for not proceeding with the operation. Mucosectomy is easier in familial polyposis than in ulcerative colitis. In ulcerative colitis the presence of severe proctitis renders the outcome of mucosectomy uncertain, since it practically precludes complete excision of the rectal mucosa without injury to the smooth muscle cuff. As we have seen ("Transsection of the Rectum"), retention of only a short length of pelvic cuff goes a long way toward simplifying mucosectomy.

The number of aids to rectal mucosectomy that have been tried experimentally or clinically, such as chemical débridement [24, 38], curettage [26], and the surgical ultrasonic aspirator [32] is evidence of its difficulty. Actually none of these devices seems more effective than simple blunt-scissor dissection preceded by infiltration with isotonic saline containing a vasoconstrictive drug.

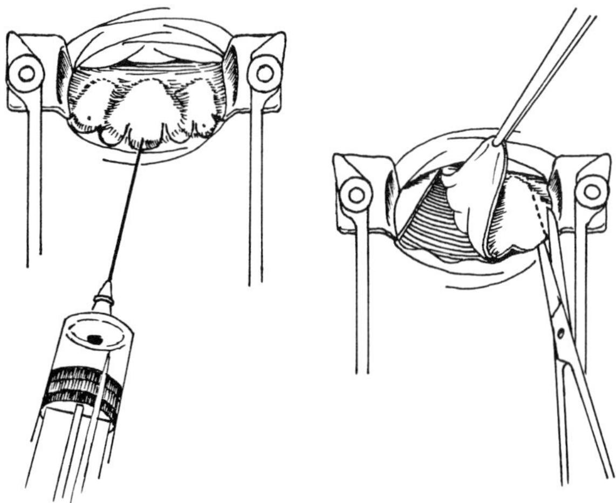

Fig. 15.1. Submucosal infiltration and mucosectomy

The Ileal Reservoir

The Kock continent ileostomy reservoir [36] inspired the S-shaped ileal reservoir introduced by Parks and Nicholls in 1978 [55]. The Parks pouch consisted of three juxtaposed segments of ileum, each segment about 15 cm long, and a 5-cm "spout" protruding at the distal end (Fig. 15.2). Out of 20 patients so treated, ten were able to evacuate spontaneously and the remainder had to use a transanal catheter [56]. This disadvantage was attributed [19] – inaccurately as we shall see – to the fact that the middle segment of the S was antiperistaltic.

The J-shaped pouch introduced by Utsunomiya [78] was formed by folding the terminal ileal segment upward, bringing its extremity, closed by a row of staples, into contact with the next ileal segment, and constructing a side-to-side ileo-ileal anastomosis (Fig. 15.3). The side-to-end anal anastomosis was between the lower convexity of the folded segment (i. e., the apex of the J) and the anal canal. With this procedure, evacuation was invariably spontaneous and was more complete than that reported with Parks' S pouch, but median daily stool frequency was slightly higher [79].

The isoperistaltic lateral reservoir (H pouch) devised by Fonkalsrud [18, 19], similar to an arrangement previously proposed by Peck [57], was fashioned from two isoperistaltic ileal segments placed side by side (Fig. 15.4). Fonkalsrud found that it produced less stasis and achieved a more regular defecatory pattern than did the S-shaped reservoir, of which he had previous clinical experience [17].

Although Dozois [14] bestowed on the J-shaped res-

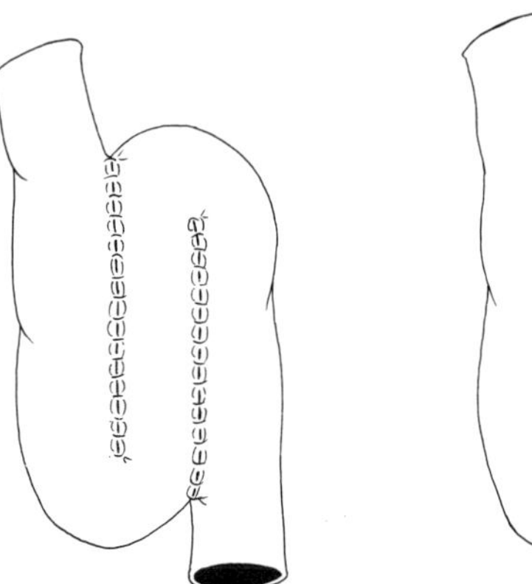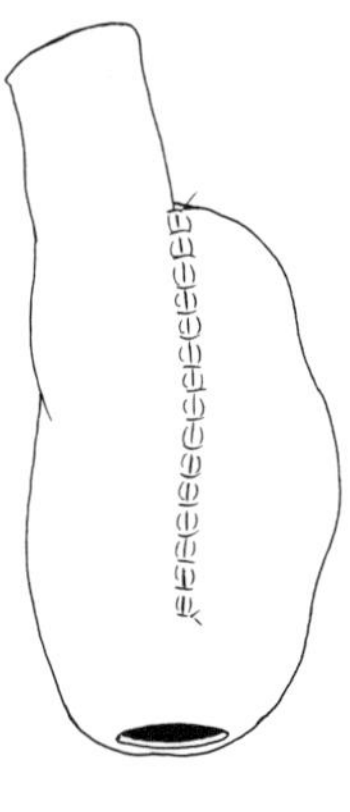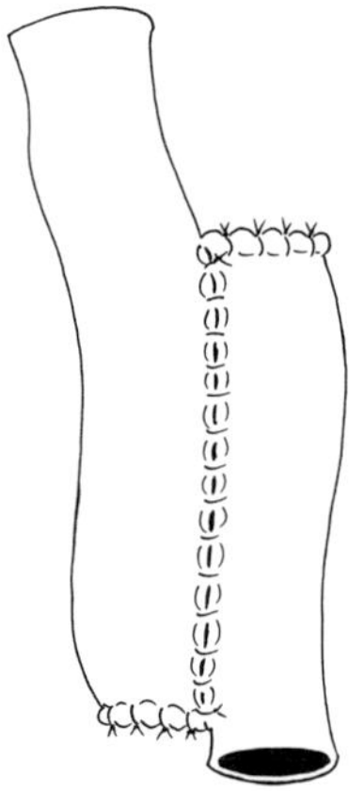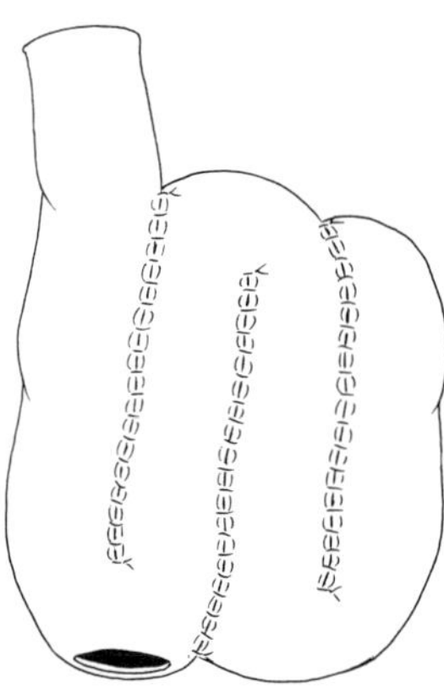

Fig. 15.2 *(left)*. The Parks or S reservoir formed from three segments of ileum, each segment 15 cm long, placed side by side. A 5-cm spout is left protruding at the distal end

Fig. 15.3 *(right)*. Utsanomiya or J reservoir, formed by folding the terminal ileal segment upward. The lower convexity of the folded segment is sutured to the pectinate line

Fig. 15.4 *(left)*. The Fonkalsrud or H reservoir formed from two isoperistaltic ileal segments placed side by side

Fig. 15.5 *(right)*. The W reservoir formed from four segments of ileum, each segment 15 cm long, placed side by side

ervoir the accolade of a favorable report from the Mayo Clinic (based on 369 ileal pouch-anal anastomoses done there during 1981–1984, 356 using the J and 13 the S reservoir), this can probably not be regarded as the final verdict.

We know now that the difficulty in evacuating the S pouch was not due to antiperistaltism of the middle segment of the S, but to the initial use of an excessively long outflow tract. When Rothenberger et al. [63, 64], Bubrick et al. [8], Cohen et al. [11], and Rohner [61] shortened the outflow tracts of their S pouches by 2–3 cm, they observed that spontaneous evacuation improved at the expense of self-catheterization. Out of seven patients whom Liljeqvist and Lindquist [40] regarded as "failed S pouches" because of repeated fecal soiling and the need for self-catheterization, six achieved efficient evacuation and four became completely free from leakage after a corrective operation to shorten the outflow tract.

An inverse correlation between pouch size and stool frequency has been noted. Already in patients with straight IAA (i. e., with no pouch) Heppell et al. [29] observed that the greater the capacity of the neorectum, the fewer were the bowel movements. In two series of patients treated by Taylor et al. [74], a straight IAA group with their smaller neorectal capacity had a higher stool frequency than a group who had undergone IAA with J-pouch construction. Nicholls and Pezim [50] found that after closure of the protective ileostomy, two-loop pouches were significantly smaller (197 ml) than three-loop pouches (416 ml), and that the patients with the two-loop pouches defecated more frequently (five to six times in 24 h) than those with the three-loop pouches (three to four times in 24 h). Stool frequency was significantly lower (median, five times in 24 h) in 17 patients with three-loop pouches, than in 22 patients with two-loop (J or H) pouches (median, seven times in 24 h) studied by Nasmyth et al. [46] 12 months after closure of the diverting ileostomy.

In an attempt to achieve greater pouch capacity, and in consequence lower stool frequency, Nicholls and Pezim [50] designed a four-loop (W) pouch (Fig. 15.5) consisting of four juxtaposed ileal segments and compared its performance with that of the three-loop pouch. Not only did stool frequency fall, as had been hoped, but in addition the four-loop pouches were evacuated more comfortably and more completely than those with only three loops. These investigators concluded that a large reservoir is preferable to a small reservoir.

The different designs for ileal reservoirs and the techniques of their construction, are described and reviewed by Schoetz et al. [66], Williams and Johnston [83], and Herfarth and Stern [31].

Protective Ileostomy

The unavoidable hazards of the mucosectomy and the technical difficulties of the anastomosis make establishment of a protective, temporary ileostomy practically mandatory (Fig. 15.6). Nevertheless, immediate restoration of ileoanal continuity may be possible in certain selected cases and in the hands of surgeons with special experience in the execution of IAA. Out of 200 patients in whom Metcalf et al. [44] performed proctocolectomy with ileal pouch-anal anastomosis, all but nine were given temporary diverting ileostomies. Although the outcome was successful in eight of the nine, Metcalf and her colleagues stressed that they "still hesitate to recommend this approach."

The technique of choice is a hermetically sealed terminal ileostomy, as illustrated by Turnbull and Weakley [77]. The distal end, closed over a tube that permits radiological verification before take-down of the ileostomy [61], is fixed to the deep abdominal wall below the ileostomy. Alternatively, after the surgeon has gained experience, and if he or she is satisfied with the anastomosis, a lateral ileostomy can be established, taking care to "terminalize" it partially by suturing the afferent loop to two-thirds of the cutaneous orifice, to the detriment of the efferent loop. The chief advantage of this second method is that it simplifies later closure of the ileostomy by a peristomal incision, whereas with the first method it is generally necessary to reutilize the median or paramedian incision. A technique of loop ileostomy closure with intestinal stapling devices has been described by Kestenberg and Becker [35].

The temporary protective ileostomy should be maintained for 8–12 weeks [15, 27, 44]. It can be closed safely if rectal examination confirms suppleness of the suture line, absence of dehiscence or extrinsic infiltration, and good sphincter tone, and if radiographic opacification of the pouch shows satisfactory sphincter control during filling, good expansion, healing of the pouch-anal-anastomosis, and no leakage. The patient should be advised to wear a protective pad during the days immediately following closure because of the risk of uncontrolled temporary fecal leakage by day or by night. Medication to delay intestinal transit is often indicated.

Indications and Contraindications

In general, only subjects under the age of 60 years, psychologically robust, and not obese should be considered for IAA. Any suspicion of Crohn's disease is an absolute contraindication. Nicholls et al. [49] reported two patients, misdiagnosed as ulcerative colitis at the time of the reservoir operation,

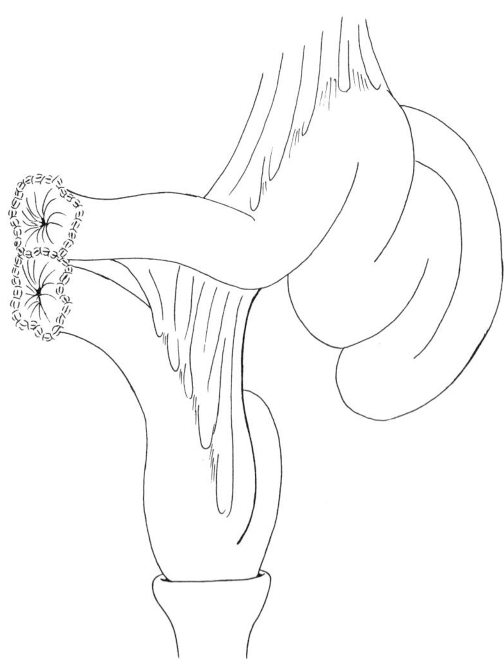

Fig. 15.6. Ileoanal reservoir covered by a protective ileostomy

whose pouches had to be removed when they were found to have Crohn's disease.

Ulcerative colitis, now a surgical condition, is one of the two major indications, but only if the rectum is little affected (especially by cicatricial lesions causing fibrosis or stenosis) and is free from cancer. Anal or perianal disease such as fistula or chronic abscess, or sphincter hypotonicity due to aging, trauma, or neurological disease are contraindications. IAA should not be done as an emergency for fulminating colitis or toxic megacolon, which require a three-stage operation. Indications for operation are further discussed by Coran et al. [12].

That familial polyposis coli is an indication for IAA now seems to be almost unanimously accepted, at least in patients who have multiple rectal polyps at initial presentation or severe rectal polyposis developing after ileorectal anastomosis [33]. Polyposis coli is associated with a very real risk of the development of rectal cancer, although the risk has been evaluated differently by different investigators. Moertel et al., in a study in 1971 [45], found that cancer developed in 59% of 143 patients followed for 23 years after colectomy and ileorectosigmoidostomy, and reached the formal conclusion that "procedures which allow retention of the cancer-prone rectal mucosa must be discarded as therapeutically inadequate." Watne et al. [81], who were of opinion that cancer of the rectum is a persistent threat for the patient with polyposis coli, reported an incidence of cancer in the retained rectum of 22% with a median follow-up of 14 years after colectomy and ileoproctostomy, and were "very optimistic about the ileoanal endorectal pull-through procedure," especially for younger children. Bussey, in contrast, in 1975 [10], found a cumulative cancer risk of only 3.6% after 25 years. In 58 Danish polyposis patients, Bülow [9] noted a 3.5% risk of rectal cancer at 5 years after colectomy and ileorectal anastomosis and 13.3% at 10 years, figures which, in view of the fact that most of these patients were under 30 years of age, should be regarded as far from reassuring. In a review based on experience at the Familial Polyposis Registry of the Cleveland Clinic Foundation, Jagelman [33] expressed the belief that, although the risk of rectal cancer is real, it does not warrant removal of the rectum in all patients with familial polyposis coli. For him the procedure of choice in most patients is ileorectal anastomosis, with IAA as second choice before proctocolectomy and ileostomy.

Results

Operative and Postoperative Mortality

In many of the published series the operative mortality is nil. In 839 operations reported by nine surgeons at a recent symposium, only one postoperative death had been recorded [84].

Postoperative Morbidity

The incidence of *small bowel obstruction,* about 10% [15, 75, 84], closely approximates the incidence previously reported in total colectomy, irrespective of the method of reestablishing continuity. Fonkalsrud [21] encountered 19 obstructive episodes in 77 patients who had undergone IAA with a lateral isoperistaltic ileal reservoir – partial obstruction to the reservoir outlet in 16 patients and intestinal obstruction due to adhesions in three patients. Intestinal obstruction that developed in three patients operated on by Coran et al. [12] was successfully treated by an enterolysis. *Pelvic sepsis* arising between the reservoir and the rectal cuff has been described in 10%–15% of patients [54, 84]. Half respond satisfactorily to antibiotics, but in the other half surgical drainage is necessary, and in nearly 50% of these latter the pouch has to be excised and a permanent ileostomy created. Pelvic sepsis occurred in 22% of

50 straight IAA patients operated on by Taylor et al. [75], but in only 14% of 113 patients in whom they performed J-pouch IAA. *Partial breakdown of the ileoanal suture* is common (about 12%). If protected by a temporary ileostomy, it has no serious consequences, but it often leads to *anastomotic stricture.* This, however, is amenable to correction by dilatation or digital stretching and, in contrast to severe pelvic infection, does not seem to react adversely on function [15, 27, 43, 84]. *Peritonitis* has been reported in 4.3% of cases and intestinal obstruction in 7% at the time of closure of the ileostomy [15].

Functional Results

Continence has, on average, been judged acceptable, only a minority of patients suffering involuntary fecal loss, and it improves with time. Reviewing functional results in 157 patients, Metcalf et al. [43] and Dozois [14] made a distinction between seepage (minor staining) and soilage (requiring a protective pad). At a mean interval of 375 days after ileostomy closure, seepage was observed in 23% of the patients by day and in 47% at night, and soilage in 2% and 5%, respectively. At 9 months the daytime figures were 31% for seepage and 5% for soilage, and at 18 months 19% and 0%, respectively. Patients under 50 years of age and those with polyposis coli had better continence than patients over 50 and those with ulcerative colitis.

Difficulty in *spontaneous evacuation* of the S-pouch was overcome, as we have seen (see "The Ileal Reservoir"), by shortening the outflow tract. Even so, some patients have to massage their suprapubic region in order to precipitate defecation; others have difficulty in evacuating flatus and have to adopt a special position to do so. Spontaneous evacuation of the J-pouch, in contrast, seems to present no problems.

Stool frequency varies with the type of pouch (see "The Ileal Reservoir"), but is never less than three to four times by day and once at night. Like continence, it improves with time, as is reflected by the rate of consumption of antidiarrheal remedies which, in a study by Dozois and de Calan [15], were being taken by 46% of patients after 9 months and by only 29% after 18 months. The improvement is probably due to a progressive increase in the volume of the ileal pouch. In follow-up studies ranging from 2 to 35 months after operation, Becker et al. [5] and Stryker et al. [73] noted that stool frequency was related to pouch capacity, to the rapidity of pouch filling, and to the completeness of pouch evacuation.

Manometric, electric, and motility studies conducted by Becker [4] and Stryker et al. [71] concluded that IAA does not interfere with anal sphincter function or with jejunoileal motility. Kawarasaki et al. [34], in a study in dogs with side-to-side isoperistaltic ileal reservoirs, noted that, as the reservoir dilated during the 8 weeks after its construction, stool frequency decreased from 18 to five times per 24 h, and electric activity in the muscle of the reservoir returned to near normal.

Urogenital Sequelae

Although a long rectal muscle cuff (see "Transection of the Rectum") had no advantage in respect of fecal continence, it may have obviated urogenital sequelae by forming a kind of "protective wall." No urogenital sequelae were in fact reported by Parks et al. [56] or Parks [54]. Out of 77 patients followed by Fonkalsrud [20, 21] after IAA with different lengths of rectal muscle cuff, none experienced bladder dysfunction or abnormal sexual function.

Metcalf et al. [43] and Dozois [14] reported retrograde ejaculation (but not impotence) in 9% of 96 male patients who had had IAA with rectal transsection 2–4 cm above the pectinate line. This finding would seem to point to a lesion of the pudendal nerve, yet the surgical dissections performed during the ileoanal procedure never approach that structure. The same comment was made by Stryker et al. [72] in seeking an explanation for electromyographic abnormalities, consistent with denervation of the external anal sphincter, which they had detected in patients with major fecal soilage after IAA. Damage to the pudendal nerve, they suggested, might have occurred perioperatively as a result of excessive traction on the nerve, of compression, or of inflammation, or might have antedated the IAA.

No conclusion is possible at present, but additional studies aimed at eliminating the possibility of such complications in a patient group comprising a large element of young men are clearly indicated. Retrograde ejaculation was also noted by Taylor et al. [75] and Becker and Raymond [6].

Six out of 92 women in Dozois' [16] series had normal pregnancies at term, five of them per vaginam. Neal et al. [47] encountered mild dyspareunia in two out of 13 women but no case of impotence in 19 men. No urinary complications have been reported, although Neal et al. [47] found a significant increase in bladder capacity in one case.

Inflammation of the Ileal Reservoir ("Pouchitis")

Pouchitis has been reported to occur in some 10%–20% of patients who have undergone IAA, and to be readily corrected by oral administration of metronidazole [6, 54]. It is more common after IAA done for ulcerative colitis than after IAA done for familial polyposis coli [6]. It may be that it also exists in a more serious form. Franceschi et al. [23] have described a pouchitis-like syndrome caused by a solitary mucosal ulcer that developed in the J-type ileal reservoir of a man with familial polyposis coli who had undergone IAA. The ulcer healed after antibiotic therapy.

Although experience with the Kock pouch is in this respect encouraging, the real incidence of pouch infection is not known, and the possibility that masked or latent infection may produce grave complications at a much later date should be kept in mind. A case might even be made for giving prophylactic courses of metronidazole in the presence of pain, changes in stool frequency, or fever. In one of our patients, an S pouch perforated spontaneously 3 years after the operation and had to be excised. Two female patients who had undergone IAA with S pouches on account of familial polyposis coli, and who had never had recourse to catheterization, suffered attacks of intestinal obstruction, which could conceivably have reflected latent reservoir infection. One of these patients was operated on for obstruction at another hospital 1 year after her IAA. The intestine was distended up to the pouch orifice, and the surgeon was surprised at the absence of kinking or banding. The second patient was sent into our hospital as an emergency by a surgeon who had diagnosed intestinal obstruction from mechanical causes. In view of the radiological findings – distension of the whole of the small intestine – the pouch was drained through a transanal tube, and the symptoms cleared up. Perhaps they would have responded to the same simple therapy in the other patient too. Possibly the cause of the trouble in both cases was acute atony of the pouch secondary to latent pouchitis. It is too early, however, to link these complications specifically with pouch morphology.

Long-Term Metabolic Effects

How the body will tolerate the ileal neorectum as the years pass is as yet unknown. Possible long-term metabolic consequences have been envisaged by Nilsson et al. [51] and Cohen et al. [11]. A metabolic assessment was done by Nicholls et al. in 1981 [48] in 14 patients who had had IAA more than 6 months previously: levels of plasma electrolytes, serum albumin, calcium, phosphorus, and red cell folate were normal; there was no case of Vitamin B_{12} malabsorption as judged by the Schilling test, although four patients had marginally low values; inflammation of the reservoir mucosa was associated with abnormally high counts of fecal aerobic bacteria. Further reassurance comes from earlier experience with the continent ileostomy, as Kock et al. [37] have pointed out.

Recurrence of Rectal Polyps

Recurrence of rectal polyps was discussed in connection with retention of rectal mucosa above the pectinate line ("Rectal Mucosectomy").

Revisional Surgery

Under revisional surgery mention may be made of: the excellent result obtained by Pescatori and Parks [59] with posterior transmucosal myotomy of the small bowel for outlet obstruction of the reservoir and spasms of the efferent limb; Fonkalsrud's [21] corrective operations, such as shortening or removing the reservoir, shortening the rectal muscle cuff, and relieving outlet obstruction or obstruction due to adhesions; Liljeqvist and Lindquist's [40] shortening of the reservoir outflow tract already described under "The Ileal Reservoir"; reestablishment of a permanent ileostomy, with or without pouch excision, reported as having been required in some 5% of IAA cases [83]; and resection of the upper end of the ileal reservoir, distended as a result of partial obstruction of the reservoir, in 19 of 82 patients who had undergone IAA with an H pouch [70].

It is gratifying to reflect that, thanks to the technical improvements described in the previous section, these surgical adjustments will gradually cease to be required.

Conclusions

IAA now has a well-established place in the surgical management of disorders of the mucosa of the colon and rectum. This statement should, however, be qualified by the following cautionary remarks:

- It should be explained to patients before operation that the intention is to provide them with an acceptable alternative solution, but that they cannot count on their functions becoming completely normal.
- The operative technique is difficult, and even in experienced hands the morbidity is high, as is shown by the "learning curve" [83] characteristic of all institutions that have introduced the operation. Therefore the procedure should not become generalized but should be practiced eclectically by specially trained surgical teams.
- There is still uncertainty as to the best technique for reestablishing intestinal continuity and, in particular, as to the optimal length of rectal muscle cuff. The short muscle cuff favors good function and minimizes infection. But does it also, as does the long cuff, preclude urogenital sequelae?
- The long-term evolution is not yet known. Extrapolation from the results obtained with the Kock pouch is not entirely reassuring. One cannot but wonder if complications such as spontaneous perforation or obstruction due to atony of the pouch will not occur with disturbing frequency in the medium or long term. Regeneration of mucosa between the ileal reservoir and the muscle cuff, perhaps causing secondary functional difficulties, is another potential source of anxiety.

Despite these reservations, one fact seems to emerge clearly in the light of the new perspectives, namely, that in benign diseases of the mucosa of the colon and rectum (with the exception of Crohn's disease), the rectal sphincter must at all costs be respected. This recommendation is addressed not only to surgeons but also to physicians, who should know that an expectant therapeutic attitude that might lead to sacrifice of the rectal sphincter in ulcerative colitis or familial polyposis coli must henceforth be regarded as a medical error.

References

1. Bacon HE (1971) Present status of the pull-through sphincter-preserving procedure. Cancer 28: 196–203
2. Beart RW Jr, Dozois RR, Kelly KA (1982) Ileoanal anastomosis in the adult. Surg Gynecol Obstet 154: 826–828
3. Beart RW Jr, Dozois RR, Wolff BG, Pemberton JH (1985) Mechanisms of rectal continence: lessons from the ileoanal procedure. Am J Surg 149: 31–34
4. Becker JM (1984) Anal sphincter function after colectomy, mucosal proctectomy, and endorectal ileoanal pull-through. Arch Surg 119: 526–531
5. Becker JM, Hillard AE, Mann FA, Kestenberg A, Nelson JA (1985) Functional assessment after colectomy, mucosal proctectomy, and endorectal ileoanal pull-through. World J Surg 9: 598–605
6. Becker JM, Raymond JL (1986) Ileal pouch-anal anastomosis: a single surgeon's experience with 100 consecutive cases. Ann Surg 204: 375–383
7. Black BM, Walls JT (1967) Combined abdomino-endorectal resection: reappraisal of a pull-through procedure. Surg Clin North Am 47: 977–982
8. Bubrick MP, Jacobs DM, Levy M (1985) Experience with the endorectal pull-through and S pouch for ulcerative colitis and familial polyposis in adults. Surgery 98: 689–698
9. Bülow S (1984) The risk of developing rectal cancer after colectomy and ileorectal anastomosis in Danish patients with polyposis coli. Dis Colon Rectum 27: 726–729
10. Bussey HJR (1975) Familial polyposis coli. Family studies, histopathology, differential diagnosis and results of treatment. John Hopkins University Press, Baltimore, pp 73–74
11. Cohen Z, McLeod RS, Stern H, Grant D, Nordgren S (1985) The pelvic pouch and ileoanal anastomosis procedure: surgical technique and initial results. Am J Surg 150: 601–607
12. Coran AG, Sarahan TM, Dent TL, Fiddian-Green R, Wesley JR, Jordan FT (1983) The endorectal pull-through for the management of ulcerative colitis in children and adults. Ann Surg 197: 99–105
13. Cranley B, McKelvey STD (1982) The pelvic ileal reservoir: an experimental assessment of its function compared with that of normal rectum. Br J Surg 69: 465–469
14. Dozois RR (1985) Ileal J' pouch-anal anastomosis. Br J Surg 72 [Suppl]: 80–82
15. Dozois RR, de Calan L (1985) Rectocolite ulcéro-hémorragique: alternatives chirurgicales à l'iléostomie conventionnelle de Brooke. Gastroenterol Clin Biol 9: 687–689
16. Dozois RR, de Calan L (1985) Recto-colite ulcéro-hémorragique: alternatives chirurgicales à l'iléostomie de Brooke. Med Hyg 43: 267–274
17. Fonkalsrud EW (1980) Total colectomy and endorectal ileal pull-through with internal ileal reservoir for ulcerative colitis. Surg Gynecol Obstet 150: 1–8
18. Fonkalsrud EW (1981) Endorectal ileal pullthrough with lateral ileal reservoir for benign colorectal disease. Ann Surg 194: 761–766
19. Fonkalsrud EW (1982) Endorectal ileal pullthrough with ileal reservoir for ulcerative colitis and polyposis. Am J Surg 144: 81–87
20. Fonkalsrud EW (1984) Endorectal ileoanal anastomosis with isoperistaltic ileal reservoir after colectomy and mucosal proctectomy. Ann Surg 199: 151–157
21. Fonkalsrud EW (1985) Endorectal ileal pullthrough with isoperistaltic ileal reservoir for colitis and polyposis. Ann Surg 202: 145–152
22. Fonkalsrud EW, Ament ME (1978) Endorectal mucosal resection without proctectomy as an adjunct to abdominoperineal resection for nonmalignant conditions: clinical experience with five patients. Ann Surg 188: 245–248
23. Franceschi D, Chen PF, Yuh JN (1986) Solitary J' pouch ulcer causing pouchitis-like syndrome. Dis Colon Rectum 29: 515–517
24. Fujiwara T, Kawarasaki H, Fonkalsrud EW (1984) Endorectal ileal pullthrough procedure after chemical debridement of the rectal mucosa. Surg Gynecol Obstet 158: 437–442
25. Grant D, Cohen Z, Mchugh S, McLeod R, Stern H (1986) Restorative proctocolectomy. Clinical results and manometric findings with long and short rectal cuffs. Dis Colon Rectum 29: 27–32
26. Hampton JM (1976) Rectal mucosal stripping: a technique for preservation of the rectum after total colectomy for chronic ulcerative colitis. Dis Colon Rectum 19: 133–135
27. Handelsmann JC, Fishbein RH, Hoover HC Jr, Smith GW, Haller JA Jr (1983) Endorectal pull-through operation in adults after colectomy and excision of rectal mucosa. Surgery 93: 247–253
28. Heimann TM, Bolnick K, Aufses AH (1986) Results of surgical treatment for familial polyposis coli. Am J Surg 152: 276–278
29. Heppell J, Kelly KA, Phillips SF, Beart RW Jr, Telander RL, Perrault J (1982) Physiologic aspects of continence after colectomy, mucosal proctectomy, and endorectal ileo-anal anastomosis. Ann Surg 195: 435–443
30. Heppell J, Weiland LH, Perrault J, Pemberton JH, Telander RL, Beart RW Jr (1983) Fate of the rectal mucosa after rectal mucosectomy and ileoanal anastomosis. Dis Colon Rectum 26: 768–771
31. Herfarth C, Stern J (1986) Die kontinenzerhaltende Proktocolektomie. Chirurg 57: 263–270
32. Hodgson WJB, Funkelstein JL, Woodriffe P, Aufses AH Jr (1979) Continent anal ileostomy with mucosal proctectomy: a bloodless technique using a surgical ultrasonic aspirator in dogs. Br J Surg 66: 857–860
33. Jagelman DG (1986) Choice of operation in familial adenomatosis coli. Ann Chir Gynaecol 75: 71–74
34. Kawarasaki H, Fujiwara T, Fonkalsrud EW (1985) Electric activity and motility in the side-to-side isoperistaltic ileal reservoir. Arch Surg 120: 1045–1047
35. Kestenberg A, Becker JM (1985) A new technique of loop ileostomy closure after endorectal ileoanal anastomosis. Surgery 98: 109–111
36. Kock NG (1969) Intra-abdominal "reservoir" in patients with permanent ileostomy: preliminary observations on a procedure resulting in fecal "continence" in five ileostomy patients. Arch Surg 99: 223–231
37. Kock NG, Myrvold HE, Nilsson LO, Philipson BM (1985) Achtzehn Jahre Erfahrung mit der kontinenten Ileostomie. Chirurg 56: 299–304
38. Kojima Y, Sanada Y, Fonkalsrud EW (1982) Evalua-

tion of techniques for chemical debridement of colonic mucosa. Surg Gynecol Obstet 155: 849–854

39. Kraske P (1885) Zur Exstirpation hochsitzender Mastdarmkrebse. Verh Dtsch Ges Chir 14: 464

40. Liljeqvist L, Lindquist K (1985) A reconstructive operation on malfunctioning S-shaped pelvic reservoirs. Dis Colon Rectum 28: 506–511

41. Lisfranc J (1826) Mémoire sur l'excision de la partie inférieure du rectum devenue carcinomateuse. Rev Med Fr 2: 380

42. Martin LW, Le Coultre C, Schubert WK (1977) Total colectomy and mucosal proctectomy with preservation of continence in ulcerative colitis. Ann Surg 186: 477–480

43. Metcalf AM, Dozois RR, Kelly KA, Beart RW Jr, Wolff BG (1985) Ileal "J" pouch-anal anastomosis: clinical outcome. Ann Surg 202: 735–739

44. Metcalf AM, Dozois RR, Kelly KA, Wolff BG (1986) Ileal pouch-anal anastomosis without temporary, diverting ileostomy. Dis Colon Rectum 29: 33–35

45. Moertel CG, Hill JR, Adson MA (1971) Management of multiple polyposis of the large bowel. Cancer 28: 160–164

46. Nasmyth DG, Williams NS, Johnston D (1986) Comparison of the function of triplicated and duplicated pelvic ileal reservoirs after mucosal proctectomy and ileo-anal anastomosis for ulcerative colitis and adenomatous polyposis. Br J Surg 73: 361–366

47. Neal DE, Williams NS, Johnston D (1982) Rectal, bladder and sexual function after mucosal proctectomy with and without a pelvic reservoir for colitis and polyposis. Br J Surg 69: 599–604

48. Nicholls RJ, Belliveau P, Neill M, Wilks M, Tabaqchali S (1981) Restorative proctocolectomy with ileal reservoir: a pathophysiological assessment. Gut 22: 462–468

49. Nicholls RJ, Moskowitz RL, Shepherd NA (1985) Restorative proctocolectomy with ileal reservoir. Br J Surg 72 [Suppl]: 576–579

50. Nicholls RJ, Pezim ME (1985) Restorative proctocolectomy with ileal reservoir for ulcerative colitis and familial adenomatous polyposis: a comparison of three reservoir designs. Br J Surg 72: 470–474

51. Nilsson LO, Kock NG, Lindgren I, Myrvold HE, Philipson BM, Ohren C (1980) Morphological and histochemical changes in the mucosa of the continent ileostomy reservoir 6–10 years after its construction. Scand J Gastroenterol 15: 737–747

52. Nissen R (1933) Demonstrationen aus der operativen Chirurgie, no 39. Berlin Surgical Society. Zentralbl Chir 60: 888

53. Parc R, Frileux P, Tiret E, Huguet C, Levy E, Loygue J (1985) Coloproctectomie, proctectomie muqueuse distale, anastomose iléo-anale avec réservoir (36 cas). IXème Journées Francophones d'Hépatologie et de Gastroentérologie, Brussels

54. Parks A (1982) Ileo-anal pouch operation. In: Heberer G, Denecke H (eds) Colo-rectal surgery. Springer, Berlin Heidelberg New York, pp 105–106

55. Parks AG, Nicholls RJ (1978) Proctocolectomy without ileostomy for ulcerative colitis. Br Med J 2: 85–88

56. Parks AG, Nicholls RJ, Belliveau P (1980) Proctocolectomy with ileal reservoir and anal anastomosis. Br J Surg 67: 533–538

57. Peck DA (1980) Rectal mucosal replacement. Ann Surg 191: 294–303

58. Pemberton JH, Heppell J, Beart RW Jr, Dozois RR, Telander RL (1982) Endorectal ileoanal anastomosis. Surg Gynecol Obstet 155: 417–424

59. Pescatori M, Parks AG (1984) Transmucosal myotomy of the small bowel after ileoanal anastomosis. Dis Colon Rectum 27: 316–318

60. Ravitch MM, Sabiston DC Jr (1947) Anal ileostomy with preservation of the sphincter: a proposed operation in patients requiring total colectomy for benign lesions. Surg Gynecol Obstet 84: 1095–1099

61. Rohner A (1985) L'anastomose iléo-anale: alternative à l'iléostomie définitive? Schweiz Rundsch Med Prax 36: 942–946

62. Rothenberger DA, Vermeulen FD, Christenson CE, Balcos EG, Nemer FD, Goldenberg SM, Belliveau P, Nivatvongs S, Schottler JL, Fang DT, Kennedy HL (1983) Restorative proctocolectomy with ileal reservoir and ileoanal anastomosis. Am J Surg 145: 82–88

63. Rothenberger DA, Wong WD, Buls JG, Goldberg SM, Christenson CE (1984) Restorative proctocolectomy with ileal reservoir and ileoanal anastomosis for ulcerative colitis and familial polyposis. Dig Surg 1: 19–26

64. Rothenberger DA, Buls JG, Nivatvongs S, Goldberg SM (1985) The Parks S ileal pouch and anal anastomosis after colectomy and mucosal proctectomy. Am J Surg 149: 390–394

65. Safaie-Shirazi S, Soper RT (1973) Endorectal pullthrough procedure in the surgical treatment of familial polyposis coli. J Pediatr Surg 8: 711–716

66. Schoetz DJ Jr, Coller JA, Veidenheimer MC (1985) Alternatives to conventional ileostomy in chronic ulcerative colitis. Surg Clin North Am 65: 21–33

67. Schraut WH, Block GE (1982) Ileoanal anastomosis with proximal ileal reservoir: an experimental study. Surgery 91: 275–281

68. Schraut WH, Rosemurgy AS, Wang CH, Block GE (1983) Determinants of optimal results after ileoanal anastomosis: anal proximity and motility patterns of the ileal reservoir. World J Surg 7: 400–408

69. Soave F (1964) Hirschsprung's disease: a new surgical technique. Arch Dis Child 39: 116–124

70. Stone MM, Lewin K, Fonkalsrud EW (1986) Late obstruction of the lateral ileal reservoir after colectomy and endorectal ileal pullthrough procedures. Surg Gynecol Obstet 162: 411–417

71. Stryker SJ, Borody TJ, Phillips SF, Kelly KA, Dozois RR, Beart RW Jr (1985) Motility of the small intestine after proctocolectomy and ileal pouch-anal anastomosis. Ann Surg 201: 351–356

72. Stryker SJ, Daube JR, Kelly KA, Telander RL, Phillips SF, Beart RW Jr, Dozois RR (1985) Anal sphincter electromyography after colectomy, mucosal rectectomy, and ileoanal anastomosis. Arch Surg 120: 713–716

73. Stryker SJ, Phillips SF, Dozois RR, Kelly KA, Beart RW Jr (1986) Anal and neorectal function after ileal pouch-anal anastomosis. Ann Surg 203: 55–61

74. Taylor BM, Beart RW Jr, Dozois RR, Kelly KA, Phillips SF (1983) Straight ileoanal anastomosis vs ileal pouch-anal anastomosis after colectomy and mucosal proctectomy. Arch Surg 118: 696–701

75. Taylor BM, Beart RW Jr, Dozois RR, Kelly KA, Wolff BG, Ilstrup DM (1984) The endorectal ileal pouch-anal anastomosis: current clinical results. Dis Colon Rectum 27: 347–350

76. Telander RL, Perrault J (1980) Total colectomy with rectal mucosectomy and ileoanal anastomosis for chronic ulcerative colitis in children and young adults. Mayo Clin Proc 55: 420–433
77. Turnbull RB, Weakley FL (1967) Atlas of intestinal stomas. Mosby, St Louis, p 207
78. Utsunomiya J, Iwama T, Imajo M, Matsuo S, Sawai S, Yaegashi K, Hirayama R (1980) Total colectomy, mucosal proctectomy, and ileoanal anastomosis. Dis Colon Rectum 23: 459–466
79. Utsunomiya J, Oota M, Iwama T (1986) Recent trends in ileoanal anastomosis. Ann Chir Gynaecol 75: 56–62
80. Valiente MA, Bacon HE (1955) Construction of pouch using "pantaloon" technic for pull-through of ileum following total colectomy: report of experimental work and results. Am J Surg 90: 742–750
81. Watne AL, Carrier JM, Durham JP, Hrabovsky EE, Chang W (1983) The occurrence of carcinoma of the rectum following ileoproctostomy for familial polyposis. Ann Surg 197: 550–554
82. Waugh JM, Turner JC Jr (1958) A study of 268 patients with carcinoma of the midrectum treated by abdominoperineal resection with sphincter preservation. Surg Gynecol Obstet 107: 777–783
83. Williams NS, Johnston D (1985) The current status of mucosal proctectomy and ileo-anal anastomosis in the surgical treatment of ulcerative colitis and adenomatous polyposis. Br J Surg 72: 159–168
84. Williams NS (1986) Restorative proctocolectomy with ileal reservoir: symposium. Int J Color Dis 1: 2–19
85. Wolfstein IH, Bat L, Neumann G (1982) Regeneration of rectal mucosa and recurrent polyposis coli after total colectomy and ileoanal anastomosis. Arch Surg 117: 1241–1242

16 Rectovaginal Fistulas

M.-C. Marti

Rectovaginal fistulas are located above the dentate line and should therefore be distinguished from ano-vaginal fistulas. These lesions are rare and account for less than 5% of all anorectal fistulas. They result in very severe and distressing vaginal symptoms which vary according the underlying disease: fecal soiling and smell, discharge, vaginitis, passage of flatus and even feces especially during diarrhea, discharge of mucus or blood.

Etiology

A rectovaginal fistula may result from a great variety of lesions as summarized in Table 16.1. Published statistics give very different incidences of the various etiologies due mainly to the referral pattern of particular surgeons or hospitals. Obstetrical injuries are responsible for 11%–88% of rectovaginal fistulas [9, 14, 16]. Prolonged labour may induce necrosis of the rectovaginal septum. Nowadays such lesions are rare in Western countries but still frequent in medically undeveloped countries.

Inflammatory bowel diseases are responsible for 2%–22% of rectovaginal fistulas. Crohn's disease seems to be much more responsible in causing fistulas than is colitis due to the transmural involvement [1, 7, 8, 25].

Irradiation of pelvic cancer, mainly utero-cervico-vaginal cancers, may result in proctitis complicated by necrosis and fistula. Lesions should be carefully biopsied to rule out recurrent cancer as they may occur 6 months to 2 years after therapy. Contact therapy with high local dosage is more frequently responsible for fistulas than external irradiation.

Clinical Evaluation

Complete gynecological and anorectal examination is necessary to confirm the presence of a fistula; to determine the size, extension, and location of the tract; to assess the state of the sphincter; to determine the presence of an underlying disease. Therefore, vaginal examination, proctoscopy, sigmoido-or colonoscopy, barium enema, fistulograms, and numerous biopsies should be performed.

Table 16.1. Etiology of rectovaginal fistulas

Infection	Anal gland Bartholin's abscess
Inflammatory bowel disease	Crohn's disease Colitis
Obstetrical trauma	Childbirth injury Prolonged labor with septum necrosis
Operative trauma	Vaginal or rectal procedures
Trauma	Violence Impalement Forceful coitus Foreign bodies Dilator after vaginal plasty
Hematological disorders	Leukemia Agranulocytosis
Irradiation injury	External irradiation Curietherapy for cervix or endometrium carcinoma
Tumor	Uterine, cervical, vaginal, rectal cancers Endometriosis Giant condyloma
Congenital disorders	

Table 16.2. Classification of rectovaginal fistulas

	Level in the anorectum	Level in the vagina
Low fistula	Slightly above dentate line	Inside vaginal fourchette
Mid fistula	Between low and high fistula	
High fistula	In the mid-rectum	Behind or near the cervix

Classification

Rectovaginal fistulas can be classified according their location and their size (Table 16.2). Exact location is useful in determining if repair can be performed by a perineal or a transabdominal approach. A fistula is "small" if less than 0.5 cm in diameter; "medium" if it is 0.5–2.5 cm, and "large" if over 2.5 cm in diameter.

Treatment

Medical Treatment

Spontaneous or nonsurgical healing of a rectovaginal fistula depends on its etiology, its size, and its extent. It occurs in half the cases of small rectovaginal fistulas which are secondary to obstetrical trauma [19]. In these cases, local treatment, removal of foreign bodies (especially stitches after repair of an episiotomy or a perineal tear resulting in episioproctotomy), dietetic measures, and prescription of bulk-forming agents may be useful in achieving spontaneous healing. In cases of inflammatory bowel disease, aggressive medical treatment is usually unsuccessful. Furthermore, irradiation- or neoplasm-induced fistulas never heal spontaneously.

Surgical Treatment

Preoperative Conditions

Surgery should be attempted only if the condition of the patient is optimal. This means that the underlying disease has been aggressively treated with steroids, sulfalazine, antibiotics, antidiarrheal agents, and hyperalimentation. Local tissues should be as normal as possible.

A temporary left iliac terminal colostomy may be necessary to achieve these conditions. Thereafter, surgery must be planned after an interval of several weeks to a few months in cases of traumatic rectovaginal fistulas [14] or after 1 year or more in patients with fistulas which have been caused by irradiation [13].

With or without colostomy, a bowel preparation is mandatory: the large bowel and rectum should be absolutely empty. No feces should be in contact with sutures for at least 7–10 days. Vaginal preparation with mechanical cleansing regimens and local disinfectants should be carried out. Perioperative broad-spectrum antibiotics are recommended to prevent delayed healing, fistula recurrence, and cellulitis. The bladder should be drained by urethral catheter or suprapubic cystocatheter.

Table 16.3. Surgical procedures for correction of rectovaginal fistulas

Local repairs
Fistulotomy and drainage
Laying open followed by primary suture
Inversion of fistula
Excision of fistula with layer closure ± muscle interposition through
- Vaginal approach
- Rectal approach
- Combined rectovaginal approach
- Perineal approach
- Transsphincteric approach of Mason

Sliding flap advancements
Mucosa and partial thickness of the internal sphincter (Laird)
Anterior rectal wall (Noble)
Segmental internal sphincter (Belt)
Endorectal

Sphincter-preserving transabdominal repairs
Mobilization, division, layer closure without bowel resection
± interposition of omentum
Pull-through procedures
Low anterior resection (with hand suture or stapler)
Transsacral resection – anastomosis
Sleeve anastomosis (Parks)
Onlay patch anastomosis (Bricker)

Abdominoperineal resection
Colostomy

Approaches

Several approaches are possible; the choice depends on the height of the tract, the quality of local tissue, the underlying disease, and the chosen technique. Rectal, vaginal, perineal, abdominal, transsphincteric, and transsacral approaches are possible, singly or, mainly, in combination. Possible techniques are listed in Table 16.3.

Local Repairs

Fistulectomy and Drainage

Fistulectomy and drainage is the procedure of choice for anovaginal fistula but results in severe and definitive incontinence in cases of rectovaginal fistulas. Simple fistulotomy should not be advocated for rectovaginal fistulas any longer.

Laying Open Followed by Primary Suture

This technique is mainly used by gynecologists for complete perineal tears or episioproctotomy [9, 11, 19, 21]. The entire rectovaginal tract is excised which means resection of all the sphincters and pe-

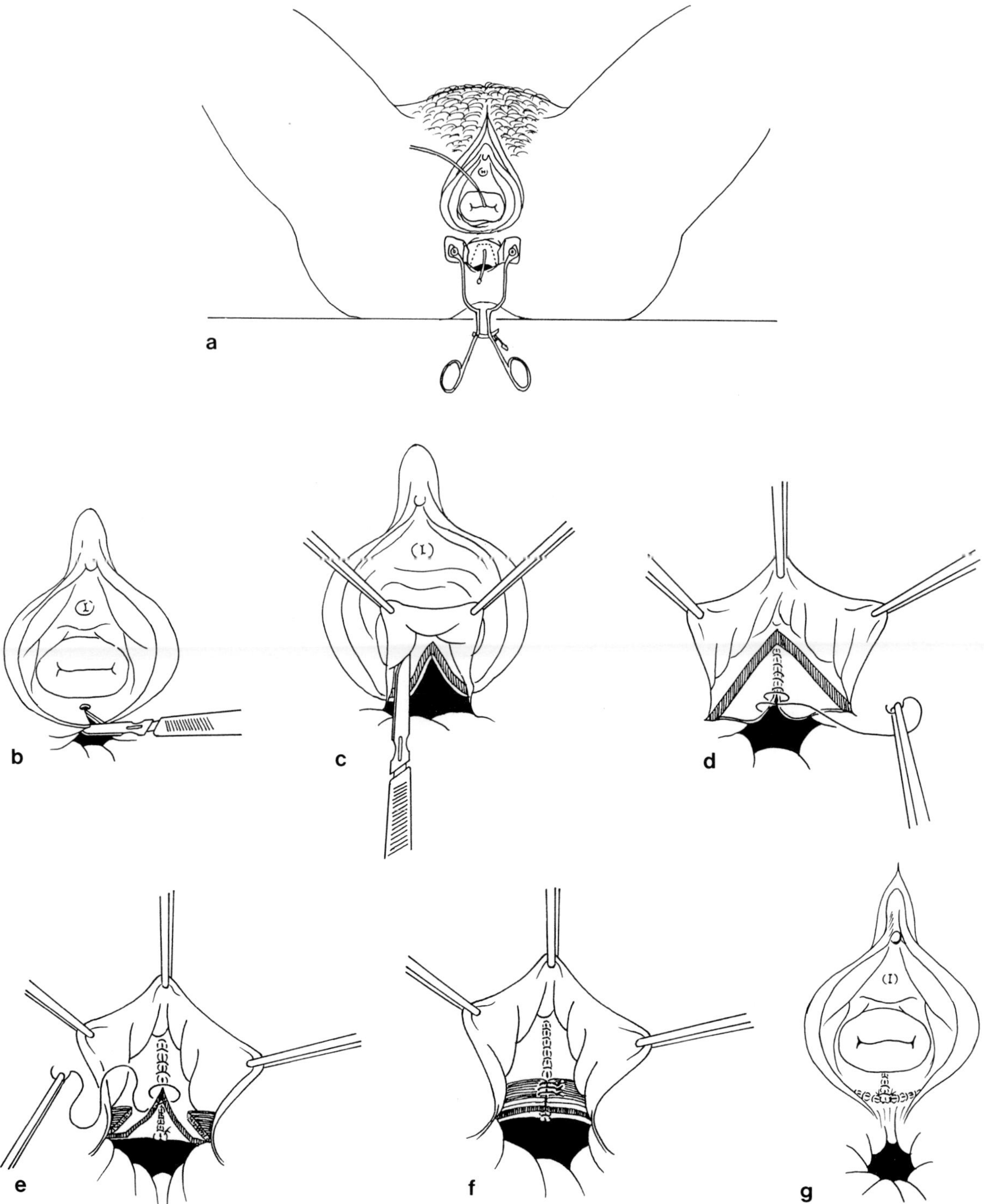

Fig. 16.1 a–g. Laying open of a rectovaginal fistula. **a** Catheterization of the fistulous tract; **b** opening of the tract; **c** mobilization of the vaginal mucosa; **d** suture of anal mucosa; **e** suture of internal sphincter and rectal musculature; **f** suture of external sphincter; **g** closure of mucosal and skin wounds to reconstruct perineal body

rineal body (Fig. 16.1). After mobilization and dissection of anorectal and vaginal walls, the wound is closed layer by layer with absorbable suture material. The anorectal wall is closed; external and internal sphincters are sutured with monofilament absorbable material; fat, vaginal and anal skin are closed.

There are no reports of long-term follow-up, but immediate 100% successful repair has been reported by Given [9] and Hibbard [14].

Musset [21] has used a technique of laying open followed by secondary suture. The first step is an episioproctotomy without colostomy. After healing of any infectious tract, 6–8 weeks after the first step, reconstruction of the rectovaginal septum is performed, no dissection of the sphincter muscles is necessary, and, using a Reverdin needle, retracting edges of the sphincter may be sutured together.

Stitches are withdrawn on the 7th day. Published results are very good: more than 96% of cases are totally cured, even those that have already been treated by various other procedures without success.

Inversion of Fistula

Small low rectovaginal fistulas surrounded by healthy tissue may be treated by inversion. Using a vaginal approach, a circular incision is made around the vaginal opening (Fig. 16.2). The flaps of vaginal mucosa are mobilized. Several purse-string sutures are placed to obliterate and invert the fistula into the bowel. The mucosa is closed with continuous or separate stitches.

Local Excision With Layer Closure

Excision of the fistulous tract followed by layer closure has been tried using a vaginal approach (Fig. 16.3) or a rectal approach [12]. Disadvantages of these methods of local repair resulting in high recurrence rate are the excessive tension on the suture line due to insufficient mobilization and to direct apposition of rectal and vaginal sutures. To prevent apposition of suture lines, a vascularized flap of muscle or fatty tissue can be interposed.

Goligher [11] proposed a transperineal approach with broad dissection of the rectovaginal septum. After the fistula is divided, the fistulous opening on

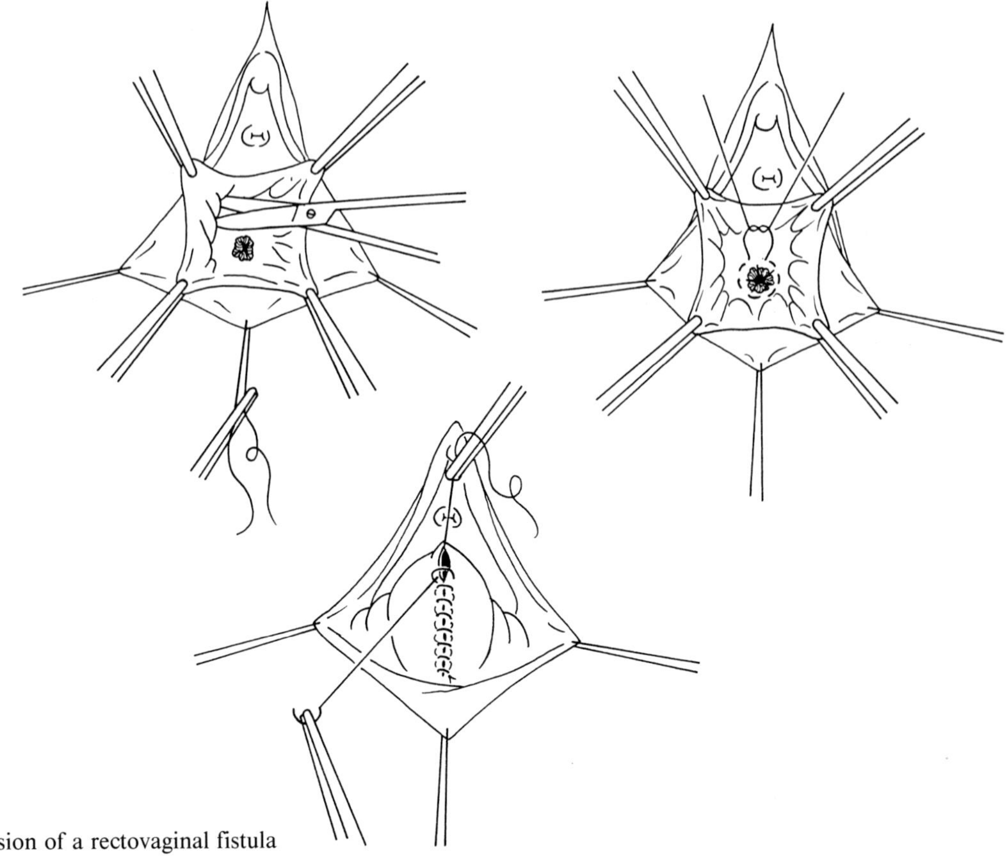

Fig. 16.2. Inversion of a rectovaginal fistula

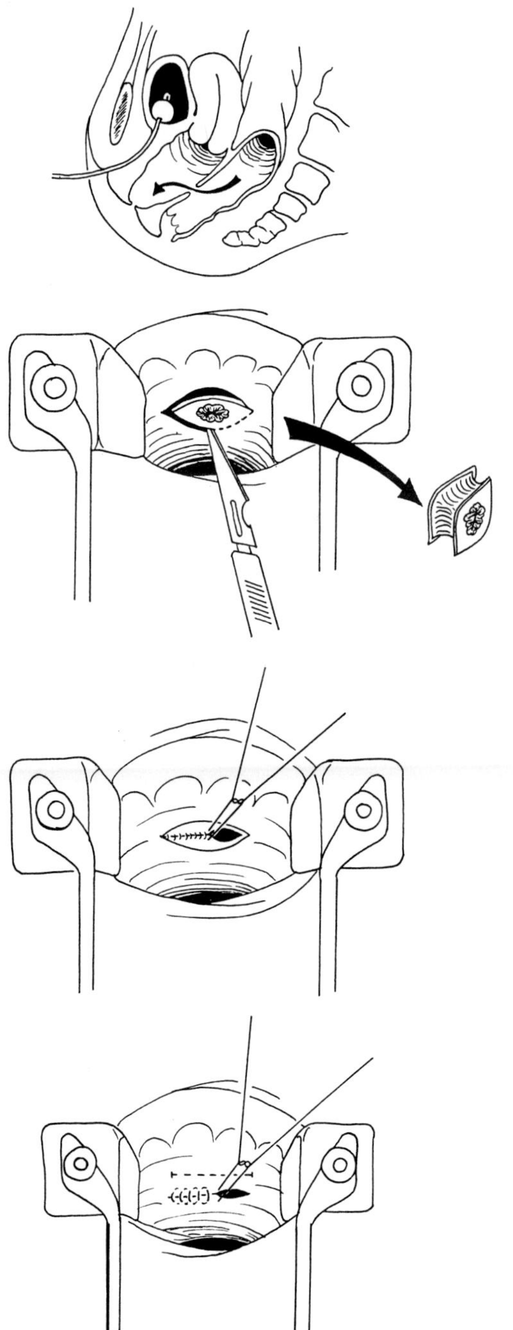

Fig. 16.3. Local excision of a rectovaginal fistula with layer closure

the rectal and vaginal mucosa is closed by interrupted sutures without tension. The muscular layers are closed to ensure interposition between the mucosa sutures. If possible, the rectum and vagina are slightly rotated in opposite directions to prevent direct apposition of the suture lines.

Results using this layer closure are very variable.

Lescher and Pratt [16] report a 84% recurrence rate, and Given [9] reports a 30% recurrence rate. Hibbard [14] achieved primary healing in 14 cases. Such a repair should not be attempted for a high rectovaginal fistula. Nevertheless, Lawson [15] could successfully repair 42 out of 53 high fistulas by opening the pouch of Douglas to facilitate closure of the fistula.

Transsphincteric Approach

The transsphincteric approach described by Mason [18] to treat rectoprostatic fistulas has also been used to treat rectovaginal fistulas. This approach may be useful to treat a mid or high fistulous tract without opening the abdominal cavity.

Flap Advancements

Several methods have been described using mucosal flaps [10, 20, 22, 24]. Advancement of the anterior rectal wall was already used by Noble in 1902 [22]. Belt [2] and Goldberg [10] use an anorectal flap consisting of mucosa, submucosa, and circular muscle (Fig. 16.4). The base of the flap should be twice the width of the apex to prevent interference with blood supply. The flap is about 7 cm in length, but at least 4 cm above the fistula. After raising the flap, the muscular layers are mobilized laterally and sutured without tension on the midline. The perineal body and the rectovaginal septum are reconstructed by interrupted sutures of absorbable material. Any excess flap, including the rectovaginal fistula, is excised. The vagina is left open to allow drainage. Using this procedure, primary healing was achieved by Goldberg in 22 out of 25 patients.

Sphincter-Preserving Transabdominal Repairs

Local repairs and flaps advancements cannot be used to cure high rectovaginal fistulas whatever origin they may have. In the case of a fistula caused by irradiation, tissue quality is so bad that suturing is impossible. In these cases, an abdominal approach may be necessary.

In the most simple procedure, the rectovaginal septum is mobilized from above, the fistulous tract is divided; the apertures or defects in the rectal and vaginal walls are closed by interrupted sutures. Well-vascularized tissue, mainly omentum, is interposed. Such a procedure is possible if the quality of local tissue is nearly normal [3, 9, 11]. It is impossible in cases of irradiation change, inflammatory bowel disease, carcinoma, or diverticulitis. In these

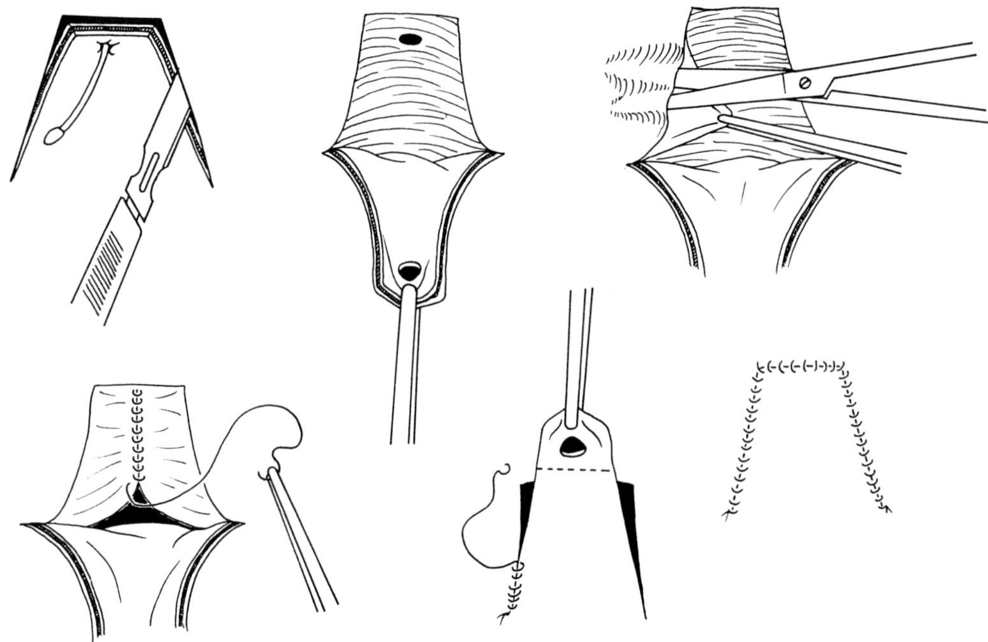

Fig. 16.4. Rectoanal flap advancement

cases, a resection of at least the rectosigmoid may be required. If the anal sphincter can be preserved, continuity should be restored by a pull-through procedure [6], a very low anterior resection with hand or stapled suture, a sleeve anastomosis, or even a combined abdominotranssacral reconstruction [17].

To prevent recurrence of the fistulous tract and anastomotic dehiscence, the bowel suture line must be at a far lower level than the vaginal closure, the proximal bowel must be free of disease and have an optimal blood supply, and tissue should be interposed between rectum and vagina. Several procedures have been described. Omentum pedicles based on the right gastroepiploic artery have been used [3, 11]. A flap of tissue including the bulbocavernous muscle and the adjacent labial fat or Martius graft has been interposed [9, 13, 18]. Gracilis muscle has been transferred from the thigh, and also flaps of the rectus abdominis muscle have been advocated [13]. The use of the long adductor, sartorius, or gluteus maximus muscles have also been reported [5, 9].

Parks [23] has described a technique of sleeve anastomosis. He used it to treat five postirradiation rectovaginal fistulas. After mobilization the recum is divided at the level of the rectovaginal fistula. The remaining rectal mucosa is stripped off the underlying muscle from the anus as far as the dentate line. The lower part of the rectum is totally denuded leaving a muscular stump or cuff. The healthy proximal colon is threaded through the muscle sleeve covering the fistula; the anastomosis is performed through the anus at the level of the dentate line.

Onlay Patch Anastomosis

An onlay patch anastomosis has been devised by Bricker [4] and used with success in five patients suffering from radiation-induced rectovaginal fistula. The rectosigmoid colon is mobilized and the rectovaginal fistula is exposed (Fig. 16.5). The sigmoid colon is divided; the distal part is turned down and anastomosed to the excised edges of the fistulous opening in the rectum. With the proximal part, an end-iliac colostomy is established. At the second stage, after healing has been radiologically and endoscopically established, the proximal colostomy is mobilized and sutured end-to-side to the intrapelvic loop of the rectosigmoid.

Bricker [4] states that this procedure has several advantages over the other methods of repair: the whole rectum need not be mobilized; the presacral space is not opened, preventing hemorrage from presacral venous plexus and neurological damage; continence will not be altered. The risk of leakage still exists as the turned down sigmoid has also been irradiated.

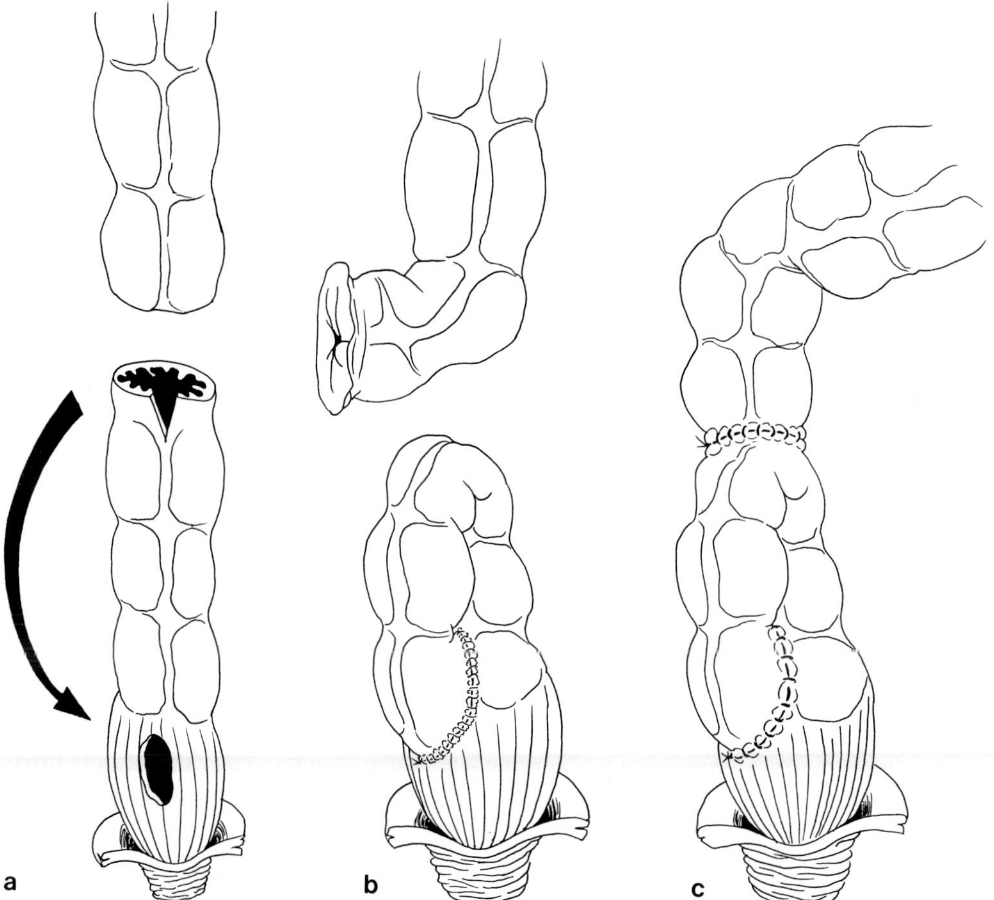

Fig. 16.5a–c. Onlay patch anastomosis to treat a high rectovaginal fistula

Abdominoperineal Resection

In cases of extensive carcinoma with fistula arising from the rectum, from the uterus, or from the vagina, major surgery may be necessary. Abdominoperineal resection or even pelvic exenteration may be indicated. In active and extensive inflammatory bowel disease, proctectomy and or colectomy may be required [7].

Other Procedures

Poor-risk patients may be treated by a total diverting colostomy. In elderly patients who are unable to manage a colostomy, a colpocleisis may be proposed forming a common chamber from the vagina and the rectum [9, 13].

Optimal Choice of Procedure

The optimal choice of procedure depends on the location, the size, and the etiology of the fistula, the possible involvement of adjacent organs, and the patient's general condition. Local repair can be attempted in good-risk patients (obstetrical and traumatic fistula). A protective colostomy may be necessary to reduce risk of leakage. Resection and the onlay patch technique should be considered for irradiation-induced fistulas. In cases of inflammatory bowel disease, no repair should be attempted unless the disease is in remission.

Carcinomatous fistula can only be treated by extensive surgery; if the patient's condition is too poor to sustain a major operation, definitive terminal colostomy must be planned.

References

1. Beecham CT (1972) Recurring recto-vaginal fistula. Am J Obstet Gynecol 40: 323
2. Belt RL, Belt RL Jr (1969) Repair of anorectal vaginal fistula utilizing segmental advancement of the internal sphincter muscle. Dis Colon Rectum 12: 99–103
3. Bentley RJ (1973) Abdominal repair of high rectovaginal fistula. J Obstet Gynecol Br Commonw 80: 364–367
4. Bricker EM, Johnston WD (1979) Repair of postirradiation rectovaginal fistula and stricture. Surg Gynecol Obstet 148: 499–506
5. Byron RL, Ostergard DR (1969) Sartorius muscle interposition for the treatment of radiation-induced vaginal fistula. Am J Obstet Gynecol 104: 104–107
6. Cuthbertson AM, Buzzart AJ (1973) Pullthrough resection of the rectum with vagino-cystoplasty for repair of a rectovesicovaginal fistula. Aust NZ J Surg 43: 72–78
7. Faulconer HT, Muldoon JP (1975) Rectovaginal fistula in patient with colitis. Dis Colon Rectum 18: 413–415
8. Givel JC, Hawker P, Allan RN, Alexander-Williams J (1982) Enterovaginal fistulas associated with Crohn's disease. Surg Gynecol Obstet 155: 494–496
9. Given FT (1970) Rectovaginal fistula: a review of 20 years' experience in a community hospital. Am J Obstet Gynecol 108: 41–46
10. Goldberg SM (1980) Rectovaginal fistula. In: Goldberg SM, Gordon PP, Nivatvongs S (eds) Essentials of anorectal surgery. Lippincott, Philadelphia, pp 316–332
11. Goligher JC (1975) Rectovaginal fistula and irradiation proctitis and enteritis. In: Goligher JC (ed) Surgery of the anus, rectum and colon. Thomas, Springfield
12. Greenwald JC, Hoexter B (1978) Repair of rectovaginal fistula. Surg Gynecol Obstet 146: 443–445
13. Graham JB (1965) Vaginal fistulas following radiotherapy. Surg Gynecol Obstet 120: 1019–1030
14. Hibbard LT (1978) Surgical management of rectovaginal fistulas and complete perineal tears. Am J Obstet Gynecol 130: 139–147
15. Lawson J (1972) Rectovaginal fistulae following difficult labour. Proc R Soc Med 65: 283–286
16. Lescher TC, Pratt JH (1967) Vaginal repair of the simple rectovaginal fistula. Surg Gynecol Obstet 124: 1317–1321
17. Marks G (1976) Combined abdominotranssacral reconstruction of radiation injured rectum. Am J Surg 131: 54–59
18. Mason AY (1974) Transsphincteric surgery of the rectum. Prog Surg 13: 66–97
19. Mattingly RF (1977) Anal incontinence and rectovaginal fistulas. In: Te Linde RW (ed) Operative gynecology, 5 edn. Lippincott, Philadelphia
20. Mengert WF, Fish SA (1955) Anterior rectal wall advancement: technic for repair of complete perineal laceration and rectovaginal fistula. Obstet Gynecol 5: 262–265
21. Musset R (1978) Fistules rectovaginales. Encycl Med Chir Paris Techniques chirurgicales 4.4.06.41870
22. Noble GH (1902) A new operation for complete laceration of the perineum designed for the purpose of eliminating danger of infection from the rectum. Trans Am Gynecol Soc 27: 357
23. Parks AG, Allen CL, Frank JD, McPartlin JF (1978) A method of treating postirradiation rectovaginal fistulas. Br J Surg 65: 417–421
24. Russel TR, Gallagher DM (1977) Low rectovaginal fistulas. Approach and treatment. Am J Surg 134: 13–18
25. Tuxen PA, Castro AF (1979) Rectovaginal fistula in Crohn's disease. Dis Colon Rectum 22: 58–62

17 Prostatorectal Fistulas

P. Graber

Introduction

Prostatorectal fistula is a rare condition. Major clinical descriptions are not found in the literature where the problem is mostly dealt with in the form of case reports. This has not always been so. The earliest known observation of such a fistula was described by Wagnerum in 1685, and the first attempts at surgical closure were made early in the last century, namely by Ashley Cooper in 1823. Surgical treatment of the condition was always regarded as difficult and involving many obstacles and complications. This situation can be explained in part by the paucity of suitable technical aids at the time, but it must also be borne in mind that these historical cases had little in common with those encountered today. At the present time we are usually confronted with single fistulas in a more or less healthy terrain, whereas in the past the patients presented with complicated fistulas marked by sinuosities and irregularities, and accompanied by abscesses with multiple openings. These fistulas were mostly of tuberculous origin, whereas tuberculosis has nowadays given place to traumatic and, above all, iatrogenic lesions [6].

Physiopathology

The prostate is separated from the rectum by a double wall consisting of the prostatic body itself and the fascia of Denonvilliers, or rectovesical septum, which is an extension of the peritoneal fold of Douglas. This barrier is practically impassable by tumors, and it is rare for it to be invaded by rectal carcinomas in the one direction or by prostatic tumors in the other. However, to some extent the two organs share a common vascular system. The veins of the middle rectum empty into the periprostatic plexus, which in turn drains into the internal iliac vein. Lymphatic drainage of both organs is in the same direction, with convergence toward the hypogastric and iliac ganglia. The fascia of Denonvilliers – which resists invasion by tumors – can therefore be evaded by an infection. This explains the occurrence of suppurating prostatitis and especially of tuberculosis associated with prostatorectal fistulas.

The occurrence and, above all, persistence of a prostatorectal fistula are dependent on the coincidence of a number of factors (Fig. 17.1), in particular an empty prostatic capsule or one with a pathological content, and an obstacle to urinary flow. The consequent urinary pressure keeps the fistula open and results in drainage from the prostate toward the rectum and not – as the alternative term "rectoprostatic" would indicate – in the opposite direction. The rare exceptions are in boys with anorectal agenesis and communication of a rectal fistula at the level of the utricle. In newborn infants with this malformation the meconium and feces are excreted via the urinary tract.

Pathogenesis

Surgical Complications

The most common cause of disorders of the prostatic capsule is a surgical operation (Table 17.1). The fibrous capsule surrounding the prostate thickens with age and also as a result of nodular hyperplasia – the so-called adenoma – of the central part of the organ. During a "prostatectomy" operation the adenoma is split either with the finger or with the handle of the resectoscope at a readily identifiable level and is thus separated from the capsule. The aim of the operation is to leave an empty and regularly shaped prostatic capsule. In patients with inflammatory affections such as prostatitis or, in particular, cancer, cleavage of the adenoma is difficult or even impossible since these disorders originate in the peripheral part of the organ before in-

Table 17.1. Etiological classification of rectoprostatic fistulas

Complications of surgery or X-ray therapy	65–80%
Injuries	15%
Abscess	5–10%

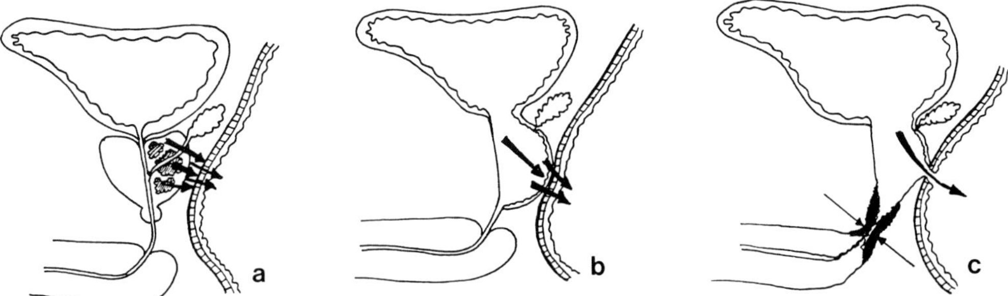

*Fig. 17.1. **a** Prostatic segment with pathological content;   **b** empty prostatic segment;   **c** urethral stenosis below the prostatic segment

vading its center. When this is the case, the rectal wall is often accidently perforated by instruments used in attempts to remove adherent portions of tissue. This complication often remains undiscovered during the operation and is subsequently hidden by the bladder catheter. Urine is seen to be escaping via the rectum only after the latter has been withdrawn [5].

This anatomical risk is greatest in radical operations for cancer. In radical prostatectomy, unlike the adenomectomy described, the whole of the gland is excised along with the capsule and the seminal vesicles. The level of dissection passes behind the prostate and along the fascia of Denonvilliers on the anterior aspect of the rectum as far as the urethra. The intervention terminates in a vesicourethral anastomosis at this level. The topographical risks associated with radical surgery are tempered by the good visibility of the anterior wall of the rectum. In the case of a lesion – provided the rupture does not exdeed 1–2 cm in size – it can be repaired by means of a primary suture. Another rectal lesion described in patients undergoing curative treatment for cancer of the prostate is actinic necrosis due to interstitial radiotherapy [4]. In this combined approach, the prostate is exposed surgically, and elements producing short-range radiation are inserted to create an intense and homogeneous irradiation field. The fistulas observed are the result of local overdosage. On account of the nature of the terrain involved, their treatment poses a difficult problem.

Endoscopic Surgery

Rectal lesions are only a rare occurrence in endoscopic surgery of the prostate. Even when there is no definite level of cleavage, directional control is fully maintained, so that transurethral resection is effective as a palliative treatment of cancers of the prostate. However, accidents may occur during the positioning of instruments. Thus the importance of the urethral angulation at the bulbomembranous level is often overlooked. An instrument introduced forcibly without regard for this physiological angulation will head straight toward the rectum and may perforate it at the level of the prostatic apex. Again, in the presence of a carcinomatous block past which a rigid instrument must occasionally be forced, perforation of the rectum is by no means a rare event. This complication is revealed immediately by the evacuation of rinsing fluid via the rectum.

Infectious Fistulas

Small accidental fistulas will probably heal spontaneously provided urinary flow is not obstructed by urethral stenosis. The narrowing of the urethra is, however, not a complication but usually the principal etiological factor. In fact, the high urinary pressure prevents healing of the prostatitis, while intraprostatic urinary reflux causes permanent reinfection. The infected material is mainly retained in the posterior lobe whose efferent canals are long and narrow. Abscesses may occur in the immediate proximity of the rectum, with inherent danger of perforation. The causative organisms are usually those of the intestinal flora.

Diagnosis

Clinical Examination

The diagnosis of prostatorectal fistula is primarily clinical. The patient sees the loss of urine via the rectum immediately after micturition, or he discharges gas and occasionally solids along with his urine. The severity of these symptoms naturally depends on the size of the fistula. The clinical examination begins with perineal inspection for the presence of other possible fistular openings indicative of a complex system. The elasticity of the tissues, and particularly the tone of the anal sphincter, may be impaired by inflammatory fibrosis. A prostato-rectal fistula is located 5–6 cm from the anal verge and can normally be found by rectal palpation. A vesical tube inserted prior to the examination can sometimes be palpated directly across the rectum. Rectal palpation will furnish information not only on the diameter and localization of the fistula, but also on the shape and mobility of the residue of the prostatic capsule. Persistent adenomatous foci, cancerous nodules, or dullness indicating an undrained abscess will jeopardize any attempt at repair.

Radiological Diagnosis

The clinical diagnosis is completed by a radiological examination which includes retrograde urethrocystography and an anterograde exposure during micturition. Retrograde filling of the bladder is carried out with a 10% contrast medium solution given by a syringe applied directly to the external urethral meatus. The cystograms so obtained provide information on the morphology and volume of the bladder as well as on the configuration of the prostatic compartment. Urethrography performed during micturition allows the functioning of the bladder-neck to be studied and above all enables a distal urethral stenosis to be excluded. The passage of contrast medium between the prostatic urethra and the rectum cannot, however, be visualized in all cases. Small fistulas are occasionally obstructed by inflammatory edema. A large fistula, on the other hand, can result in the escape of contrast medium into the rectum, with consequent failure to visualize the bladder. Clearly the topography of a complex fistular system must be studied by fistulography using a viscous contrast medium.

Endoscopy

The diagnostic procedure of greatest value, especially in patients with postoperative fistulas, is urethral endoscopy. Introduction of a urethrocystoscope makes direct visualization of the fistular opening possible. In cases with retraction due to scarring, the anterior wall of the rectum must be lifted with the finger in order to bring the fistula into the visual field of the instrument. Endoscopy furnishes information on the state of the prostatic capsule, which is often deformed by scarring and by the residue of the adenoma. Although endoscopy of the rectum and anus does not help greatly in patients with low fistulas, it is clear that a complete examination of the anal canal must precede any attempt at repair of a complex fistular system.

Differential Diagnosis

The classical urinary symptomatology of prostatorectal fistulas may be modified by previous prostatic surgery. Prostatectomy namely supresses the bladder-neck and the anatomical separation between the latter organ and the prostatic urethra is abolished. Urine can penetrate freely into the prostatic urethra and passage of urine through the fistula thus becomes permanent. In this situation it becomes difficult to distinguish between a urethral and a vesicorectal fistula.

A similar problem arises in severe posttraumatic situations in which the origin of a urinary leak is not always obvious. The leak can namely be ureteral, vesical, or urethral, either exclusively or in combination. In the face of a problem of this kind, it is essential to carry out an i. v. urography in order to obtain an overall picture of the upper urinary tract. A CT scan can also yield valuable topographical information on injured pelvic compartment.

Treatment

Conservative Treatment

Conservative measures can be tried in patients with small prostatorectal fistulas in whom spontaneous healing is possible. Such measures are formally indicated in patients with small perforations occurring during endoscopy which are recognized immediately. The following are recommended:

- Urethral catheter (20 French) with continuous drainage
- Antibiotic therapy directed against all gram-negative and anaerobic pathogens
- An "astronaut" diet for 2 weeks

Healing generally ensues within 10–15 days. It must be confirmed radiologically.

Conservative Treatment With Colostomy

As a general rule, prostatorectal lesions caused by endoscopic procedures have a greater tendency to spontaneous healing than those due to open surgery [8]. In the presence of a defect with an opening exceeding 5 mm in size, conservative treatment can be tried, but it is essential to perform a colostomy beforehand for temporary exclusion of the rectosigmoid. Local therapeutic measures are the same as described above, with permanent surveillance of the proper functioning of the urethral catheter together with broad-spectrum antibiotic cover. Restoration of sigmoid continuity can be envisaged within 6 weeks after clinical healing and radiological confirmation of fistular closure [9].

Surgical Treatment: The Mason Procedure [7]

General Description

Transsphincteric exposure permits surgery under direct vision of the rectum. If normal anatomy is restored in layers by accurate suture, the muscles heal and the patient retains normal defecation and complete anal continence. Careful preoperative preparation is essential since many of these patients are in a poor general condition. A preliminary, excluding, left colostomy is mandatory to ensure complete separation of the urinary and fecal pathways.

Operative Technique

After mechanical cleansing of the large bowel the patient is placed in a prone position on the operating table. The pelvis is elevated by a roll or bolster. Skin incision begins at a point just to the left of the sacrococcigeal junction and extends down to the anal verge posteriorly in the midline (Fig. 17.2). The underlying muscles can be divided into an inner and an outer tube. The outer tube is a muscle complex made up of the levator ani, the puborectalis, and the external sphincter. Although the exact nomenclature of the various muscles need not concern the operating surgeon, it is essential to mark each layer by identifying sutures before dividing them (Fig. 17.3). The necessity for this marking will become evident when the anatomy has to be restored. The nerve supply lies lateral to the line of division and is not damaged during the operation. The inner visceral tube bears the autonomic nerves and consists of the rectum and the anal canal. The distal end is made up of the inner sphincter.

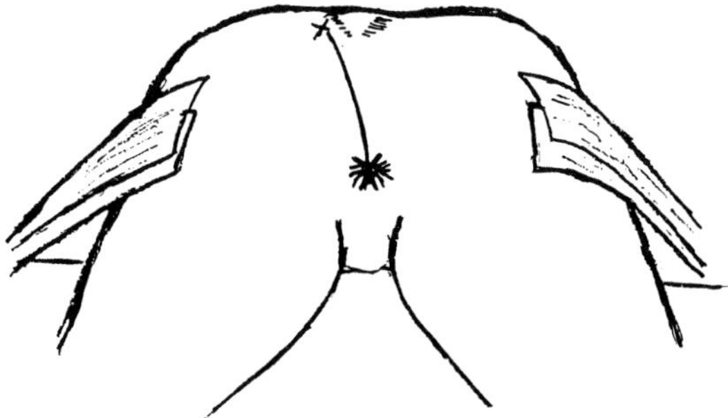

Fig. 17.2. Patient's position and skin incision

The posterior transrectal and transsphincteric approach provides an ideal exposure to prostatorectal fistulas (Fig. 17.4). The rectal mucosa is freed from the underlying rectal muscle. The scar tissue is removed, and the edges of the muscular coats of the rectum are freshened. The prostatic capsule is defined, and each layer is sutured separately using polyglycolic acid suture material (Fig. 17.5).

The intervention is completed by a careful anatomical reconstruction of the inner visceral tube and outer muscular layer (Fig. 17.6). A drain is inserted to empty the pararectal space between the inner and outer tubes.

Postoperative Management

The exposure is well tolerated even by old and poor-risk patients. Infection occurs in about 20% of cases and is mostly limited to the upper part of the wound overlying the ischiorectal fat. Minor dehiscence and small temporary fistulas have a good tendency to spontaneous healing. The urethral catheter is normally removed after 2 weeks and the temporary colostomy closed after 6 weeks.

Surgical Treatment of Multiple Pelvic Traumata

All patients presenting with multiple pelvic traumata involving communication between the rectum and the urinary tract – whether due to an open impalement fracture or a bullet wound – require surgical treatment as a matter of urgency, the aim being débridement of devitalized tissue, hemostasis, and drainage. Generally speaking, surgery terminates with a double diversion, namely an excluding colostomy on the one hand and a urethral catheter of generous caliber on the other. Reconstruction is not indispensable in this early operative phase, and in any case it should not be attempted unless the pa-

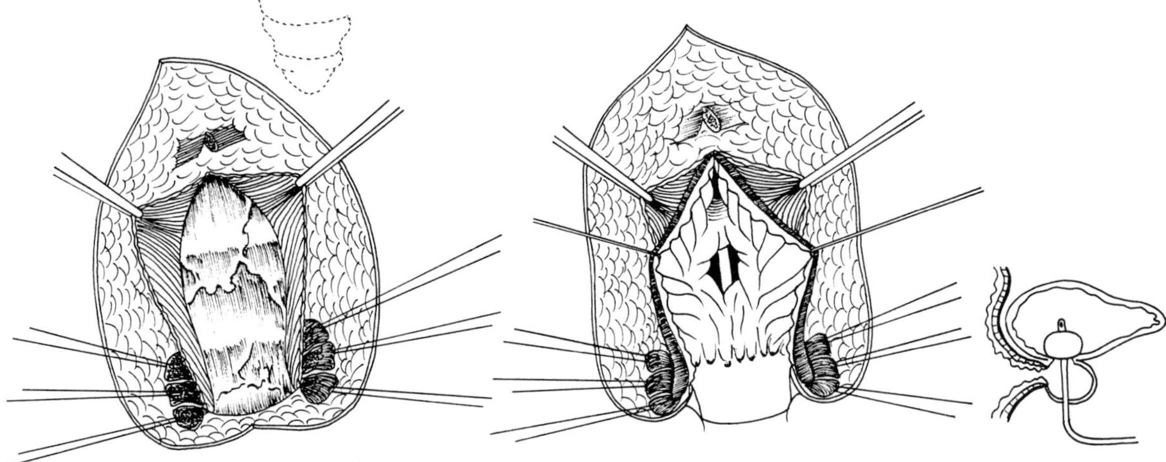

Fig. 17.3. Outer tube

Fig. 17.4. Inner tube and fistula

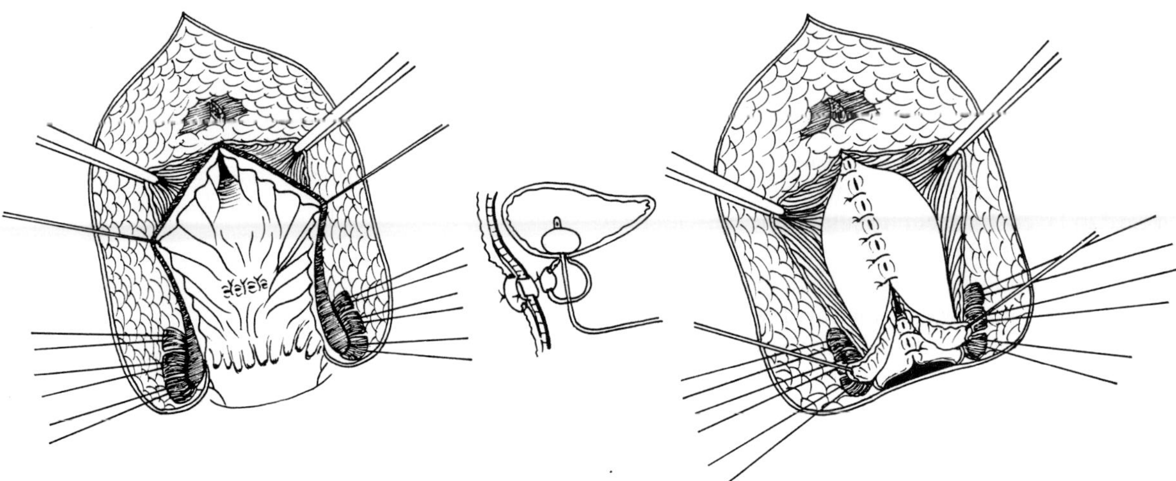

Fig. 17.5. Closure of fistula

Fig. 17.6. Closure of inner and outer tubes with reconstruction of sphincter

tient's general condition allows prolongation of the surgery by several hours, and the latter can be performed under favorable technical conditions, notably as regards the exposure and illumination. The success of primary repair depends essentially on the quality of the tissues and the size of the defect to be repaired. It is imperative that none of the sutures is under tension, a principle easier to adhere to on the rectal than on the urethral wall. It is namely difficult or even impossible to repair the urethra by the normal procedure of end-to-end suturing when the defect is larger than 2 cm. The edges of the defect can be brought together by mobilizing the distal urethra, a procedure requiring separation of the urethral bulb from the cavernous body. The proximal stump can be reached by lowering the prostatovesi-

cal mass, a technique calling, however, for supplementary access in the form of suprapubic cystotomy.

A relatively simple method of reconstructing the proximal urethra is the "pull-through" described by Badenoch. This begins with attachment of the well-mobilized distal stump to a urethral tube which is then introduced into the previously dilated prostatic segment up to the width of a finger. The tube and the invaginated urethra are held in this position either by subpubic traction or by suturing. Union of the urethral tissue is complete in about 2 weeks, after which time the supporting tube can be withdrawn.

Another possible method of primary urethral repair consists of marsupialization of the proximal stump by insertion of a flap of scrotal [3] or perineal [2] skin. Both methods demand a very fine technique, however, and are rarely suitable for primary repair in a severely injured patient. The results of reconstructions involving primary closure of a rupture are difficult to compare and depend as much on parasurgical factors as on the technique used. In the mid-term, however, complications occur frequently. On the urinary side they take the form of stenosis, incontinence, and infections, while the most common anal symptom is incontinence. Another, almost unavoidable, consequence of major pelvic injury is sexual impotence of neurovascular origin.

Treatment of Infected Fistulas

In patients with fistulas of infectious origin, any attempt at repair must be preceded by very careful preparation. This involves control of the bacterial infection, drainage of all infected material contained in prostatic or periprostatic abscesses and microabscesses, and finally correction of any urethral stenosis obstructing the free flow of urine [7]. The antiinfectious therapy does not aim at sterilization of the urine which is impossible under the circumstances – but at the establishment of a terrain free of local or general signs of inflammation. If the infection persists, any foci within the prostatic capsule must be eliminated by endoscopic resection. Infected material outside the capsule must be dealt with via the perineum, namely by drainage through a surgical incision, though this has the disadvantage of creating an area of scar tissue. In some cases these abscesses are encapsulated, in which case they should be emptied by puncture and repeated irrigation. As far as correction of the urethral stenosis is concerned, this is at present achieved by two methods: a short stenosis, rare in these patients, is accessible to simple repair by endoscopic urethrotomy, while a long and irregular stenosis calls for a two-stage operation with initial marsupialization of the narrowed portion of the urethra followed by definitive reconstruction 2–3 months later after complete healing of the local lesions.

Early or Late Correction?

The right time for surgical intervention after diagnosis of a prostatorectal lesion depends on the etiology. Ruptures due to pelvic traumata naturally call for immediate attention. At the other extreme, fistulas that are well epithelialized can be tolerated for years without serious consequences for the patient, and complications often occur only when surgical closure is attempted. As for lesions of iatrogenic origin, it is not always easy to decide on the best moment for correction. Attempts at repair during open prostatectomy are rarely successful. At worst, transfixing sutures located within the prostatic capsule under conditions of poor visibility can even aggravate the situation as a result of ischemic necrosis. Independently of any surgical procedure, conservative measures including vesical drainage antibiotic therapy, and a residue-free diet must be adopted immediately. If these fail, the terrain must be prepared by exclusive colostomy before definitive surgical repair of the lesion is undertaken.

References

1. Badenoch AW (1950) A pull-through operation for impassable traumatic stricture of the urethra. Br J Urol 22: 404–408
2. Blandy JP, Singh M, Tresidder GC (1968) Urethroplasty by scrotal flap for long urethral strictures. Br J Urol 40: 261–267
3. Johanson B (1953) Reconstruction of the male urethra in strictures. Acta Chirurg Scand [Suppl] 176
4. Jordan GH, Lynch DF, Warden SS, McCraw JD, Hoffmann GC, Schellhammer PF (1985) Major rectal complication following interstitial implantation of 125 iodine for carcinoma of the prostate. J Urol 134: 1212–1214
5. Kilpatrick FR, Mason AY (1969) Post-operative rectoprostatic fistula. Br J Urol 41: 649–654
6. Kuss R, Chatelain C, Jardin A, Gorin JP (1973) Traitement des fistules prostato-rectales après chirurgie de la prostate. (Intérêt de l'abord postérieur trans-anosphintérien et transrectal). J Chir (Paris) 105 (2): 109–124
7. Mason AY (1974) Transsphincteric surgery of the rectum. Prog Surg 13: 66–97
8. Olsson CA, Willscher MK, Krane RJ, Austen G Jr (1976) Management of prostatic fistulas. Urol Surv 25: 135–143
9. Vidal Sans J, Palou Redorta J, Pradell Teigell J, Banus Gassol JM (1985) Management and treatment of eighteen recto-uretral fistulas. Eur Urol 11: 300–305

18 Polyps

P. Meyer

Introduction

This chapter deals with adenomatous polyps of the colon and rectum. These benign tumors are of great clinical importance because they are considered to be precancerous [96]. Nearly all colorectal cancers develop from previously benign adenomatous polyps [34, 44, 91]. The transformation of benign adenomas into malignant growths is a well-established fact and is known as the adenoma-carcinoma sequence in the literature [26, 38, 92, 93].

Definition

The term "polyp" is not synonymous with adenoma but is defined as any projection of tissue into the lumen of the digestive tract. By definition, multiple polyps number between 5 and 100 in the colon and rectum [91]. In 25%-30% of cases, there is more than one polyp; of these, 19% have 3-10, the majority 2-5, and only 2% more than 10 [124, 133]. Polyposis coli is the condition in which there are more than 100 polyps [14, 91, 133]. For further details see Chap. 33.

Pathology

The polyps most frequently encountered in the colon and rectum (98%) are generally epithelial in nature (see Table 18.1). They are either adenomatous or hyperplastic [5]. Hyperplastic polyps are not considered as being precancerous and, unlike adenomas, their role in the genesis of cancer is considered improbable [71, 83].

Hyperplastic Polyps

Hyperplastic polyps (metaplastic polyps, focal polypoid hyperplasia [2, 69, 90]) are frequent and found predominantly in the rectum. In fact, 90% of the polyps less than 5 mm in diameter are hyperplastic [2, 38, 71, 125]. They are often associated

Table 18.1. Classification of polypoid tumors of the colon

I. Epithelial tumors
  A. Hyperplastic (metaplastic polyps)
  B. Adenomas
    1. tubular (adenomatous polyps)
    2. villous
    3. tubulovillous (papillary)
  C. Adenomatosis
    1. familial polyposis
    2. Gardner's syndrome
    3. Turcot's syndrome

II. Nonepithelial tumors
  A. Smooth muscle tumors (leiomyomas)
  B. Vascular tumors
    1. hemangiomas
    2. lymphangiomas
  C. Lipomas

III. Hamartomas
  A. Peutz-Jeghers polyps and polyposis
  B. Juvenile polyps and polyposis
    1. Juvenile polyps in childhood
    2. Juvenile polyposis syndromes
    3. Cronkhite-Canada syndrome
  C. Neurofibromas and ganglioneuromas

IV. Inflammatory of reactive tumors
  A. Inflammatory pseudopolyps
  B. Lymphoid polyps
  C. Lipoid granulomas and barium granulomas

V. Miscellaneous tumors

with colorectal carcinoma, and their presence mandates further screening [19, 62, 72].

Macroscopically, these polyps are small (<3 mm), sessile, and rarely pedunculated, in contrast to adenomas. They are also paler in appearance and less friable.

Histologically, they contain elongated and tortuous glands. The cells contain a basal nucleus, and atypical cells are absent. The dividing cells never extend past the inferior portion of the crypts. The basement membrane is thickened [69, 90] and there is no new glandular formation as seen in adenomas [75, 84]. On the other hand, there is no hyperplasia in even the smallest adenoma [71].

Adenomatous Polyps

Three types of adenomatous polyps can be distinguished by their architectural arrangement, which is never pure [124]. The cellular characteristics are the same for the three types [99].

Tubular Adenomas

These adenomas consist in up to 75% glandular tubules.
Macroscopically, the intestinal mucosa exhibit a deep red growth of tissue, sessile when small or pedunculated. The pedicle, a pale rose color, is made up of normal mucosa because it is formed by the peristaltic movement of the intestine. When the stalk is long and thin, the polyp is generally benign [81].
Microscopically [83] there is a proliferation of tubular glands with dysplastic cells. The nuclei are large, hyperchromatic, and no longer in a basal position. There is a cytoplasmic basophilia and a net decrease in mucin production. In addition, villous elements are seen. The transition between the adenoma and normal mucosa is sharply delineated. The cardinal sign of nonmalignancy is the lack of infiltration of the muscularis mucosa by the tubular glands, however distorted the former may be. In fact, any breach in the muscularis mucosa must be regarded as a sign of malignancy. Invasion of the muscularis mucosa implies a risk of dissemination via the adjacent lymphatic plexus [20, 37, 38, 126].
In case of breach of the muscularis mucosae, the pathologist may be confronted by a somewhat difficult differential diagnosis in trying to distinguish those cases of "pseudoinvasion" (epithelial misdisplacement) from carcinoma. Pseudoinvasion is characterized by the presence of mucin containing glands, generally cystic, in the submucosa. Accompanying signs of inflammation, hemorrhage, and hemosiderin deposits are the hallmarks of these ischemic lesions. This benign condition may be mistaken for malignant invasion. Pseudoinvasion is found in 6% of the adenomas and 38% of them when there is synchronous cancer [36, 48]. It is most commonly seen with polyps having a somewhat long pedicle, and might be due to repeated torsion causing ischemic lesions.
There is a clear relationship between the size and type of polyp. Whereas 90% of adenomas smaller than 1 cm are tubular, only 54% of those whose size is between 1.1 and 2 cm and 18% greater than 3 cm are tubular [57].

The incidence of early invasive carcinoma in tubular adenomas is 3.4%–5% [34, 36, 44, 124].

Villous Adenomas

Numerous long villous projections make up 75% of these adenomas.
Macroscopically, these tumors, which are normally sessile, are soft with a consistency of velvet, and are cauliflower in shape.
Microscopically, one distinguishes numerous frond-like projections, resembling small bowel villi. They are lined by an atypical neoplastic epithelium with numerous goblet cells. The cardinal sign of malignancy is the breach of the muscularis mucosae by the dysplastic cells proliferation.
Villous adenomas are less frequent than tubular adenomas. They account for 4%–10% of all colorectal adenomas. They predominate in men, with a ratio of about 3:2, and are more often encountered between the sixth and seventh decades [4, 53, 113]. They occur predominantly in the rectum [53, 113].
There is a clear relationship between the size and type of adenomas. Whereas only 0.8% of adenomas smaller than 1 cm are villous, 3.8% of those whose size is between 1.1 cm and 2 cm, 26% of those between 3.1 cm and 4 cm, and 40% larger than 4 cm are villous [57].
The incidence of early invasive carcinoma in villous adenomas is between 30% and 70% [3, 44, 104, 113, 134]. Moreover, they are more often associated with synchronous adenomas and synchronous or metachronous cancer than other adenomas [34, 113].

Tubulovillous Adenomas
(mixed villous and adenomatous polyps,
villo-glandular adenoma, papillary adenoma)

While an adenomatous polyp never consists entirely of a single element, tubulovillous adenomas contain a markedly mixed structure with more than 25% of the adenoma being composed of elements which differ from the dominant form. Only 9% of polyps less than 1 cm are tubulovillous adenomas, whereas 42% of the polyps ranging in size from 1.1 to 2 cm, 67% of those from 2.1 to 3 cm, and 44% larger than 4 cm are tubulovillous adenomas [57]. The incidence of malignancy is 17%, which is intermediate between that of tubular adenomas and villous adenomas. The incidence depends on the villous elements, the size of the polyp, and whether or not the polyp is sessile [44].

152   P. Meyer

Malignant Polyps

By definition, all polyps are dysplastic growths, consisting of cellular atypia. Morson and Sobin [94] have defined three degrees of dysplasia: mild, moderate, and severe. Severe dysplasia is the equivalent of carcinoma in situ. According to these authors, this terminology should be abandoned so as not to be confused with colorectal cancer. Such confusion in terminology risks inappropriately excessive treatment, i. e., surgical resection [94]. In effect, severe dysplasia (carcinoma in situ) is an invasion of the mucosa by atypical cellular elements, but without breach of the muscularis mucosa. The risk of metastases is minimal. A complete resection of the offending polyp may be considered to be curative [123, 138, 143]. Complete resection implies that removal of the stalk and the base has been complete and that no areas of dysplasia remain; otherwise, recourse to more radical surgery is recommended [138, 143].

In cases where severe dysplasia breaches the muscularis mucosa and reaches the submucosa, one refers to early invasive carcinoma [26]. This is seen in approximately 2%-8% of adenomas [17, 52, 123, 143]. This growth carries the theoretical risk of reaching surrounding lymphatics and therefore spreading to distant tissues [37]. Some authors have found metastases in 5%-33% of their cases [20, 24, 37, 65, 67, 70, 80, 108, 109, 123], whereas others have found none [76, 98, 100, 103, 121, 143]. The risk of dissemination is at the heart of the controversy as to whether endoscopic resection is sufficient treatment, or whether more aggressive surgery is required [137]. This therapeutic problem also applies to polypoid carcinoma, a polyp that is composed of entirely malignant cells with no vestige of adenomatous tissue [39, 143].

Epidemiology

The incidence of adenomatous polyps varies according to geography, age, and sex. Although most often seen in Whites [15], the frequency of this lesion is more closely related to life style and in particular to diet. Neither race nor climate seem to be important risk factors [144].

Western Europe, North America, and Australia have the highest rates of adenomatous polyps, whereas the indigenous populations of Africa and Japan have very low rates, with this disease being virtually unheard of in Black South Africans [7, 50, 57, 59, 99, 144]. Individuals from these low-risk populations aquire an intermediate incidence of the disease after emigrating to countries where adenomatous polyps are seen more frequently, and after having adopted a Western life style and diet; examples are the Black population of North America and Japanese of Hawaï [22, 127].

The incidence of adenomas in Europeans and Americans is estimated to be 7%-12.5%. This estimate was found to be similar, whether diagnosed by sigmoidoscopy [88], double-contrast barium enema [136], or autopsy findings in a normal population [30].

Epidemiological studies have revealed that a diet poor in fiber and rich in fat predisposes to the appearance of both adenomas and carcinomas of the colon and rectum [11, 51, 63, 86]. These findings have been corroborated by animal studies [114, 115, 130]. Bile acids, directly dependant on the quantity of fat ingested, have also been incriminated, as increased levels have been associated with a higher rate of adenomas [59]. Recently, it has been shown that the most important element is the proportion of deoxycolic acid to lithocolic acid [106, 107].

Other predisposing factors cited have been, in particular, a family history of either colorectal [78, 79] or gynecological [9, 60] cancer, atherosclerosis [23], nulliparous women [43, 112], and age [15].

The maximum incidence of adenoma is seen between the ages of 60 and 70 years [15, 57]. The age distributions of adenomas and carcinomas are different. The mean ages for adenomas are 58.1 years in England [99] and 61.0 years in Germany [57]. The mean ages for carcinomas are 62.1 [99] and 64 years [57]. Age is also seen to influence the site of distribution. In those patients less than 65 years old, adenomas are most frequently found in the distal half of the colon, both sexes affected equally; 75% of polyps are found in the last 25 centimeters [15, 57]. In men over 65 years and women over 75 years, adenomas are found most often in the proximal half of the colon [29, 129].

Overall there is a net male predominance, 63% in men versus 37% in females [57]. This sex distribution persists despite varying incidence: 58% in men versus 47% in women over 50 years in the USA [118], and 43% of men versus 32% of women in Norway for the same age group [29].

Prevention and Screening

Primary prevention of adenomas, based on epidemiological studies, aims at discovering and therefore modifying the principal risk factors, especially dietary ones. Secondary prevention of adenomas consists of screening for and the subsequent ablation of polyps. Screening consists of searching for occult blood in feces, colonoscopy or double contrast barium enema complementing rectosigmoidoscopy. Polyp ablation includes endoscopic resection and more complete surgical removal depending on the given situation. The effectiveness of secondary prevention has been shown by Gilbertsen [46], whose study demonstrated that endoscopic resection of colonic polyps reduced by 85% the risk of ensuing rectal cancer. In addition, those tumors discovered during proctosigmoidoscopy were still at an early stage of growth.

Screening

The presence of occult blood in the stool is associated with the presence of an ulcer or erosion [49]. The discovery of occult blood is made by means of chemical methods based on the fact that hemoglobin modifies the color of guaiac. This reaction is not specific, and up to 75%–85% false positives are seen in both polyps and cancers [8, 54], especially in the absence of dietary restrictions. The number of false negatives is unknown, but is probably elevated in the case of polyps. However, the loss of blood is no greater in patients with polyps than those without [28]. Ribet [117] reports a sensitivity of 15% and a specificity of 90% for the diagnosis of adenoma when a search for occult fecal blood is made on six occasions on three different days. Heinrich [55] has proposed a screening plan consisting of 2 days abstention from meat and vitamin C, then three to six tests for occult blood using the most sensitive chemical methods available based on the guaiac test. If the test proves positive, three to six further tests for occult blood are made using immunochemical tests. If these are positive, confirming the presence of blood, then either a complete colonoscopy or a double contrast barium enema should be performed. This approach has the advantage of avoiding unnecessary endoscopic or radiological investigations.

While it is obvious that all symptomatic patients (blood in the stool, changes in bowel habit) should undergo a complete screen including a complete colonoscopy and/or a double-contrast barium enema, the handling of asymptomatic patients remains a problem [140]. Winawer [139] has recommended a screen for all patients over 40 years of age during any medical examination for whatever the cause. These patients should undergo annual guaiac tests as well as rectosigmoidoscopy every 3–5 years, preferably with a long fiberoptic endoscope. For asymptomatic patients at high risk of developing an adenoma, and therefore colorectal cancer, it is essential that the screening described above be performed on a regular basis. What remains controversial is the frequency of regular checkups, whether annually or every 3–5 years.

The high risk group includes patients with ulcerative colitis of the entire colon for more than 7 years, patients with ulcerative colitis localized to the left colon for more than 15 years, a past history of either adenoma or cancer of the colon, and genital cancer in women [139]. Equally at risk are those patients with a genetic predisposition. They are divided into two groups: the first being those with polyposis including familial polyposis coli and Gardner's Syndrome, the second being patients without polyposis and includes the colonic cancer syndrome including gastrointestinal cancers, adenocarcinomatosis and Muir's Syndrome. The main characteristics of these cancers is that they afflict a family, with transmission being autosomal dominant; the patient is generally younger than the usual population of patients with colonic cancer; and several primary growths are seen either in the same organ or in different organs [139]. Patients who have previously had an adenoma removed or have undergone a colonic resection for cancer are also considered at increased risk because between 10%–25% will be found to have recurrent adenomatous polyps [13, 120]. The risk of developing a metachronous malignancy is 37%–64% in patients with adenomatous polyps [13, 27, 120, 135]. From 30% to 59% of the patients having undergone a polypectomy will have a recurrence at a later date [56, 68, 101, 102, 131]. Bussey [13] has shown that in patients with a single adenoma the risk of multiple malignancies was 2%; when there were 5 adenomas, this risk increased to 23%. In fact the number of polyps is directly associated with an increased risk of developing new polyps at a later date [56, 131]. Polyps with high degree of atypia are more often associated with new polyp development, and in 81% of the cases these new polyps develop at the same site as the initial growth [101].

The frequency and type of screening differs from author to author. However, it seems generally agreed upon that asymptomatic patients over

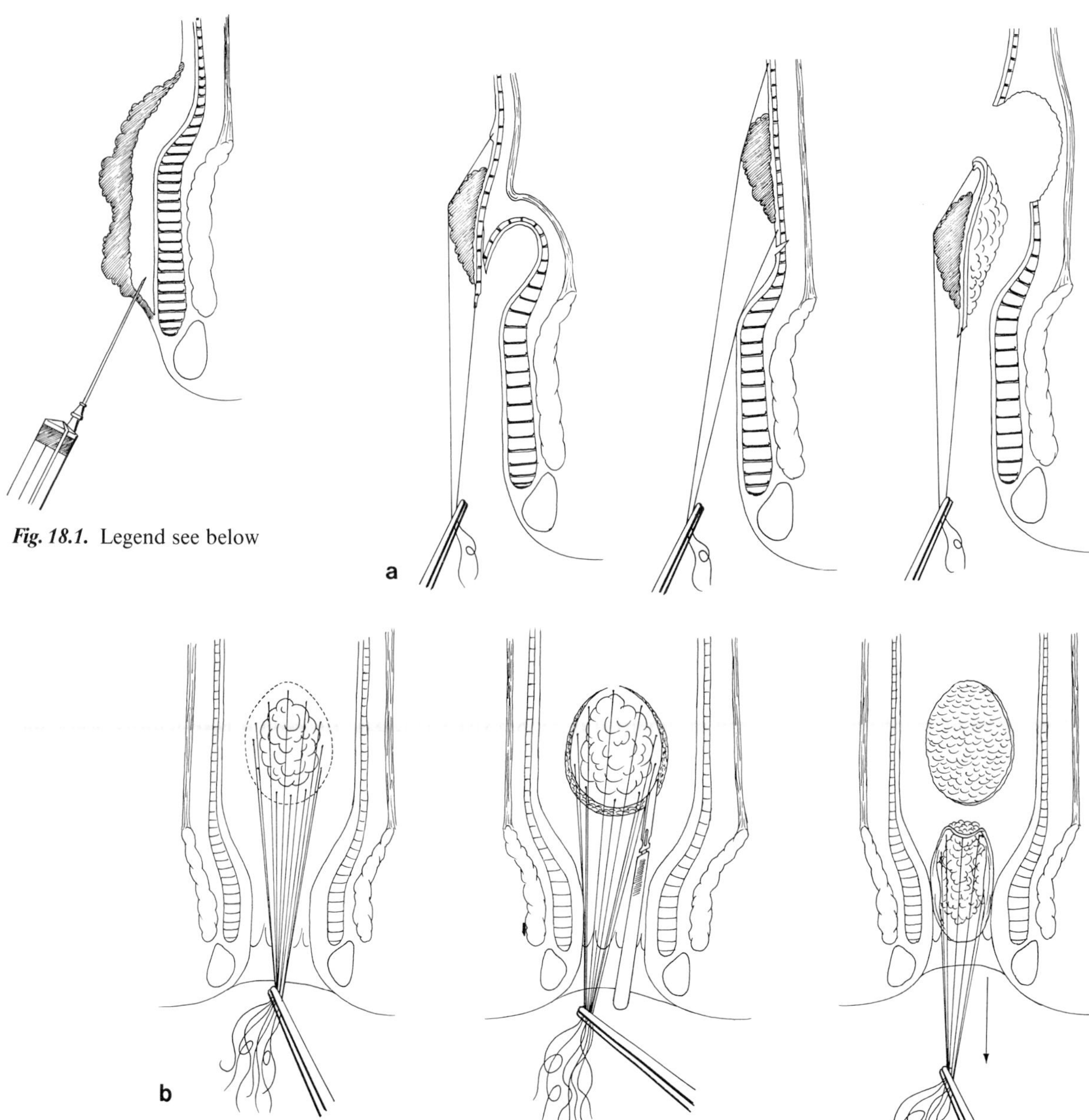

Fig. 18.1. Legend see below

Fig. 18.1. Submucosal excision of a villous adenoma according to Park's technique: submucosal space is infiltrated with saline to lift the lesion

Fig. 18.2a, b. Local tumor excision using the "parachute" technique from Francillon in frontal *(a)* and sagittal view *(b)*. Stitches are placed all around the lesion. The stitches are pulled under traction and the lesion is excised. Excision is conducted outside of the traction sutures to ensure adequate safety margins and in depth through the entire thickness of the rectal wall, if necessary

not only total colectomy because of the risk of future malignancy, but also prophylactic hysterectomy. It should be noted that Agrez [1] found a family history in 13% of the patients with metachronous cancers. A subtotal colectomy has been proposed by Lillehei and Wangensteen [74] for those patients presenting with a cancer associated with polyps. This attitude has been corroborated by other authors [10, 33, 40, 120] given the unusually high incidence of synchronously and metachronously diagnosed cancers. Rosenthal and Baranowski 120] have proposed a total colectomy in all patients with an adenomatous polyp associated with a carcino-

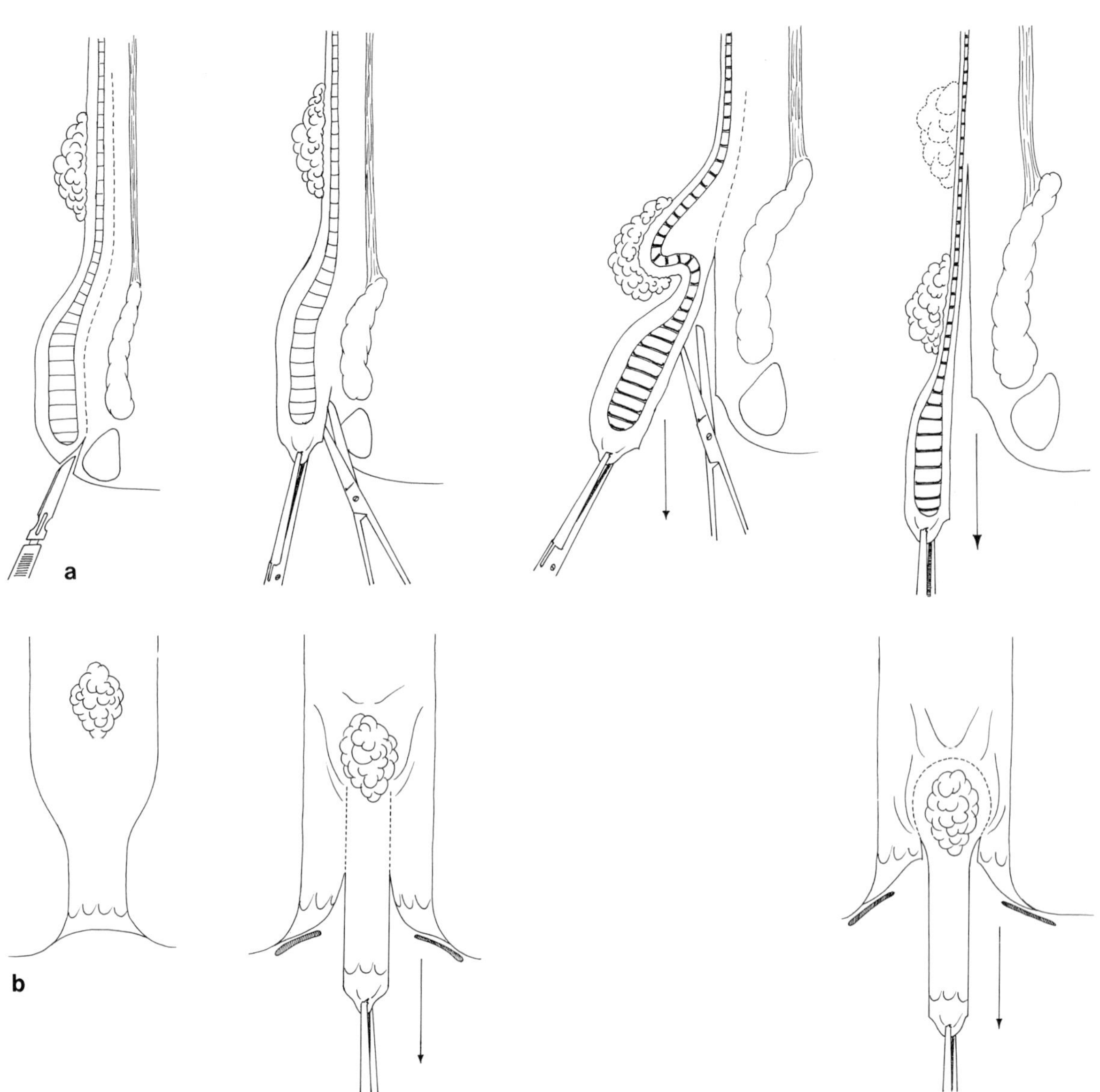

Fig. 18.3a, b. Faivre's procedure. Tumor excision by using a traction flap. *a* Frontal and *b* sagittal views. Excision begins at anal margin. The flap encompasses the internal sphincter and is pulled under traction to allow down mobilisation of the lesion which may be progressively exteriorized. A full thickness excision may be realized

ma. Scarborough [122] recommends a total colectomy when a single polyp is discovered in two or three segments of colon. Several authors agree with this approach in cases of synchronous cancer, especially when there are associated polyps [25, 40, 73, 120, 126]. The different situations confronting the surgeon (multiple polyps with or without synchronous cancer affecting one or several segments of bowel) make this a complex therapeutic problem. Prophylactic total colectomy should only be considered in those patients with a small operative risk [18].

Local Excision of Rectal Tumors

Local excision is only possible in that portion of the rectum which is extraperitoneal. The guidelines mentioned previously must be scrupulously observed: no biopsy but rather complete excision, a thorough histological examination, involvement of the submucosa implying the same risk of dissemination as with colonic polyps.

Currently there are three surgical options for removing adenomas and adenocarcinomas of the rectum, namely: the submucosal resection described

158   P. Meyer

by Parks [111] (Fig. 18.1), the excision popularized
by Francillon (a technique known as a "parachute")
[42] (Fig. 18.2), and Faivre's "lambeau tracteur" [35]
(Fig. 18.3). These different approaches to the extraperitoneal rectum may be performed under spinal,
epidural, or caudal anesthesia. General anesthesia
is not required. Preoperative preparation seems
necessary to reduce the risk of surgical complications. Therefore, a thorough mechanical cleansing
of the gastrointestinal tract and the use of braod
spectrum antibiotics covering both aerobic and anaerobic microorganisms in the preoperative period
is recommended. Postoperatively, the rectum
should be kept empty by the use of a low residue
diet [82].

The technique described by Parks (Fig. 18.1) calls
for the infiltration of the submucosa with a solution
of saline combined with a vasoconstrictor (either
adrenaline or vasopressin) which will facilitate the
dissection. When the submucosa is infiltrated with
tumor, the detachment normally seen on infiltration
is lost. This increases the risk of either an incomplete excision or an excision which does not respect
the appropriate planes of dissection. This situation
requires alternative techniques which assure complete excision [110].

Local excision popularised by Francillon [42]
(Fig. 18.2) permits, in contrast to Parks' technique,
the removal of a ring of rectal tissue which includes
all the layers of the wall of the rectum. The newly
formed rectal orifice is then resutured after meticulous hemostasis. The Faivre's "lambeau tracteur"
[35] (Fig. 18.3) also calls for a complete excision of
all the layers of rectal wall. The advantage over
Francillon's approach is that there is less anal dilatation. Electrotherapy, laser, and cryotherapy have
no place in the curative treatment of rectal adenomas; their use is only in palliative surgery [82].

References

 1. Agrez MV, Ready R, Ilstrup D, Beart RW (1982) Me-
    tachronous colorectal malignancies. Dis Colon Rec-
    tum 25/6: 569–574
 2. Arthur JF (1968) Structure and significance of meta-
    plastic nodules in the rectal mucosa. J Clin Pathol
    21: 735–743
 3. Bacon HE, Eisenberg SW (1971) Papillary adenoma
    or villous tumor of the rectum and colon. Ann Surg
    174: 1002–1008
 4. Begelow B, Winkelman J (1964) Polyps of the colon
    and rectum. A review of 12 years' experience and re-
    port of unusual case. Cancer 17: 1177–1186
 5. Behringer GE (1970) Changing concept in the histo-
    pathologic diagnosis of polypoid lesions of the co-
    lon. Dis Colon Rectum 13: 116–128
 6. Berci G, Panish JF, Chapiro M, Corlin R (1974)
    Complications of colonoscopy and polypectomy. Re-
    port of the Southern California Society for Gastroin-
    testinal Endoscopy. Gastroenterology 67: 584–585
 7. Berg JW, Howel MA (1974) The geographic patholo-
    gy of bowel cancer. Cancer 34: 807–814
 8. Brandstatter G, Kratochvil P (1978) Early diagnosis
    of colonic-rectal neoplasms by detecting occult
    blood in the feces. Wien Med Wschr 128: 209–210
 9. Bremond A, Collet P, Lambert R, Martin JL (1984)
    Breast cancer and polyps of the colon. A case-con-
    trol study. Cancer 54: 2568–2570
10. Brief DK, Brener BJ, Goldenkranz R, Alpert J, Yalof
    I, Parsonnet V (1983) An argument for increase use
    of subtotal colectomy in the management of carcino-
    ma of the colon. Am Surg 49: 66–72
11. Burkitt DP (1978) Colonic-rectal cancer: Fiber and
    other dietary factors. Am J Clin Nutr 31: 558–564
12. Burns FJ (1980) Synchronous and metachronous
    malignancies of the colon and rectum. Dis Colon
    Rectum 23: 578–589
13. Bussey HJR (1978) Multiple adenomas and carcino-
    mas. Major Probl Pathol 10: 72–80
14. Bussey HJR, Morson BC (1978) Familial polyposis
    coli. In: Lipkin M, Good RA (eds) Gastrointestinal
    tract cancer. Plenum, New York, pp 275–294
15. Chapman I (1963) Adenomatous polypi of large in-
    testine: incicence and distribution. Ann Surg 157:
    223–226
16. Christie JP (1977) Colonoscopic excision of large ses-
    sile polyps. Am J Gastroenterol 67: 430–438
17. Christie JP (1984) Malignant colon polyps-cure by
    coloscopy or colectomy? Am J Gastroenterol 79:
    543–547
18. Chu DZJ, Giacco G, Martin RG, Guinee VF (1986)
    The significance of synchronous carcinoma and pol-
    yps in the colon and rectum. Cancer 57: 445–450
19. Clark JC, Collan Y, Eide TJ, Esteve J, Ewen S, Gibbs
    NM, Jenson OM, Koskela E, MaClennan R, Simp-
    son JG, Stalsberg H, Zaridze DG (1985) Prevalence
    of polyps in an autopsy series from areas with varing
    incidence of large bowel cancer. Int J Cancer 36:
    179–196
20. Colacchio TA, Forde KA, Scantlebury VD (1981)
    Endoscopic polypectomy: inadequate treatment for
    invasive colorectal carcinoma. Ann Surg 194:
    704–707
21. Coopers HS (1983) Surgical pathology of endoscopi-
    cally removed malignant polyps of the colon and
    rectum. Am J Surg Pathol 7: 613–622
22. Correa P, Duques E, Cuello C, Haenszel W (1972)
    Polyps of the colon and rectum in Cali, Columbia.
    Int J Cancer 9: 86–96
23. Correa P, Strong JP, Johnson WD, Pizzolato P,
    Haenszel W (1982) Atherosclerosis and polyps of the
    colon. Quantification of precursors of coronary heart
    disease and colon cancer. J Chron Dis 35: 313–320
24. Coutsoftides T, Sivak MV, Benjamin SP, Jagelman D
    (1978) Colonoscopy and the management of polyps
    containing invasive carcinoma. Ann Surg 188:
    638–641
25. Cunliffe WJ, HasletonPS, Tweedle DEF, Schofield
    PF (1984) Incidence of synchronous and metachro-
    nous colorectal carcinoma. Br J Surg 71: 941–943
26. Day DW, Morson BC (1978) Pathology of adenomas.
    In: Morson BC (ed) The pathogenesis of colorectal

cancer. Volume 10. Major problems in pathology. Saunders, Philadelphia, pp 43-57
27. Dowling K, Watne A, Foshag L, Vargish T (1985) Management of nonfamilial adenomatous polyps and colon cancers. Surgery 98: 684-688
28. Dybdahl JH, Daae LNW, Larsen S, Myren J (1984) Occult faecal blood loss determined by a 51Cr method and chemical tests inpatients referred for colonoscopy. Scand J Gastroenterol 19: 245-254
29. Eide TJ, Stalsberg H (1978) Polyps of the large intestine in Northern Norway. Cancer 42: 2839-2848
30. Ekelund G (1963) On cancer and polyps of the colon and rectum. Acta Pathol Microbiol Scand 59: 165-170
31. Ekelund G, Phil B (1974) Multiple carcinomas of the colon and rectum. Cancer 33: 1630-1634
32. Elliot MJ, Louw JH (1979) A 10 year survey of large bowel carcinoma at Groote Schieur Hospital with particular reference to patients under 30 years of age. Br J Surg 66: 621-624
33. Enker WE, Dragacevics S (1978) Multiple carcinomas of the large bowel: A natural experiment in etiology and pathogenesis. Ann Surg 187: 8-11
34. Enterline HT, Evans GW, Mercado-Lugo R (1962) Malignant potential of adenomas of colon and rectum. JAMA 179: 322-330
35. Faivre J (1980) Die transanale Elektroresektion mit Hilfe eines analen Zuglappens bei Tumoren des Rektums. Proktologie 2: 77-80
36. Fechner RE (1973) Adenomatous polyps with submucosal cysts. Am J Clin Pathol 59: 498-502
37. Fenoglio CM, Kaye GI, Lane N (1973) Distribution of human lymphatics in normal, hyperplastic and adenomatous tissue: its relationship to metastases from small cancers in pedunculated adenomas. Gastroenterology 64: 51-66
38. Fenoglio CM, Lane N (1974) The anatomic precursor of colorectal carcinoma. Cancer 34: 819-823
39. Fenoglio CM, Pascal RP (1982) Colorectal adenomas and cancer: pathologic relationships. Cancer 50: 2601-2608
40. Fogler R, Weiner E (1980) Multiple foci of colorectal carcinoma: Argument for subtotal colectomy. NY State J Med 80: 47-51
41. Franchini A, Giardimo R, Cola B (1982) Multiple tumors of the large bowel. Ann Gastroenterol Hepatol 18: 309-311
42. Francillon J, Moulay A, Vignal J, Tissot E (1974) L'exérèse par voie basse des cancers de l'ampoule rectale. Nouv Press Med 3: 1365-1366
43. Fraumeni JF, Lloyd JW, Smith EM, Wagoner JK (1969) Cancer mortality among nuns: role of martial status in etiology of neoplastic disease in women. J Natl Cancer Inst 42: 455-468
44. Fruhmorgen P, Matek W (1983) Significance of polypectomy in the large bowel. Endoscopy 15: 155-157
45. Fucim C, Spencer RJ (1986) An appraisal of endoscopic removal of malignant colonic polyps. Mayo Clin Proc 61: 123-126
46. Gilbertsen VA, Nelms JM (1978) The prevention of invasive cancer of the rectum. Cancer 41: 1137-1139
47. Greenburg AG, Saik RP, Coyle JJ, Peskin GW (1981) Mortality and gastrointestinal surgery in the aged. Arch Surg 116: 788-791
48. Greene FL (1974) Epithelial misdysplacement in adenomatous polyps of the colon and rectum. Cancer 33: 206-217
49. Griffith CDM, Turner DJ, Saunders JH (1981) False-negative results of hemoccult test in colorectal cancer. Br Med 283: 472
50. Haenszel W, Correa P (1971) Cancer of the colon and rectum and adenomatous polyps. Cancer 28: 14-24
51. Haenszel W, Berg JW, Segi M, Kurihara M, Locke FB (1973) Large-bowel cancer in Hawaiian Japanse. J Natl Cancer Inst 51: 1765-1779
52. Haggit RC, Glotzbach RE, Soffer EE, Wruble LD (1985) Prognosis factors in colorectal carcinomas arising in adenomas: implications for lesions removed by endoscopic polypectomy. Gastroenterology 89: 328-336
53. Halney PH, Hines MO, Ray JE (1971) Villous tumors. Experience with 217 patients. Am Surg 37: 190-197
54. Heeb MA, Ahlvin RC (1978) Screening for colorectal carcinoma in a rural area. Surgery 83: 540-541
55. Heinrich HC (1982) Frühdiagnostik kolorektaler Polypen und Karzinome durch chemischen und/oder immunochemischen Okkultblut-Nachweiss in Stuhl. Med Klin 77: 797-801
56. Henry GL, Condon RE, Schulte WJ, Aprahamian C, DeCosse JJ (1975) Risk of recurrence of colon polyps. Ann Surg 182: 511-515
57. Hermanek P, Karrer K, Sobin LH (1983) Statistics of adenomas. In: Hermanek P, Karrer K, Sobin LH (eds) Atlas of colorectal tumors. Butterworths, London, pp 58-59
58. Hermanek P, Karrer K, Sobin LH (1983) Early detection, screening. In: Hermanek P, Karrer K, Sobin LH (eds) Atlas of colorectal tumors. Butterworths, London, pp 134-136
59. Hill MJ (1974) Bacteria and ethiology of colonic cancer. Cancer 34: 815-818
60. Howell MA (1976) The association between colorectal cancer and breast cancer. J Chron Dis 29: 243-261
61. Jarvinen HJ, Ovaska J, Mecklin JP (1988) Improvements in the treatment and prognosis of colorectal carcinoma. Br J Surg 75: 25-27
62. Jass JR (1983) Relation between metaplastic polyp and carcinoma of the colorectum. Lancet 1: 28-30
63. Jensen OM, MaClennan R (1979) Dietary factors and colorectal cancer in Scandinavia. Israël J Med Sci 15: 329-334
64. Johnson SM (1978) Colonoscopy and polypectomy. Amer J Surg 136: 313-316
65. Kodaira S, Teramoto T, Ono S, Takizawa K, Katsumata T, Abe O (1981) Lymph node metastases from carcinomas developing in pedunculated and semipedunculated colorectal adenomas. Aust NZ J Surg 51: 429-433
66. Kodaira S, Ono S, Purri P, Takizawa K, Kotake K, Tsuyuki A, Okuda M, Abe O (1981) Endoscopic polypectomy of the large bowel: management of cancerbearing polyps. Int Surg 66: 311-314
67. Kraus FT (1965) Pedunculated adenomatous polyp with carcinoma in the tip and metastasis to lymph nodes. Dis Colon Rectum 8: 283-286
68. Kronborg O, Hage E, Adamsen S, Deichgraeber E (1983) Follow-up after colorectal polypectomy. II. Repeated examinations of the colon every six

months after removal of sessile adenomas and adenomas with the highest degrease dysplasia. Scand J Gastroenterol 18: 1095-1099

69. Lane N, Lev R (1963) Observations on the origin of adenomatous epithelium of the colon. Cancer 16: 751-764

70. Lane N, Kaye GI (1967) Pedunculated adenomatous polpy of the colon with carcinoma, lymph node metastases, and suture line recurrence. Report of a case and discussion of terminology problems. Am J Clin Pathol 48: 170-182

71. Lane N, Kaplan H, Pascal RP (1971) Minute adenomatous and hyperplastic polyps of the colon: Divergent pattern of epithelial growth with specific associated mesenchymal changes. Gastroenterology 60: 537-551

72. Lane N, Fenoglio CM (1976) Observations on the adenoma as precursor to ordinary large bowel carcinoma. Gastrointest Radiol 1: 111-119

73. Leborgne J, Heloury Y, Leneel JC, Lenne Y, Malvy P (1984) Les cancers multiples colo-rectaux. Réflexions. A propos de 12 observations. Med Chir Dig 13: 605-612

74. Lillehei RC, Wangensteen OH (1955) Bowel function after colectomy for cancer, polyps and diverticulitis. JAMA 159. 163-170

75. Lipkin M (1974) Phase 1 and phase 2 proliferative lesions of colonic epithelial cells in diseases leading to colonic cancer. Cancer 34: 878-888

76. Lipper S, Kahn LB, Ackerman LV (1983) The significance of microscopic invasive cancer in endoscopically removed polyps, of the large bowel. Cancer 52: 1691-1699

77. Lockart-Mummery HE, Heald RJ, Chir M (1972) Metachronous cancer of the large intestine. Dis Colon Rectum 15: 261-264

78. Lovette E (1976) Family studies in cancer of the colon and rectum. Br J Surg 63: 13-18

79. Lynch HT, Lynch PM (1979) The cancer family syndrome. A pragmatic basis for syndrome identification. Dis Colon Rectum 22: 106-110

80. Manheimer LH (1965) Metastases to the liver from a colonic polyp. Report of a case. N Engl J Med 272: 144-145

81. Marshak RH (1965) The pedunculated adenomatous polyp. Am J Dig Dis 10: 958-967

82. Marti MC (1985) Transanal surgical treatment of rectal tumors. Acta Chir 52: 321-324

83. Maskens AP (1979) Histogenesis of adenomatous polyps in the human large intestine. Gastroenterology 77: 1245-1251

84. Maskens AP, Dujardin-Loits RM (1981) Experimental adenomas and carcinomas of the large intestive behave as distinct entities. Cancer 47: 81-89

85. McDermott FT, Hughes ESR, Pihl E, Johnson WR, Price AB (1985) Local recurrence after potentially curative resection for rectal cancer in a serie of 1008 patients. Br J Surg 72: 34-37

86. McMichael AJ, McCall MG, Hartshorne JM, Woodings TL (1980) Patterns of gastro-intestinal cancer in European migrants to Australia: the role of dietary change. Int J Cancer 25: 431-437

87. Moertel CG, Bargen JA, Dockerty MB (1958) Multiple carcinomas of the large intestine: A review of the literature and a study of 261 cases. Gastroenterol 34: 85-98

88. Moertel CG, Hill JR, Dockerty MB (1966) Routine proctoscopic examination. Second look. Mayo Clin Proc 41: 368-374

89. Moreaux J, Catala M (1985) Les cancers multiples du côlon et du rectum. Fréquence et résultats du traitement chirurgical. Gastroenterol Clin Biol 9: 336-341

90. Morson BC (1962) Some pecularities in the histology of intestinal polyps. Dis Colon Rectum 5: 337-344

91. Morson BC, Bussey HJR (1970) Predisposing causes of intestinal cancer. Curr Prob Surg 2: 1-50

92. Morson BC (1974) The polyp-cancer sequence in the large bowel. Proc R Soc Med 67: 451-457

93. Morson BC (1974) Evaluation of cancer of the colon and rectum. Cancer 34: 845-849

94. Morson BC, Sobin LH (1976) Histological typing of intestinal tumors. Geneva, World Health Organization, 13-58

95. Morson BC, Bussey HJR, Samoorian S (1977) Policy of local excision for early cancer of the colorectum. Gut 18: 1045-1050

96. Morson BC (1983) Markers for increased risk of colorectal cancer. In: Sherlock P, Morson BC, Veronesi BL (eds) Precancerous lesions of the gastrointestinal tract. Rosen, New York, pp 255-259

97. Morson BC (1984) The evolution of colorectal carcinoma. Clin Radiol 35: 425-431

98. Morson BC, Whiteway JE, Jones EA, Macrae FA, Williams CB (1984) Histopathology and prognosis of malignant colorectal polyps treated by endoscopic polypectomy. Gut 25: 437-444

99. Muto T, Bussey HJ, Morson BC (1975) The evolution of cancer of the colon and rectum. Cancer 36: 2251-2270

100. Muto T, Kamina J, Sawada T, Kusama S, Itai Y, Ikenaga T, Yamashiro M, Hino Y, Yamaguchi S (1970) Colonoscopic polypectomy in diagnosis and treatment of early carcinoma of the large intestine. Dis Colon Rectum 23: 68-75

101. Nava H, Carlsson G, Petrelli NJ, Herrera L, Mittelman A (1987) Follow-up colonoscopy in patients with colorectal adenomatous polyps. Dis Colon Rectum 30: 465-468

102. Neugut AI, Johnsen CM, Forde KA, Treat MR (1985) Recurrence rates for colorectal polyps. Cancer 55: 1586-1589

103. Nivatvongs S, Goldberg SM (1978) Management of patients who have polyps containing invasive carcinoma removed via colonoscope. Dis Colon Rectum 21: 8-16

104. Orringer MB, Eggleston JC (1972) Papillary (villous) adenomas of the colon and rectum. Surgery 72: 378-381

105. Overholt BF (1975) Colonoscopy: a review. Gastroenterology 68: 1308-1320

106. Owen RW, Thompson RH, Hill MJ, Wilpart M, Malinguet P, Roberfroid M (1987) The importance of the ratio of lithocholic to deoxycholic acid in large bowel carcinogenesis. Nutr Cancer 9: 68-71

107. Owen RW, Dodo M, Thompson RH, Hill MJ (1987) Fecal steroids and colorectal cancer. Nutr Cancer 9: 73-80

108. Palacios R, Wellman K (1966) Adenomatous polyps of the colon with adenocarcinoma and pulmonary metastases. Gastroenterology 51: 82-86

109. Panish JF (1979) Management of patients with poly-

poid lesions of the colon. Am J Gastroenterol 71: 315–324

110. Parks AG, Nicholls RJ (1983) Perianal endorectal operative techniques. In: Todd IP, Fielding LP (eds) Operative surgery. Colon, rectum and anus, 4th edn. Butterworths, London, pp 316–326

111. Parks AG, Stuart AG (1973) The management of villous tumors of the large bowel. Br J Surg 60: 688–695

112. Potter JD, McMichael AJ (1983) Large bowel cancer in women in relation to reproductive and hormonal factors: a case-control study. J Natl Cancer Inst 71: 703–709

113. Quan SHQ, Castro EB (1971) Papillary adenomas (villous tumors). A review of 215 cases. Dis Colon Rectum 14: 267–280

114. Raicht RF, Cohen BI, Fazzini EP, Sarwal AN, Takahashi M (1980) Protective effect of plant sterols against chemically induced colon tumors in rats. Cancer Res 40: 403–405

115. Reedy BS, Weisburger JH, Wynder EL (1974) Effect of dietary fat level and dimethylhydrazine on fecal acid and neutral sterol excretion and colon carcinogenesis in rats. J Natl Cancer Inst 52: 507–511

116. Reilly JC, Rusin LC, Theverkauf FJ (19829 Colonoscopy: its role in cancer of the colon and rectum. Dis Colon Rectum 25: 532–538

117. Ribet A, Escourrou J, Frexinos J, Delpu J (1980) Screening for colorectal tumors-results of two years experience. Cancer Detect Prev 3: 449–461

118. Rickert RR, Auerbach O, Garfinkel L, Hammond EC, Frasca JM (1979) Adenomatous lesions of the large bowel. An autopsy study. Cancer 43: 1847–1857

119. Rider JA, Kirsner JB, Moeller HC, Palmer WL (1959) Polyps of the colon and rectum. JAMA 170: 633–638

120. Rosenthal I, Baronofsky ID (1960) Prognostic and therapeutic implications of polyps in metachronous coli carcinoma. JAMA 172: 37–41

121. Rossini RP, Ferrari A, Coverlizza S (1982) Colonoscopic polypectomy in diagnosis and management of cancerous adenomas: an individual and multicentric experience. Endoscopy 14: 124–127

122. Scarborough RA (1960) The relationship between polyps and carcinoma of the colon and rectum. Dis Colon Rectum 3: 336–342

123. Shatney CH, Lober PH, Gilbertsen VA, Sosin H (1974) The treatment of pedunculated adenomatous colorectal polyps with focal cancer. Surg Gynecol Obstet 139: 845–850

124. Shinya H, Wolff WI (1979) Morphology, anatomic distribution and cancer potentional of colonic polyps. An analysis of 7000 polyps endoscopically removed. Ann Surg 190: 679–683

125. Shinya H (1982) Colonoscopy: diagnosis and treatment of colonic diseases. Igaku-Shoin, New York

126. Soullard J, Potet F (1975) La prévention des cancers recto-coliques. Arch Fr Mal App Dig 64: 197–200

127. Stemmermann GN, Yatani R (1973) Diverticulosis and polyps of the large intestine. Cancer 31: 1260–1269

128. Thomson JS (1977) Treatment of sessile villous and tubovillous adenomas of the rectum. Experience of St. Mark's Hospital. 1963–1972. Dis Colon Rectum 20: 467–472

129. Vatn MH, Stalsberg H (1982) The prevalence of polyps of the large intestine in Oslo: An autopsy study. Cancer 49: 819–825

130. Wattenberg LW, Loub WD (1978) Inhibition of polycyclic aromatic hydrocarbon-induced neoplasia by naturally occurring indoles. Cancer Res 38: 1410–1413

131. Waye JD, Braunfeld S (1982) Surveillance intervalles after colonoscopic polypectomy. Endoscopy 14: 79–81

132. Weir JA (1975) Colorectal cancer. Metachronous and other associated neoplasma. Dis Colon Rectum 18: 4–5

133. Welch CE, Hedberg SE (1975) Polypoid lesions of the gastrointestinal tract, 2nd edn. Saunders, Philadelphia

134. Welch JP, Welch CE (1976) Villous adenomas of the colo-rectum. Am J Surg 131: 185–191

135. Welch JP (1981) Multiple colorectal tumors. Am J Surg 142: 274–280

136. Welin S (1967) Results of the Malmö technique of colon examination. JAMA 199: 369–371

137. Wilcox GM, Anderson PB, Colacchio TA (1986) Early invasive carcinoma in colonic polyps. A review of the literature with emphasis on the assessment of the risk of metastasis. Cancer 57: 160–171

138. Winawer SJ, Witt TR (1981) Cancer in a colonic polyp, or malignant colonic adenomasis polypectomy sufficient? Gastroenterology 81: 625–626

139. Winawer SJ (1981) Preventive screening and early diagnosis. In: DeCosse JJ (ed) Clinical surgery international: large bowel cancer. Churchill Livingstone, Edinburgh, pp 46–62

140. Winawer SJ, Sherlock P (1982) Surveillance for colorectal cancer in average-risk patients, familial high-risk groups, and patients with adenomas. Cancer 50: 2609–2614

141. Wolff WI, Shinya H (1973) A new approach to the management of colonic polyps. Adv Surg 7: 45–67

142. Wolff WI, Shinya H (1973) A new approach to colonic polyps. Ann Surg 178: 3

143. Wolff WI, Shinya H (1975) Definitive treatment of malignant polyps of the colon. Ann Surg 182: 516–524

144. Wynder EL, Reddy BS (1974) Metabolic epidemiology of colorectal cancer. Cancer 34: 801–806

19 Malignant Anal Tumors

G. Pipard

Definition

The main subject of this chapter is the malignant invasive anal tumor, for information on benign tumoros conditions the reader should refer to the appropriate chapters of this volume. In the anal canal and the external anal margin (perianal skin) non-malignant conditions include fibrous polyps, hidradenoma of the perianal glands, condyloma acuminatum, keratoacanthoma, and leukoplakia without atypia. At the level of the anorectal junction inflammatory, hyperplastic, and juvenile polyps of the mucosa are to be distinguished from carcinoma [6, 29].

Lesions at the border between benign and precancerous conditions i.e., leukoplakia with atypia [5], bowenoid papulosis [83], and precancerous lesions such as adenomatous polyps of the anorectal junction [29], carcinoma in situ [26], Bowen's disease [82] of the anal canal, and Paget's disease of the anal margin [47] are likewise treated elsewere in this volume.

Embryology and Anatomy

The anatomical and histopathological classification of malignant tumors of the anal region is confused because of their complex embryological origin [34]. The results of many existing clinical studies cannot be compared in detail because of the divergent opinions as to the precise limits between the anal canal and the anal margin. However, the differences in pathological features, treatment, and prognosis of malignant tumors of the anal canal and the true external anal margin indicate that a distinction of these tumors is mandatory, especially wehen conservative treatment modalities are being considered.

The anal region is of mixed embryological origin [34, 41, 43] endodermal in its proximal part and ectodermal in its distal part. The junction of the hindgut with the proctodeum, an external depression, is at the level of the cloacal membrane during embryonal and fetal life, and after the disappearance of this the area is called the "transitional" zone of the anus. This zone corresponds macroscopically with the columns of Morgagni or valves of the anus. Their inferior limit is called the dentate (pectinate) line. When observed histologically, there is no clear boundary but a real transitional zone with intermingled characteristics of cuboidal rectal mucosa and modified squamous epithelium. Transitional epithelium can extend for up to 20 mm above the dentate line and contain islands of squamous cells within it thus providing the explanation for the presence of squamous cell carcinoma in the proximal anal canal.

Anal Canal

The proximal limit of the anal canal is represented by the anorectal ring at the superior part of the columns of Morgagni or by the upper limit of the external anal sphincter muscle [33, 69]. At this level the rectal mucosa with its deep glands of Lieberkühn is replaced by an epithelium of the transitional type.

The supra pectinate anal canal, called the transitional zone, is a slightly more reddish color than the rectal mucosa and shows the columns and sinus of Morgagni. The anal ducts or anal glands originate at this level.

The distal limit of the anal canal is for some authors the dentate line, e.g., Hardcastle and Bussey [38] (St. Mark's Hospital, London), Greenall et al. [35] (Memorial Sloan Kettering Center, New York), and Al Yurf et al. [1] (Cleveland Clinic). Tumors arising in the part of the anus distal to the dentate line (the pecten), with its mucosa of nonkeratinizing squamous cells, are described by these authors as tumors of the anal margin. For others, e.g., Beahrs [4] (Mayo Clinic, Rochester), Papillon [58] (Centre Leon Berard, Lyon), Cummings et al. [15] (Princess Margaret's Hospital, Toronto), the distal limit of the anal canal is the junction of the pecten with the perianal skin, called the anal verge. Their definition of the true external anal margin coincides with the definition of the perianal skin in the Union Internationale Contre le Cancer (UICC) classification [39] and the definition of the anal margin in the international histological classification of the World Health Organization [53].

Thus the distal limit of the anal canal is subject to controversy and the anatomical boundary used to distinguish the anal canal from the anal margin will influence the relative incidence of tumors allotted by various authors to each region: for those using the anal verge as the distal limit of the anal canal only 15% of anal cancers arise in the anal margin, whereas 30% of the anal tumors arise in this site when the dentate line is chosen as the distal limit of the canal.

Perianal Skin (Anal Orifice, External Anal Margin)

There are few indications regarding the lateral extent of the external anal margin. The principle described by Beahrs [4] has been adapted in general: carcinoma arising from the perianal area outside the anal verge in a region defined by a circle 6 cm in diameter, with the anal orifice as the center, is regarded as carcinoma of the external anal margin. Figure 19.1 reproduces the recommendations of the UICC relative to the anatomical limits of the anal canal and the perianal skin. In this chapter all references relating to this problem are discussed according to these proposed limits. The *anal canal* is subdivided into supra- and infrapectinate parts. The perianal skin is defined as the skin distal to the anal verge.

Pathology

The complexity of the anal anatomy is expressed in the pathological classification of tumors in this region. The macroscopic limits of the various parts of the anal region are well described, but the histological borders are much less precise. Erratic islands of a neighboring epithelial type can be frequently found and explain the absence of specific tumor types for each topographic subsite. The international histological classification proposed by the World Health Organization [53], shown in Tables 19.1 and 19.2, has gained wide acceptance.

Tumors of the epithelial and nonepithelial types and malignant melanoma form the main groups. The epithelial tumors are classified into squamous, basaloid, mucoepidermoid, glandular, and undifferentiated carcinoma types. The various tumor types may occur as pure or mixed. Examination of a tiny biopsy specimen can lead to an erroneous interpretation. It is recommended that a tumor be classified according to the predominant cell type.

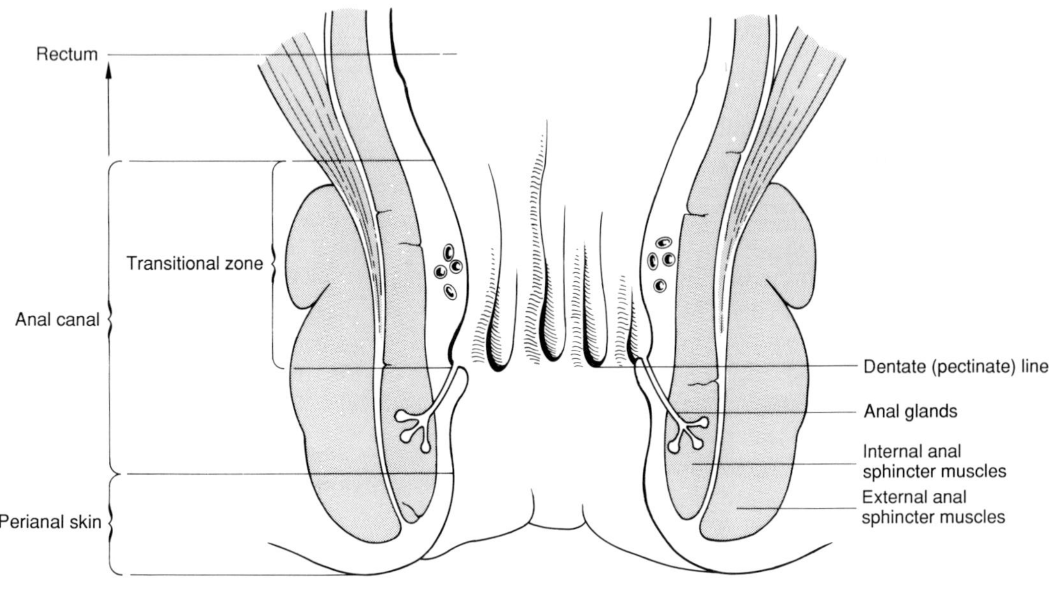

Fig. 19.1. The limit of the anal canal and the perianal skin according to the recommendations of the UICC. [Hermanek and Sobin 1987]

Table 19.1. International histological classification of tumors of the anal canal

I. Epithelial tumors
   A. Benign
   B. Malignant
      1. Squamous cell carcinoma
      2. Basaloid carcinoma
      3. Muco-epidermoid carcinoma
      4. Adenocarcinoma
         a. adenocarcinoma of rectal type
         b. adenocarcinoma of anal glands
         c. adenocarcinoma within anorectal fistula
      5. Undifferentiated carcinoma
      6. Unclassified carcinoma
II. Nonepithelial tumors
III. Malignant melanoma
IV. Unclassified tumors
V. Secondary tumors
VI. Tumor-like lesion

Table 19.2. International histological classification of tumors of the anal margin

I. Epithelial tumors
   A. Benign
   B. Malignant
      1. Squamous cell carcinoma
      2. Basal cell carcinoma
      3. Others
   C. Bowen's disease
   D. Paget's disease
II. Nonepithelial tumors
III. Unclassified tumors
IV. Secondary tumors
V. Tumor-like lesions
   A. Condyloma acuminatum
   B. Giant condyloma
   C. Pseudo-epitheliomatous hyperplasia
   D. Fibrous polyp (anal tag)
   E. Others

Tumors of the Anal Canal

Epithelial Tumors

Squamous Cell Carcinoma

Carcinoma in situ (Tis) occurs in the anal canal. Biopsy proof must be obtained to eliminate coexisting invasive carcinoma. Most of the malignant invasive tumors in the anal canal are of the nonkeratinizing type, often poorly differentiated [7, 28, 29] like carcinomas of the uterine cervix. The keratinizing type of squamous cell carcinoma arises predominantly from the skin of the anal orifice, but can be seen in the infrapectinate part of the anal canal [35]. Histological, grading and its implications for prognosis were emphasized by Hardcastle and Bussey [38], Loygue et al. [48], and Boman et al. [7] in analyses of surgical series.

Basaloid Carcinoma

Basaloid carcinomas are to be considered as a variety of the epidermoid type. They are termed as cloacogenic or transitional by some authors [31, 41]. Publications in the 1950 s by Grinvalsky and Hellwig [37], updated by Gillespie [31], regarding tumor appearance at electron microscopy illustrate the complexity of terminology. Various degrees of differentiation which have prognostic implications have been described [25, 30]. The predominant cell type is used to classify these tumors which frequently feature a mixed pattern with squamous components. Because of this, the percentage of tumors termed basaloid, transitional, or cloacogenic cancers in the published series varies widely from 10% to 50% [3, 7, 12, 15, 36], Cummings et al. [15] indicated 90% of the squamous type and 10% of the basaloid variety; Salmon et al. [73] reported 19 basaloid and 183 squamous cell carcinoma. When histology was reviewed in our series (Widgren, unpublished data), in one-third of the patients some change was made in the diagnosis of the pathological subtype, as was the case in other series [75]. Consequently the histopathological subtype should not be a criterion for treatment decisions, especially with respect to radiotherapy. Basaloid carcinoma do not seem to have better prognosis [7] than squamous cell carcinoma [35]. The rate of cancer deaths was the same in the series of Merlini and Eckert [51] for the squamous and basaloid subtypes.

Mucoepidermoid Carcinoma

Mucoepidermoid carcinomas are rare tumors thought to derive from the anal duct glands. These glands exhibit, near their opening into the sinus of Morgagni, an epithelial lining of the transitional type, but deeper down they are lined by cylindrical muciparous cells. This type of carcinoma is an intimate mixture of squamous, mucoid, and intermediate cell [29].

Adenocarcinoma

An authentic adenocarcinoma of the anal canal, related to ectopic islands of glandular mucosa, must be distinguished from the eventual adenocarcinomas arising from the anal duct glands or occasionally from a fistula [50]. Histochemical determination may be useful. This pathological condition is very rare. Merlini and Eckert [51] reported on nine patients suffering from adenocarcinoma of the anal canal glands in a series of 106 patients with anal tumors during the period 1942–1983, 66% of them died from cancer despite management with radical surgery. In the Department of Radiotherapy at the University Hospital of Geneva only two cases of true adenocarcinoma originating in the anal canal were observed from 1976 to 1987. True adenocarcinomas originating in the anus are to be distinguished from adenocarcinomas of the lower rectum extending to the anus.

Undifferentiated Carcinoma

Some of the undifferentiated carcinomas seem to be of the small cell type. A neuroendocrine origin comparable to small cell carcinoma of the lungs has been suggested. The prognosis is poor [7], with a high probability of distant metastases.

Tumors of the Nonepithelial Type

Rhabdomyosarcoma, Leiomyosarcoma, and Fibrosarcoma

Useful indications can be found in the review by Gebbers and Laissue [29]. The rarity of these conditions is illustrated by only two cases seen over a 40-year period at the University Hospital of Lausanne [51].

Malignant Melanoma

Malignant melanoma occurs in the vicinity of the pectinate line and is a polypoid or nodular tumor [13, 68, 75]. In about 30% of cases it is without pigmentation and at presentation is often already greater than 4 cm. It is a rare tumor and is said to constitute 12% of anal cancers. Its prognosis is disastrous.

Carcinoma in Associated Lesions

Dysplasia with atypia must be distinguished from regenerative hyperplasia [29]. Carcinoma associated with Crohn's disease and ulcerative colitis [67] has been reported, as has multicentric carcinoma [63].

Tumors of the Perianal Skin (Anal Orifice, External Anal Margin)

The *keratinizing squamous cell type* is predominant. *Basal cell carcinoma* of the perianal skin is a very rare disease [54]. Papillon et al. [60] observed three cases among 45 patients with carcinoma of the perianal skin. The natural history is local ulceration without metastasis.

Morphology and Extension of Malignant Tumors of the Anus

Morphology and Local Extension

Most of the carcinomas of the anal canal are infiltrating tumors with little propensity for exophytic growth due to the absence of intestinal lumen when the anus is in the resting position. At the beginning a small ulceration or fissure with slightly exophytic, but indurated, margins is present. Later on, the mucosa breaks down and a more or less deep ulceration, fixed to the underlying sphincter and giving rise to bleeding, can be detected. Only a few tumors near the anorectal junction are of the polypoid type. They also have an infiltrative base. Confusion with hemorrhoids is very common. In the middle and higher proximal part of the anal canal, tumors can remain without mucosal ulceration for a large part of their clinical history. At the beginning this type of carcinoma presents as a submucosal nodular infiltration. In more advanced stages the sphincter muscles are deeply invaded although there is little mucosal ulceration. The permeation of malignant cells takes place toward the rectal submucosa. Infiltration of 2–3 cm of the lower rectum is a frequent observation. Late presentation with extensive circular infiltration, stenosis, and incontinence has been seen. Beside this infiltration of rectal submucosa and sphincter muscles, extension to neighboring organs such as the vagina, bladder, and prostate has been reported in 15%–20% of cases [58]. The inferior part of the rectovaginal septum is the site most frequently involved. As the tumor grows, it causes narrowing of the vagina, but the vaginal mucosa is not ulcerated for a very long time. In our series, destruction of the vaginal mucosa has been seen in only one patient who had a tumor larger than 4 cm at presentation, the diagnosis of an anal tumor was established due to vaginal infection and bleeding. The vulva is nearly always spared. In addition to the visual examination, palpation of the infiltrating tumor beneath the perineal skin provides significant information on tumor extension.

In men, the prostate and the posterior urethra can be infiltrated which, in advanced cases, gives rise to a neoplastic pelvic blockage. Laterally the ischiorectal fossa is gained by the tumor and suppuration or fistulas with clinically subacute symptoms can be seen.

About 40% [58], 60% [44] of the tumors of the anal canal are of the proximal type. Carcinomas arising in the middle and lower part of the anal canal are more likely to exteriorize across the external anal orifice, but the visible external part of the tumor is nearly always smaller than the proximal palpable infiltration. In general, there is no difficulty, at least when the initial extent of the tumor is evaluated under general anesthesia, to differentiate these tumors of the middle and lower anal canal with exophytic or ulcerative extension to the perianal skin from carcinomas of the anal orifice itself, as defined in the anatomical staging system of the UICC illustrated in Fig. 19.1. The exteriorized tumors of the anal canal involve, in general, only part of the circumference of the anal orifice, contrary to carcinomas originating in the perianal skin which have a tendency to become circumferential.

The rare tumors of the mucoepidermoid or glandular types developing in conjunction with anal duct glands or fistulas have a clinical progression similar to the distal type.

Lymphatic Spread

Lymphatic dissemination of anal carcinomas takes place in two directions: by the pelvic route and by the inguinal route [29, 34]. There are numerous connections in the submucosal lymphatic network of the anal region, and the description of the main routes of spread in relation to the exact tumor topography in the anal canal or the anal margin are somewhat theoretical, especially when fairly advanced tumors are considered. Lymph node metastases are related to the size, topography, histology, and grade of the primary tumor [7, 28, 48, 75], but in each individual case there may be a surprising discordance between huge primary tumors and freedom of metastatic spread to the regional lymph nodes.

Inguinal Nodes

The section of the anus distal to the dentate line is drained to the superficial inguinal nodes. The frequency with which these nodes are reported to be involved varies somewhat. The most recent publications indicate involvement in about 10% of cases: Nigro [55] saw inguinal node involvement in four out of 104 patients; Cantril et al. [11] in seven out of 39 patients; Salmon et al. [73] in 23 out of 183 patients, five with bilateral and 18 with unilateral inguinal node involvement at presentation. In general, the involvement is unilateral and a single lymph node in the lower internal quarter of the inguinal fold is palpable. In our series we observed six out of 68 patients with synchronous inguinal involvement, five patients with unilateral and only one with bilateral involvement. We saw metachronous inguinal metastases in four out of 68 patients followed up for at least 24 months, twice with primary tumor recurrence and twice without any local failure in the anal canal.

Pelvic Nodes

The route via the mesorectum, the superior hemorrhoidal and inferior mesenteric vessels is considered to be the main route of spread for tumors of the middle and proximal anal canal. Large surgical series show 25%–30% [7, 28, 35, 37, 44, 48] of lymph nodes involved in this direction. When analyzing the specimens of abdominoperineal resection for anal canal cancer, Loygue et al. [48] found pararectal lymph nodes involved in 20%–25% of tumors less than 4 cm in diameter, in 31% of tumors 4–6 cm in size, and in 56% of tumors greater than 6 cm in diameter. Low-grade tumors showed less tendency for lymphatic spread; 9% of well-differentiated carcinomas, in contrast to 47% of undifferentiated tumors, showed regional mesenteric lymph node involvement. Pararectal node involvement was found with 25% of carcinomas arising in the proximal part of the anal canal. Tumors of the distal canal had a negligeable percentage of metastatic mesenteric nodes, but pelvic nodes were positive with 25% of carcinomas infiltrating the rectovaginal wall.

Frost et al. [28] found pelvic node involvement in patients whose tumors had just reached the submucosal layers of the anal epithelium. Deep infiltration of the anal sphincter muscles was linked to a high percentage of node metastases in their series.

Metastatic lymph nodes are usually close to the primary tumor, a few centimeters above the dentate line. Very careful clinical examination of this area is strongly recommended by Papillon [58]. In our conservatively treated series of locally advanced anal canal cancers of more than 4 cm diameter, pretherapeutic computerized tomographic (CT) scans showed images of enlarged perirectal nodes in only three out of 29 patients. This is very low when compared with histopathological results of radical surgical series. But this CT image criterion of enlarged, grossly involved nodes as opposed to invisible, only potentially microscopically involved nodes can be helpful in treatment decisions, especially when conservative primary radiation therapy versus radical surgery is being discussed. In a series of 37 patients locally controlled by radiotherapy between 1971 and 1973 [58], a failure rate of 24.3% was seen in pelvic lymph nodes when the perirectal nodes had not been irradiated. In 30 patients, seen between 1974 and 1978 in whom the primary tumor and the posterior pelvis had been irradiated, the failure rate in the pelvic nodes dropped to 6.6% [58]. Thus metastatic deposits in lymph nodes were shown to be radiosensitive.

The other route of pelvic lymph drainage is via the middle hemorrhoidal vessel and via the ischiorectal fossa to the hypogastric iliac nodes. Data on the incidence of synchronous involvement of the lateral pelvic nodes are scarce in surgical literature [76, 81]. In our experience from 1976 to 1987 only three cases of synchronous lateral pelvic nodes were seen in a total of 95 patients: one patient had enlarged iliac nodes at initial CT, the other had an isolated hypogastric node recurrence without any symptom of recurrence at the site of the primary tumor. Another patient had concomitant inguinal and iliac nodes on presentation. Schraut et al. [76] reported on seven out of ten patients with tumors more than 4 cm in diameter who had positive hypogastric and/or obturator nodes when dissection was extended to these areas at the time of initial radical surgery.

In their series of 59 patients treated by radical surgery, Stearns and Quan [81] found 45 patients with pelvic lymphadenectomy in addition to the abdomino perineal resection. Fifteen out of 45 had metastases to hypogastric and/or obturator nodes. One-third of the 15 positive patients survived.

Carcinomas of the perianal skin have an essentially inguinal lymphatic spread. Spread to the pelvic nodes is reported when local conservative treatment by excision or irradiation fails and radical surgery is necessary for salvage [1]. No pelvic nodes were observed by Beahrs [4] and Schraut et al. [76] in superficial small tumors of the perianal skin.

Distant Metastases

Carcinoma of the anus is predominantly a locoregional disease, and metastatic spread to distant organs is a rare condition when control of the primary tumor and its regional lymph nodes is obtained. About 5%–10% of patients with distant metastases at initial work-up have been reported [4, 35,

38]. We have observed only one patient with initial metastasis to the liver and synchronous bilateral inguinal lymph nodes. Nigro [55] observed four out of 104 patients with this condition, all of when died within less than 18 months.

Death due to metastatic disease without recurrence of the primary tumor was observed in the Geneva series in only two out of 68 patients. All the other recorded distant metastasis were combined with locoregionally uncontrolled cancer. Lung, liver, bone, and peritoneum are at risk.

Classification and Staging

The UICC TNM 1987 Classification

Classification of tumors with respect to their extension at the moment of diagnosis should permit establishment of prognostic factors, treatment guidelines, and comparison of treatment results. A new classification based on clinical examination and completed by the results of radiographic imaging and endoscopy was proposed for anal cancers by the UICC in 1987 [39]. Tables 19.3 and 19.4 show this clinical classification with its various categories for tumors, nodes and metastases. Anal canal cancers (ICD-O 154.2) and cancers of the perianal skin (ICD-O 173.5) are clearly separated. The latter are classified as skin tumors of the trunk originating in the perianal skin.

The 1987 UICC classification of anal canal cancers introduces tumor size as a classification criterion for the first time. The previous UICC classification had given rise to criticism, particularly when a conservative treatment approach was planned. The precise degree of sphincter infiltration- with respect to the external and internal sphincter – was difficult to assess by clinical examination. Small tumors of the proximal anal canal which rapidly involved the lower rectum had to be classified T3. Carcinomas distal to the dentate line and extending slightly toward the skin of the anal orifice did not have the bad prognosis of T3 tumors. Tumors infiltrating the external sphincter and classified as T2 might have been less easy to cure by conservative methods than some tumors clinically staged as T3. These considerations are of the utmost importance when nonsurgical series have to be reported and analyzed

The new 1987 classification identifies tumors of less than 2 cm, tumors from 2 to 5 cm, tumors above 5 cm, and tumors invading adjacent organs. Invasion of sphincter muscles alone does not classify for T4. The 1987 classification also specifies that the

Table 19.3. UICC/TNM classification of malignant tumors - anal canal (ICD-O 154.2). (From [39])

T - Primary Tumor
    TX Primary tumor cannot be assessed
    TO No evidence of primary tumor
    Tis Carcinoma in situ
    T1 Tumor 2 cm or less in greatest dimension
    T2 Tumor more than 2 cm but not more than 5 cm in greatest dimension
    T3 Tumor more than 5 cm in greatest dimension
    T4 Tumor of any size invades adjacent organ(s), e. g., vagina urethra, bladder (involvement of the anal sphincter muscle(s) *alone* is not classified T4)

N - Regional Lymph Nodes
    NX Regional lymph nodes cannot be assessed
    NO No regional lymph node metastasis
    N1 Metastasis in perirectal lymph node(s)
    N2 Metastasis in unilateral internal iliac and/or inguinal lymph node(s)
    N3 Metastasis in perirectal and inguinal lymph nodes and/or bilateral internal iliac and/or inguinal lymph nodes

M - Distant Metastasis
    MX Presence of distant metastasis cannot be assessed
    MO No distant metastasis
    M1 Distant metastasis
        The categories M1 and pM1 may be further specified according to the following notation:
        Pulmonary PUL
        Osseous OSS
        Hepatic HEP
        Peritoneum PER
        Lymhnodes LYM
        Others OTH

Table 19.4. UICC/TNM classification of malignant tumors - skin tumors - trunk including anal margin and perianal skin (ICD-O 173.5). (From [39])

T- Primary Tumor
    TX Primary tumor cannot be assessed
    TO No evidence of primary tumor
    Tis Carcinoma in situ
    T1 Tumor 2 cm or less in greatest dimension
    T2 Tumor more than 2 cm but not more than 5 cm in greatest dimension
    T3 Tumor more than 5 cm in greatest dimension
    T4 Tumor invades deep extradermal structures, e. g., skeletal muscle or bone

N - Regional Lymph Nodes
    The regional lymph nodes are the ipsilateral inguinal nodes
    NX Regional lymph nodes cannot be assessed
    NO No regional lymph node metastasis
    N1 Regional lymph node metastasis

M - Distant Metastasis
    MX Presence of distant metastasis cannot be assessed
    MO No distant metastasis
    M1 Distant metastasis
        Any metastasis to other than regional lymph nodes is considered M1

rectum there is, to our knowledge, no publication on results of endorectal sonography in the diagnosis of perirectal metastatic nodes of anal canal cancer.

Other Classifications

Institutions traditionally using radiotherapy as a primary conservative treatment modality, such as the Fondation Curie [71], the Centre Leon Berard [58] where external irradiation of anal cancer has been routine practice since the early 1960s, have alsways used their own simple clinical classification based on tumor size. Tumors are classified with respect to their maximal size: less than 4 cm, from 4 to 6 cm, and more than 6 cm, movable or fixed with respect to adjacent organs or structures. Involvement of the perianal skin and tumor extension to the lower rectum does not classify for T 3. Papillon [58] proposed the Centre Leon Berard classification which has been used in Geneva since 1976. This clinical classification takes in to account almost all the factors needed for a conservative treatment decison:

- T 1 and T 2 are small tumors up to and including 4 cm in diameter. Their limited local extent permits conservative treatment by radiation with a high probability of cure and good functional results.

regional lymph nodes of the anal canal are the inguinal, perirectal, and internal iliac lymph nodes. Physical examination, endoscopy, and radiological imaging are the procedures advised for assessment of the various TNM categories.

Only inguinal nodes are easy to evaluate, with the possibility of cytological proof by fine needle puncture or histological proof by excision. Careful palpation of the mesorectum in the vicinity of the primary anal tumor in order to disclose lymph nodes is a clinical procedure which gives valuable information, especially when performed under general anesthesia [58]. A bipedal lymphangiogram does not give information on perirectal and hypogastric nodes.

Currently the best imaging tool seems to be the CT which, in some patients, shows grossly enlarged perirectal and pelvic nodes compared with patients with the probability of only microscopic lymph node deposits. Contrary to adenocarcinoma of the

- T3 are tumors of more than 4 cm in diameter, movable, with no ulceration of the vaginal mucosa, and no direct extension to genital or urological structures. These tumors are primarily operable, but have a high probability of cure with primary radiotherapy with sphincter preservation.
- T4a are tumors with ulceration of the vaginal mucosa and with an accrued risk of rectovaginal fistula when treated conservatively by radiotherapy.
- T4b are massive tumors with direct extension and/or fixation to neighboring organs other than the rectum, perianal skin, and vagina. These tumors have much less probability of being definitely cured by conservative radiotherapy with acceptable functional results, and there is also an undue risk of occult tumor progression in postirradiation fibrotic areas which is very difficult to monitor by clinical examination and even repeated tissue probes. These repeated probes can even promote painful postradiaton necrosis. Massive T4b tumors in the Centre Leon Berard classification are often not primarily operable. Combined preoperative chemoradiotherapy followed by planned radical surgery seems to be the standard [59] treatment, and new modalities without surgery, such as radical chemoradiotherapy with or without secondary scar excisions, are an investigational approach.

Epidemiology

Incidence

Anal cancer is said to be 20–30 times less common than colorectal cancer [2, 84] and constitutes 2%–5% of all cancers of the terminal intestine. These figures are to be modified in countries with a high incidence of anal cancers, e.g., northeastern Brasilia and India where the incidence of anal cancer is close to the incidence of cancer of the uterine cervix, penis and vulva. Exogenic factors such as viral infection by herpes simplex and some categories of human papilloma virus [64, 85] have been thought to contribute to the pathogenesis of anal cancer.

Age and Sex

In Europe and North America the mean age of patients is 58–60 years [3, 7, 35, 59]. Carcinoma of the anal canal is more frequent in females [2, 73, 84] the sex ratio being 2–5:1 in favor of women. Papillon and Montbarbon [59] indicate a sex ratio of 4.7:1 in 332 patients seen from 1971 to 1986, Salmon et al. [73] 5.5:1 based on 183 cases seen from 1968 to 1979. In selected areas such as San Francisco [2, 11] the female/male ratio is 1:1, and in some hospitals the ratio is even inverted. In the Geneva patient group observed from 1976 to 1985, there were 52 women and 16 men. Mean age was 65 years with a range of 35–92, with 26 out of the 68 patients being 70 years or older. Cancer of the external anal margin, when defined as cancer of the perianal skin, distal to the anal verge, is more frequent in men [1, 7, 35, 52] with a sex ratio of 1:3 in favor of males.

Associated Lesions and Predisposing Factors

The presence of nonmalignant perianal conditions, such as hemorrhoids, condyloma acuminatum [45, 85], chronic fistulas [50], leukoplakia [5], psoriasis, chronic abscess, chronic pruritus, herpes, effects of previous irradiation [78], and lichen sclerosus et atrophicus [80] have been claimed as frequently associated lesions in cancer of the perianal skin but much less in cancer of the anal canal.
Extramammary Paget's disease [47] and Bowen's disease [82] merit special attention. These noninvasive intraepithelial conditions may predispose to invasive cancer or be associated with cancer of the anus or visceral neoplasms. In the series of Greenall et al. [35], who defined the distal limit of the canal by the dentate line, 60% of the patients with cancer of the anal margin had one or more of these conditions, compared to only 6% of patients with anal canal cancer. Papillon [58], who defined the limit of the anal canal at the anal verge, observed these associated conditions in very few patients with cancer of the anal canal. For practical purposes it can be said that the frequent association of benign and precancerous conditions with anal cancer requires biopsy of any doubtful lesion on this area.
To understand better the etiological factors of anal cancers, the sexual history of both male and female patients needs to be elucidated. Case reports and epidemiologic al studies suggest that a possible predisposing factor to anal cancer is venereal disease. Condylomata is a venereally transmitted disease,

and its association with anal carcinoma is strong. Malignant transformation in condyloma acuminatum has been described [45]. The giant condyloma of Buschke-Loewenstein [9] is histologically a true squamous carcinoma. Syphilis has also been suggested. In large epidemiological studies Dahlin et al. [18] and Austin [2] demonstrated a higher than expected incidence of anal cancers in unmarried males. The homosexual popultion is possibly at particular risk of anal cancer, as suggested by the data obtained by Cantril et al. [11].

Clinical Symptoms and Diagnostic Procedures

Clinical manifestation of anal cancer is often late and nonspecific. At diagnosis most tumors are 3–4 cm or more in diameter. Sometimes an inguinal node is the first clinical manifestation. It is rare that anal cancer is disclosed in a hemorrhoidectomy specimen or at routine clinical examination. The interval between first clinical symptoms and diagnosis is in general several months. In our patients with anal canal cancer, 52 out of 68 had tumors 4 cm or more in diameter at initial diagnosis. Bleeding as a first symptom is not constant: it is seen in about 50% of the patients.

Frequently clinical symptoms related to deep infiltration of advanced lesions, such as change in bowel habits, pelvic pain, discomfort in the sitting position, and presence of a perineal mass, are the reasons for consultation. When these symptoms are associated with intermittent bleeding, an erroneus diagnosis of hemorrhoids – which are sometimes present in addition to the cancer – is often made. Delay in diagnosis prejudices the success of conservative treatment.

The clinical examination represents an essential step in the treatment approach, especially when conservative treatment by irradition is under discussion. In general, the genupectoral position is advised. The exact extension in the craniocaudal direction has to be stated with precision. It can be of appreciable value to the radiotherapist when the superior pole of the tumor is marked by a metal seed, preferably inserted at the boundary between tumor and healthy mucosa. The circumferential tumor extension has to be stated relative to the decubitus or genupectoral position of the patient. The maximal diameter of the tumor should be measured.

The infiltrative part of the tumor is evaluated by palpation of the ischiorectal fossa and the perineum. The possibility of moving the tumor with respect to underlying structures has to be stated. For anterior tumors in female patients, vaginal inspection to disclose mucosal ulceration is mandatory.

The precise description is best completed by an individual anatomical scheme established at the time of the first clinical examination. This basic evaluation of the extent of the tumor should be done, whenever possible, by the surgeon and the radiotherapist in a joint session. This perineal and pelvic examination to disclose contiguous tumor extension should be completed by palpation of the mesorectum in the presacral area and by palpation of the lateral pelvic walls for eventual metastatic lymph node involvement. If the evaluation of extent of the tumor is difficult due to excessive pain or stenosis, general anesthesia has to be planned. Routine clincal examination includes evaluation of the inguinal nodes, especially at the medial part of the inguinal folds.

CT scans give additional information on the mesorectal and hypogastric nodes. Endoscopic examination shows the tumor morphology and allows for a diagnostic biopsy: when conservative irradiation is the therapy of choice, the biopsy should have the aim of assessing the diagnosis but should not be performed with excisional intent. The amount of radiotherapy to be given after a simple biopsy or incomplete excisional surgery is the same, but functional results are worse in the latter case.

A routine CT scan of the liver does not seem necassary, initial liver metastases are an exception. Sonography of the liver can be done in high-risk patients with lymph node involvement or high-grade tumors.

Biological markers of anal tumors are lacking. Determination of carcinoembryonal antigen level as for adenocarcinomas of the colon and rectum does not give useful information of tumor regression or local and distant recurrence. In our experience, even with massive liver metastases, this biological marker remained under the clinically sigificant level. Recently a radioimmunological assay for squamous cell carcinoma antigen expression in serum has been introduced [65]. Sensitivity in this series was 78% and specificity 92%.

All the other routine radiographic and biological examinations have to be considered on an individual basis depending on the choice of treatment modality. It must be emphasized that a clinical examination which results in a precise tumor description is one of the most important steps whenever conservative radiotherapy is under discussion. The final decision between radical surgery and radiation boost after an initial sequence of radiation or radiochemotherapy – to be considered as a test of radiosensitivity – is based on the clinical response of the tumor.

Conservative Treatment Modalities of Cancers of the Anal Canal

Several conservative treatment modalities can be discussed: local excision and various methods of external and interstitial radiotherapy.

Local Excision

There is hardly any indication for conservative local excision in infiltrative carcinoma of the anal canal. Greenall et al. [35], in a collected series of 889 patients with anal cancer, found 10% of them treated by local excision, 41% of whom had local recurrence. Table 19.5 shows results of local excision for carcinoma of the anal canal. Local excision alone can be performed as a curative treatment modality only in very early lesions of the lower anal canal. Local excision with a 1–1,5 cm safety margin is suitable for lesions below the dentate line, which do not significantly encroaching upon it, measure less than 2 cm in diameter, and are not more than microinvasive at the histopathological examination.

In the Mayo Clinic series [7], in which the authors strictly adhered to these indication criteria of tumor invasion confined to the anal epithelium and subepithelial connective tissue with comfortable safety margins of the surgical specimen, 12 out of 13 patients were definitely locoregionally controlled by local excision, the one recurrence was salvaged by radical surgery. These observations showed that regional lymph node metastases were nonexistant in this very early tumor group. The cases reported were of the squamous cell carcinoma type. Local mangement was unsuccessful in two patients with tumor invading through the musculature [7]. In the experience of Frost et al. [28], only small, 1–2 cm, superficial tumors had a low rate of lymph node invasion (one out of 13) on the surgical specimen, whereas there were lymph node metastases associated with 57% of tumors of 5–6 cm with only superficial invasion.

Small tumor size is not always related to the superficial depth of invasion [28]. Tumors as small as 0.5 cm in diameter have been reported to infiltrate the external sphincter muscle, emphasizing the potential risk of lymph node dissemination and the danger of locoregional recurrence. When deep invasion was seen despite a tumor size of 1–2 cm in the series of Frost et al. [28], 75% of patients (three out of four) had node metastases. Schraut et al. [76] reported on seven patients with anal canal cancer treated by local excision: five with small microinvasive lesions were cured, two with deep tumor invasion failed.

Carcinomas of small diameter situated at the level of the dentate line can result in substantial anal stricture when locally excised with safety margins; thus they are not suitable for local excision for topographic reasons, even when only superficially localized to the submucosal layer. Special surgical techniques with regard to reconstruction of partial sphincter muscle and puborectalis muscle defects

Table 19.5. Local excision for carcinoma of the anal canal

Reference	Patients treated (n)	Patients treated by LE[a]	Survivors at 5 years	Local recurrences (n)	Distant limit of canal
Boman et al. 1984 [7]	188	2 DI	NI	2/2	DL
		12 SF	12/12	1/12	
Clark et al. 1986 [12]	67	3 IR	NI	NI	AV
		9 TR	NI	4/9	
Greenall et. al. 1985 [35]	126	11	5/11	7/11	DL
Pyper and Parks 1985 [69]	57	4 AL	NI	NI	DL
		4 SL	3/4	1/4	
Schraut et al. 1983 [76]	31	2 DI	NI	2/7	AV
		5 SF	5/7	0/5	
	469	52	74%	37%	

[a] Lesions described as: SF, superficial; DI, deeply invasive; SL, small lesion; AL, advanced lesion; IR, incompletely resected; TR, totally resected.
LE, local excision; DL, dentate line; AV, anal verge; NI, not indicated.

have been described with good functional results [61, 62]. Thus it can be stated that it is not a lack of surgical skill in repairing sphincter defects but a high probability of microscopic residual tumor deposits in the excised area and a high probability of nontreated cancer in the regional lymph nodes which are the reasons why local excision alone is rarely recommended in carcinoma of the anal canal.

Alternative conservative treatment modalities such as primary curative radiotherapy should be discussed when radical surgery is thought to be an overtreatment. The indication of local excision alone in anal canal cancer is a difficult treatment decision. Blind local destructive methods, such as fulguration by electrocoagulation, application of liquid nitrogen, or laser, are no longer indicated when radiotherapy is available, even when done with palliative intent.

Local Excision and Postoperative Irradiation

No reliable indications on the role and success of postoperative radiotherapy in incompletely locally excised carcinoma of the anal canal can be drawn from the surgical reports as the anal canal lesions are mostly grouped with the perianal cancers in the local excision groups. Surgical tumor debulking with postoperative radiotherapy for positive margins has to be strongly advised against in cancer of the anal canal. Clinical examination in the early postoperative period is not reliable in the evaluation of the extent of residual tumor. When incomplete local excision and postoperative irradiation are mentioned [28, 76], poor tolerance of radiation and high rates of minor and major local complications are documented. In our series there was one severe case of radionecrosis requiring amputation and one case of partial sphincter leakage with protrusion of the rectal mucosa in patients who had undergone wide but incomplete local excision and were subsequently referred for postoperative irradiation. The very difficult question of the optimal time interval between such unfortunate tumor debulking and "rescue" irradiation has to be raised. There is actually no clinically reliable test or imaging procedure to document the potential of the tumor to recruit nondividing cells into the proliferative state and accelerate the cell cycle. In the absence of documented guidelines, the answer would be in favor of as short an interval as possible between inadequate tumor surgery and irradiation. Unfortunately incomplete reepithelialization of the

excised mucosa before starting irradiation can give rise to local infection and poor short- and long-term tolerance to radiotherapy.

Radiotherapy

Radiotherapy with the aim of curing infiltrating carcinoma of the anal canal has been used since 1921, particularly in Europe. Major contributions have been made by the Fondation Curie in Paris. In Anglo-Saxon countries radical surgery is the traditional treatment policy and until very recently only inoperable patients were handed over by surgeons, with regret, to radiotherapy. Interstitial implants, external irradiation, and a combination of both are employed as definite treatment modalities with a conservative aim.

Interstitial Implants and External Irradiation Limited to the Anal Canal Without Treatment of the Mesorectal Nodes

Interstitial implants of radium 226 were already being used for anal cancer in the 1930s. In 1960 Courtial et al. [14] reported a 36% 5-year survival rate for 60 patients with small or moderately advanced anal cancers treated by interstitial radium. Devois and Decker [20] and Dalby and Pointon [19] also did pioneering work. Severe cases of radionecrosis were reported, probably due to a lack of precise dosimetry and nonoptimal implant techniques [8]. Papillon [58] showed better tolerance by fractionation of the implants. Since the early 1960s curietherapy alone has mostly been discontinued to be replaced by external megavoltage irradiation alone or combined with interstitial implants.

The use of artificial isotopes, e. g., iridium 192 [42], implantation of empty source carriers, dosimetry by computer, and recently available remote afterloading machines have renewed the interest in interstitial implants. An interstitial implant alone, without external irradiation, is a local therapeutic measure and rarely indicated. Owing to the rapid fall-off in the absorbed radiation dose at the periphery of the implant, regional lymph nodes are not affected by these interstitial treatments. When interstitial implants are used alone for infiltrative large or undifferentiated tumors with a high probability of mesorectal lymph node involvement, these techniques are to be considered suboptimal with bad treatment results. Papillon and Montbarbon [59] reported an 18.6% pelvic node failure rate when using local treatment of the anal canal without irradiation of the presacral pelvic area. These failures dropped to 6.1% after 1974 when local anal irradiation was accompanied by posterior pelvic radiotherapy. Interstitial implants alone have comparable indications to local excision in anal canal carcinoma.

In the Geneva Department of Radiotherapy, a fractionated interstitial implant alone has been used only twice in 10 years for the treatment of invasive squamous cell carcinoma of the anus: once with success in an 80-year-old patient who had been treated by conventional external irradiation and radium insertions for a squamous cell carcinoma of the uterine cervix 30 years previously, and once without success in another patient not fit for any surgical procedure who had been irradiated for an unknown perineal disease by superficial orthovoltage 25 years previously.

For didactic reasons it has to be emphasized that, with the patient in the lithotomy or genupectoral position, a small direct perineal irradiation field using external beams, e. g., cobalt, electrons, low-energy photons of linear accelerators, or betatrons, allows for treatment of the anal canal alone without valuable thearapeutic contribution to the lymph node-bearing mesorectal areas. These direct perineal fields of external irradiation can be compared to other local procedures such as interstitial implants alone or wide local excision.

Combination of External Irradiation
and Interstitial Implants

The optimal indication for interstitial implants seems to be in combination with external irradiation in a sequential treatment approach initated by Papillon [58]. External radiation is directed to all tissue volumes in the perineum and pelvis presumed to harbor microscopic and macroscopic tumor. This part of the treatment is given first in fractionated treatment sessions. Papillon advises a 3000-cGy minimal dose in ten sessions over 17 days to a direct perineal field with the patient in the lithotomy position. The maximal dose to the perineal skin is 4200 cGy [59]. Perineal irradiation is supplemented by 1800 cGy in six fractions to the lymph node-bearing mesorectum via a transsacral field. After a 6–8-week rest period, an interstitial implant of iridium 192, 1500 cGy, is applied to the area of the primary tumor. Scar biopsy is not attempted. The main advantage of interstitial implants is the strictly local effect of this type of radiation, saving the neighboring normal tissue from high total doses. If this type of conservative radiotherapy

fails, radical rescue surgery can be performed with good healing conditions.

Locoregional results and survival figures obtained by external irradiation and interstitial iridium 192 are very favorable. Papillon and Montbarbon [59] recently reported on 222 patients treated with a conservative aim by cobalt and interstitial iridium from 1971 to 1984. The patients were followed up for at least 3 years. Among them were 159 patients followed up for 5 years. The disease-free survival rate was 64.6% at 3 years and 64.1% at 5 years; 14% of the patients died from intercurrent disease and 20% died of anal cancer. The 5-year survival rate was 76.2% for tumors of 4 cm or less and 58.3% for tumors larger than 4 cm at presentation. Of the patients alive at 5 years in the 4 cm or less group, 82% had normal sphincter function, as did 70.6% in the larger than 4 cm group Severe postirradiation complications were seen in 2.2% of the 5-year survivors.

In Geneva we used a technique similar to that advocated by Papillon in 39 patients from October 1976 to October 1985. Combined chemotherapy was not emloyed in this group of patients. Minimal follow-up of the whole group was more than 24 months in September 1987 [66]. Local control with normal sphincter function was 75% in the 4 cm or less tumor group and rose to 87.5% after rescue surgery for primary tumor recurrence or severe complications. In patients with locally more advanced, larger than 4 cm, tumors the corresponding treatment results were 69% of primary local control and 78.3% after salvage surgery. In our institution 18.8% of patients with small tumors, 4 cm or less, and 26.1% of patients with tumors larger than 4 cm died of local anal cancer and/or distant metastases. Radiation necrosis, without tumor recurrence, requiring radical surgery was observed in two out of 39 patients. One patient with necrosis of the perianal skin could be managed by conservative surgery. This amounts to 7.7% of patients who required surgery for complications. Table 19.6 summarizes these results.

Radical External Irradiation Alone

External irradiation alone is used as a definite primary curative treatment. The main experience with this type of conservative treatment approach has been gained by the Fondation Curie [73], Princess Margaret's Hospital [15], the Hôpital Tenon [3], and the Institut Gustave Roussy [24]. Other reports come from San Francisco [11, 21] and Geneva [71]. Various arrangements for irradiation portals by me-

Table 19.6. Combined external irradiation and interstitial iridium 192 without chemotherapy for anal canal cancer

Reference	Patients (n)	ExtRT (Gy)	[192] Ir (Gy)	Dose to inguinal region if NO (Gy)	Local control (RT/after rescue APR) (%)	Survival at 5 years (%)	Late complications (grade III) (%)
Papillon and Montbarbon 1987 [59] (Centre Leon Berard)	159[a]	30	15–20	–	Tumor ≤ 4 cm: 82.5/87.3 Tumor > 4 cm: 70.6/73.9 NS	76.2[a] 58.3[a] $p < 0.05$	2.2
Pipard 1989 [66] (Geneva University Hospital)	39[b]	30	15–20	–	Tumor ≤ 4 cm: 75/87.5 Tumor > 4 cm: 69/78.3	81[b] 73.9[b]	7.7

[a] Minimum follow-up ≥ 5 years,
[b] Minimum follow-up ≥ 2 years,
ExtRT, external radiotherapy; RT, radiotherapy; APR, abdominoperineal resection.

gavoltage machines have been described by the above institutions. In general, doses of up to 40–45 Gy are directed at tissues possibly harboring infraclinical tumor deposits, and doses of up to, 60–65 Gy are directed at the macrosopic tumor bulk by means of a boost to reduced tissue volumes.

In the series of the Fondation Curie only very early tumors were treated by irradiating a perineal field. Fields to the total pelvis and the inner part of the inguinal folds have mostly been described, thus taking into account the pelvic and inguinal lymph node problem. Daily doses of 180–200 cGy are given. In the series of Cantril et al. [11], ten out of 38 patients required a break in treatment because of poor acute tolerance to radiation. Cummings et al. [15] documented poor acute tolerance to high-dose continuous external irradiation even without combined chemotherapy. The Toronto regimen [15] is 50 Gy in 4 weeks, with a 250 cGy daily fraction dose. Split-course regimens allowing for recovery of the acute skin and bowel reactions have therefore been described.

Table 19.7 shows local control and survival figures of the published series using external megavoltage irradiation without chemotherapy for anal canal carcinoma. Local control with sphincter preservation by primary irradiation is about 80% in small (T1, T2) tumors and about 60% in larger (T3, T4) tumors. It must be emphasized that rescue surgery is not always feasible in psychologically and medically disabled elderly patients. In patients fit for rescue surgery final local control is about 85% in small and 70% in large anal canal tumors.

The rate of major complications requiring surgery was 8% in the Fondation Curie from 1968 to 1982.

Table 19.7. Radical external irradiation without chemotherapy for cancer of the anal canal

Reference	Patient (n)	Dose to primary tumor (Gy)	Dose to inguinal region (Gy)	Local control (%)	Survival at 5 years (%)	Late complications (grade III) (%)
Eschwege et al. 1985 [24]	64	60	–	T1–T2: 91 T3: 72 T4: 66 All: 81	T1–T2: 72 T3–T4: 35 All: 46	14
Cantril et al. 1983 [11]	88	60–70	–	80	79	5
Cummings et al. 1984 [15]	25	50	25–30	60	85	12
Salmon et al. 1984 [73]	158	50–65	50	Tumor < 4 cm: 76 Tumor 4–6 cm: 57 Tumor > 6 cm: 25	Tumor < 4 cm: 70 Tumor 4–6 cm: 57 Tumor > 6 cm: 33	8

Eschwege [24] indicated 14% major complication rate, with all cases observed during the first 2 years after irradiation. Cantril et al. [11] reported a local control rate of 26 out of 32 at 5 years, two patients suffered from radiation necrosis. Cummings et al. [15] indicated three major complications in 25 patients treated by radical radiation alone.

Five-year survival covers a wide range of 33%–85%, depending essentially on initial tumor size and presence of synchronous inguinal and pelvic metastatic lymph nodes. Acknowledging the fact that some patients in the radiation therapy series would never have been in curative surgical statistics, these results are at least as good if not better than those obtained by primary mutilating surgery.

Combined Radiochemotherapy

Combined radiation and chemotherapy for anal cancer has been performed for more than 10 years but remains a wide field of investigation. Published series are small. Mostly follow-up is too short for final conclusions. Neither the optimal combination and sequence of chemotherapy, nor the optimal dose and portal arrangement of radiation therapy has been agreed upon unanimously. There are no results of a randomized trial comparing the same irradiation technique with or without chemotherapy available. Institutional series comparing results obtained by radiation alone and subsequently by concomitant radiochemotherapy show some advantage of the combined modality [15, 35, 59, 66].

Anal carcinoma presents initially in more than 90% as a locoregional disease; chemotherapy is used for an additive or sensitizing effect with local radiotherapy. Various active drugs with moderate efficacy have been described, including bleomycin, doxorubicin, mitomycin, *cis*-platinum [72]. Laboratory data have shown additive effects only for mitomycin and radiation [70]. Although superadditive effects have been suggested for 5-fluorouracil and radiation, independent action could not be excluded [10].

The acute toxicity of combined radiochemotherapy includes leukopenia, thrombocytopenia, proctitis, perineal dermatitis, diarrhea, stomatitis, temporary hair loss. This toxicity is mild to moderate in patients treated with up to 30 Gy, with more severe acute enteroproctitis and perineal reactions in those treated with higher radiotherapy doses [15, 35, 55, 56].

Among the various radiochemotherapy modalities, three main working hypotheses can be distinguished: Preoperative chemoradiation, Definitive chemoradiation, and Chemoradiation and interstitial implants.

The most representative series published for each of them are shown in Table 19.8.

Preoperative Chemoradiation

Preoperative chemoradiation involves a significantly reduced amount of external irradiation combined with one or two cycles of chemotherapy followed by abdomino perineal resection. More recently, based on numerous negative surgical specimens, scar excisions or multiple biopsies have been performed [46, 52, 55, 74].

In 1974 Nigro et al. [56] published a report on the use of 5-fluorouracil (1000 mg/m^2/24 h continuous infusion for 4 days) and mitomycin (15 mg/m^2 i. v. bolus on day 1) concomitantly with 30 Gy over 3 weeks external irradiation as a preoperative measure. A 4-days course of 5-fluorouracil was repeated after the end of radiotherapy. Despite the reduced irradiation dose, tumor-free operative specimens raised the question as to the usefullness of radical surgery and the possibility of a conservative approach in cases of a clinical disappearance of the tumor.

The tumor disappeared clinically about 6 weeks after the induction therapy in 97 out of 104 patients in the collected series of the Wayne State University [55]. Microscopic examination of the radical surgery specimen or of the excised scar showed no more tumor in 83 out of 93 patients, 11 undergoing no biopsy at all. Despite a negative scar biopsy, recurrence occurred in seven out of 61 patients, four of whom could be rescued by delayed radical surgery.

The original protocol of Nigro has been modified by several investigators [15, 35, 40, 59, 66, 79]. But there are remarkably consistent favorable results. In the series of the Memorial Sloan Kettering Center [35], radiation therapy began 2–3 days after chemotherapy. A second course of chemotherapy was not given. Greenall et al. [35] reported on 11 out of 18 conservatively treated patients after initial chemoradiotherapy. The corrected 5-year survival rate was 88%, comparing favorably with the 58% obtained in the previous radical surgery series at the same institution. About half of the patients retained normal anal function. Beside some severe acute reactions requiring inpatient care in Nigro's series, no severe late complications are indicated. When looking for factors related to residual disease in the scar specimen, tumor size of more than 5 cm was the most suggestive.

Table 19.8. Radiochemotherapy for anal canal carcinoma

Reference	Patients (n)	RT to primary and pelvic nodes (Gy)	RT to inguinal nodes (Gy)	5-FU, Mito-C courses (n)	Local control (%)	APR (%)	Survival (%)	Follow-up
Preoperative chemoradiation								
Nigro 1984 [55]	104	30	30	1 syn + 1 asyn	85	28	85	2–11 years
Michaelson et al. 1983 [57]	37	30	30	1 asyn	81	49	78	5–74 months
Definitive chemoradiation								
Cummings et al. 1984 [15]	30	50[a] 25+25[b]	25–30	2 syn	93	6	90	8–50 months
John et al. 1987 [40]	22	30–50[c]	30–40	2 syn	100	0	100	17–62 months
Sischy 1985 [79]	29	55–57[d]	45	2 syn	90	3	90	1–9 years
Dunst et al. 1988 [22]	21	30–50[e]	30–45	2 syn	78	19	76	2–25 months
Chemoradiation and interstitial iridium 192								
Papillon and Montbarbon 1987 [59]	70 (T3)	30+15 Ir	–	1 syn	87	NI	NI	3–10 years
Pipard 1989 [66]	29 (T3)	30–40+15 Ir	30–40	1 syn	79	10	86	2–7 years

[a] FUMIR continuous – no interruption in chemoradiation.
[b] FUMIR split – a break of several weeks after 25 Gy and subsequent field reduction for another 25 Gy.
[c] No split.
[d] Split after 30–45 Gy for better acute tolerance.
[e] Improved local control compared to 66% local control of 77 nonrandomized T3 tumors treated without concomitant chemotherapy.
5-FU, 5-fluorouracil; Mito-C, mitomycin-C; APR, abdomino perineal resection; NI, not indicated for this subgroup; syn, asyn, synchronous or asynchronous administration of chemotherapy with respect to radiotherapy; RT, radiotherapy; Ir, interstitial implant of iridium 192; Gy, gray (1 Gy = 100 cGy = 100 rads).

Definitive Chemoradiation

Definitive chemoradiation involves a moderately reduced amount of radical external irradiation combined with chemotherapy: 50–55 Gy combined with two chemotherapy courses, if necessary in a split-course regimen for better acute tolerance, are given. In general, the volume of the irradiation field has to be reduced after 30–40 Gy. Scar excision is not always performed, and radical surgery is reserved for tumor recurrence or severe complications. The main purpose is to obtain the same results with moderate total doses of external irradiation and synchronous chemotherapy as with very high-dose external irradiation of 65 Gy alone. The University of California's experience published by John et al. [40] describes 22 out of 22 patients who were locally tumor free, additional radiochemotherapy was administered in three. None had died of cancer after a 17–62-month follow-up. The adverse effects were represented in the patients of John et al. by various degrees of acute dermatitis, diarrhea and reversible hematological disorders. No severe late complications were reported.

The Princess Margaret's Hospital series [15] shows that primary local tumor control rose from 60% to 90% when chemotherapy (5-fluorouracil, mitomycin) was added to radiotherapy (FUMIR) (28 out of 30 patients controlled), but survival figures did not change significantly when comparing patients irradiated with or without concomitant chemotherapy. In the Toronto Fumir regimen acute intestinal, perineal, and hematological toxicity required prolonged inpatient care and resulted in several modifications to the continuous radiochemotherapy regimen: a 4-week break (FUMIR split), radiation boost after 25 Gy through small fields, omission of the second course of chemotherapy in some patients. Five out of 30 patients required surgery for late complications. Sischy [79] published favorable results and had to advise split-course irradiation because of bad acute tolerance after 3–4 weeks of irradiation. Dunst et al. [22] have given preliminary favorable results using external irradiation combined with two synchronous chemotherapy cycles.

Chemoradiation and Interstitial Implants

The combination of chemoradiation and in interstitial implants involves a significantly reduced amount of external irradiation, combined with one cycle of chemotherapy, and followed by an interstitial implant. No scar excision is performed. Surgery is reserved for rescue operations. It has been documented in the chemoradiotherapy plus "scar excision" reports that there was more frequent residual disease after treating large tumors with combined radiochemotherapy despite impressive clinical tumor shrinkage or even disappearance. Excision of the total amount of initial tumor-bearing tissue for microscopic examination is not possible when the aim of treatment is optimal sphincter preservation. Local recurrence despite negative biopsy controls has been reported. Thus biopsy of the initial tumor site is not fully reliable in advanced anal canal cancers.

The interstitial iridium implant gives additional localized irradiation to the whole initial tumor bed, while sparing surrounding healthy tissue better than external irradiation. This was the working hypothesis, based on the pioneering work of Papillon, adopted in our institution in July 1980 for anal canal cancers larger than 4 cm at the greatest diameter. The dose of external irradiation was 3000–4000 cGy in 15–20 fractions of 200 cGy per day. A very simple irradiation technique was used whereby parallelly opposed fields were irradiated with the patient lying in the prone position. The potentially lymph node-bearing pelvis up to the level of S1/S2 and the perineal primary tumor with a distal safety margin of 2 cm were included in simple rectangular fields. The medial part of the inguinal folds was not shielded in these fields.

During the 1st week of external irradiation concomitant chemotherapy was given: 0.4 mg/kg (maximal dose 20 mg) mitomycin, on day 1 and 800–1000 mg/m^2 5-fluorouracil on days 1–5 by means of 24 h drop infusions. A second course of chemotherapy was not given. After a 6-week rest period interstitial iridium was inserted for an additional dose of 1500–2000 cGy; 7 cm standard-length needles were used. The number of active lines varied from five to twelve needles, according to the initial tumor volume. In 29 patients, all having tumors greater than 4 cm at initial presentation and followed up in September 1987 after at least for 24 months, the local control rate was 79.3%. After radical rescue surgery local control was 89.6% (26 out of 29 patients); 13.8% of patients died from cancer, 10.3% of intercurrent diesease; 75,8% were alive without evidence of disease. No severe complications requiring surgery were observed. Mild fibrosis essentially limited to the tissue area implanted by iridium, but not impairing sphincter function, and occasional bleeding due to telangiectasia were minor sequelae in 20.6% of the patients treated [66].

Papillon and Montbarbon [59] reported an 87% local tumor control rate in tumors greater than 4 cm (T3 in the Centre Leon Berard Classification) when giving concomitant radiochemotherapy and iridium compared to 74% in their T3 cobalt/iridium series without chemotherapy.

In summary, primary conservative treatment using the various radiation modalities with or without combined chemotherapy results in survival figures comparable to those obtained by primary radical surgery. Preservation of useful sphincter function is possible in the majority of patients treated for small tumors and in about half of the patients treated for more advanced tumors over 4–5 cm at the greatest diameter. Sphincter conservation by irradiation is more hazardous for patients with tumors of more than 6–8 cm at presentation. Severe complications are rare with modern radiotherapeutic techniques.

Mutilating Treatment of Cancers of the Anal Canal

Abdominal perineal resection is the surgical procedure of choice. In some instances external irradiation represents a planned preoperative modality. External irradiation may also be advised as a postoperative modality when microscopic tumor clearance is felt to be improbable or when extensive lymph node metastasis are found.

Abdominoperineal Resection

For patients with invasive tumors of the anal canal and for patients with in situ or microinvasive carcinoma larger than 2 cm in diameter, abdominoperineal resection is the procedure agreed upon by most surgeons. Greenall et al. [35] stated that it is recommended as the standard procedure against which all others must be compared. As to the technical aspects of the operation, the perineal line of

Table 19.9. Potentially curative abdominoperineal resection for carcinoma of the anal canal

Reference	Patients (n)	APR (n)	Local recurrences (%)	Survival at 5 years (%)	Distal limit of canal
Boman et al. 1984 [7]	188	118	27	71	AV
Clark et al. 1986 [12]	67	41	58	NI	AV
Frost et al. 1984 [28]	172	109	27	62	AV
Greenall et al. 1985 [35]	144	103	21	58	DL
Hardcastle and Bussey 1968 [38]	92	83		48	DL
Loygue et al. 1980 [48]	124	33		53	AV
Merlini and Eckert 1985 [51]	69	69		23	AV
O'Brien et al. 1982 [57]	21	21		38	DL
Pyper and Parks 1985 [69]	57	37		42	DL
Schneider and Schulte 1981 [75]	49	33	32	29	AV
Schraut et al. 1983 [76]	31	24	54	54	AV
	1014	671		48	

APR, abdominoperineal resection; NI, not indicated; AV, anal verge; DL, dentate line.

resection should reach the ischial tuberosity on either side and should include removal of the contents of the ischiorectal fossa, in addition to the standard abdominoperineal resection used for rectal adenocarcinoma.

The experience of Schraut et al. [76] suggests that hypogastric and obturator lymph node dissection is useful. This type of extended surgery has the potential of accrued genitourinary morbidity. As to the need and benefits of such extended surgical procedures, the data are insufficient to allow a conclusive statement. Occasional long-term survivors among patients with hypogastric node involvement in addition to regional mesorectal nodes have been reported [76]. Stearns and Quan [81] reported on five out of 15 patients found to have positive nodes in the iliac lymphadenectomy specimen who had survived for more than 5 years. Posterior vaginectomy is recommended by Goligher [33] although others are more conservative when the rectovaginal septum is free of disease.

Retrospective evaluation of the results of radical surgery shows considerable variation in 5-year survival figures: from 23% to 71%. Case selection; separate treatment evaluation of particularly bad prognostic groups; exclusion of patients treated for palliation only; presentation of results as absolute, corrected, or actuarial data; nonagreement relative to the distal limit of the anal canal – dentate line or anal verge – make comparison of surgical series difficult. Percentage survival is about 50% at 5 years when more recent publications are reviewed. Survival after radical surgery is related to tumor size, grading, depth of invasion, and node involvement [7, 28, 35, 48, 69, 75, 76, 78, 81]. Table 19.9 summarizes the most recently published surgical results.

It is useful to notice that major surgery is not applicable to 15%–20% of patients because of their poor medical or psychological condition. An operative mortality of 3%–8% is to be taken into account.

Preoperative External Irradiation

When radiation treatment was used in huge tumors not suitable for primary radical surgery, shrinkage and even total disappearance of the tumor could be confirmed in the operative specimen [56, 59]. There does not seem to be a striking difference in the radiosensitivity of the various histopathological types of anal cancer; in particular, radioresistance in cloacogenic, transitional, or basaloid carcinoma could not be confirmed. A favorable response to moderate doses of irradiation (30–55 Gy) with conversion of fixed tumors to technically operable ones was observed by Papillon and Montbarbon [59] who reporte on 11 out of 21 negative surgical specimens after preoperative irradiation of 3000 cGy in 10 fractions, and a survival rate of 52% was seen in these patients at 3 years. An additional 14% died of intercurrent disease during the 3-year follow-up period. In the Geneva series, two patients with anal canal cancer and pelvic lymph nodes on pretherapeutic CT or lymphangiogram had no remaining tumor when planned radical surgery was performed after preoperative irradiation. Salmon et al. [73] reported on 4500–6500 cGy preoperative irradiation and found nine out of 25 resection specimens without tumor. Eighteen out of 25 patients were without recurrence at 3 years, in four the tumor had recurred.

Barthelemy et al. [3] published a series of 31 preoperative irradiations: crude survival in T3 and T4 tumors was 52% at 5 years. Eschwege et al. [24] Frost et al. [28], and Cantril et al. [11] observed similarly favorable responses to 4000–4500 cGy preoperative irradiation with subsequent low local recurrence rates after radical surgery.

Moderate preoperative irradiation 3000 cGy in ten fractions or a slightly higher and more protracted external irradiation of 4000–4500 cGy in 20–23 fractions, seems to be of benefit in locally advanced tumors. Advantages in local control and subsequent advantages in survival figures compared to surgery alone are highly probable. Preoperative irradiation may represent a test of radiosensitivity. An indication for radical surgery in large tumors can eventually be converted to a conservative treatment policy if the tumor has disappeard 4–6 weeks after the end of preoperative irradiation. In these cases, additional irradiation may represent, especially in poor-surgical risk patients, a worthwhile alternative treatment modality.

Colostomy before preoperative irradiation is, in general, not necessary. Occasionally colostomy may be needed in very advanced tumors with complete narrowing of the anal canal presenting with permanent incontinence or severe obstruction.

Postoperative Irradiation

Radiation as a postoperative adjunct is proposed by Glanzmann [32] on the basis of an analysis of unsatisfactory results of radical irradiation alone. Surgeons who agree upon locoregional failures after radical surgery also advise postoperative irradiation in deeply infiltrating, poorly differentiated and lymph node-positive tumors. In the publication by Frost et al. [28], the postoperative recurrences in node-positive patients dropped from 25% to 17% when radiation was given after surgery. Similarly favorable effects were seen by Schneider and Schulte [75].

Treatment of Lymph Nodes in Cancers of the Anal Canal

Synchronous Inguinal Nodes

Prophylactic lymph node dissection of the groin is not advised, despite its theoretical advantage [81], keeping in mind the considerable morbidity associated with this procedure.

When pathological inguinal nodes are present, radical groin dissection or step-by-step dissection followed by postoperative irradiation is indicated as a therapeutic measure to avoid cancer progression into a fixed and ulcerating groin mass. Inguinal synchronous lymph node metastases, even when locally controlled, are prognostically a serious problem. Fewer than 20% of the patients have survived 5 years in surgical publications [28, 35, 44, 49, 69, 75, 81]. In our series, six out of 68 patients had synchronous inguinal metastases, five patients in unilateral and one patient with bilateral nodes. All nodes were movable and treated by a simple exision of macroscopically enlarged nodes. Radical inguino crural node dissection was not attempted as a primary surgical procedure. Node excision was followed by postoperative radiation therapy to the involved groin and the homolateral intrapelvic nodes up to the common iliac nodes. Radiation of 45 Gy was given to the lateral pelvic nodes and 60 Gy to the involved inguinal area. A combination of cobalt and electrons was used. No prophylactic irradiation was given to the opposite inguinal fold. All synchronous inguinal metastases were controlled, and we observed only one patient with a moderate leg edema. No pathological fracture of the femoral head was seen in our patients. None of our patients had local recurrence in the inguinal fold or the iliac nodes. Two out of six died of liver and pulmonary metastases to the locoregionally controlled cancer. The remaining 66% are alive with no evidence of disease.

Papillon and Montbarbon [59] reported on 11 out of 19 5-year survivors (57.8%) in their patients presenting with synchronous inguinal metastases. They employed inguinal irradiation after more or less extended groin dissection.

Metachronous Inguinal Nodes

Metachronous lymph node metastases are well documented in the inguinal region only. Their prognosis seems more favorable than that of synchronous nodes: The 5-year survival rate in surgical series is indicated as being from 40% to 70% [35, 49, 57]. We have observed four out of 68 patients in this condition: two without recurrence of the primary tumor and two with concomitant recurrent cancer in the irradiated anal canal. Two out of four are alive with no evidence of disease. Two have died of cancer.

We recommend simple node excision and postoperative irradiation if possible. If the inguinal fold has already been irradiated during primary irradiation, more extensive node surgery is required with a high probability of lymphedema. When fixed metachronous nodes are detected, preoperative irradiation and/or intra-arterial chemotherapy selectively directed toward the involved side can be discussed.

Pelvic Nodes

The 5-year survival rates are low, about 30% [4, 7, 35, 48, 69, 81], when metastatic pelvic lymph nodes are discovered in the radically excised specimen. Node-negative patients have much better local control and survival figures of up to 70%. These are strong arguments in favor of postoperative irradiation whenever radical surgery was the primary treatment decision.

On the other hand, when primary conservative irradiation is given, the treatment fields have to encompass the presacral and hypogastric node areas, even in patients with nonenlarged nodes on the CT scan. When enlarged pelvic nodes are seen by this imaging device, radical surgery is advised after preoperative radiochemotherapy. Despite numerous arguments in favor of the radiosensitivity of pelvic nodes, comparable to the radiosensitivity of the primary anal canal cancer, radical irradiation alone or combined with chemotherapy remains an investigational approach in these patients with enlarged pelvic nodes.

Recurrences of Anal Canal Cancer

After Primary Radical Surgery

The median time to pelvic and perineal recurrence after radical surgery is about 10–15 months with a wide range of 2–96 months. Rescue surgery and radiation therapy combined recently with chemotherapy have been used, but prognosis is very poor, only scarcely better for pelvic recurrences than for distant metastases. Greenall et al. [35] reported on 67 patients with recurrences of anal canal cancer who survived 7–9 months (range 1–48 months). In general, rescue by irradiation after failure of radical surgery is rarely successful. No patient was rescued by irradiation in the publications of Glanzmann [32] and Merlini and Eckert [51]. Boman et al. [7] reported on five out of 21 survivors at 5 years after irradiation for postoperative recurrence. Diagnosis of recurrence in the operated patient is in general late.

The best current approach seems to be a combination of radiation and chemotherapy whenever repeated surgery is not indicated.

After Irradiation With a Conservative Aim

The median time to local recurrence after radical irradiation is reported to be 2 years [59, 66, 73]. In our series the latest recurrence after conservative external irradiation combined with interstitial iridium was observed at 18 months. Papillon and Montbarbon [59] registered all local recurrences within 2 years. In the Fondation Curie publication [73] on results by external irradiation alone, the cumulative recurrence rate at 2 years was 87%. Radical rescue surgery is an excellent treatment modality for local recurrence after conservative irradiation. In our group of 68 patients irradiated with the aim of conservation from October 1976 to October 1985, 14 out of 68 failed locally. Two patients were in too bad medical condition for rescue surgery. Two patients refused surgery for psychological reasons and died. Among the ten remaining patients fit for surgery five were saved. Five patients died of cancer despite surgery. The favorable results of rescue surgery after radiotherapy failure in anal canal cancer are mentioned in other series: five out of six patients were saved in the report of Cantril et al. [11]. The healing conditions after rescue surgery were good in nearly all our patients treated by moderate external irradiation and interstitial iridium. Two out of ten patients had a perineal sinus for a prolonged time.

**Treatment of Carcinoma of the Perianal Skin
(Anal Orifice, External Anal Margin)**

Treatment guidelines from the literature are difficult to establish. The rarity of carcinoma of the perianal skin and the divergent opinions relative to the distal limits of the anal canal make comparison between the results of various treatment modalities hazardous. The anatomical location of the lesion seems to be of prognostic and therapeutic significance to many authors. It is believed [1, 23, 44, 60] that, although they arise in adjacent areas, squamous cell carcinomas of the perianal skin and the anal canal are very different and, except for the fact that they are malignant, they have little in common, whether considered from the clinical, surgical, or histological points of view.

In their publications Papillon et al. [60], Cummings et al. [16], and Cutuli et al. [17] consider only tumors within a 6-cm radius of the anal verge, as does Beahrs [4] in agreement with the current 1987 UICC recommendations. On the contrary, Greenall et al. [35] and AI Jurf et al. [1] give the treatment results for all tumors distal to the dentate line as results for tumors of the anal margin.

Essentially, the treatment policy has to face the local tumor problem with special attention to the inguinal nodes. Distant metastases in locoregionally controlled patients are uncommon: none of the patients died from distant metastases alone in the series of Greenall et al.; Cummings et al. and Cutuli et al., and only one out of 35 patients died in the report of Papillon et al. Carcinomas of the perianal skin are said to have a more favorable outcome than anal canal cancers. They are identified at an earlier stage, they are well differentiated, and give rise to no or few metastases in the pelvis.

Lymph node extension to the inguinal folds is, on the contrary, a therapeutic challenge. It can appear years after the treatment of the primary carcinoma, grow very fast, fix underlying tissues, and ulcerate the skin.

Local Excision

Eby and Sullivan [23] reviewed the current concepts of local excision in carcinoma of the anus. In a collected series of 320 patients (limit of the anal margin not always clearly specified with respect to the anal verge and dentate line), they found 25% treated by local excision and 75% by abdomino perineal resection. The overall 5-year survival rate for patients managed with local excision was 64.7% compared to 49.4% for patients treated by primary abdominoperineal resection.

Carcinoma of the perianal skin can be managed by local excision and, if there is a recurrence, conservative reexcision may be advisable [1, 35]. Flaps or skin grafts allow for wide safety margins and prevent closure under tension.

In the publication by Schraut et al. [76] 11 out of 16 cancers of the perianal skin were cured by local excision, but it is noteworthy that these patients had in situ or microinvasive carcinoma, and 80% of the patients without palpable inguinal nodes survived 5 years. Five other patients with perianal skin carcinoma were treated by radical surgery.

The same favorable results were obtained for small and superficial lesions by Beahrs [4]. In the report by Al Jurf et al. [1] nine out of 13 patients were locally controlled by conservative excision or reexcision. Long-term surveillance is indicated since late recurrences, up to 14 years, were reported after initial excision.

When there is a recurrence after conservative surgery, rescue by reexcision is supported by Greenall et al. [36]: nine out of 10 recurrences of carcinoma of the anal margin could be rescued by a second surgical procedure, and a 90% 5-year survival rate was observed in these patients. When more than half the anal circumference is involved, local excision is discouraged because of bad functional results, and more radical surgery is advised [1]. Deeply invasive tumors recurred in the experience of Schraut et al. [76] and had to be treated by abdomino perineal resection.

Schulz et al. [77] reported favorable tumor control by local excision and postoperative irradiation in six out of seven patients presenting with T2 or T3 squamous cell carcinoma of the perianal skin.

Table 19.10 summarizes some of the published results. Local excision shows favorable results as a primary treatment procedure in small superficially invasive squamous cell carcinoma of the perianal skin. In more advanced tumors local excision followed by radiotherapy can be tried, but tolerance of the perineum to high doses of radiation is poor, and post-treatment ulcers or sclerosis may outweigh the potential functional benefit of such a combined procedure.

Radiotherapy and Combined Radiochemotherapy

Results of external radiotherapy as a primary treatment modality have been reported by the authors from the Centre Leon Berard, the Princess Marga-

Table 19.10. Local excision with curative intent for carcinoma of the perianal skin (anal margin, anal orifice)

Reference	Patients (n)	Primary LE (n)	LE for recurrent lesion (n)	Local control (n)	Survival at 5 years (%)	Distal limit of canal
Eby and Sullivan 1969 [23] (collected series)	81	81			65	
Al Yurf et al. 1979 [1]	17	10	3	7/10 2/3	80 66	DL
Frost et al. 1984 [28]	20	20		8/20	66	AV
Greenall et al. 1985 [35]	48	31		18/31	68	DL
Greenall et al. 1986 [36]	11		10	9/10	90	DL
Pyper and Parks 1985 [69]	13	11		NI	50	DL
Schraut et al. 1983 [76]	16	11		2/11	80	AV
	164	13	62	71		

LE, local excision; NI, not indicated; AV, anal verge; DL, dentate line.

ret's Hospital and the Fondation Curie [16, 17, 60]. Use of an interstitial iridium implant is rare since the anatomical conformation of the perianal region does not allow for a perfect geometry of the implant. Convergent implant lines have a high potential of overdosage and subsequent necrosis. More recently, chemotherapy with concomitant external irradiation has been used. Papillon et al. [60] have suggested 40 Gy in 2½ weeks combined with chemotherapy since 1978, Cummings et al. [16] have advised 50 Gy in 4–8 weeks with chemotherapy for advanced lesions. The Fondation Curie [17] has published results with a more protracted irradiation scheme of 65 Gy in 6–8 weeks. The local cure rate by radiotherapy is high in T1 and T2 tumors: 80%–100% (13 out of 13 in the series of Cummings et al. [15], 20 out of 24 in the publication by Papillon et al. [60], and nine out of 11 in the report by Cutuli et al. [17]).

Tumors which are larger than 5 cm or deeply infiltrative have local failure rates of about 30% after radiotherapy. In the radiotherapy series, 32%–48% of patients treated had T3 or T4 tumors, five-year survival rates are about 50% in the radiotherapy series, including all tumor stages. Local failure after radiotherapy could be successfully treated by surgery in more than half of the patients (four out of six in Toronto [16], two out of five in Lyon [60], and three out of four in Paris [17]). Complications after radiotherapy were in most cases mild and included perineal fibrosis and telangiectasia in 25%–30% of cases. Severe complications were rare: 3%–10%, re-

quiring colostomy for necrosis or intervention for femoral head fracture [17]. Radiotherapy is a good treatment approach for tumors smaller than 5 cm. Large tumors may need a combined treatment approach with pre- or postoperative irradiation.

Special histological types of tumors, such as the very rare mucoepidermoid tumors, adenocarcinomas, and verrucous carcinomas, should be treated by surgery first [60].

Treatment of Lymph Nodes in Cancer of the Perianal Skin

Lymph node extension to the inguinal folds can be a therapeutic problem. About 20% of the patients suffering from carcinoma of the perianal skin present with synchronous inguinal nodes. For movable nodes a therapeutic combination of irradiation in a pre- or postoperative sequence is advised. Homolateral intrapelvic nodes up to the common iliac level should be included in the radiation field. A CT scan provides a useful investigative tool for exploration of the deep inguinal, femoral, and iliac nodes. When synchronous inguinal metastasis are properly managed, mostly by limited surgery and irradiation, prognosis is not too poor: two out of seven, one out of three, and two out of four patients, presenting with synchronous inguinal nodes have died of the disease in radiotherapy series [16, 17, 60]. In the very troublesome situation of fixed or ulcerated nodes, intra-arterial chemotherapy or intravenous chemotherapy concomitant with radiotherapy could be tried in order to make secondary surgery possible.

After treatment of the primary tumor of the perianal skin, nodes can appear metachronously very late in the follow-up period. In the Fondation Curie's report [17] three out of three patients with metachronous inguinal nodes died of the disease, as did three out of four in the series by Papillon et al. [60]. Because of the bad outcome of these metachronous node metastases, the "watch and see" policy for treatment of the inguinal folds seems to be indicated only in patients with very small and superficial carcinoma of the perianal skin. Patients with tumors of 5 cm or more should have prophylactic inguinal irradiation or diagnostic inguinal node sampling when prophylactic irradiation is felt not to be suitable [60]. This is a very different, i. e., much more aggressive, treatment policy for the inguinal problem in perianal skin cancer in comparison to the same problem in anal canal cancer.

Conclusions and Proposals for Treatment Algorithms for Carcinoma of the Anal Canal and the Perianal Skin

The rarity of the disease, which occurs in less than 5% of all the terminal intestine, is a significant factor in the failure to establish a standardized method for classification and treatment. Detailed classification by size, site, and degree of differentiation of the lesions and correlation of the results with the different methods of treatment give insufficient data for acceptable statistical conclusions.

Based on the review of recent literature and 10 years' personal experience it can be said that carcinoma of the anal canal may be treated, in the majority of cases, in a conservative manner by primary radiotherapy with or without chemotherapy. Various types of fractionation and various irradiation techniques constantly show high percentages of local control when the primary tumor and the mesorectal nodes are irradiated in an adequate fashion. Only the acute reactions of the healthy tissues and the percentage of late radiation sequelae seem to be somewhat different depending on treatment portals, size of tumor, and protraction of radiotherapy. All patients can be accepted for radiotherapy. Only patients with poor tumor regression after irradiation, persistent ulceration, fistulas, and enlarged pelvic nodes on the CT scan should be submitted to radical surgery after preoperative irradiation. Figure 19.2 shows a treatment proposal for anal canal

Table 19.11. Carcinoma of the perianal skin – treatment proposal

Tis, microinvasive T	Excision
T1, T2, T3	Excision + 45–50 Gy postoperative RT (verrucuous, mucoepidermoid and pseudocondylomatous carcinoma should always be excised) or 5-FU + mitomycin + 50–60 Gy RT (one to two synchronous courses in a split-course regimen)
T3 > 10 cm in diameter	Surgery with skin graft + postoperative RT
T4	Abdominoperineal resection + postoperative RT or 5-FU + mitomycin + 40–50 Gy RT + / – Iridium + / – Surgery (individualize)
NO	Prophylactic inguinal node sampling (nod radical node dissection) or elective inguinal irradiation 45–50 Gy if primary tumor > 5 cm
N1 (+)	Surgery + postoperative RT

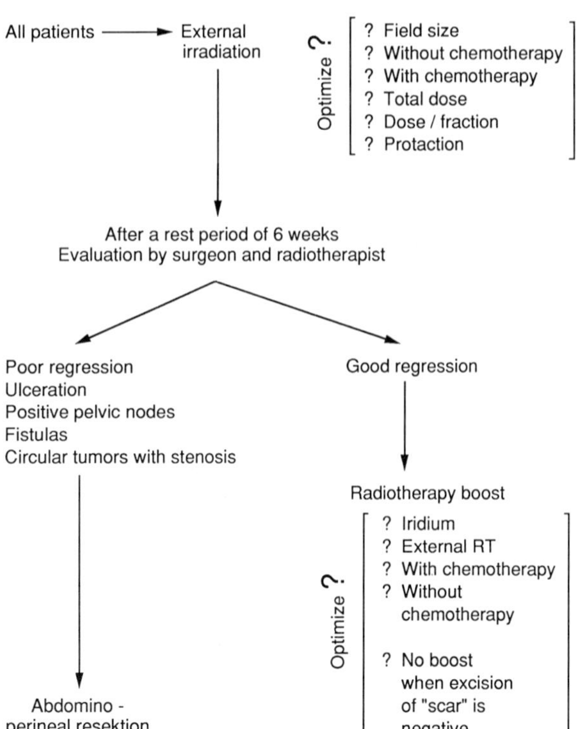

Fig. 19.2. Cancer of the anal canal – treatment proposal. The question *marks* show the numerous questions left unanswered when trying to optimize radiotherapy of anal canal carcinoma. Randomized trials with international collaboration are required

carcinomas. In the right margin of this table are shown the numerous questions left unresovled when optimization of primary radiotherapy for anal canal carcinomas is to be discussed.

In small tumors of the anal canal elective irradiation of the clinically normal (NO) inguinal folds does not seem necessary. In advanced carcinoma of the anal canal prophylactic irradiation of the inner part of the inguinal fold is advisable. Synchronous metastatic inguinal nodes are to be managed by surgery and irradiation.

Table 19.11 shows a treatment proposal for carcinoma of the perianal skin. Small T1 and T2 tumors can be treated by local excision if they are only microinvasive. Postoperative external irradiation has to be discussed in invasive tumors or in the case of doubtful surgical margins. In rare tumors, such as tumors of the mucoepidermoid is verrucous types, local excision is preferable to irradiation.

When primary radiotherapy is used for T3 invasive carcinoma of the perianal skin, concomitant chemothcrapy seems to improve the local control rate. T4 tumors are indications for a combined radiosurgical approach.

The policy for treatment of inguinal nodes is guided by the risk of late metachronous metastases in this region, which are often very difficult to manage. Clinically normal (NO) inguinal nodes should receive elective irradiation or be submitted to biopsy sampling in all invasive carcinoma of the perianal skin.

In conclusion, optimal treatment of malignant tumors of the anus requires a team approach. Primary tumors and nodes must be managed according to their respective stage. Initial work-up, treatment decision, and follow-up need close collaboration among the surgeon, radiotherapist, and medical oncologist.

References

1. Al Jurf AS, Turnbull RB, Fazio VW (1979) Local treatment of squamous cell carcinoma of the anus. Surg Gynecol Obstet 148: 574–578
2. Austin DF (1982) Etiological clues from descriptive epidemiology: squamous carcinoma of the rectum or anus. Natl Cancer Inst Monogr 62: 89–90
3. Barthelemy N, Loygue J, Parc R et al. (1986) Etude d'une serie de 204 cas de cancer du canal anal traités de 1972–1982, Société Française de Radiologie. J Eur Radiother 7: 133–140
4. Beahrs OH (1979) Management of cancer of the anus. Am J Roentgenol 133: 791–795
5. Bender MD, Lechago J (1976) Leukoplakia of the anal canal. Dig Dis Sci 21: 867–872
6. Bensaude A, Nora J (1968) Differential diagnosis of carcinoma of the anal margin. Proc R Soc Med 61: 624–626
7. Boman BM, Moertel CG, O'Connell MJ, Scott M, Weiland LH, Beart RW (1984) Carcinoma of the anal canal. A clinical and pathologic study of 188 cases. Cancer 54: 114–125
8. Boulis Wassif S, Caspers RJL (1983) Die Therapie des analen Karzinoms. Colo-Proctology 4: 228–231
9. Buschke A, Löwenstein L (1925) Über karzinomähnliche Condylomata Acuminata des Penis. Klin Wochenschr 4: 1726–1728
10. Byfield JE, Barone RM, Sharp TR, Frankel SS (1983) Conservative management without alkylating agents of squamous cell anal cancer using cyclical 5-FU alone and X-ray therapy. Cancer Treat Rep 67: 709–712
11. Cantril ST, Green JP, Schall GL, Schaupp WC (1983) Primary radiation therapy in the treatment of anal carcinoma. Int J Radiat Oncol Biol Phys 9: 1271–1280
12. Clark J, Petrelli N, Herrera LM, Helmann A (1986) Epidermoid carcinoma of the anal canal. Cancer 57: 400–406
13. Cooper PH, Millis SE, Allen MS (1982) Malignant melanoma of the anus. Report of 12 patients and analysis of 225 additional cases. Dis Colon Rectum 25: 693–703
14. Courtial J, Fernandez Colmeiro JM (1960) Les indications et les résultats de la roentgenthérapie et de la curiethérapie dans les cancers du canal anal. Arch Mal Appar Dig 49: 43
15. Cummings B, Keane TJ, Thomas G, Harwood A, Rider W (1984) Results and toxicity of the treatment of anal canal carcinoma by radiation therapy or radiationtherapy and chemotherapy. Cancer 54: 2062–2068
16. Cummings BJ, Keane TJ, Hawkins NV, O'Sullivan B (1986) Treatment of perianal carcinoma by radiation or radiation plus chemotherapy. Int J Radiat Oncol Biol Phys 12 [Suppl 1]: 170
17. Cutuli B, Fenton J, Labib A, Bataini JP, Mathieu G (1988) Anal margin carcinoma: 21 cases treated at the Institute Curie by exclusive conservative radiotherapy. Radiother Onocl 11: 1–6
18. Dahlin JR, Weiss NS, Klopfenstein LL, Cochran LE, Chow WH, Daifuku R (1982) Correlates of homosexual behavior and the incidence of anal cancer. Jama 247: 1988–1990
19. Dalby JE, Pointon RS (1961) The treatment of anal carcinoma by interstitial irradiation. Am J Roentgenol 85: 515–520
20. Devois A, Decker R (1960) La curiepuncture du cancer de l'anus. Arch Fr Mal App Dig 49: 54–67
21. Dogett SW, Green JP, Cantril ST (1986) Efficacy of radiation alone for limited squamous cell carcinoma of the anal canal. Int J Radiat Oncol Biol Phys 12: [Suppl 1] 170–171
22. Dunst J, Wolf N, Sauer R (1988) Radiochemotherapie des Analkanalkarzinoms: Frühergebnisse des Erlanger Krankengutes. In: Wolf N (ed) Fortschritte in der Proktologie. Zuckerschwerdt, Munich (in press)
23. Eby LS, Sullivan ES (1969) Current concepts of local excision of epidermoid cancer of the anus. Dis Colon Rectum 12: 332–337
24. Eschwege F, Lasser P, Chavy A et al. (1985) Squamous cell carcinoma of the anal canal: treatment

by external beam irradiation. Radiother Oncol 3: 145-150

25. Fenger C (1979) The anal transitional zone. Location and extent. Acta Pathol Microbiol Immunol Scand (A) 87: 379

26. Fenger C, Nielsen VT (1986) Intraepithelial neoplasia in the anal canal. Acta Pathol Microbiol Immunol Scand (A) 94: 393-349

27. Fenger C, Nielsen VT (1986) Precancerous changes in the anal canal epithelium in resection specimen. Acta Pathol Microbiol Immunol Scand (A) 94: 63-69

28. Frost DB, Richards PC, Montague ED, Giacco GG, Martin RG (1984) Epidermoid cancer of the ano-rectum. Cancer 53: 525-530

29. Gebbers JO, Laissue JA (1984) Pathologie der Anal-tumoren. Schweiz Rundschau Med (Praxis) (27): 847-862

30. Ghavamzadeh M, Widgren S (1979) Les carcinomes du canal anal. Schweiz Med Wochenschr 109 (17): 646-652

31. Gillespie JJ, MacKay B (1978) Histogenesis of cloacogenic carcinoma. Hum Pathol 9: 579-587

32. Glanzmann C (1978) Radiotherapie in der Behandlung von Analkarzinomen. Strahlentherapie 154: 174-178

33. Goligher JC (1984) Surgery of anus, rectum and colon. Baillière-Tindall, Eastbourne

34. Gray's anatomy, 36th ed (1980) Churchill Livingstone, Edinburgh

35. Greenall MJ, Quan SHQ, DeCosse JJ (1985) Epidermoid cancer of the anus. Br J Surg 72 [Suppl]: 97-103

36. Greenall MJ, Magill GB, Quan SHQ, DeCosse JJ (1986) Recurrent epidermoid cancer of the anus. Cancer 57: 1437-1441

37. Grinvalsky HT, Helwig EB (1956) Carcinoma of the anorectal junction. Cancer 9: 480-488

38. Hardcastle JD, Bussey HJR (1986) Results of surgical treatment of squamous cell carcinoma of the anal canal and anal margin at the St. Mark's Hospital 1928-1966. J R Soc Med 61: 629-630

39. Hermanek P, Sobin LH (eds) (1987) TNM classification of malignant tumors, UICC, 4th edn. Springer, Berlin Heidelberg New York

40. John MJ, Flam M, Lovalvo L, Mowry PA (1987) Feasibility of non-surgical definitive management of anal canal carcinoma. Int J Radiat Oncol Biol Phys 13: 299-303

41. Keihr S, Hickey RC, Martin RG et al. (1972) Cloacogenic carcinoma of the anal canal. Arch Surg 104: 407-415

42. Keiling R, Grunewald JM, Achille E (1973) Radiotherapie des cancers malpighiens de l'anus: la curietherapie interstitielle à l'iridium 192 des epitheliomas du canal anal. J Radiol Electrol Med Nucl 54: 634-635

43. Klotz RG, Pamukoglu T, Souillard DH (1967) Transitional cloacogenic carcinoma of the anal canal. Clinicopathological study of 373 cases. Cancer 20: 1727-1747

44. Kuehn PG, Eisenberg H, Reed JF (1968) Epidermoid carcinoma of the perianal skin and anal canal. Cancer 22: 932-938

45. Lee SH, MacGregor DH, Kuziez MN (1981) Malignant transformation of perianal condyloma accuminatum. Dis Colon Rectum 24: 462-467

46. Leichmann L, Nigro N, Vaitkevicius VK (1985) Cancer of the anal canal: model for preoperative adjuvant combined modality therapy. Am J Med 78: 211-215

47. Lock MR, Katz DR, Parks A, Thomson JPS (1977) Perianal Paget's disease. Postgrad Med J 53: 768-772

48. Loygue J, Laugier A, Parc A, Weisgerber G (1980) Cancer épidermoide de l'anus. A propos de 149 observations. Chirurgie 6: 710-716

49. Marti MC, Pipard G (1986) Die epidermoiden Karzinome des Analkanals. Chir Gastro-Enterolog. mit interdiszi plinearen Gesprächen 2: 57-66

50. McAnally AK, Dockerty MB (1949) Carcinoma developing in chronic draining cutaneous sinuses and fistula. Surg Gynecol Obstet 188: 87-96

51. Merlini M, Eckert P (1985) Malignant tumors of the anus. Am J Surg 150: 370-372

52. Michaelson RA, Magill GB, Quan SHQ et al. (1983) Preoperative chemotherapy and radiationtherapy in the management of anal epidermoid carcinoma. Cancer 51: 390-395

53. Morson BC, Sobin LH (1976) Histological typing of intestinal tumors. International histological classification of tumours, No. 15. World Health Organization, Geneva, pp 67-69

54. Nielsen OV, Jensen SL (1981) Basal cell carcinoma of the anus - a clinical study of 34 cases. Br J Surg 68: 856-857

55. Nigro MD (1984) An evaluation of combined therapy for squamous cell carcinoma of the anal canal. Dis Colon Rectum 27: 763-766

56. Nigro MD, Vaitkevicius VK, Considine BJ (1974) Combined therapy for cancer of the anal canal: a preliminary report. Dis Col Rectum 17: 354

57. O'Brien PH, Jenrette JM, Wallace KM, Metcalf JS (1982) Epidermoid carcinoma of the anus. Surg Gynecol Obstet 155: 745-751

58. Papillon J (1982) Rectal and anal cancers. Springer, Berlin Heidelberg New York

59. Papillon J, Montbarbon MD (1987) Epidermoid carcinoma of the anal canal. Dis Col Rectum 30: 324-334

60. Papillon J, Renard L, Pipard G (1985) Le cancer de la marge de l'anus. J Eur Radiother 6: 29-34

61. Parks A (1981) Squamous carcinoma of the anal canal. Ann Gastroenterol Hepato 17: 103-107

62. Parks A, Thompson JPS (1977) Per anal endorectal operative technique in operative surgery. In: Todd IP Colon, rectum and anus. Butterworth, London, pp 157-167

63. Parturier-Albot M, Prevost AG, Albot G, Bolgert M (1982) Les cancers multicentriques de la région anorectale. Ann Gastroenterol Hepatol, 18: 227-235

64. Penn I (1986) Cancers of the anogenital region in renal transplant recipients - analysis of 65 cases. Cancer 58: 611-616

65. Petrelli N, Shaw N, Bhargava A, Herrera L, Sischy B, Daufelet J, Mittelman A (1987) Squamous cell carcinoma (SCC) antigen - a marker in patients with primary squamous cell carcinoma of the anal canal. Proceedings of the American Society of Clinical Oncology. Atlanta, May 17-19, 1987 Abstr 724

66. Pipard G (1989) Combination therapy of anal carcinoma. In: Sauer R (ed) Diagnostic imaging and radiation oncology, volume interventional therapy - brachycurietherapy. Springer, Berlin Heidelberg New York (in press)

67. Preston DM, Fowler EF, Lennard-Iones JE, Hawley

PR (1983) Carcinoma of the anus in Crohn's disease. Br J Surg 70: 346–347
68. Pyper PC, Parks TG (1984) Melanoma of the anal canal. Br J Surg 71: 672–673
69. Pyper PC, Parks TG (1985) The results of surgery for epidermoid carcinoma of the anus. Br J Surg 72: 712–714
70. Rockwell S (1982) Cytotoxicities of mitomycine-C and X-rays to aerobic and hypoxic cells in vitro. Int J Radiat Oncol Biol Phys 8: 1035–1039
71. Rohner A, Schopfer P, Paunier JP, Garcia J (1984) Le cancer de la region anale. Med et Hyg 32: 1127
72. Salem PA, Habboubi N, Anaissie E, Brihi ER, Issa P, Abbas JS, Khalyl MF (1985) Effectiveness of cisplatin in the treatment of anal squamous cell carcinoma. Cancer Treat Rep 69: 891–893
73. Salmon RJ, Fenton J, Asselain B, Mathieu G, Girodet J, Durand JC (1984) Treatment of epidermoid anal canal cancer. Am J Surg 147: 43–48
74. Schlag P (1986) Aspekte operativer und multimodaler Therapie beim Analkarzinom. Chirurg 57: 488–492
75. Schneider TC, Schulte WJ (1981) Management of carcinoma of anal canal. Surgery 90: 729–733
76. Schraut WH, Wang C, Dawson PJ, Block GE (1983) Depth of invasion, location and size of cancer of the anus dictate operative treatment. Cancer 51: 1291–1296
77. Schulz U, Bamberg M, Gross E, Niebel W (1982) Die kombinierte chirurgisch-radiologische Therapie der Plattenepithelkarzinome des Analkanals und der perianalen Haut. Strahlentherapie 158: 327
78. Singh R, Nime F, Mittelmann A (1981) Malignant epithelial tumors of the anal canal. Cancer 48: 411–414
79. Sischy B (1985) The use of radiation therapy combined with chemotherapy in the management of squamous cell carcinoma of the anus and marginally resectable adenocarcinoma of the rectum. Int J Radiat Oncol Biol Phys 11: 1587–1597
80. Sloan PJM, Goepel G (1981) Lichen sclerosus et atrophicus and perianal carcinoma: a case report. Clin Exp Dermatol 6: 399–402
81. Stearns MV, Quan SH (1970) Epidermoid carcinoma of the anorectum. Surg Gynecol Obstet 131: 953–957
82. Strauss RJ, Fazio VW (1979) Bowen's disease of the anal and perianal area: a report and analysis of twelve cases. Am J Surg 137: 231–234
83. Wade TR, Kopf AW, Ackermann AB (1979) Bowenoid papulosis of the genitalia. Arch Dermatol 115: 306–308
84. Young JL, Percy CL, Asire AJ (1981) Surveillance, epidemiology and end results: incidence and mortality data 1973–1977. Natl Cancer Inst Monog 57: 1066
85. Zachow KR, Ostrow RS, Bender M, Watts S, Okagaki T, Pass F, Faras AJ (1982) Detection of human papillomavirus DNA in ano-genital neoplasia. Nature 300: 771–772

20 Rectal Tumors

J.-C. Givel

Introduction

In frequency of occurrence, carcinoma of the colon and rectum ranks second among the cancers in the developed countries [42]. There is a marked predominance of lesions located in the rectum (the last 15 cm of the large intestine). If we exclude neoplasms of the rectosigmoid, these cancers represent around one-third of all colorectal tumors. Although occurring predominantly at an advanced age, this type of cancer is sometimes found in younger patients, even where no predisposing risk factors are present. However, most of those affected are over 60 years of age, occurrence being most frequent during the 7th decade (60–69 years). The proportion of patients younger than 30 years of age is given as between 1% and 4%, depending on the author. A slight preponderance of the disease in males has been noted.

Pathology

Allmost all malignant tumors of the rectum are adenocarcinomas. Four types can be distinguished on the basis of their histological differentiation:

- Well differentiated
- Moderately differentiated
- Poorly differentiated
- Mucoid

The first two are by far the most frequent, making up 80% of these cancers. They grow slowly and produce metastases only at a later stage. The poorly differentiated and mucoid lesions exhibit considerably more malignant behavior. They make up 20% of these tumors, develop more quickly, and have a more marked tendency to metastasize. Their prognosis is significantly less favorable. A certain correlation exists between histological differentiation and local spread, the great majority of tumors of stage A in the Dukes classification showing either good or moderate differentiation. This means that the majority of cancers diagnosed at an early stage, while still confined to the rectal wall, are of moderate malignancy, a factor which contributes to a more favorable prognosis [36].

Various anatomical and biological parameters help to predict the behavior of a cancer of the rectum. Malignancy is an intrinsic tumoral factor and does not necessarily bear a direct relationship to size. A small tumor of poor differentiation, measuring 2 cm in diameter, is much more malignant than a well-differentiated adenocarcinoma of 5-cm caliber.

Dukes proposed a simple and widely accepted grading of the adenocarcinomas based on the pathological examination of surgical specimens [7]. It takes into account two significant prognostic factors: extent of spread and occurrence of lymphatic metastases. The classic Dukes' grading makes a distinction between three stages:

- A: Growth confined to the rectum, absence of any extrarectal spread or lymphatic metastases
- B: Spread by direct continuity into extrarectal tissues; absence of lymphatic metastases
- C: Lymphatic metastases (irrespective of local spread)

Several modifications of Dukes' classification have been suggested, in particular by Astler and Coller (Fig. 20.1) [2].

Grades B and C have been subdivided into two groups in order to allow a more precise differentiation of local spread and lymphatic metastases:

- B1: Local extension into the muscularis propria and subserosa, with the serosa unaffected
- B2: Extension up to or through the serosa
- C1: Only the glands close to the primary tumor are affected
- C2: More extended lymphatic metastases, involving the glands up to the main ligature on the local vessels

Finally, a grade D has been added to describe distant metastases, in particular hepatic ones.

Among the numerous other classifications of the degree of extension of a rectal tumor, mention must be made of those of the Union Internationale Contre le Cancer (UICC) and the American Joint

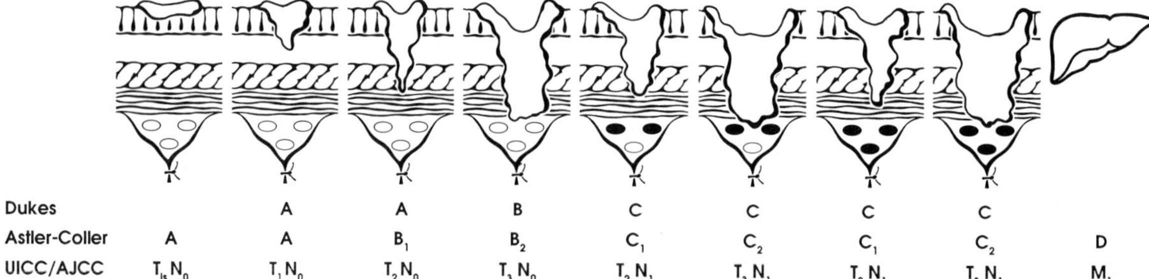

Fig. 20.1. Correlation of Dukes, Astler-Coller and UICC/AJCC tumor classifications

Committee on Cancer (AJCC) [1, 18]. They define the extension of the primary tumor, its regional lymph node metastasis, and any distant metastases (Table 20.1).

On the basis of these definitions, the AJCC recommend a distinction to be made between five stages (Table 20.2).

The majority of tumors develop from existing adenomatous polyps or villous adenomas which have undergone secondary malignant transformation (see Chap. 18). The invasive cancer typical of an early stage takes the form of an exophytic sessile mass,

Table 20.1. TNM classification of colorectal tumors

T – Primary Tumor

TX	Primary tumor cannot be assessed
T0	No evidence of primary tumor
Tis	Carcinoma in situ
T1	Tumor invades submucosa
T2	Tumor invades muscularis propria
T3	Tumor invades through muscularis propria into subserosa or into nonperitonealized pericolic or perirectal tissues
T4	Tumor perforates the visceral peritoneum or directly invades other organs or structures

Note: Direct invasion in T4 includes invasion of other segments of the colorectum by way of the serosa, e. g., invasion of the sigmoid colon by a carcinoma of the cecum.

N – Regional Lymph Nodes

NX	Regional lymph nodes cannot be assessed
N0	No regional lymph node metastasis
N1	Metastasis in one to three pericolic or perirectal lymph nodes
N2	Metastasis in four or more pericolic or perirectal lymph nodes
N3	Metastasis in any lymph node along the course of a named vascular trunc

M – Distant Metastasis

MX	Presence of distant metastasis cannot be assessed
M0	No distant metastasis
M1	Distant metastasis

Table 20.2. Staging of colorectal tumors

Stage 0	Tis	N0	M0
Stage I	T1	N0	M0
	T2	N0	M0
Stage II	T3	N0	M0
	T4	N0	M0
Stage III	Any T	N1	M0
	Any T	N2, N3	M0
Stage IV	Any T	Any N	M1

deep red or purple in color, indurated and of heterogenous consistency. It is raised above the normal surrounding mucosa, which is pink and soft, has an irregular surface which is raspberry-like in appearance and bleeds easily on contact. The lesion is mobile with respect to the rectal wall. Its consistency represents the most important diagnostic criterion, often allowing a benign lesion to be distinguished from a malignant tumor by palpation. Malignant polyps ulcerate as they grow, the ulceration predominating at the center of the lesion, which progressively acquires a crater-like appearance. As the parietal invasion by the tumor advances, the neoplasm loses its mobility. Some tumors are relatively flat, showing a greater tendency to grow into the wall than to protrude into the intestinal lumen. Many cancers of the rectum are already ulcerated at the time of diagnosis, with marked evidence of parietal invasion [36].

Carcinomas of the rectum may spread in three ways:

- By local continuity
- By lymphatic dissemination
- By venous spread

A distinction should be made at a local level between tumors limited to the rectal wall and those extending beyond it. The two types differ significantly, both in terms of their prognosis and their tendency to local or remote spread.

Lymphatic dissemination takes place along one of the three main rectal drainage channels, occurring in the upward direction in 99% of cases. The affected glands are found in the mesorectum, attached to terminal arterial branches in the immediate proximity of the tumor. The significance of the lymphatic metastases depends on their histological differentiation and local spread.

Venous invasion leads to the formation of malignant thrombi, whose embolization results in distant metastases. Intravascular penetration by the tumor generally occurs at the point where the veins emerge into the bowel wall. Venous invasion increases as a function of the degree of malignancy and depth of tumor spread. However, its prognosis is not as unfavorable as that associated with lymphatic dissemination [36].

Cancers of the rectum may give rise to metastases as far as the liver or the lungs, less frequently the bones.

Thus the prognosis of a rectal tumor does not depend only on its distant dissemination, but also on its local spread and the presence of lymphatic or venous invasion. These characteristics are identified during a histological examination of the resected specimen. The pathological examination involves taking a biopsy of the primary lesion at the point of its deepest parietal penetration and dissecting it to identify each gland and venous structure. The reliability of the examination depends largely on the care with which it is carried out.

In addition to adenocarcinomas, various other rare malignant tumors may occur in the rectum. Epithelial lesions include tumors of the endocrine cells (most often carcinoids), epidermoid carcinomas, sometimes associated with an adenocarcinoma, and metastases of tumors of other organs. These originate mainly in the stomach, but may also occur in the breasts, the prostate, the ovaries, the bladder, the kidneys, the uterine cervix, and the lungs. Nonepithelial neoplasms may include a lymphoma, a tumor of the smooth muscle - neurogenic or lipomatous - or a secondary site of a plasmocytoma [33].

Symptoms

The symptoms caused by a cancer of the rectum are discussed principally in Chap. 2. Rectal bleeding, diarrhea, modified motions, discharge of mucus, false need to defecate, and abdominal pain are the symptoms most commonly encountered in patients suffering from a rectal tumor. Bleeding generally accompanies defecation; the blood is sometimes mixed with the stools, and it may be impossible to distinguish it from that originating from hemorrhoids. Abdominal pain may be due to an intestinal obstruction, the result of a stenosing lesion giving rise to a progressive ileus. At an advanced stage, local pain suggests direct invasion of adjacent structures, with infiltration of nerve tissue. An advanced condition is characterized by obstruction of the ureters, an iliac venous thrombosis, and fistulization towards other organs, in particular the intestines, the bladder, the vagina and uterus, or the abdominal wall. A prostate tumor may also invade the rectum and ulcerate it. It is sometimes difficult to establish the differential diagnosis between a rectal lesion and a cancer of the prostrate.

Examinations

It is common practice to divide the rectum into thirds (lower, middle, and upper). The majority of tumors are located in the lower third (6 cm) and are therefore easily accessible to digital palpation. Lesions situated to within 10-12 cm of the anal verge (lower two-thirds of the rectum) may also be palpated.

Diagnosis is therefore most frequently based on rectal palpation, and most lesions come to light during a thorough clinical examination. Apart from determining the dimensions of the tumor, such an examination allows it to be located with respect to adjacent structures, thus providing an essential criterion for the choice of treatment. The digital examination may also include palpation of any enlarged nodular structures at the back of the rectum, a procedure which does not require any special skill on the part of the examining physician. Although infrequent, the discovery of such glands provides important information, especially if local excision of the primary tumor is planned. In certain cases, endoscopy or a barium enema allows a diagnosis to be made. A rigid sigmoidoscopy visualizes any upper rectal lesions, locates them with respect to the anal verge and allows a biopsy to be taken for pathological examination. The well-known histological heterogeneity of rectal tumors makes it advisable to take several biopsies of a lesion.

Endorectal ultrasonography provides valuable information about the depth of parietal invasion by the tumor, the direction of extrarectal invasion, and possible attack of neighboring organs, thus contributing to a significant improvement in the quality of the preoperative staging. It allows each layer of the rectum, as well as possible periorganic glands, to be visualized. It allows an objective correlate to be established for the clinical grading based on tumor mobility determined by rectal palpation, as stated by Mason in 1976 [29]:

I   Tumor mobile with respect to the underlying rectal muscles
II Tumor mobile but not clearly distinguishable from the rectal wall
III Tumor and rectal mobilites reduced by partial fixation
IV Tumor and rectal wall fixed

Endorectal ultrasonography is also useful for follow-up checks on patients after resection with an anastomosis. Coupled with a CT scan, this examination allows lesions of the smallest size to be detected [15].

Colonoscopy or a double-contrast barium enema allow the entire colon system to be examined, so that concurrent lesions of different localization (polyps, tumors) are not missed. Examinations of this kind should be performed systematically before the operation, unless an obstructive rectal lesion requires them to be carried out subsequently.

It is essential to determine the extent of the disease by means of an exhaustive preoperative examination. This allows the most appropriate choice of treatment, depending on factors such as local spread, and the general state of health and age of the patient. A general check-up should rule out possible distant dissemination of the disease. Enlargement or heterogeneity of the liver, as well as the presence of possible ascites or any abdominal mass located away from the primary lesion should be looked for. Palpation of the region of the rectum or vagina sometimes reveals peritoneal invasion. Apart from clinical examination, metastases are also brought to light by standard radiography of the thorax, hepatic ultrasonography, or transverse tomography of the abdomen, as well as by an immunoscintigraphic examination.

Treatment

The treatment of cancer of the rectum represents a subject of considerable debate. There exist numerous methods of treatment which sould be discussed on the basis of various criteria. Surgery remains the main form of treatment for this disease. It offers a wide variety of techniques, ranging from total resection to local excision. Various nonsurgical approaches, applied alone or in conjunction with surgical methods, have recently been developed. They include radiotherapy, chemotherapy, and immunotherapy.

The numerous factors involved in a discussion of methods of treatment for cancer of the rectum include tumor localization (distance separating the lesion distally from the anal verge), the type of lesion (macroscopic appearance, size, circumferential spread, possible fixation, histological differentiation, existence of presacral adenopathies, degree of ploidy), the age, sex, morphology, and general physical and mental condition of the patient. Fixed pelvic tumors are associated with a poor prognosis. It is highly likely that a residual disease will remain after excision, and there exists a high probability of anastomotic recurrence. Abdominoperineal resection of the rectum (APR) thus probably represents the best operation here. The indication for preoperative radiotherapy should be carefully examined in such cases. Histological differentiation and the degree of lymphocytic infiltration in the vicinity of the tumor are two factors of equal importance. A high degree of differentiation and marked lymphocytic infiltration both suggest a favorable prognosis. With regard to degree of ploidy, it appears increasingly well established that diploid tumors are associated with a better prognosis than aneuploid ones.

Surgical Treatment

There has been no significant improvement in the survival rates for rectal cancer patients after treatment for several decades. In contrast, the operational mortality after excision of a rectal tumor has been significantly reduced. From around 10% in 1950, it dropped to 2.5% in 1972. This progress is due to the improvement of anesthesia/reanimation techniques, of prophylactic antibiotic treatment as well as the use of effective methods of preparing the large bowel. Significant advances have also been made in the area of surgical technique. The main ones relate to the increase in the number of interventions of the resection/anastomosis type, allowing the sphincter to be preserved, both after radical tumor resection and after local treatment, with a parallel reduction of extensive abdominoperineal resections. The advent of circular staplers allowing the creation of very low end-to-end anastomoses has played a significant role in this respect. The importance of this development varies from one center to another. At St. Mark's Hospital, London, 85% of patients with rectal cancer had an abdominoperineal resection in 1950 as against 45% in 1975. Currently, the majority of patients operated on for rectal cancer have either resection/anastomosis or a local excision. It is rather improbable that these numbers will increase in the future because they have reached the limits fixed principally by the extension and localization of the tumor. The number of resection/anastomoses has increased most for the middle third of the rectum (between 12 and 8 cm from the anal verge). Recent pathological data have shown that a distal spread beyond 1 cm is exceptional, occurring in fewer than 3% of cases. This has permitted the length of intestine resected caudally from a tumor to be considerably reduced. An examination of the appearance of the tumor (ulcerated, infiltrative) should therefore precede all decisions regarding the length of bowel to resect.

The wish to avoid a colostomy at all costs and to restore bowel continuity should never be satisfied at the expense of oncological safety by reducing the resected edges free of the tumor. The distance separating the anal verge from the lower edge of the tumor is of major importance in this respect. It must be examined with great care by the surgeon.

An extended tumor of the middle third of the rectum, immediately associated with recurrence, requires a synchronous combined excision of the rectum to avoid its persistence or recurrence in the vicinity of the anastomosis. In contrast, it does not always make sense to perform an extended resection with a very distal anastomosis in the case of an advanced disease with significant metastatic dissemination. Various papers have shown that the prognosis for an extended resection anastomosis for cancer of the middle third of the rectum is no worse than that for total excision of the rectum. The 5-year survival rates after either of these interventions for cancer of the middle third of the rectum, with the same Dukes' grading and of identical histological differentiation, are similar. Patients with tumors of Dukes' grade B with moderate differentiation have a 5-year survival rate of around 61% after resection/anastomosis and 69% after APR.

Excision of a tumor of the rectum may be performed by means of various techniques of resection and anastomosis:

- Abdominoperineal resection (APR)
- Low anterior resection
- Coloanal anastomosis
- Abdominoanal pull-through resection
- Abdominosacral resection
- Transsacral excision
- Transsphincteric excision
- Transanal excision

Hartmann's operation and a colostomy represent two useful complementary procedures, essentially representing temporary or palliative treatment. Three local parasurgical techniques should be briefly mentioned in this context:

- Electrofulguration
- Destruction by cryosurgery
- Coagulation by laser

APR is reserved mainly for very low or advanced tumors, where good functional results and/or low recurrence rates cannot be achieved by anus sparing procedures.

The operation is performed on a patient in the lithotomy position by two teams operating in a synchronous manner. The anus is first of all stitched by means of two perianal purse-string sutures. The exact site of the future colostomy is located the day before the operation and marked, for instance by a stitch.

A median peri- and subumbilical laparotomy incision allows good abdominal access in the majority of cases. After having ruled out intraperitoneal tumor dissemination, the intestinal loops are gathered up and held in the upper abdomen, by means of packs, for example. The sigmoid loop and rectum are mobilized, starting along the left paracolic groove. The mobilization must be performed along a length sufficient to permit the proximal colon to project out at the point of the future colostomy. The left ureter is defined during this procedure.

The peritoneal incision is continued as far as the base of the bladder. The surgeon thus slides his left hand under the inferior mesenteric vessels, and the peritoneum is slit in an identical way on the right. The mesenteric vascular pedicle is ligated and severed as high up as possible. The lateral peritoneal incisions are subsequently joined at an anterior point. The retrorectal cavity is dissected using scissors and the fingers, while applying traction to the rectosigmoid in the anterior direction. Dissection starts in the region of the sacral promontory. The presacral cavity is relatively avascular and usually easy to locate. After its location and incision, the right hand may be introduced into it and the cleavage followed by the finger. The rectum should thus be exposed as far as the tip of the coccyx, in front of the presacral fascia, avoiding injury to the presacral veins. If a fixed tumor makes this procedure difficult, it is advisable for the abdominal surgeon to wait until his perineal colleague meets up with him to ensure being at the correct level, rather than proceeding blindly. In any case, this site corresponds to the usual point where the two surgeons meet.

Let us now turn to the anterior dissection. The posterior wall of the bladder and the seminal vesicles (or the uterus and posterior vaginal wall in females) should be exposed by combined dissection using the scissors and fingers. The fascia of Denonvilliers is incised to sever the rectum totally from the prostate and the seminal vesicles. Dissection continues distally as far as the lower edge of the prostate. The urethra (containing a vesical catheter) may thus be palpated. In females, the posterior wall is pushed forwards as far as the point where it is to be excised.

Subsequently, the lateral ligaments of the rectum and the median hemorrhoidal arterias must be divided successively to the right and then the left. A long pair of scissors allows the surgeon to bypass the zone distal to these structures. After division, the ligaments and arteries are clamped, severed, and ligated.

The rectum is thus completely separated at its front, side, and back. Only a number of fibrous structures of minor importance still remain and are severed without special precautions.

The sigmoid is severed proximally, in general using a GIA stapler, to allow establisment of the colostomy. A cutaneous and subcutaneous cylinder of 2–3-cm diameter is excised at the site marked for the colostomy prior to incision. Its diameter should correspond more or less to that of the sigmoid. The anterior aponeurosis of the large right muscle of the abdomen is incised in cruciate fashion, and the underlying muscle fibers are then divided longitudinally to expose the peritoneum, which is cut with the scissors. The orifice thus created must permit the passage of two fingers. It should be checked that no lesion of the epigastric vessels has occurred during this procedure. If this does happen, a careful hemostasis must be performed.

A clamp is introduced via the colostomy orifice into the abdominal cavity to grasp the colon, which is ready to be lifted out. It should pass through the wall without excessive pulling. The distal end of the sigmoid is then wrapped, for instance, with a glove. The left proximal colon may be fixed to the peritoneal wall by a number of anchoring points. Finally, the pelvic floor is reconstructed by joining the available peritoneal edges, and the laparatomy incision is sutured section by section.

After resection of the redundant projecting colon at the stoma, the colon wall is anastomosed to the skin, the orifice being delimited by eight separate points of nonabsorbable monofilament 4/0.

The perineal dissection ideally starts as soon as the abdominal surgeon judges the lesion to be resectable. An elliptical incision is made outside the anal sphincter, including a sufficient margin of perianal skin. The edges of the latter are joined and placed on several Kocher forceps. The dissection is deepened into the adipose tissue of the ischiorectal fossa, careful hemostasis being applied to each vessel encountered. The inferior hemorrhoidal vessels are thus ligated and severed. An orthostatic dilator is placed into position as soon as the depth of the dissection allows it. The section is continued forwards by incising the deep transverse muscle of the perineum. In the reverse direction, the presacral cavity is accessed by incising the anococcygeal raphe in front of the tip of the coccyx. Care should thus be taken to perform the dissection a sufficient distance in front of the sacrum, as a movement too close to the bone risks injury to the presacral fascia and thus a severe hemorrhage. At all events, a point too far towards the front should not be chosen, owing to the risk of perforating the rectum. With this in mind, the abdominal surgeon should help to guide the perineal surgeon along the right path. The rectum and anus are thus entirely exposed along the posterior midline. A finger is then slid above the levator muscles of the anus, on each side. These muscles are then divided close to the pelvic wall, using scissors or an electric lancet.

It sometimes happens than one or both lateral ligaments of the rectum are separated as far as the perineum. Care should then be taken not to injure a ureter in the course of this procedure. The proximal rectum may finally be removed from the pelvis. While applying traction to it, the remaining attachments of the rectouretal muscle and of the fascia in the vicinity of the ureter are severed by scissors. The ureter should be located and injury to it avoided during this procedure.

The perineum is finally thoroughly rinsed, suction drainage tubes are placed in position, and the skin is sutured. There is no point in joining up or suturing the remaining fragments of the levator muscles.

In females, it is generally necessary for abdominoperineal resection of the rectum and anus to include resection of the posterior wall of the vagina. The perineal closure is continued until the fourchette is reconstituted.

The complications associated with the SCE operation most frequently involve a ureteric, vesical, or urethral lesion.

Extended operations involving an anastomosis may be considered on the basis of various techniques.

They permit a major procedure to be performed while preserving the sphincters. They differ more in the method used to produce the anastomosis than in the extent of the abdominal dissection. Anterior resection is the most frequently performed operation of this type.

In a high anterior resection, the anastomosis is made by an abdominal route, above the line of reflection of the peritoneum. A low anterior resection is characterized by an anastomosis located below the line of peritoneal reflection. Other methods require colorectal or coloanal anastomoses, which are performed via the peranal route, i.e., by a pull-through operation involving a rectocolectomy by the abdominotransanal route with total rectal excision and removal of the mucosa of the anal canal. Various anastomoses may also be considered via an abdominosacral route.

A low anterior resection requires complete mobilization of the rectum from the sacral concavity, and division of the lateral ligaments and the median hemorrhoidal arteries. The anastomosis is performed at the level of the rectum, distal to the line of peritoneal reflections. The operation cannot be called a low anterior resection if these criteria are not respected!

The patient is placed in the lithotomy position or in the dorsal recumbent position. If required, the former allows a reconstruction to be performed with the aid of an EEA stapler, a coloanal anastomosis to be created, or even an APR to be performed.

The initial stage is identical to that described for the abdominoperineal resection. Depending on the length of the rectosigmoid junction, it is not necessary to systematically mobilize the left colon as far as the splenic flexure. As soon as operatibilty is confirmed, the mesorectum must be separated. Clamps are placed behind the rectum and the mesentery incised in front of it. Applying traction to the proximal colon allows better separation of the mesentery from the posterior rectal wall. A clamp with grips is applied about 5 cm below the distal edge of the tumor. The intestine is then incised distal to the clamp, and anchorage points are placed on the distal rectum. The long Allis forceps may be used to define the severed edges of the rectum. As soon as the specimen has been resected to its proximal point, an end-to-end anastomosis is created. It is preferable to use suture material of an absorbable type; however, the exact type used is less important than the technique. This latter varies, depending on the surgeon, between use of a single layer of purse-string sutures to link separated points, involving an important muscle layer and a minimal thickness of

mucosa, and an anastomosis with two layers of stitching, i.e., muscular and mucosal. For a low anastomosis, it is preferable first to leave all the posterior sutures in place and to tie them subsequently. The two commissures as well as the anterior wall are constructed in a second stage. One suture on each layer is sufficient in the majority of cases, even though some surgeons prefer to lower and fix the anterior peritoneum in the region of the anastomosis. The pelvic floor is not restored. Extensive lavage of the true pelvis is subsequently performed.

Certain authors recommend placing and even suturing a piece of the greater omentum around the anastomosis [16, 21]. This procedure may be performed by mobilizing a piece of the omentum, taking care to avoid interrupting the vascular supply.

A low anterior anastomosis may also be performed by using a circular stapler introduced via the anus. This allows an end-to-end anastomosis with two series of staples and resection of two intestinal sections while ensuring that an adequate intestinal lumen is maintained. Staplers with the following calibers are available: 25, 28, and 31 mm. The patient should be placed in the lithotomy position, allowing easy access to both anus and abdomen. The surgical procedure is initially identical to that described above for manual anastomosis. After excision of the bowel segment containing the tumor, the distal end of the remaining colon is prepared for the anastomosis. All adipose tissue must be meticulously removed from a bowel section of between 1 and 2 cm. A circular purse-string suture is placed at a point on the free intestinal edge. A nonabsorbable, sufficiently resistant monofilament should be used. Prolane 0 is eminently suited for this purpose.

The distal rectum is prepared in an identical manner below the tumor, and the mesentery is removed. Appropriate forceps, allowing introduction of the circular purse-string suture, are placed at a sufficient distance below the tumor.

Unfortunately, this instrument often cannot be used for anastomoses situated very low in the pelvis. In such cases, therefore, a transparietal purse-string suture must be placed by hand. Dental forceps are initially placed on the bowel, distal to the tumor. A flexible intestinal or vascular clamp is applied onto the distal rectum stump and used for traction. In this way, by using dental forceps only, the bowel is cut continuously in the distal direction while placing the purse-string at a point on its free edge.

With experience, the surgeon should thus be able to choose a stapler of suitable size. The largest dimension available (31 mm) should always be tried. The sigmoid colon usually has the smallest lumen, but its caliber can generally be increased by using a dilator. In the case of colic spasm, intravenous administration of 2 mg glucagon, or a Fowley catheter may be of use [17, 32]. The perineal surgeon gradually dilates the anus and introduces the lubricated instrument into the rectum. The abdominal surgeon then guides it in the forwards direction, while his perineal colleague always has a tendency to work towards the sacrum. When the stapler anvil has passed the distal rectum stump, the instrument is opened to its maximal extent and the distal end separates from the rod. The purse-string suture placed on the distal stump is then pulled tight and tied. By using the Allis forceps, for example, the proximal bowel is subsequently gradually slid over the anvil until it covers it completely. The proximal purse-string suture is then tied. The sequence of knots on the two ends of the bowel may be inverted, the aim being to initially tie the end which is most difficult. The strands of the purse-string suture are thus cut close to the knot, and the perineal surgeon thightens the wing nut to join up the two parts of the stapler. The abdominal surgeon ensures that no tissue is located between the anvil and rod. The safety catch is then removed, and pressure is applied to the handles to complete the anastomosis and suture the intestinal parts by means of the clips and cutters. The anvil is then again moved a short distance away from the rod, and the instrument is withdrawn from the anus by a smooth rotation applied by the abdominal surgeon.

The rings of tissue from the two ends of the colon are finally removed from the rod and examined after cutting the ends of the purse-string sutures, ensuring that they are intact. If this is not the case, the anastomosis must either be repeated or reinforced by means of additional sutures. Its permeability is tested by placing water into the true pelvis and observing any bubbles appearing when air is insufflated into the rectum after clamping the proximal colon. If this method is successful and there is no sign of a leak, no additional suture points are required.

A new generation of circular terminoterminal staplers has recently been introduced. They are characterized essentially by a more harmonious shape of anvil, which may be easily detached, and by an angulation in the rod. A pointed trocar may also be fixed at the end of the rod; it can penetrate and pass through an obstructed end.

The main complication in colon surgery is anastomotic dehiscence, responsible for between a third and a half of all deaths in the postoperative period. This rate varies considerably according to different authors, ranging between 5% and 30%. Various factors suggest that it is often linked to surgical technique. The most frequent causes are excessive tension of the anastomosed bowel ends, insufficient vascularization, a local hematoma, and an abscessed accumulation draining into the colon during the postoperative period at the point of the anastomosis [11, 41]. The true incidence of dehiscence after low anterior resection is in fact greater than is suggested by the postoperative course, since most cases remain infraclinical and are revealed only by systematic monitoring enemas [31]. In contrast, it is always difficult to know if the rate of dehiscence is lower here than after conventional manual suturing, since the results available on this subject vary considerably from author to author [10].

Even if the splenic flexure needs only rarely to be mobilized when performing a low anterior anastomosis, it must always be ensured that the proximal colon is sufficiently detached to prevent any tension at the suture line. The fixation of the great omentum around the anastomosis also reduces the risk of dehiscence. If these precautions are observed, a low anterior anastomosis needs to be temporarily protected by a proximal colostomy only in exceptional cases. If signs of sepsis, of significant losses of blood, of a systemic condition, or of poor nutrition are present, this step is, however, frequently indicated.

When the patient's chances of survival are slim, an APR or an operation of the Hartmann type will frequently be preferred. The patient will find it easier to cope with a sigmoidal colostomy than a double-ended transverse colostomy.

The perioperative complications in this case are the same as those associated with APR. The postoperative management after low anterior resection is identical to that required for all surgery of the colon. In the postoperative period, a hemorrhage, a dehiscence, or, after some delay, an anastomotic stenosis frequently occurs [27]. A pelvic abscess or a fecal fistula is encountered less frequently.

Any anastomotic recurrence usually develops in the 2 years following the resection. The affected patient may be totally asymptomatic, but suspicious signs may be revealed by palpation, endoscopy, or endorectal ultrasonography. The symptoms may be as varied as bleeding; a modification of the caliber of the stools; or pain in the pelvis, abdomen, or sacrum. A biopsy usually confirms the diagnosis, which may also be made on the basis of a barium enema or a CT scan. Numerous patients with local recurrence show no evidence of disseminated disease. The only hope of cure in such cases is to perform another resection, which frequently involves APR. Before taking this step, however, a check should be made to ascertain whether the patient presents the symptoms of disseminated disease [26].

Various other techniques of anastomosis after low anterior resection have been described. Thus, some surgeons practice side-to-end anastomoses, above all if there is a significant disparity between the calibers of the two organs to be joined.

Coloanal (transanal) anastomosis was developed by Parks in 1972 [39, 40]. It allows the colon to be joined to the anal canal by transanal suture. The patient is placed in the Trendelenburg position. The rectum is mobilized by the abdominal approach and is completely resected. After introducing an anal dilator, the colon is lowered down to the proximal point of the anal canal and sutured to its distal stump, sometimes to that of the rectum, by separated points. The mucosa of the remaining stump should be exised as far as the pectinate line, the ideal site for the anastomosis. A short cylinder of muscle from the lower rectum and the upper anal canal is used to sheathe the last 2–3 cm of the colon, protecting this region from a possible dehiscence.

A variant of the above technique is to create a J-pouch above the anastomosis [22]. Defecation is less frequent, but spontaneous discharge sometimes presents problem [38].

The abdominoanal *pull-through* operation is generally reserved for anastomoses located at least 7 cm from the anal verge. However, this procedure is little used today, as various more recent methods are preferred. There are several modifications of the basic technique, all having a common underlying principle [45]. After resection of the tumor, the remaining colon is drawn down, pulled through the anus to project several centimeters beyond the rectum edge, with or without eversion of the parietal cylinders. Between 7 and 10 days later, when sufficient adhesion has been established between the colon and the distal anorectal stump, the projecting colon is excised. Continence is poorer than after a coloanal anastomosis of the kind described by Parks [37, 38]. The operational mortality associated with this procedure is extremely low.

Abdominosacral (coccygeal) resection represents an approach to rectal surgery first described at the end of the nineteenth century but recently modified by Localio and Stahl [23] and Mason [28]. Compared with the transsacral resection, it offers the advantage of a more complete dissection of the lymphatic structures.

It combines an abdominal dissection with a sacral approach, by means of two techniques:

1. *Localio and Stahl [23].* The patient is placed on the right side, and rectal excision is performed via the abdomen. The perineal surgeon penetrates the retrorectal cavity via a transverse incision above the sacrum and excision of the coccyx. The anastomosis is performed after lifting the colon and the distal rectal stump out through the sacral wound.

2. *Mason [28].* Transsphincteric modification: the retrorectal cavity is accessed by posterior division of the levator muscles of the anus and sphincter. The latter is reconstructed after completion of the anastomosis.

In a *transsacral (Kraske) excision,* the patient is placed in the jackknife position, with the buttocks spread out. A median incision is made between the edge of the anal verge and the base of the sacrum. The passage through the subcutaneous tissue reveals the levator muscles of the anus and the coccyx. The levators are divided to expose the back wall of the rectum. The coccyx is excised from its muscular attachments, disarticulated, and resected. If this provides insufficient access, a complementary resection of the lower part of the sacrum base must be performed. However, the third sacral vertebra must be preserved at all costs, as otherwise continence may be endangered. The rectum is then completely mobilized, taking care not to injure its anterior part where it adheres to the vagina or prostate. The peritoneum may be divided from the anterior side of the rectum, which may thus be pulled downwards and the superior hemorrhoidal vessels divided. The bowel is severed at the desired point and the anastomosis created by means of separated points, using one or two layers. In certain circumstances, an anastomosis by means of a circular stapler may be considered [19]. The presacral cavity is then drained during the reconstruction.

Temporary incontinence is often observed after this operation. This heals up spontaneously within several weeks in the absence of nerve lesions.

The indication for this intervention must exclude a malignant condition. It should be reserved for benign lesions, polyps, or superficial tumors of small dimensions, since sufficient excision of the adipose and lymphatic tissue surrounding the rectum is difficult.

The *transsphincteric excision* used for removing certain superficial cancers of limited extent located very low in the rectum has been updated by Mason. It can be used alone or in association with an abdominal approach (cf. abdominosacral resection, p. 195).

The patient is placed in the flexed jackknife position. The levator muscles of the anus and external sphincter are incised completely along the median posterior line. The rectum is separated in depth and subsequently opened, allowing an excellent visualization of its median and distal parts. Although tumors of the posterior rectum wall can be most easily exposed in this way, those with posterior or lateral localization can also be seen after complete mobilization of the rectum. Repair of the sphincter usually gives satisfactory functional results.

This method has the drawback of not allowing an associated extended excision of the lymphatic tissue, so that it is often used merely as a palliative measure for patients in a poor general state of health. Mason has described an alternative to this technique. It allows an anastomosis to be performed by the same route after an abdominoanal pull-through procedure at a very low point.

Transanal (local) excisions have recently attracted renewed interest. Even if an extensive resection is the treatment of choice for most rectal carcinomas, local techniques may be considered in some situations. Apart from surgical excision and electrofulguration, vaporization by laser or contact radiotherapy may be performed via the transanal route. Excisision has the advantage over other techniques of providing a specimen for a definitive pathological examination.

The indication for local treatment is more difficult to decide than mastering the technique. It should, after all, permit total excision of the tumor. If the histological examination of the specimen confirms that removal has been complete and that the lesion is well or moderately differentiated, no supplementary treatment is required. The cancers of choice for this technique are of small diameter (less than 3 cm), exophytic, mobile, and well differentiated [3, 20]. The first three criteria are generally determined by preoperative rectal palpation, but valuable additional data are obtained by endorectal ultrasonography. Seventy percent of tumors confined to the rectum may be identified purely by means of rectal palpation. Enlarged retrorectal glands are palpated in only 50% of subjects in whom pathological examination subsequently shows glandular invasion in the surgical specimen.

Local excision may be performed via a surgical proctoscope (depending on localization and size of the tumor). It is often preferable to enlarge the anus and to keep it wide open by means of a suitable dilator. The tumor is inspected and and anchoring suture placed distal to it. Infiltration of the submucosa with a solution containing adrenaline facilitates dissection and reduces the hemorrhage. The tumor, delimited about 1 cm from its edges, is excised together with a complete parietal disc. The rectum is sutured as the dissection proceeds, each point being used in turn to apply traction. The indications for this method of treating malignant tumors are very limited. If the histological examination of the excised specimen reveals invasion of the intestinal wall, the arteries, or lymph vessels, an extensive resection must be performed immediately.

Hartmann's operation can be useful as a palliative measure in the case of an advanced rectal tumor. It involves the excision of the upper two-thirds of the rectum and the adjacent sigmoid, with establishment of a terminal left iliac colostomy and closure of the retained distal rectal stump at the level of the pelvic floor. Hartmann's operation was the surgical intervention of choice for carcinomas of the upper and middle third of the rectum before anterior resection became a reliable method. It is now indicated for rectal cancers only when an anterior resection or an abdominoperineal excision is out of the question. The possibility of secondary restoration of digestive continuity by means of staplers has renewed interest in this old method.

A simple colostomy represents another palliative surgical method for rectal neoplasms. It may be terminal, established generally in the left iliac fossa, or have two ends, left iliac and right transverse. In the case of tenesmus or incontinence due to obstruction by a nonresectable rectal tumor causing the patient considerable discomfort, a colostomy may transform the quality of life. A surprising improvement of the general and local state of health is often observed after such an intervention. Attachment of the tumor to adjacent structures may be due mainly to the inflammation, which is, however, reduced or sometimes even disappears after draining the underlying bowel due to diversion of the flow of matter. Sometimes, a tumor excision may even be subsequently considered.

However, a routine colostomy should not be performed in the presence of an advanced malignancy with extensive metastases or peritoneal carcinosis. Where no acute obstruction is present, the patient will be less comfortable with a stoma, and it is unlikely that he or she will live long enough to gain much benefit from it. In fact, there is no evidence to show that a colostomy has prolonged life in such cases.

Certain patients intially presenting a disseminated disease may benefit, in terms of survival, from surgical excision of their metastases. A solitary lesion of the liver or lungs, or multiple metastases of a single hepatic lobe may be treated in this way. Unfortunately, these are rare cases, corresponding to 5%–10% of patients with hepatic metastases. Some work has shown that a hepatic resection, even a major one, does improve the changes of survival.

Even though they are very painful, especially when occurring in the pelvis, local recurrences cause death only in rare cases. Only exceptionally is a local recurrence encountered without concurrent metastases. Excision of such recurrences, if at all possible, has thus little chance of improving the patient's life expectancy: the 5-year survival rate after apparently complete excision of the local recurrence is of the order of 5%–10%. An excision is possible only in 10%–20% of patients with local recurrence. If this situation is to be improved, the recurrences must be detected earlier and removed as soon as possible.

Treatment by Electrofulguration

The objective of electrofulguration is to destroy a tumor and an adjacent strip of normal tissue, both at the periphery and in depth, by coagulation. This procedure may be considered when the tumor involves less than 50% of the circumference of the rectum, when it is mobile, exophytic and well or moderately differentiated, when the patient presents disseminated disease with metastases, or when the aim is to provide effective palliative treatment. It may also be used in the presence of a debilitating disease, or when the patient refuses or is unfit for a colostomy. This method is relatively contraindicated for a circumferential lesion which is poorly differentiated or highly anaplastic, a highly ulcerated tumor, a neoplasm extending above the line of peritoneal reflection or before it in females. One of the major drawbacks of this technique is that it does not provide a specimen which can be used for pathological examination [24, 25].

Regular follow-up checks are indispensable. It is probable that, in the majority of cases, the procedure must be repeated after a longer or shorter interval. Monthly checks should be made over a period of about 6 months. A biopsy is taken or possibly a repeated electrofulguration performed on each occasion.

This method requires locoregional or general anesthesia. The patient is placed in the jackknife position if the lesion is anterior, in the lithotomy position if it is mainly posterior. After anal dilation, a surgical proctoscope of suitable diameter and length is introduced. A standard surgical diathermy machine with a sharp end is used. Its point is introduced into the tumor tissue as the coagulating current is applied. The procedure is repeated until the entire area of the tumor has been treated. The necrotic tissue is removed by means of forceps or a curette. The operation is completed when normal tissue (muscle wall or perirectal fat) is exposed. Its duration varies according to the dimensions and depth of penetration of the tumor: it may be between 1 and 2 h. For large lesions, several sessions may be required.

The most frequent complication of this method is the postoperational rise of body temperature, which may reach 39°–40°. This phenomenon occurs frequently, often the evening after the intervention. A broad-based antibiotic is therefore administered preoperatively and for 48–72 h after the intervention. Sometimes, a hemorrhage occurring during coagulation may necessitate a blood transfusion. A rectal stenosis may be observed, mainly when the tumor extension involves more than 50% of the circumference of the rectum. In females, a rectovaginal fistula may complicate the removal of a lesion located on the anterior wall of the rectum.

Treatment by Cryosurgery

Cryosurgery is used by certain authors as a palliative method for patients presenting an inoperable tumor of the rectum or a recurrence after an operation [12, 13].

Treatment by Laser Photocoagulation

Photocoagulation by laser is also indicated as a palliative treatment for cancer of the rectum [4, 30]. In contrast, it has no place in the treatment of curable cancers of this organ. For nonremovable stenosing tumors or when hemorrhage presents a major problem, the laser allows a sufficient lumen to be restored as well as effective hemostasis. It can often obviate a colostomy. This aim is frequently achieved, given that the patients suitable for laser photocoagulation do not have a long life expectancy. Among the complications of the method, perirectal abscesses and intestinal perforation have been reported. However, they occur rarely.

This technique has probably a certain future for the above indications, particularly in conjunction with the use of endorectal ultrasonography for preoperational staging. It will doubtless gradually supplant electrofulguration and cryosurgery for the treatment of rectal cancer without resection. However, the technique requires considerable experience on the part of those who perform it, as well as relatively sophisticated equipment.

Complementary Treatments

Complementary treatments for cancer of the rectum essentially comprise radiotherapy, chemotherapy, and immunotherapy. Even though surgical techniques have improved and become more refined, it hardly seems likely that surgery alone will be able to significantly improve the survival rate of patients suffering from rectal cancer. This has, in fact, remained the same for the last 30 years. There are two reasons for this failure:

- The wellknown tendency of malignant gastrointestinal tumors to form metastases
- The relatively long period elapsing between onset of the disease and its diagnosis in most cases

Consequently, recent therapeutic research has concentrated on the following:

- Seeking adjuvant treatments, selecting patients, and forecasting their response to treatment
- Nonsurgical treatments, alone or in combination, for treating recurrences

The role of *radiotherapy* in the treatment of rectal adenocarcinomas remains a subject of controversy. Should we expect benefits from adjuvant radiotherapy? If so, are these due to a reduction of the incidence of local recurrence or to an improvement in the survival rate? Which dosages and optimal diets should be selected? Should a tumor be irradiated preoperatively, postoperatively, or both together [34]? External readiotherapy for treating rectal carcinomas as a complement to surgery may be applied either before or after the operation.

Preoperative treatment aims to reduce the extent of the tumor growth, allowing a complete secondary excision to be considered. Another of its objectives is to limit the chances of dissemination of viable tumor cells during surgery [43]. It should therefore be reserved for tumors which are fixed or deeply ulcerated or when indurated glands are palpated in the presacral cavity. Various recent studies show that preoperative radiotherapy does not significantly prolong survival but does reduce the rate of local recurrences. A statistical significant reduction of the incidence of affected glands in irradiated patients has also been shown. This method has thus been shown to be of undeniable benefit for treating patients with nonresectable tumors.

The optimal dosage for preoperative treatment is between approximately 40 and 45 Gy, administered over a period of 4–6 weeks. The operation is performed 6–8 weeks after termination of radiotherapy. The morbidity and mortality associated with surgery under these conditions have not increased. If the dosage does not exceed 45 Gy, there is, in particular, no increase in the incidence of anastomotic dehiscence [8].

Postoperative radiotherapy can make use of a complete pathological report obtained from a previously excised specimen. Knowing the extent of the disease, the exact area of treatment can be determined. For patients with tumor growth corresponding to the Dukes' stages associated with a high risk of local recurrence (B2 or C), radiotherapy may significantly reduce the risk of pelvic recurrence.

Numerous randomized prospective studies are currently being undertaken. It already seems clear that postoperative radiotherapy is not tolerated as well as the preoperative type. The former procedure should therefore be reserved, for the moment, for tumors corresponding to the Dukes' stages showing poor differentiation or associated with a poor prognosis. Treatment should start 1–2 months after the operation, to allow for sufficient cicatrization and reduce the risk of recurrence. The dosage administered to the tumor bed should be around 60 Gy.

The complications of this treatment are well known: urinary infection, diarrhea, cutaneous and cicatricial lesions, and lesions of the small bowel. One of the concerns expressed in the application of radiotherapy is the possibility of injury to the small bowel. The likelihood of such a complication is considerably reduced if doses do not exceed 50 Gy. A number of techniques have been suggested to minimize radiation to this relatively vulnerable organ by excluding the small bowel from the pelvis. These include construction of an omental envelope, the use of a synthetic absorbable or nonabsorbable mesh sling, a breast prosthesis, and a synthetic polymer mold [6, 9]. The age and general state of health of the patient should thus also play a role in the indications for radiotherapy.

Palliative radiotherapy may also be administered to patients with a painful recurrence after surgical excision.

Finally, interstitial radium implantation, as described by Papillon [35, 37], should not be forgotten. It certainly plays a role for carefully selected patients with a relatively small tumor of the rectum.

Rectal carcinoma is extremely resistant to chemotherapeutic agents. Practically all suitable drugs have been tested. Only some of them have proved effective and are still being used. 5-Fluorouracil (5-FU) and 5-fluorodeoxyuridin (5-FUDR) are the most promising in this respect. The nitro acids and mitomycin C have also proved useful in treating cancer of the rectum [46].

Several papers praise the merits of combining chemotherapy with radiotherapy. Unfortunately, there is still a lack of convincing evidence showing an improvement in the survival rate or a reduction of recurrences in patients given these treatments. There is no doubt that several prospective studies currently underway should, in the near future, provide answers to numerous questions which are still open in this subject [14, 44].

No study has yet shown any absolute proof of the effectiveness of immunotherapy for treating cancers of the rectum, even if the use of marked monoclonal antibodies represents a promising ray of hope in this respect [5].

References

1. American Joint Committee on Cancer (1983) Manual for staging of cancer. Lippincott, Philadelphia
2. Astler VB, Coller FA (1954) The prognostic significance of direct extension of carcinoma of the colon and rectum. Ann Surg 139: 846–851
3. Biggers OR, Beart RW Jr, Ilstrup DM (1986) Local excision of rectal cancer. Dis Colon Rectum 29: 374–377
4. Bown SG, Barr H, Mathewson K, Hawes R, Swain CP, Clark CG, Boulos PB (1986) Endoscopic treatment of inoperable colorectal cancers with the Nd YAG laser. Br J Surg 73: 949–952
5. Delaloye B, Bischof-Delaloye A, Volant JC, Pettavel J, von Fliedner V, Buchegger F, Mach JP (1985) First approach to therapy of liver metastases in colo-rectal carcinoma by intra-hepatically infused I-131 labeled monoclonal anti-CEA antibodies. Eur J Nucl Med 11– A37
6. De Luca FR, Ragins H (1985) Construction of an omental envelope as a method of excluding the small intestine from the field of postoperative irradiation to the pelvis. Surg Gynecol Obstet 160: 365–366
7. Dukes CE (1932) The classification of cancer of the rectum. J Pathol 35: 323–332
8. Duncan W (1985) Adjuvant radiotherapy in rectal cancer: the MRC trials. Br J Surg 72: 559–566
9. Dürig M, Steenblock U, Heberer M, Harder F (1984) Prevention of radiation injuries to the small intestine. Surg Gynecol Obstet 159: 162–163
10. Everett WG, Friend PJ, Forty J (1986) Comparison of stapling and hand suture for left-sided large bowel anastomosis. Br J Surg 73: 345–348
11. Foster ME, Lancaster JB, Leaper DJ (1984) Leakage of low rectal anastomosis: an anatomic explanation? Dis Colon Rectum 27: 157–158
12. Fritsch A, Seidl W, Walzel C, Moser K, Schiessel R (1982) Palliative and adjunctive measures in rectal cancer. World J Surg 6: 569–577
13. Gage AA (1968) Cryotherapy for inoperable rectal cancer. Dis Colon Rectum 11: 36–44
14. Gastroingestinal Tumor Study Group (1985) Prolongation of the disease-free interval in surgically treated rectal carcinoma. N Engl J Med 312: 1465–1472
15. Givel JC, Spinosa GP, Chapuis G (1988) Valeur de l'ultrasonographie endorectale pour le chirurgien. Helv Chir Acta 55: 235–238
16. Goldsmith HS (1977) Protection of low rectal anastomosis with intact omentum. Surg Gynecol Obstet 144: 584–586
17. Harford FJ (1979) Use of glucagon in conjunction with the end-to-end anastomosis (EEA) stapling device for low anterior anastomosis. Dis Colon Rectum 22: 452–454
18. Hermanek P, Sobin LM (1987) TNM classification of malignant tumours, 4th edn. Springer, Berlin Heidelberg New York
19. Jacobson YG (1985) Posterior rectal resection using EEA stapler. Dis Colon Rectum 28: 681–683
20. Killingback MJ (1985) Indications for local excision of rectal cancer. Br J Surg 72: 544–556
21. Lanter B, Mason RA (1979) Use of omental pedicle graft to protect low anterior colonic anastomosis. Dis Colon Rectum 22: 448–451.
22. Lazorthes F, Fages P, Chiotasso P, Bugat R (1986) Synchronous abdominotranssphincteric resection of low rectal cancer: new technique for direct colo-anal anastomosis. Br J Surg 73: 573–575
23. Localio SA, Stahl WH (1969) Simultaneous abdomino-transsacral resection and anastomosis for mid-rectal cancer. Am J Surg 117: 282–289
24. Madden JL, Kandalaft S (1967) Electrocoagulation: a primary and preferred method of treatment for cancer of the rectum. Ann Surg 166: 413–419
25. Madden JL, Kandalaft S (1971) Clinical evaluation of electrocoagulation in the treatment of cancer of the rectum. Am J Surg 122: 347–352
26. Manson PN, Corman ML, Coller JA, Veidenheimer MC (1976) Anastomotic recurrence after anterior resection for carcinoma: Lahey Clinic experience. Dis Colon Rectum 19: 219–224
27. Manson PN, Corman ML, Coller JA, Veidenheimer MC (1976) Anterior resection for adenocarcinoma: Lahey Clinic experience from 1963 through 1969. Am J Surg 131: 434–441
28. Mason AY (1970) Surgical access to the rectum – a transsphincteric exposure. Proc R Soc Med 63: 91–94
29. Mason AY (1976) Rectal cancer: the spectum of selective surgery. Proc R Soc Med 69: 237–244
30. Mathus-Vliegen EMH, Tytgat GNJ (1986) Laser pho-

tocoagulation in the palliation of colorectal malignancies. Cancer 57: 2212–2216
31. McGonaghe BA (1985) Evaluation of the proximate-ILS circular stapler: a prospective study. Ann Surg 210: 108–114
32. Minichan DP Jr (1982) Enlarging the bowel lumen for the EEA stapler. Dis Colon Rectum 25: 61
33. Morson BC, Dawson IMP (1979) Gastro-intestinal pathology. Blackwell Scientific, Oxford
34. Pahlman L, Glimelius B, Graffman S (1985) Pre- versus postoperative radiotherapy in rectal carcinoma: an interim report from a randomized multicentre trial. Br J Surg 72: 961–966
35. Papillon J (1975) endocavitary irradiation of early rectal cancer for cure: a series of 186 cases. Cancer 36: 696–701
36. Papillon J (1982) Rectal and anal cancers. Springer, Berlin Heidelberg New York
37. Papillon J (1984) New prospects in the conservative treatment of rectal cancer. Dis Colon Rectum 27: 695–700
38. Parc R, Tiret E, Frileux P, Moszkowski E, Loygue J (1986) Resection and colo-anal anastomosis with colonic reservoir for rectal carcinoma. Br J Surg 73: 139–141
39. Parks AG (1972) Transanal technique in low rectal anastomosis. Proc R Soc Med 65: 975–976
40. Parks AG (1982) Per-anal anastomosis. World J Surg 6: 531–538
41. Schrock TR, Deveney CW, Dunphy JE (1973) Factors contributing to leakage of colonic Anastomoses. Ann Surg 177: 513–518
42. Silverman A, Desai TK, Luk GD (1988) Scope of the problem. Gastroenterol Clin North Am 17: 655–656
43. Sischy B (1987) The role of radiation therapy in the management of carcinoma of the rectum. Cont Surg 30: 13–26
44. Smith DE, Muff NS, Shetabi H (1986) Combined preoperative neoadjuvant radiotherapy and chemotherapy for anal and rectal cancer. Am J Surg 151: 577–580
45. Turnbull RB Jr, Cuthbertson A (1961) Abdominorectal pull-through resection for cancer and for Hirschsprung's disease: delayed posterior colorectal anastomosis. Clev Clin Q 28: 109–115
46. Windle R, Bell PRF, Shaw D (1987) Five year results of a randomized trial of adjuvant 5-fluorouracil and levamisole incolorectal cancer. Br J Surg 74: 569–572.

21 Retrorectal Tumors

M.-C. Marti

Definition

Retrorectal or presacral tumors are rare. The retrorectal space lies between the upper rectum and the sacrum. It is limited anteriorly by the fascia propria of the rectum, posteriorly by the presacral fascia, and laterally by the ureters and iliac vessels. It is limited inferiorly by the rectosacral fascia and it communicates superiorly with the retroperitoneal space. The rectosacral fascia isolates the retrorectal space from the supralevator space. The latter is a horseshoe-shaped space limited anteriorly by Denonvillier's fascia and below by the levator ani. The retrorectal space is made up of loose connective tissue but may contain different embryological remnants.

Classification

Various tumors may develop and can be classified according their embryological origins. Several classifications have been proposed [2, 8, 16]. The latest one is summarized in Table 21.1.

Incidence

These lesions are rare. Uhlig and Johnson [16] reviewed 63 cases occuring over a 30-year period in Portland, United States. Lovelady and Dockerty [8] reported on 127 females with extragenital pelvic tumors, including 56 ectopic kidneys, treated at the Mayo Clinic between 1910 and 1947 [9]. Jackman and Clark [4] published a report on 114 retrorectal tumors seen between 1937 and 1948. Jao et al. [5], reviewing the Mayo Clinic experience between 1960 and 1979, reported on 120 patients. In 1963 McColl [10] presented 23 cases seen at St Mark's Hospital, London. Stewart et al. [15] published 20 cases studied retrospectively in Belfast. Due to the rarity of these lesions, most surgeons will have only little experience in managing them.

Congenital lesions, mainly cysts and chordomas, account for 70%–83% of these tumors. Neurogenic, osseous, and miscellaneous tumors each account for about 10%. Malignancy occurs in 33% of cases. Cystic lesions are more frequent in women whereas chordomas predominate in men [5].

Table 21.1. Classification of retrorectal tumors

Congenital
  Epidermoid cyst
  Mucus-secreting cyst
  Teratoma
  Teratocarcinoma
  Chordoma
  Meningocele
Inflammatory
  Foreign body granuloma
  Perineal abscess
  Internal fistula
  Pelvirectal abscess
  Chronic infectious granuloma
Neurogenic
  Neurofibroma
  Neurofibrosarcoma
  Neurolemoma
  Ependymoma
  Neuroblastoma
Osseous
  Osteoma
  Osteochondroma
  Osteogenic sarcoma
  Simple bone cyst
  Giant cell tumor
  Ewing's sarcoma
  Chondromyxosarcoma
  Aneurysmal bone cyst
  Myeloma
Miscellaneous
  Metastatic carcinoma
  Lipoma
  Liposarcoma
  Fibroma
  Fibrosarcoma
  Leiomyoma
  Leiomyosarcoma
  Hemangioma
  Pericytoma
  Lymphangioma
  Hemangioendothelial sarcoma
Extraabdominal desmoid tumor

Clinical Presentation

Symptoms due to these tumors result from their site and size, and the presence of infection. Poorly localized perianal pain, rectal ache, or deep rectal pain are common clinical manifestations. The pain is frequently postural occurring when the patient is sitting or standing. Pain radiating into the legs or dysesthesia in the buttocks result from involvement of the sacral plexus.

Large tumors may interfere with the passage of stools (resulting in constipation and incomplete evacuation), with bladder function (incontinence, urinary retention, obstruction of the pelvic ureters), with normal delivery (obstructed labor and dystocia).

Cystic lesions may become infected resulting in fever, chills, and perianal suppuration. These symptoms may be confused with anal fistula and pilonidal cysts.

Differential Diagnosis

Careful clinical records are necessary to exclude other conditions possibly presenting as retrorectal tumors: suppuration into the retrorectal space resulting from complicated diverticulatis, fistulization due to Crohn's disease, and metastatic spread from genitourinary or gastrointestinal tumors. Furthermore, infected cystic lesions may be confused with recurrent and incompletely treated cryptogenic anal fistulas.

According to Jao et al. [5], five conditions may indicate a presacral cyst:

- Recurring abscess in the retrorectal space.
- Repeated operation for an "anal fistula."
- Inability to find the primary source of infection at its usual site in a crypt at the dentate margin when an anal, perianal, or rectal sinus is present.
- The presence of a postanal dimple.
- Some fixation and fullness in the precoccygeal region.

Examination

Inspection of the perianal area may reveal fecal soiling, a pouting anus, a postanal dimple, a fistulous opening, and in children an anterior meningocele. Digital examination is essential. An anterior angulation of the rectum as well as a solid or cystic soft and nontender mass can be palpated. Size, consistency, lobulation, and relationship to neighboring organs must be assessed to determine the surgical approach.

Sigmoidoscopy may be negative for small tumors. Nevertheless, it should always be performed to assess the state of the overlying mucosa and possible rectal wall involvement.

Plain X-ray films of the pelvis and sacrum may demonstrate soft tissue masses, calcifications, compression, displacement, or even destruction of the sacrum and coccyx in cases of malignancy. A fistulogram is useful to distinguish a uni- or multilocular retrorectal cyst from a complex anal fistula.

Endoanal echography associated with abdominal and endovaginal ultrasonography may be successful for small and deep-lying lesions, especially cystic ones. Ultrasonography also permits evaluation of liver metastases and hydronephrosis due to urethral compression. Ultrasound-guided needle aspiration is useful for cytology.

A CT scan gives precise anatomical details about tissue density as well as the size, surface, and relationship of the tumor to the sacrum. It is the single most useful radiological investigation.

An intravenous urogram and barium enema may reveal extrinsic compression, displacement, and possible obstruction.

Angiography gives information about vascularity of the tumors and about modification in vascular distribution of the pelvis. Results may be useful during surgical procedure but do not alter the decision to operate or interfere with the surgical approach.

Myelography is helpful in cases of meningocele.

Biopsy

The best biopsy is total surgical excision. When the lesion is considered to be inoperable and a decision regarding the possibility of adjuvant therapy is required, a biopsy is necessary. Biopsy can be performed through the posterior rectal wall or using a presacral extrarectal approach. The needle is inserted under digital endoanal control. Biopsy can also be guided by endorectal ultrasonography or CT scan.

Biopsy should not be performed when there is a cystic lesion as the associated mortality rate is 40%. If the cystic appearance is the result of an anterior sacral meningocele, biopsy or drainage through the rectum or the vagina results in an almost 100% mortality rate [11].

Surgery

As the bowel can be injured during dissection or is to be resected, preoperative large bowel preparation is mandatory. Various surgical approaches are possible depending on the size of the lesion and its nature.

Abdominal Approach

An abdominal approach should be chosen for tumors located high in the rectum where safe access from below is impossible. The sigmoid should be mobilized and the rectum stretched. The excision of the retrorectal tumor may result in massive bleeding from the middle sacral artery and from presacral vessels. Dissection should therefore be conducted step by step with careful ligation of any vessel or by using hemoclips. All nerve structures should be protected.

Posterior Approach

A posterior approach is useful for low-lying tumors and for infected cysts. The patient is placed in the prone jackknife position. The sacrum, coccyx, and anococcygeal ligament are identified through a midline, curvilinear, or horizontal incision. For small lesions, a parasacral approach without cutting the sphincter or the puborectalis sling, as discribed by York Mason (see Chap. 17), may be convenient. If necessary, the coccyx is disarticulated from the S5 vertebra and resected to allow entrance into the supralevator space. The gluteus maximus muscle can be detached on each side. When there are large tumors, the S5 and even S4 vertebrae can be excised and sacral nerves divided without fear of neurological deficit. In the case of chordoma, Localio et al. [6, 7] have even resected the sacrum at the level of S2 while retaining good sphincter and bladder function.

Bleeding may result in major complications as the vascular supply comes from above.

When there are cystic lesions, the coccyx should always be excised to prevent recurrence [14].

In cases of an infected cyst, the posterior extrarectal approach is the most convenient. If the cyst has ruptured into the rectum, the posterior approach is contraindicated and transrectal drainage should be performed. It may be necessary to perform the operation in two or more stages.

Abdominosacral Approach

The approach described by Localio et al. [6, 7] is useful for removing large retrorectal chordomas and teratomas with abdominal extension. Usually the abdominal approach is performed first and then, after closure of the abdominal cavity, the patient is placed in the jackknife postition for the sacral approach. The two stages can be combined if the patient is lying on the side. Simultaneous access from the abdomen and from the sacrum can be achieved by two teams.

The main advantage of this approach is to allow good hemostasis with primary ligature of the midsacral artery.

Transrectal Approach

If a retrorectal cyst has ruptured into the rectum, a transrectal approach may be convenient.

Intersphincteric Approach

When the lesions are small, especially single or multiple cysts, an intersphincteric approach is useful. As for the postanal repair described by Parks [12], the retrorectal space is entered using the plane between internal and external sphincter. Dissection may be performed as high as 6–10 cm from the anal verge.

Radiotherapy and Chemotherapy

Adjuvant or palliative radiotherapy may be effective in cases of soft tissue sarcomas (lymphoma, myeloma, teratocarcinoma) and chordoma [13]. No evidence of any effective chemotherapy has been reported.

Prognosis

Benign tumors and cysts can be managed by excision. Inadequate removal, especially when small cysts have not been excised, may result in recurrence.

Malignant lesions have a poor prognosis [1]. Five-year survival is rare in cases of soft tissue sarcomas or teratocarcinomas. Despite a low grade of malignancy, five-year survival free of disease is difficult to assess for chordoma because of a high incidence of metastasis.

Pearlman and Friedman [13] reported a 15%–20% survival rate at 10 years; Higinbothan et al. [3] 10% at 5 years; Localio et al. [6, 7] less than 2% and Joa et al. [5] over 75% at 5 years. A better cure rate seems to be the result of early diagnosis and treatment by a multidisciplinary surgical team including a surgeon, orthopedic surgeon, and neurosurgeon.

References

1. Farthmann EH, Fiedler L (1986) Retrorectale und präsacrale Tumoren. Der Chirurg 57: 496–501
2. Freier DT, Stanley JC, Thompson NW (1971) Retrorectal tumors in adults. Surg Gynecol Obstet 132: 681–686
3. Higinbotham NL, Phillips RF, Farr HW, et al. (1967) Chordoma. Thirty-five year study at Memorial Hospital. Cancer 20: 1841
4. Jackman RJ, Clark PL (1951) Retrorectal tumors. JAMA 145: 956–962
5. Jao SW, Beart RW, Spencer RJ, et al. (1985) Retrorectal tumors. Mayo Clinic experience, 1960–1979, Dis Col Rect, 28: 644–651
6. Localio SA, Francis KC, Rossano PG (1967) Abdominosacral resection of sacrococcygeal chordoma. Ann Surg, 166: 394
7. Localio SA, Eng K, Ranson JHC (1980) Abdominosacral approach for retrorectal tumors. Ann Surg, 191: 555
8. Lovelady SB, Dockerty MB (1949) Extragenital pelvic tumors in women. Am J Obstet Gynecol, 58: 215–216
9. Mayo CW, Baker GS, Smith LR (1953) Presacral tumors: differential diagnosis and report of case. Mayo Clin Porc, 28: 616–622
10. McColl J (1963) The classification of presacral cysts and tumors. Proc R Soc Med 56: 797–798
11. Oren M, Bennett L, Lee SH, Truex RC, Gennaro AL (1977) Anterior sacral meningocele. Dis Colon Rectum, 20: 492
12. Parks AG (1975) Anorectal incontinence, Proc R Soc Med, 68: 681
13. Pearlman AW, Friedman M (1970) Radical radiation therapy of chordoma. AM J Roentgenol, 108: 333
14. Spencer RJ, Jackman RJ (1962) Surgical managment of precoccygeal cysts. Surg Gynecol Obstet, 115: 449–452
15. Stewart RJ, Humphreys WG, Parks TG (1986) The presentation and management of presacral tumors. Br J Surg 73: 153–155
16. Uhlig BE, Johnson RL (1975) Presacral tumors and cysts in adults. Dis Colon Rectum, 18: 581–596

22 Anal Incontinence

M.-C. Marti

Definition

Fecal incontinence is a very distressing symptom which interferes severely with social life, especially in a rigidly toilet-trained society like ours. Data about the frequency of the problem are not well established, but the incidence seems greater than is generally realized [7, 49].

Fecal continence is a normal state. Continence may be defined as the ability to retain solid or liquid stools and flatus not only in various positions, but also during physical exercise, coughing, and sneezing.

Continence results from the interaction of a great number of functions: consistency of stools, coordinated activity of smooth and striated muscle in the anorectum and pelvic floor, anatomic integrity of these structures, integrity of autonomic innervation, and spinal and cerebral reflexes.

Defecation means voiding of rectal content. It is a complex procedure resulting from an increase of the intraabdominal pressure and an "unlocking" of the mechanisms of continence.

Pathogenesis and Physiology

Mechanisms of Continence and Defecation

A flap-valve mechanism is responsible for gross continence. The puborectalis sling and the mesorectum which fix the rectum to the sacrum posteriorly create a double angulation of the anorectum. The puborectalis sling is responsible for the maintenance of the angle between the anal canal and the lower rectum. This anorectal angle is about $90°-105°$ at rest, $60°-90°$ during voluntary retention of feces, and between $120°-180°$ during defecation [32, 50]. Incontinence may be the result of this angle being too wide [50, 53].

The internal and external sphincter, puborectalis sling, and levator muscles are responsible for voluntary continence and evacuation. The internal sphincter, consisting of smooth musculature, produces the resting pressure within the middle part of the anal canal. This pressure is higher in the upper part of the canal. Only 20% of the resting pressure in the region of the anal sphincter is due to the activity of the external striated sphincter [32]. Division of the external sphincter alone during surgical treatment of fistula in ano results in only minimal functional disability.

Voluntary contraction of the external sphincter and of the puborectalis muscle is only of limited value. Muscular fatigability is very important – useful voluntary contraction cannot be maintained for longer than 60 s. Under normal conditions this is sufficient to induce the anorectal reflex of Debray with an increase in rectal compliance. Abnormal distension of the internal sphincter or myotomy of more than half the length of the internal sphincter [61] results in impaired fine continence of liquids and flatus.

Visco-elasticity of the rectal wall and compliance of the rectum are under the control of the anorectal inhibitory reflex of Debray. Any inflammation or fibrotic alteration of the rectal wall results in a decreased storage capacity of the rectum, this occurs in severe proctitis [17]. After low anterior resection, the innervation pathways from the anal canal to the new reservoir are destroyed but neurotization may occur after several months [56]. Ischemia and "rectal angina" may also result in fecal incontinence [20].

Anal cushions are responsible for fine continence. As a result of their apposition, they close the anal lumen like tricuspid valves. Their destruction as well as too wide a mucosal excision not only interfere with fine continence but also destroy sensitive nerve endings and mucosal receptors.

To ensure normal continence it is necessary to have:

- Normal anatomical structures
- Adequate rectal compliance
- Enough striated muscle with good contraction and a low fatigability rate
- A smooth internal sphincter with normal function
- Conservation of the anorectal inhibitory reflex of Debray

- Unaltered medullary and cerebral reflexes
- Functional baroreceptors within levator muscles
- An adequate number of sensitive nerve endings within the anal canal mucosa
- Anal cushions of normal size (not widely excised or hypertrophied)

Functional alteration or destruction of at least one of these conditions may result in more or less severe incontinence.

Classification of Incontinence

A useful classification of the different etiologies can be established better according to the altered or destroyed mechanisms rather than according to the causes themselves (Table 22.1).

Clinical Evaluation

Medical History

The medical history should reveal how severe the effect of incontinence is on social activity and work. Previous surgical procedures on the bowel and the anorectum should be listed. Patients should be asked about the beginning of the symptoms and their recent aggravation, bowel habits, frequency and consistency of stools, usual diet, rectal prolapse [19, 61], associated neurological and metabolical dysfunction such as diabetes [70, 81], gynecological and urinary problems, difficult childbirth [13, 74], previous radiotherapy [78] and surgery.
Severity of incontinence may be graded:

Grade I   Occasional fecal soiling of underwear
Grade II   Incontinence of flatus, frequent fecal soiling, uncontrolled fecal leakage
Grade III Total incontinence
About 10% of normal control subjects present with grade I [3, 82].

Examination

Detailed anorectal examination is mandatory and may reveal:

- The severity of incontinence as suggested by the extent of soiling on a perineal pad, underwear, and the perineum.
- Scars of previous surgery, of traumatic laceration and of difficult childbirth should be noted.

Table 22.1. Etiology of fecal incontinence

Sensory problems
- Destruction of sensory receptors
- Continuous stimulation of sensory receptors

Muscular problems
- Local lesions, distension
- Tears and traumatic lesions
- Degenerative lesions

Neurological problems
- Neuropathy (diabetes)
- Peripheric lesions (nervus pudendus internus)
- Proximal lesions (spinal and caudal)

Psychoorganic problems

Alteration in rectal capacity and compliance
- Destruction (low anterior resection, pull-through, sleeve anastomosis)
- Alteration of viscoelastic properties (severe inflammatory lesions)

Prolapse, intussusception, and rectoceles

- Size of a gaping patulous anus due to denervation or stretch disruption.
- Sensitivity of the anal margin and integrity of cutaneomuscular reflex to the corrugator cutis ani and cremaster.
- Tone at rest.
- Reflex contraction when performing digital examination or pathological relaxation in homosexuals.
- Fibrosis of the anal canal and adjacent tissue.
- Voluntary contraction of the puborectalis sling resulting in an anterior translation of 2 cm.
- Presence of a rectocele or a loose rectovaginal septum.
- In women, the existence of a cystocele, uterine prolapse, too deep a Douglas' pouch, rectocele which can be found by simultaneous vaginal and rectal digital examination.
- Perineal descent in response to straining or coughing with opening of the anal canal.
- Incomplete rectal prolapse or intussusception and alteration of the anorectal angle by digital examination during straining.
- Complete rectal prolapse.

Complementary Investigations

As notices by Hughes [36], clinical evaluation is usually adequate to assess the cause and severity of the condition allowing for an appropriate plan of management. Nevertheless, complementary investigations may be useful.

Endoscopy

Endoscopy with a flexible instrument may exclude any concomitant pathology such as Crohn's disease, colitis, polyposis, carcinoma, melanosis coli. Endoscopy with a rigid instrument should be performed in every case to reveal an incomplete or complete prolapse during straining.

Balloon Proctography and Defecography

Balloon proctography is a static examination whereas defecography is a dynamic one which is useful in establishing any alteration in the anatomical structures and mechanisms of defecation [48, 50, 64].

Manometry

Manometric studies with various devices will confirm clinical findings. They are useful in evaluating some disorders selectively affecting either smooth or striated muscles. The integrity of spinal reflexes and the viscoelastic properties of the rectal wall may be checked. These studies are useful particularly if biofeedback muscular training is planned. Furthermore, they allow precise evaluation of postoperative results [66].

Electromyography

Needle electrodes facilitate accurate location of the external sphincter in the treatment of ectopic anus and in cases of severe muscular tears. Electromyography is useful in investigating various neurological disorders and altered reflexes interfering with normal continence [2, 33, 77].

Measurement of Sphincter Strength

A method for quantitative evaluation of sphincter strength has been described by Henricksen [31]. A 2-cm diameter metal ball is inserted into the rectum. The force which is necessary to withdraw the ball is measured.

Conservative Treatment

Pharmacological Treatment

Patients with a minor degree of anorectal incontinence or patients who are inoperable may be treated conservatively [7, 53]. Stool thickeners, bulk-forming agents, and high dietetic fiber intake may be routinely prescribed to obtain firm stools; evacuation will be stimulated by glycerin suppositories, Dulcolax (Thomae), or Lecicarbon (Drossapharm). These suppositories should allow evacuation of stools at predictable times of the day. Lecicarbon suppositories produce rectal distension; through repeated application, rectal volume may be increased and the sensation of rectal distension stimulated. The patient will then be "continent" until the next artificially induced bowel movement.

Physical Treatment

Muscular training is very important to stimulate muscles and to increase the muscular activity. Training may be voluntary, with or without biofeedback control of the increased endoanal pressure level, or may be performed by electrical stimulation using implanted electrodes or externally activated plugs [6, 35, 47].
Electrical stimulation seems not to result in an increase of anal tone but in a regression of muscular fatigability. If contraction can be sustained for 50–60 s (this is perhaps enough), rectal compliance and then continence are achieved.
Biofeedback, as popularized by Schuster [10, 18, 21, 24], may result in a better coordination of sphincter activity in carefully selected, motivated patients. A balloon placed within the anal canal is connected to a transducer and a graph or TV monitor. The patient may observe the anal pressure reached by sphincter contraction with or without rectal distension. Gradually the visual feedback is eliminated but checked by a trained technician. Improvement usually occurs within three to five training sessions.

Surgical Treatment

The choice of a surgical technique depends mainly on the nature and the level of the lesion responsible for incontinence. Bowel preparation is mandatory. Perioperative antibiotics should be given. In cases of complex lesions or reconstructive surgery, a protective colostomy may be indicated. Bowel movement should be restricted for 8 days by an elementary or low-residue diet and bowel motility moderators such as codeine phosphate or loperamide. After 5–8 days, normal diet is progressively reintroduced; mucilage and bulk-forming agents are given together with paraffin oil. Physical training of the sphincter should not be encouraged before day 10.

Aims of Surgical Treatment

The main aims of the various surgical techniques used are as follows [51]:

- Sphincter reconstruction
- Reduction of anal canal diameter
- Reinforcement of the occlusion mechanism
- Increase of muscular mass
- Decrease in the size of the anorectal angle at rest
- Substitutive sphincteroplasty
- Artificial sphincter implantation

Sphincter Reconstruction and Sphincteroplasty

Direct reconstruction is the procedure of choice for tears, traumatic and obstetrical laceration, or iatrogenic sphincter section. For old, established lesions secondary sphincteroplasty gives good results nowadays [4, 5, 22, 59].

In fresh lesions, reconstruction with end-to-end sphincter suture should always be tried. U or X deep stitches should be placed using slowly absorbable synthetic monofilament. Knots should be tied carefully to avoid further muscular dilaceration as healthy muscle is not able to hold a simple suture. Vaginal and anal wound edges are closed whereas skin edges are approximated to allow drainage and to prevent infection.

In old lesions repair is performed through a curvilinear incision parallel to the external sphincter, extending at least 180°–200° (Fig. 22.1). The anoderm and anal mucosa are mobilized from the scar and the underlying sphincter. The sphincter is dissected free with a wide margin. As a proper plan of dissection may be difficult to identify, dissection is started at the normal muscle and continued into the scar. Electric stimulation may be helpful for identification. Nerve branches should be preserved. Fibrotic edges of the sphincter should not be excised. After excision of th mucosal and skin scar, the anoderm is mobilized and opposed with 2–0 synthetic absorbable suture before any attempt at muscular repair.

During mobilization, muscle ends can be overlapped to reduce the anal diameter. Mattress sutures are placed within the fibrotic edges to maintain the desired aperture using 2–0 synthetic monofilament absorbable suture material. The skin wound should only be partially closed to prevent infection.

When dealing with obstetrical tears or a complicated episiotomy, it is necessary to repair not only the sphincter but also the rectovaginal septum [13, 55]. Parks [59] recommended a preliminary defunctioning colostomy to ensure primary healing. Satisfactory results have been reported without a preexisting protective colostomy [27].

Sphincteroplasty is successful in more than 90% of patients with fecal incontinence due to sphincter injury, restoring most of them almost completely to normal. Published results are listed in Table 22.2.

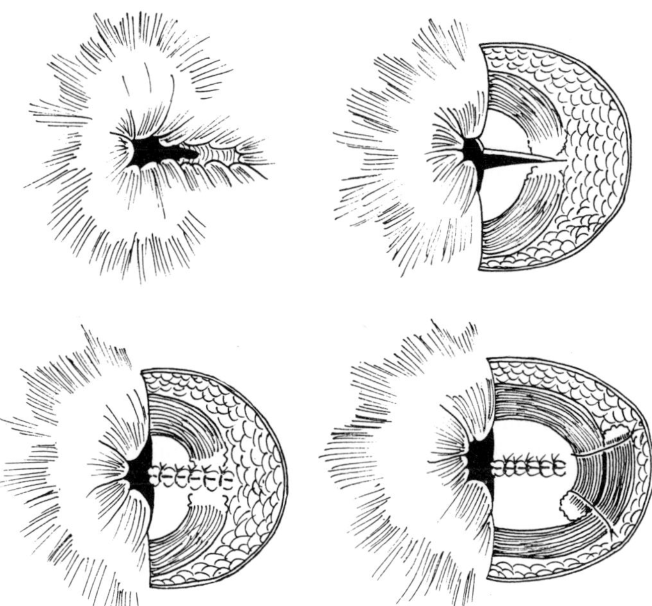

Fig. 22.1. Sphincteroplasty

Table 22.2. Results of sphincteroplasty

Reference	Patients (n)	Excellent (n)	Fair (n)	Poor (n)
Blaisdell 1957 [5]	133	42	38	20
Parks and McPartlin 1971 [60]	20	18	1	1
Goldberg et al. 1980 [25]	47	24	22	1
Sarles and Echinard 1982 [69]	18	10	5	3
Marti (unpublished)	22	21	–	1
Motson 1985 [54]	83	65	11	7
Fang et al. 1984 [22]	78	58	38	4

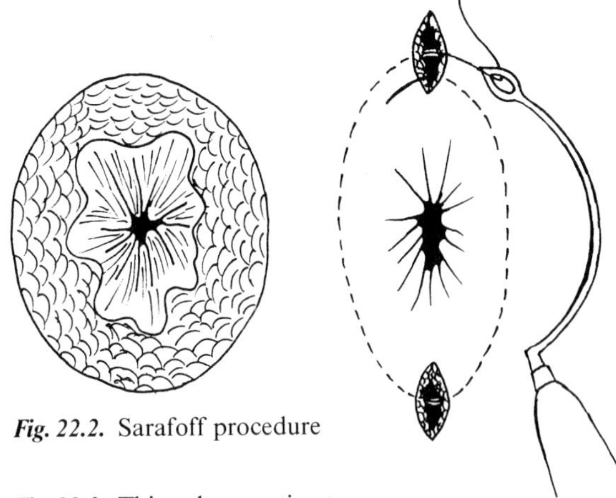

Fig. 22.2. Sarafoff procedure

Fig. 22.3. Thiersch operation ▷

Reduction of Anal Canal Diameter

A reduction in the diameter of the anal canal should help a diminished sphincter tone to achieve sufficient functional action. Several procedures have been used:

Hemorrhoidectomy

A hemorrhoidectomy such as the Milligan Morgan procedure but with high and wide mucosal excision results in a scar which narrows the lumen of the upper part of the anal canal.

Sarafoff Procedure

Initially devised to correct a Whitehead deformity with mucosal prolapse and ectropion, the Sarafoff procedure [68] produces a circular scar allowing better reduction in the size of the anal lumen (Fig. 22.2).

Thiersch Operation

Encirclement of the anal orifice with wire [26], non-absorbable suture material, fascia lata, or Teflon has been used to prevent rectal prolapse [1, 43, 45] (Fig. 22.3). This procedure creates a static barrier to the passage of rectal content, especially solid feces, but not of liquid or flatus. It does not contribute anything to the voluntary control and maintenance of continence. This procedure is frequently complicated by secondary infection and extrusion of the suture material as a foreign body.

Reinforcement of the Occlusion Mechanism

To reinforce the occlusion mechanism, Wreden [83] and Stone [76] constructed two slings of fascia lata or silk which were passed between the lower borders of the gluteus maximus muscles in front of and behind the anus, respectively (Fig. 22.4). Contraction of the buttocks put the sling under tension and compressed the anal canal. Since first publication, no further results have been published.

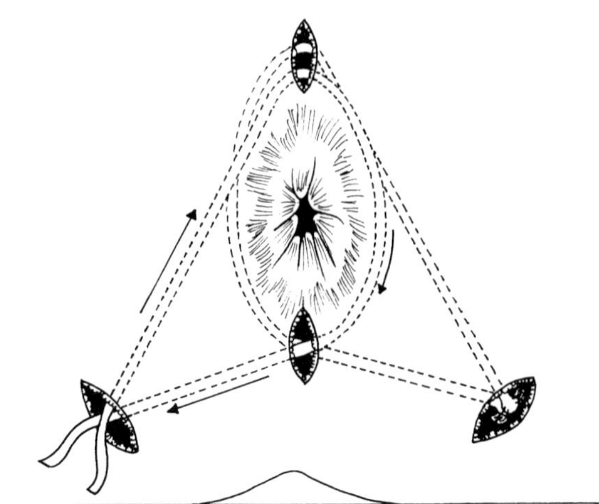

Fig. 22.4. Stone and Wreden reinforcement procedure

Muscular Grafts to Increase Muscular Mass

To supplement the sphincter muscular mass, several muscular grafts have been devised.

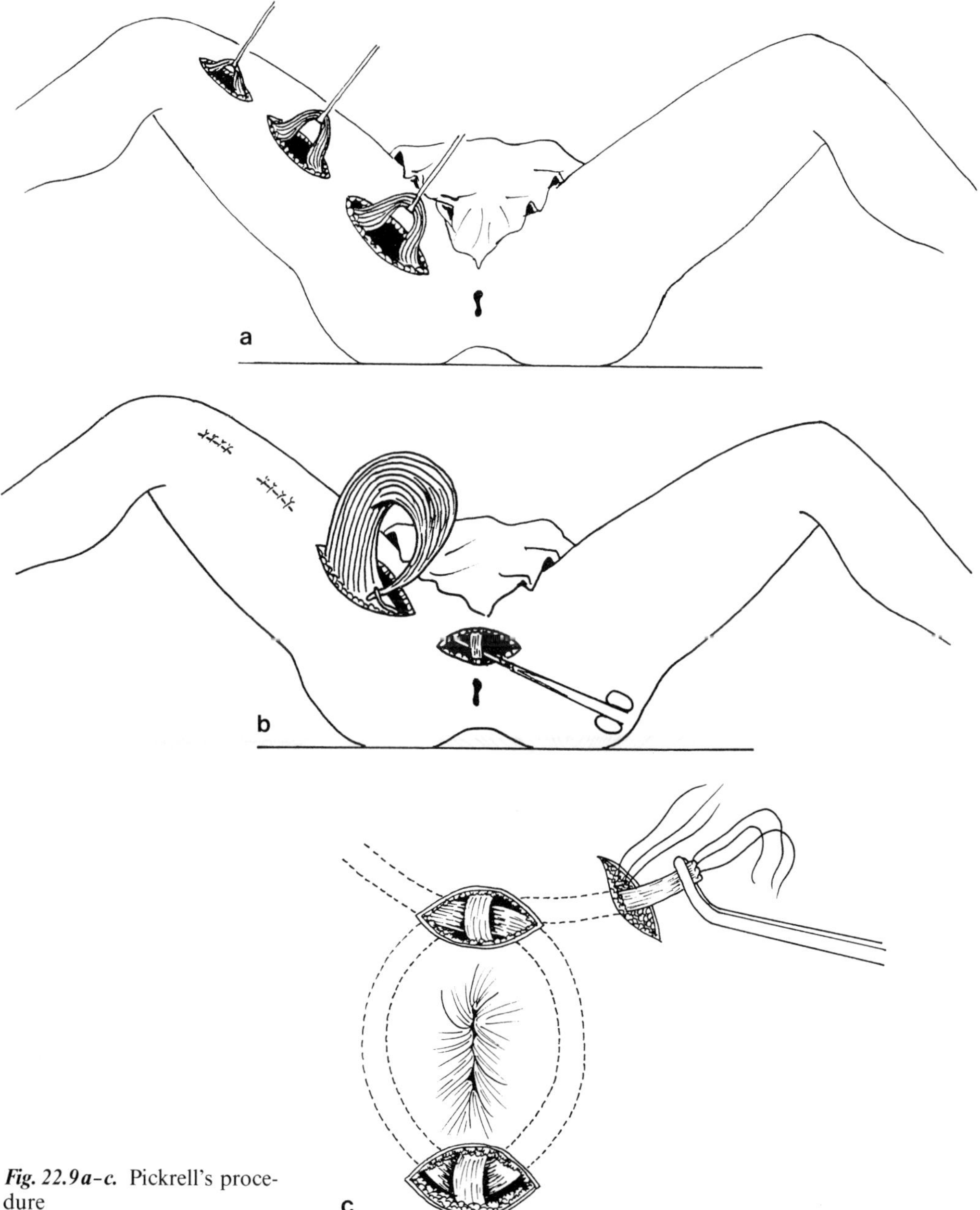

Fig. 22.9 a–c. Pickrell's procedure

tinence with internal and external sphincter dysfunction, when there is loss of the normal anorectal angle as after abdominal rectopexy, and in cases of a short anal canal (Fig. 22.10). Adequate muscle mass must be present for this operation to be successful.

Through a V-shaped incision, posterior to the anus, with its apex at the level of the tip of the coccyx, the intersphincteric plane is opened and bluntly dissected. The anal canal and internal sphincter are separated from the external sphincter up to the level of the puborectalis sling. Sharp dissection may be necessary as the puborectalis often adheres to the rectum. The dissection is continued upward in the retrorectal fatty space after division of Waldeyer's fascia to expose the upper surface of the levator ani muscles. The presacral fascia should not be opened so as to avoid massive venous bleeding.

A lattice is constructed as high as possible with polyprophylene or Maxon size O from one limb of the levator ani to the other at the level of the ileococcygeal muscle. A second lattice is inserted at the level

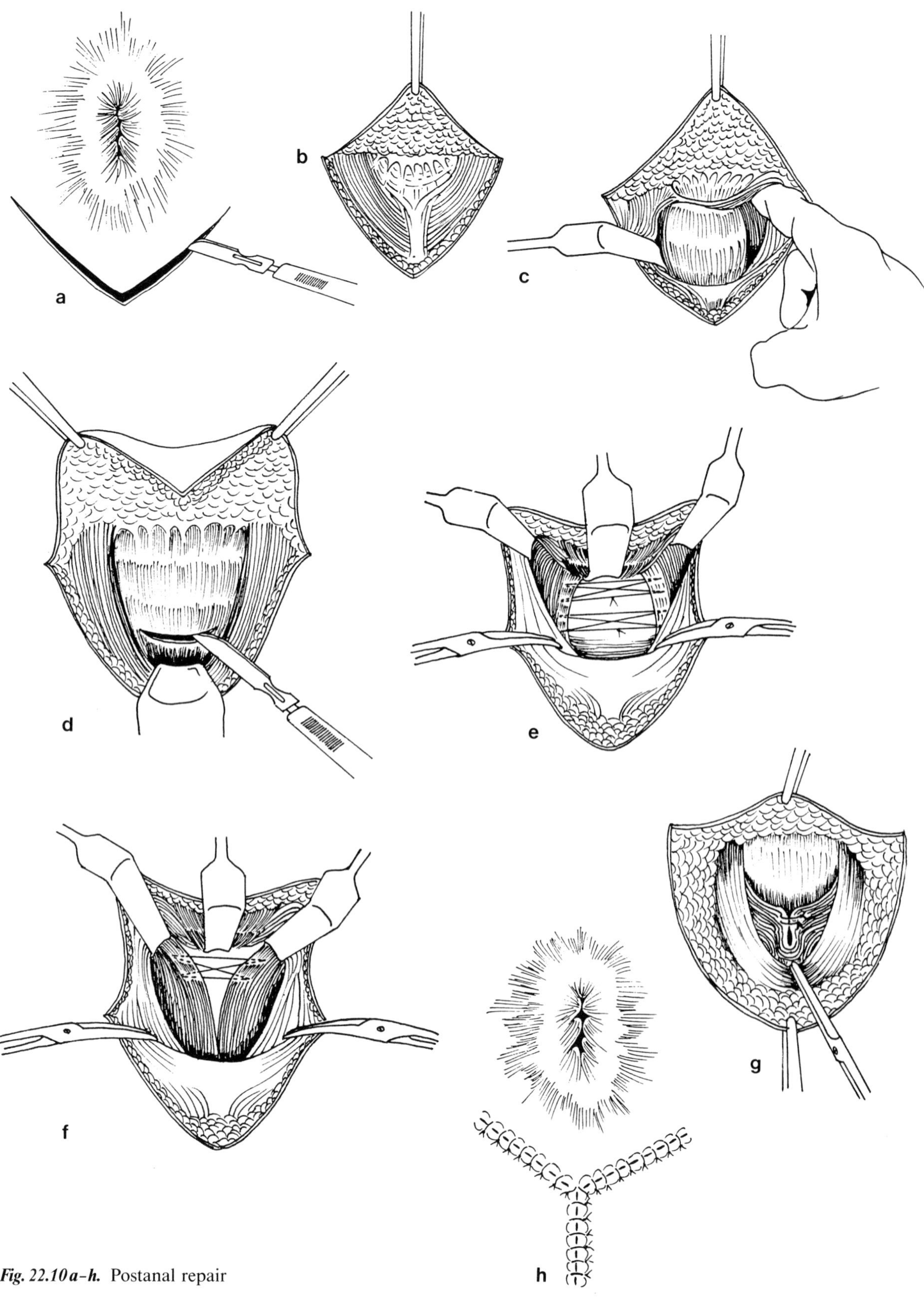

Fig. 22.10a–h. Postanal repair

Table 22.4. Results of postanal repair

Reference	Patient (n)	Completely continent (%)	Improved (%)	Not improved (%)
Parks and McCartlin 1971 [60]	183	72	12	16
Keighley 1984 [39]	89	63	21	16

of the pubococcygeal muscle. A third one is inserted in order to approximate the puborectalis muscle. Finally, the external sphincter is approximated and the skin sutured in the shape of a Y after insertion of suction drainage. The knots should not be tied too tightly to prevent ischemia and necrosis. Published results are summarized in Table 22.4.

Kottmeier's Procedure

When there is insufficient puborectalis muscle, Kottmeier [41, 42] (Fig. 22.11) has suggested the restoration of the anorectal angle by cutting the tip of the coccyx with the attachment of the pubococcygeal and iliococcygeal muscles. The released muscles reinforce the puborectalis sling. The presacral fascia should not be opened to avoid posterior herniation of the rectum. This technique was initially used to treat incontinence after correction of anal perforation. Nowadays it is also used to treat incontinence in adults after surgical correction of rectal prolapse [19].

Free Muscle Transplantation

The aim of free muscle transplantation is to place a muscle graft as a sling around the rectum and in contact with the puborectalis muscle to permit reinnervation of the transplant [28]. Such a procedure is therefore not possible in cases of neurogenic incontinence. The procedure is carried out in two stages with an interval of 2–3 weeks [29].
During the first stage the palmaris longus of the forearm or part of the sartorius muscle is denervated. During the second stage, the muscle is transplanted. The fascia should be totally removed as it would otherwise interfere with reinnervation. The skin is incised at the tip of the coccyx, the incision is continued up to the anorectal angle at the level of the muscular pelvic floor. By blunt dissection, a tunnel is created anteriorly on the muscular surface or even within the muscle up to the pubic bone

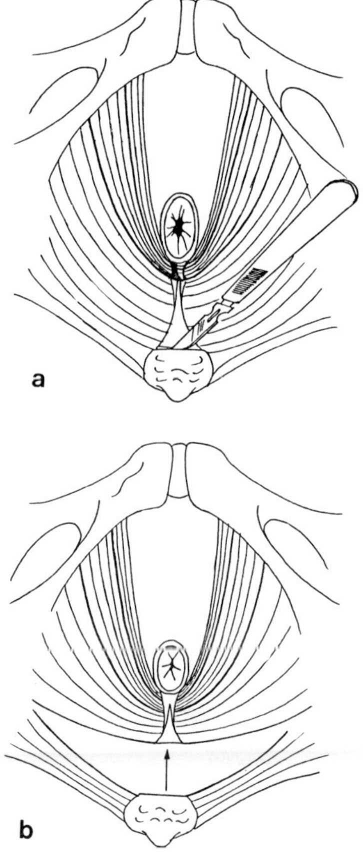

Fig. 22.11 a, b. Kottmeier's procedure

where a small incision is performed on either side. The transplant is inserted in intimate contact with the muscles and is sutured under slight tension to the periosteum of the pubis.
Positive results should not be expected before the 3rd–6th months. At 1–7 years after transplantation Hakelius [29] reported on 38 adult patients with pronounced incontinence: cure was achieved in 16 cases, marked improvement in 12, and no effect in ten.

Smooth Muscle Plasty

Schmidt [71, 72] described a surgical procedure to reconstruct a totally destroyed sphincter using a graft of pedunculated or free smooth muscle. After total mucosectomy, a segment of large bowel is wrapped around the anus to restore tone at rest. He reported on 31 patients in whom involuntary continence could be restored even during the night. According to the same concept, Holschneider [34] achieved pull-through procedures for rectal atresia with a turned up cuff.

Artificial Sphincter Implantation

Two types of artificial sphincter have been implanted. A magnetic ring similar to the device developed for obstruction of a stoma has been used to treat anal agenesis [53]. An artificial anal sphincter identical to an artificial urinary sphincter has been implanted once but needs further experimentation to evaluate it properly [11]. It seems to be useful in cases of severe neuromuscular disease.

Colostomy

In patients with total incontinence who are unable to manage their problems by conventional methods and are unfit for surgery, a colostomy may become necessary. This is the last resort for severely handicapped patients, for psychogeriatric and bedridden patients, and for patients with incontinence following radiation injury of the rectum.

Management and Selection of Appropriate Treatment

Medical history, clinical examination, and laboratory investigations are necessary to assess the severity and the etiology of incontinence. Our treatment policy is summarized in Table 22.5. Associated organ pathology should be ruled out or corrected before treatment of incontinence.

In cases of minor incontinence, conservative measures should always be tried. Electrostimulation for one or two sessions helps the patient to perceive the sphincteric action and to understand what should be achieved when contracting the perineal muscles. Muscular training of the perineal muscles should be

Table 22.5. Optimal choice of surgical procedure to treat anal incontinence

	Reconstructive procedures	Reinforcement	Substitution
Mechanical incontinence			
- Normotrophic musculature	2	1	-
- Hypotrophic musculature	-	2	1
Neurological problems	-	1	2
Aplasia and sphincter destruction	-	-	2

1, First choice procedure; 2, second choice procedure; -, useless procedure

undertaken and checked to ensure that the patient is contracting the pelvic floor and not the thigh. Physical treatment may be improved by dietetic measures and by repeated drug-induced evacuation. These measures should also be undertaken if there are changes in rectal capacity and compliance.

In patients who are incontinent after injury to the sphincters, we perform a sphincteroplasty. If muscles have been destroyed, sphincteroplasty may be complemented by muscular grafts. A free muscular transplant may only be performed if there are no signs of denervation.

If the sphincter is intact and incontinence is due to stretching of the puborectalis sling or to some partial denervation with widening of the anorectal angle, postanal repair as described by Parks [61] is the treatment of choice.

In cases of muscular denervation or extensive destruction which are not suitable for any reconstructive procedure, muscular transplantation as in Pickrell's procedure should be tried.

Definitive colostomy is the last resort and should nowadays be used only for bedridden patients and totally dependent psychiatric patients.

References

1. Aronsson H (1948) Anorectal incontinence. Acta Chir Scand 96 [Suppl 135]: 121
2. Bartolo DCC, Jarratt JA, Read MC et al. (1983) The role of partial denervation of the puborectalis in idiopathic faecal incontinence. Br J Surg 70: 664–667
3. Bennett RC, Duthie HL (1964) The functional importance of the internal anal sphincter. Br J Surg 51: 355–357
4. Blaisdell PC (1940) Repair of the incontinent sphincter ani. Surg Gynecol Obstet 70: 692–697
5. Blaisdell PC (1957) Repair of the incontinent sphincter ani. Am J Surg 94: 573
6. Bleijenberg G, Kuijpers HC (1987) Treatment of the spastic pelvic floor syndrome with biofeedback. Dis Colon Rectum 30: 108–111
7. Brocklehurst JC (1978) Management of anal incontinence. Clin Gastroenterol 4: 479–487
8. Browning GGP, Motson RW (1983) Results of Park's operation for faecal incontinence after and injury. Br Med J 286: 1873–1875
9. Bruining HA, Bos KE, Colthoff EG, Tolhurst DE (1981) Creation of an anal sphincter mechanism by bilateral proximally based gluteal muscle transposition. Plast Reconstr Surg 67: 70–73
10. Cerulli MA, Nikoomanesh P, Schuster MM (1979) Progress in biofeedback conditioning for fecal incontinence. Gastroenterology 76: 742–746
11. Christiansen J, Lorentzen M (1987) Implantation of artificial sphincter for anal incontinence. Lancet i: 244–245

12. Corman ML (1980) Follow-up evaluation of gracilis muscle transposition for fecal incontinence. Dis Colon Rectum 23: 552–555
13. Corman ML (1985) Anal incontinence following obstetrical injury. Dis Colon Rectum 28: 86–89
14. Corman ML (1985) Gracilis muscle transplantation. In: Henry MM, Swash M (eds) Coloproctology and the pelvic floor. Butterworths, London, pp 234–241
15. Corman ML (1985) Gracilis muscle transposition for anal incontinence: late results. Br J Surg 72: 521–522
16. Cunéo B, Sénèque J (1931) Reconstruction de l'appareil sphinctérien dans le prolapsus du rectum. J Chir (Paris) 38: 190–196
17. Denis P, Colin R, Galmiche JP et al. (1979) Elastic properties of the rectal wall in normal adults and in patients with ulcerative colitis. Gastroenterology 77: 45–48
18. Denis P, Colin R, Galmiche JP et al. (1983) Traitement de l'incontinence fécale de l'adulte. Résultats en fonction des données cliniques et manométriques et intérêt de la rééducation par apprentissage instrumental. Gastroentérol Clin Biol 7: 853–857
19. Deucher F, Blessing H (1974) Prolapsus and sphincter insufficiency. Prog Surg 13: 98–124
20. Devroede G, Masse S, Leger C et al. (1979) Ischemic fecal incontinence and rectal angina. Gastroenterology 76: 1121
21. Engel BT, Mikoomanesh P, Schuster N (1974) Operant conditioning of rectosphincteric responses in the treatment of fecal incontinence. N Engl J Med 290: 646–649
22. Fang DR, Nivatvongs S, Vermeulen FO et al. (1984) Overlapping sphincteroplasty for acquired anal incontinence. Dis Colon Rectum 27: 720–722
23. Goebell R (1927) Methods of forming new anal sphincter. (Kongressbericht) Arch Klin Chir 148: 612–619
24. Goldberg DA, Hodges K, Hersh T, Jinich H (1980) Biofeedback therapy for fecal incontinence. Am J Gastroenterol 74: 342–345
25. Goldberg SM, Gordon PP, Nivatvongs S (1980) Essential of anorectal surgery. Lippincott, Philadelphia
26. Goligher J (1980) Surgery of the anus rectum and colon. Baillière Tindall, London
27. Hagihara PF, Griffen WO Jr (1976) Delayed correction of anorectal incontinence due to anal sphincteral injury. Arch Surg III: 63–66
28. Hakelius L (1979) Reconstruction of the perineal body as treatment for anal incontinence. Br J Plast Surg 32: 245–252
29. Hakelius L (1985) Free muscle transplantation. In: Henry MM, Swash M (eds) Coloproctology and the pelvic floor. Butterworths, London, pp 259–268
30. Hardcastle JD, Parks AG (1970) A study of anal incontinence and some principles of surgical treatment. Proc R Soc Med 63 [Suppl]: 116–118
31. Henriksen FW, Huthouisen B (1972) Measurement of the anal sphincter through a simple method suitable for routine use. Scand J Gastroenterol 7: 555
32. Henry MM, Swash M (1985) Faecal continence, defecation and colorectal motility. In Henry MM, Swash M (eds) Coloproctology and the pelvic floor. Butterworth, London
33. Holschneider AM (1983) Elektromanometrie des Enddarms, 2nd edn. Urban and Schwarzenberg, Munich
34. Holschneider AM, Hecker WC (1981) Reverse smooth muscle plasty: a new method of treating anorectal incontinence in infants with high anal and rectal atresia. J Pediatr Surg 16: 917–920
35. Hopkinson BR, Lightwood R (1966) Electrical treatment of anal incontinence. Lancet ii: 297–298
36. Hughes E, Cuthbertson AM, Killingback MK (1983) Colorectal surgery. Churchill Livingstone, London
37. Ingelmann-Sundberg A (1951) Plastic repair of extensive defects of the anal sphincter. Acta Chir Scand 101: 155
38. Kalisman M, Sharzer LA (1981) Anal sphincter reconstruction and perineal resurfacing with a gracilis myocutaneus flap. Dis Colon Rectum 24: 529–531
39. Keighley MRB (1984) Postanal repair for fecal incontinence. J R Soc Med 77: 285–288
40. Knapp LS (1939) Plastic repair for postoperative anal incontinence. Ann Surg 109: 146–150
41. Kottmeier PK (1966) A physiological approach to the problem of anal continence through use of the levator ani as a sling. Surgery 60: 1262–1266
42. Kottmeier PK, Dziacliw K (1967) The complete release of the levator ani sling in fecal incontinence. J Pediatr Surg 2: 111–117
43. Labow S, Rubin R, Hoexter B, Salvati E (1980) Perineal repair of procidentia with an elastic fabric sling. Dis Colon Rectum 23: 467–469
44. Lennander KG (1898–1899) Sphincter ani Förstörd genom ett felgmone-plastick operation frän mm. levatores ani och mm. glutaei maxcontinentia ani. Upsala läkarefören Föth 4: 337
45. Lomas MI, Cooperman H (1972) Correction of rectal procidentia by use of a polypropylene mesh (Marlex). Dis Colon Rectum 15: 416–419
46. Loygue G, Dubois F (1964) Surgical treatment of anal incontinence. Am J Proctol 15: 361–374
47. MacLeod JH (1979) Biofeedback in the management of partial anal incontinence. Dis Colon Rectum 22: 169–171
48. Mahieu P, Pringot J, Bodart P (1984) Defecography. Gastrointest Radiol 9: 247–261, 1984
49. Mandelstam DA (1985) Faecal incontinence: social and economic factors. In: Henry MM, Swash M (eds) Coloproctology and the pelvic floor. Butterworth, London
50. Marti MC, Mirescu D (1982) Utilité du défécogramme en proctologie. Ann Gastoentèrol Hèpatol (Paris) 18: 379–384
51. Marti MC, Noethiger F (1981) Incontinence anale et chirurgie de renforcement de l'appareil sphinctérien. Schweiz Rundsch Med Prax 70: 679–682
52. Meier H, Groitl H, Willital GH (1984) Kontinensstörungen bei Kindern; diagnostisches Umgehen und therapeutische Konsequenzen. In: Farthmann E, Fiedler L (eds) Die anale Kontinenz und ihre Wiederherstellung. Urban und Schwarzenberg, Munich, pp 71–78
53. Mille R, Bartolo DCC, Locke-Edmunds JC, Mortensen NG MCC (1988) Fecal incontinence and the anorectal angle. Br J Surg 75: 101–105
54. Motson RW (1985) Sphincter injuries: indications for and results of sphincter repair. Br J Surg 72: 519–521
55. Musset R, Cottrell M, Cohen J (1963) Cure chirurgicale des déchirures obstétricales anciennes du périnée du 3e degré avec incontinence sphinctérienne anale. J Chir (Paris) 86: 661–678
56. Neill ME, Parks AG, Swash M (1981) Physiological

studies of the anal sphincter musculature in fecal incontinence and rectal prolapse. Br J Surg 68: 531–536
57. Nieves PM, Valles TG, Aranguren G, Maldonado D (1975) Gracilis muscle transplant for correction of traumatic and incontinence. Dis Colon Rectum 18: 349–354
58. Orgel MG (1985) A double-split gluteus maximus muscle flap for reconstruction of the rectal sphincter. Plast Reconstr Surg 75: 62–66
59. Parks AG (1975) Anorectal incontinence. Proc R Soc Med 68: 681–690
60. Parks AG, McPartlin JF (1971) Late repair of injuries of the anal sphincter. Proc R Soc Med 64: 1187–1189
61. Parks AG, Swash M, Urich H (1977) Sphincter denervation in anorectal incontinence and rectal prolapse. Gut 18: 656–665
62. Pickrell KL, Broadbent TR, Masters FW, Metzger JT (1952) Construction of a rectal sphincter and restoration of anal continence by transplanting the gracilis muscle. Ann Surg 135: 853–862
63. Pickrell KL, Beorgiades N, Richard EF, Morris F (1959) Gracilis muscle transplantation for the correction of neurogenic rectal incontinence. Surg Clin North Am 39: 1405
64. Preston DM, Lennard-Jones JE, Thomas BM (1984) The balloon proctogram. Br J Surg 71: 29–32
65. Prochiantz A, Gross P (1982) Gluteal myoplasty for sphincter replacement. J Pediatr Surg 17: 25–30
66. Read NW, Bannister JJ (1985) Anorectal manometry: techniques in health and anorectal disease. In: Henry MM, Swash M (eds) Coloproctology and the pelvic floor. Butterworths, London, pp 65–87
67. Richard A (1954) A propos de la communication de MM Petit-Dubaillis, Portel et Cornier sur la sphinctéroplastie anale. Mém Acad Chir 80: 303
68. Sarafoff O (1937) Ein einfaches und ungefährliches Verfahren zur operativen Behandlung des Mastdarmvorfalles. Langenbecks Arch Klin Chir 190: 219–232
69. Sarles JC, Echinard C (1982) Incontinence anale. Encyclopédie médico chirurgicale, no 40705. Paris, pp 1–8
70. Schiller L, Santa Ana CA, Schmulen CA et al. (1982) Pathogenesis of fecal incontinence in diabetes mellitus. N Engl J Med 27: 1665–1671
71. Schmidt E (1985) Spätergebnisse nach glattmuskulärem Sphinkterersatz. Chirurg 56: 305–310
72. Schmidt E (1986) Chirurgie der analen Inkontinenz. Colo Proctology 8: 218–222
73. Shoemaker J (1909) Un nouveau procédé opératoire pour la reconstitution du sphincter anal. Semaine Mèd Paris 29: 160
74. Snooks SJ, Setchell M, Swash M, Henry MM (1984) Injury to innervation of pelvic floor sphincter musculature in childbirth. Lancet ii: 546–550
75. State D, Katz A (1955) The use of superficial transverse perineal muscles in the treatment of postsurgical anal incontinence. Ann Surg 142: 262–265
76. Stone HB (1929) Plastic operation for anal incompetence. Arch Surg 18: 845–851
77. Swash M, Snooks SJ (1985) Electromyography in pelvic floor disorders. In: Henry MM, Swash M (eds) Coloproctology and the pelvic floor. Butterworths, London pp 88–103
78. Touchais JY, Paillot B, Denis P et al. (1982) Défécation impérieuse et incontinence fécale après irradiation pelvienne: étude de la distensibilité rectale chez 18 patients. Gastroenterol Clin Biol 6: 1003–1007
79. Tuttle JP (1903) In: Diseases of the anus, rectum and pelvic colon. Appleton, New York
80. Vigoni M (1960) Traitement de l'incontinence anale. Acta Chir Belg 59: 139–148
81. Wald A, Tunuguntla AK (1984) Anorectal sensorimotor dysfunction in fecal incontinence and diabetes mellitus. N Engl J Med 310: 1282–1287
82. Watts MCK J, Bennet RC, Goligher JC (1964) Stretching of anal sphincters in treatment of fissure in ano. Br Med J II: 342–343
83. Wreden RR (1929) A method of reconstructing a volontary sphincter ani: plastic operation for anal incontinence. Arch Surg 18: 841–844

23 Rectal Prolapse, Solitary Rectal Ulcer Syndrome, Descending Perineal Syndrome

E. Gemsenjäger

Definition

Rectal prolapse or procidentia is an invagination or an extrusion of the entire thickness of rectal wall into or through the anal canal. The prolapse may start at the anal verge, at the anorectal ring, or at a higher level, representing an intussusception or invagination of the anterior, the posterior, or the whole circumference of the rectal wall into the rectum or into the anal canal. The various degrees of circumferential involvement, rectal wall descent, and extrusion result in a multifaceted clinical appearance.

Etiology

Rectal prodicentia is only partially understood. It frequently occurs in patients with paralysis of the pelvic floor and of the somatic sphincter muscles in conjunction with cauda equina lesions [10], but it is quiet uncommon in paraplegic patients who also have paralysis of these muscles. Similarly, neuropathic damage to the somatic sphincter muscles, leading to pelvic floor descent and incontinence, is not regularly accompanied by rectal prolapse. Furthermore, patients with procidentia may have a normal functional state of the pelvic floor and sphincter muscles, especially young women and patients with an internal prolapse.

In some patients a temporal relationship between hysterectomy and the occurrence of the rectal prolapse has been observed (Table 23.1) (unpublished data). Indeed, the suspension stability of the uterus-vagina-pelvic floor axis may be interrupted by hysterectomy, and secondary enterocele is considered a well-known consequence of hysterectomy [17]. The gynecological enterocele is a hernia of the pouch of Douglas and may well be considered today as an internal, occult variant of rectal prolapse.

Pathophysiology

Uniform Endopelvic Appearance

Rectal prolapse can be best understood by considering its endopelvic appearance. Indeed, strikingly and invariably constant findings are encountered in the pelvic cavity at laparotomy, namely, a deep rectovaginal pouch with a largely peritonealized rectum (Figs. 23.1a; 23.2a, b; 23.8). The inferior portion of the anterior rectal wall, situated in the depth of the pouch, can easily be invaginated, then pushed into, and extruded (evaginated) through the anal canal (Figs. 23.3a, b; 23.8a). The anterior invagination promptly brings the rectal wall to a circumferential intussusception and transanal eversion (Fig. 23.1c, d), i. e., the mechanisms of sliding and intussusception are both involved when reproducing the prolapse from within the pelvis. The herniating pouch may be empty (Fig. 23.6i) or represent an enterocele (Figs. 23.3c; 23.4j, k, o).

At the starting point of the invagination a circumscribed area of fibrotic, lipomatous or edematous thickening of the subserosal tissue is often demonstrable (Figs. 23.1; 23.2a, b; 23.8b–e; 23.9g–i). (It resembles the lipomatous thickening which is frequently encountered on the anterior aspect of the esophagogastric junction in patients with a sliding hiatal hernia.) It may be a sign of chronic traumatism on the external side of the bowel wall, corresponding to the endoluminal lesion of chronic proctitis, i. e. the rectal ulcer.

The lower rectum is found deep on the pelvic floor, somewhat ascending in the posteroanterior direction (Fig. 23.2), and presenting redundant mobile bowel wall. In some instances the intussusception may even be initiated from the posterior (precoccy-

Table 23.1. Rectal prolapse and hysterectomy (prospective evaluation in 18 consecutive patients). (Unpublished data)

No hysterectomy	$n = 7$
Hysterectomy	$n = 11$

$n = 3$ No temporal relationship observed between hysterectomy (3–11 years before prolapse operation) and occurrence of rectal prolapse

$n = 8$ Symptoms of rectal prolapse observed occuring after hysterectomy (1½–5 years before prolapse operation)

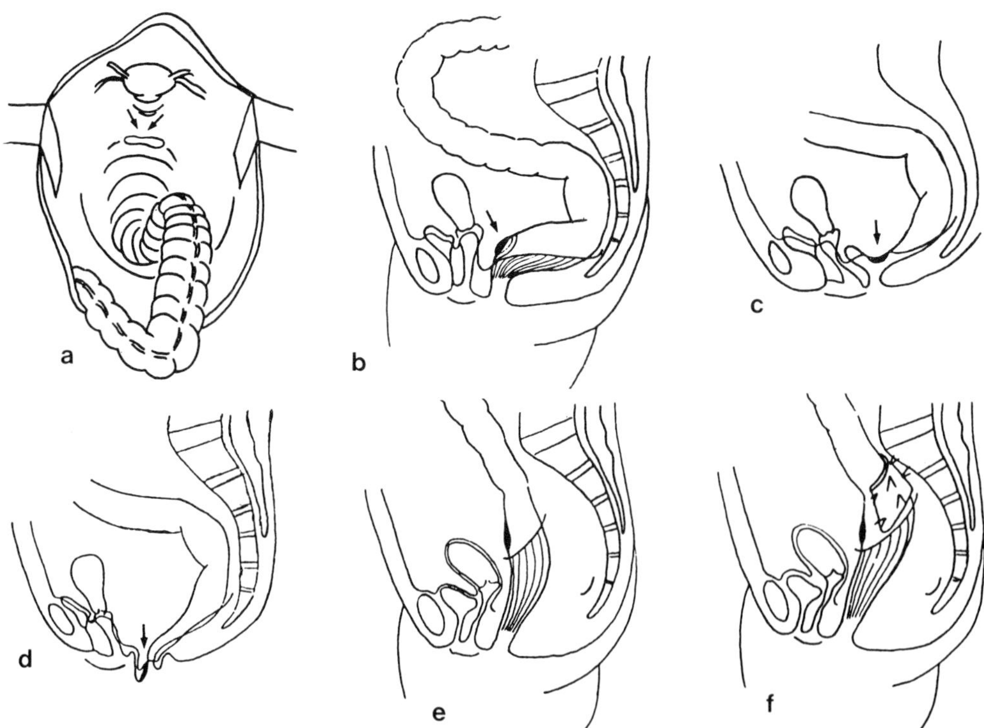

Fig. 23.1a–f. Pathophysiology of rectal prolapse and the principle of its repair. *a* Endopelvic aspect (view into the pelvis from cephalad); *b* lateral view of the deep pouch of Douglas; *c* stage of internal prolapse with rectocele formation; *d* complete (external) prolapse; *e* mobilized rectum is elevated; *f* fixation of rectum. *Arrows,* crucial point of the beginning of intussusception, with fibromatous or edematous thickening of the serosal side of the bowel wall

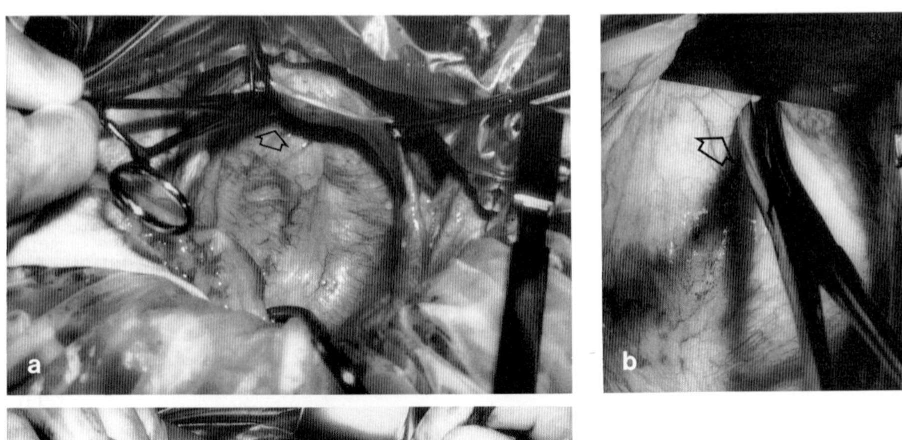

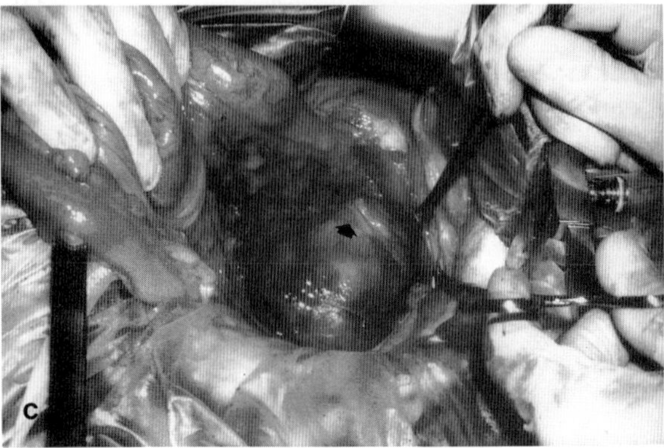

Fig. 23.2a–c. Pathophysiology of rectal prolapse. *a, b* The deep pouch of Douglas with the rectum lying displayed on the pelvic floor (see also Fig. 1a). A 67-year-old woman with complete prolapse. View from cephalad. Forceps holding tubes and cervix (supravaginal hysterectomy decades ago). Anterior rectal wall with hyperemia and edema, consecutive with chronic invagination. Pusher *(open arrows)* deep in the pouch of Douglas. *c* Bottom of pelvic cavity *(solid arrow),* with the rectum and mesorectum completely mobilized and raised (forceps holding peritoneal flap on right side) (see also Fig. 23.1e)

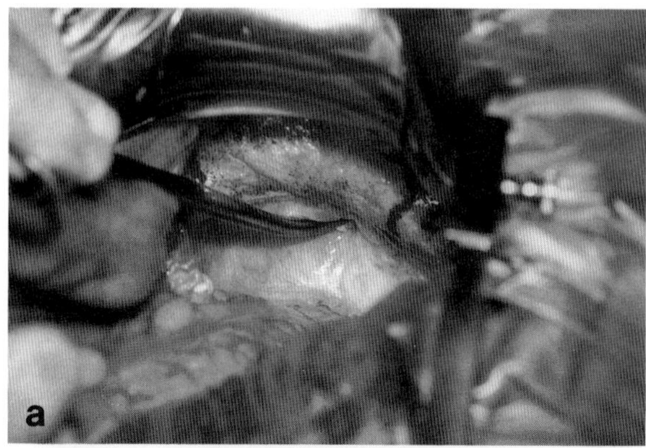

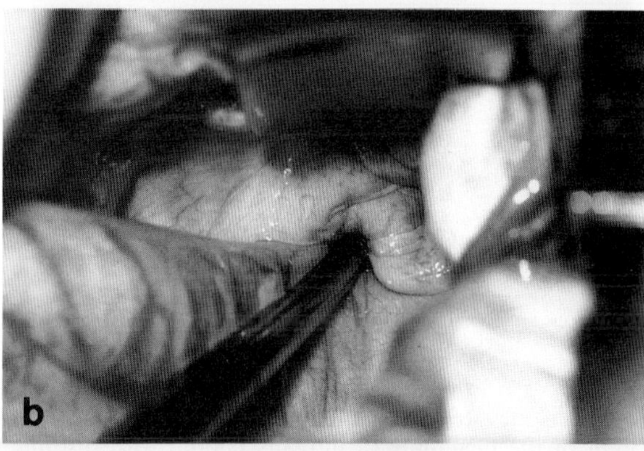

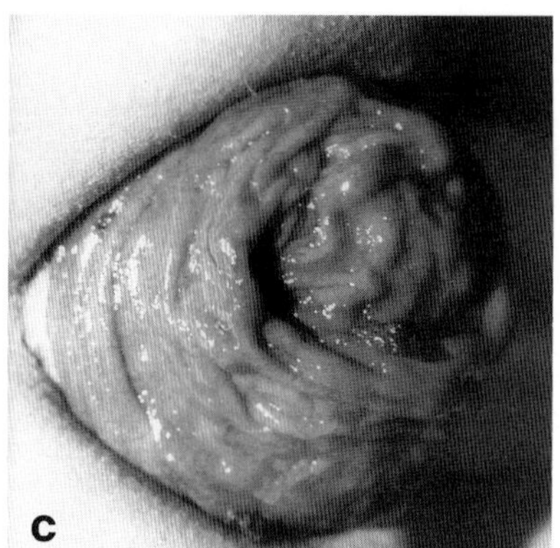

Fig. 23.3 a–c. Pathophysiology of rectal prolapse. *a, b* Intussusception of the anterior rectal wall reproduced with pusher from within the pelvis. The sliding and herniating pouch of Douglas may be of any size and may contain intestine forming an enterocele. *c* Complete prolapse, containing enterocele anteriorly, resulting in asymmetric configuration

geal) wall. We have also observed the endopelvic findings typical of rectal prolapse in one of our patients presenting with a pronounced solitary rectal ulcer syndrome (Fig. 23.7 e) in whom no rectal prolapse could be detected clinically or by defecography. A very deep pouch is occasionally found in patients without rectal prolapse who are operated on for another reason.

External Appearance

The uniform endopelvic findings of the pathological process contrast with a variety of appearances on examination from the external, perineal, and endoluminal side with respect to the following points:

- The degree of descent of the intussuscepted rectal wall: the prolapse may be complete (Figs. 23.1 d; 23.3 c; 23.4 d, g, h; 23.6 a, b, g–i) or it may remain internal (Figs. 23.1 c; 23.4 c, g–m; 23.6 c–f; 23.10) to form an occult, supra- or intraanal prolapse.
- The height and site of the beginning of the intussusception: it may be at the anal verge (Fig. 23.6 a, b) or above (Fig. 23.4 a–d, j–o; 23.10); it may be found anteriorly or in another position.

- The extrusion may occur only during defecation and on straining, or even on standing, walking, coughing.
- The functional state of the pelvic floor and of the internal and external sphincter may be found to be normal (Fig. 23.6 c) or deficient (Fig. 23.6 a, b, g), the patients with rectal prolapse being continent, or partially or totally incontinent (Table 23.2).
- The clinical and histological signs of traumatic proctitis, i.e., the solitary rectal ulcer syndrome (Fig. 23.4 e; 23.7 e–g) may or may not be present.

Table 23.2. Classification of incontinence (according to [13])

Continent	Normal continence
Partially continent	Incontinence in diarrhea, urgency, inability to control flatus, soiling
Incontinent	Gross fecal incontinence

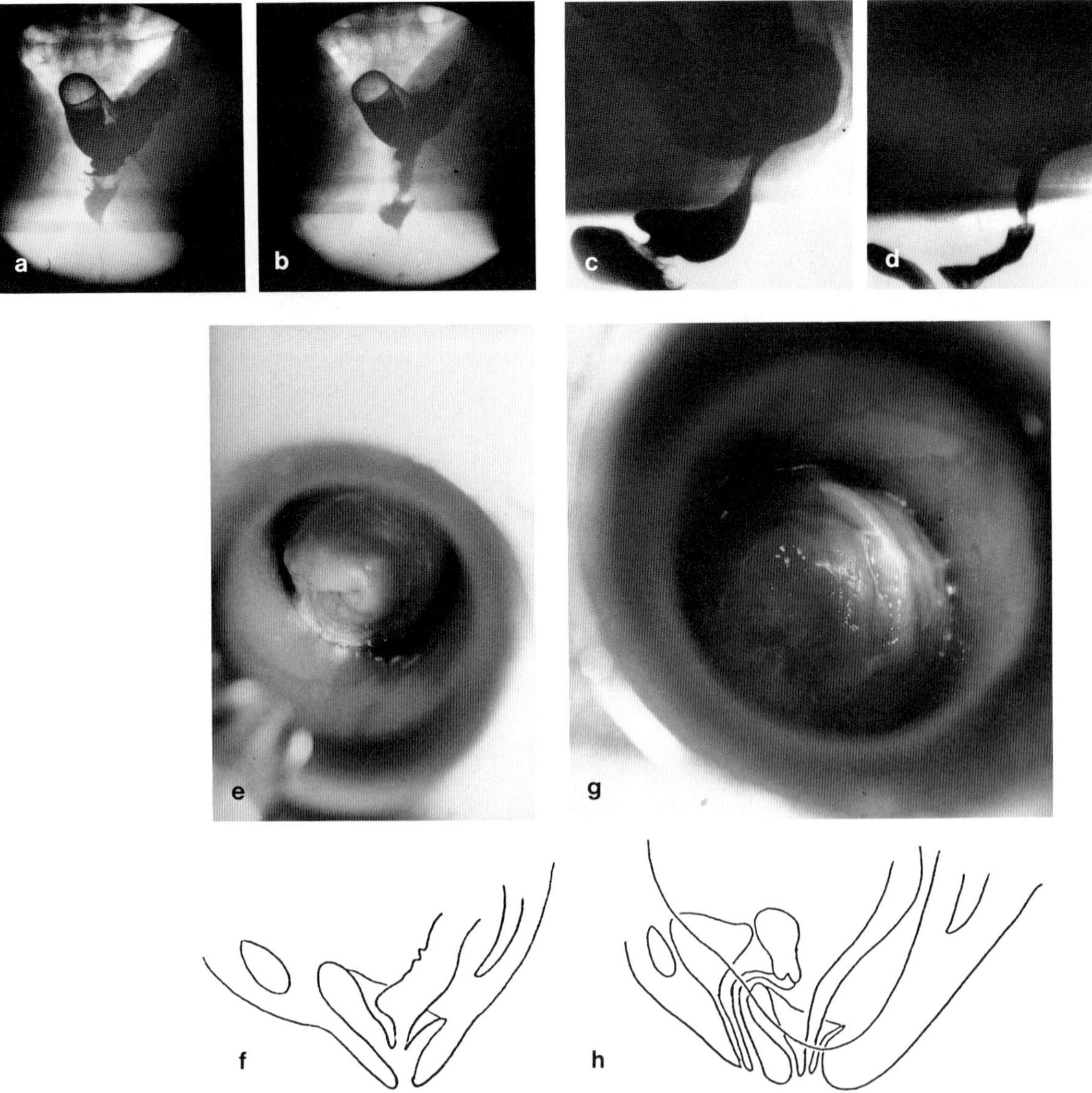

Fig. 23.4a-o. Pathophysiology and clinical appearance of rectal prolapse. *a, b* Anteroposterior view of intussusception at defecography. *c* Lateral view of intussusception with rectocele formation. Stage of internal prolapse. *d* Transanal descent of rectal wall, stage of complete (external) prolapse. *e, f* Proctoscopic view of the stage of internal prolapse of anterior rectal wall (see 23.4c). *g,*

h Proctoscopic view of beginning of complete extrusion. *a-h* A 28-year-old woman, normal continence, complete prolapse on defecation, internal prolapse on clinical examination. Symptoms of lump and pain in the perineum; mucuos discharge. The anterior mucosal folds were hyperemic and edematous. (Same patient as in Figs. 23.3b, 23.9c.) *i-o* see p. 222

Associated Pathological Conditions and Their Clinical Features

Sphincter Function, Incontinence. Descending Perineal Syndrome

Patients with rectal prolapse may be continent or may demonstrate varying degrees of functional deficiency and incontinence.

In *normal* subjects the anal canal is closed and held in position by the continuous *basal* contraction of the external and internal sphincter and of the pelvic floor muscles. The force of the somatic muscles, i. e., the external sphincter and the pelvic floor muscles, can be temporarily increased (*phasic* contraction) by voluntary or reflectory (anal reflex, increase in intraabdominal and intrarectal pressure, coughing) contraction. In patients with decreased

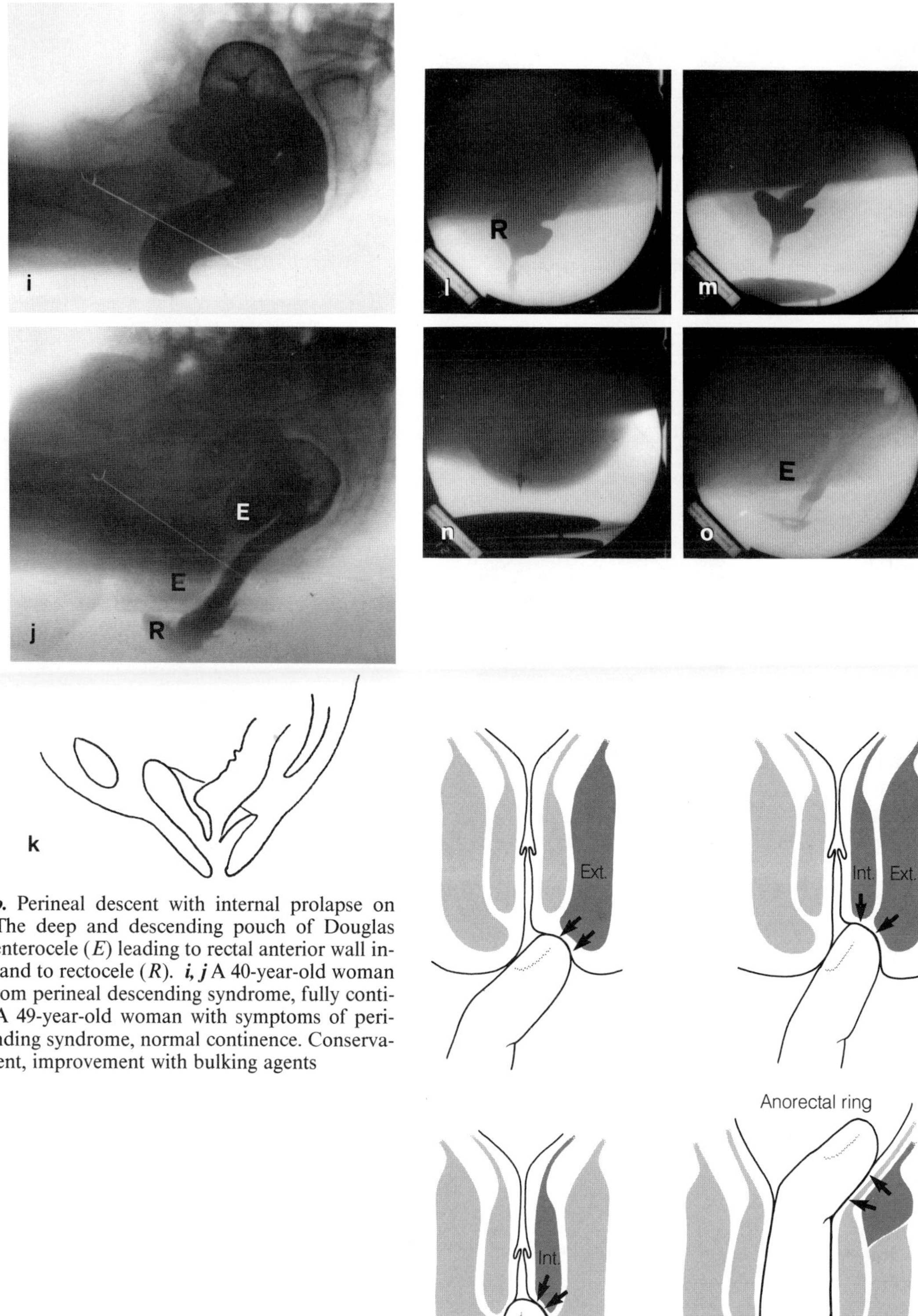

Fig. 23.4i–o. Perineal descent with internal prolapse on straining. The deep and descending pouch of Douglas acts as an enterocele (*E*) leading to rectal anterior wall invagination and to rectocele (*R*). *i, j* A 40-year-old woman suffering from perineal descending syndrome, fully continent. *l–o* A 49-year-old woman with symptoms of perineal descending syndrome, normal continence. Conservative treatment, improvement with bulking agents

Fig. 23.5. Clinical examination of sphincter function. Palpation and inspection of sphincter topography, and examination of resistance to stress at the level of the subcutaneous portion of the external sphincter and of the anorectal ring reveal the basal tonus of the somatic sphincter muscle

or absent somatic sphincter muscle function (neuropathic incontinence, paraplegy, lumbar anesthesy), the anus is still closed by the basal contraction of the *internal* sphincter. Its distension leads to a temporary relaxation with the anus gaping for a few seconds.

Deficiency of the *somatic* sphincter muscles is revealed by a weak *basal* tonus of the external sphincter and of the pelvic floor with the puborectalis sling. It leads to a shortening of the sphincter zone and to a descent of the perineum with some eversion of the anal canal on straining. At this point the external sphincter has lost its ability to invert and plug the anal canal. No or little resistance to stress is offered to the examining finger at the various levels of the external sphincter and at the anorectal ring (Figs. 23.5; 23.6g–i), the anus may gape on slight traction of the perianal skin (Fig. 23.6a, h) or on straining.

Damage to the pelvic floor muscles leads to perineal descent. In patients with a weak sphincter tone the *phasic* (voluntary or reflectory) contraction of the somatic sphincter is usually, but not always, also poor or absent. In some patients voluntary contraction is completely absent, but a definite contraction may be observed on scratching the perianal skin (positive anal reflex). In patients with a weak somatic sphincter, the anus may be closed by the internal sphincter or it may be gaping. A gaping anus reveals – in addition to a low or absent basal tone of the surrounding somatic sphincter muscles – damage to the internal sphincter or a state of permanent stretch and relaxation. As a consequence no (further) relaxation of the internal sphincter can be elicited by rectal distension in patients with rectal prolapse and incontinence (absent or reduced internal relaxation reflex) [13, 23].

Various partial sphincter deficiencies have also been detected by manometry [23]. It has been confirmed by manometry that the basal and the phasic contractions are very low or absent in incontinent or partially incontinent patients with rectal prolapse [13].

An abnormal descent of the perineum (i. e., below the plain of the ischial tuberosities during straining or the pubocyccygeal line at defecography (Fig. 23.4j, k) indicates a weak pelvic floor. It frequently occurs in patients with incontinence and prolapse. It has been demonstrated that the weakness of the pelvic floor and external sphincter is initiated by damage to the nerve supply of these muscles [3, 12, 19, 28–30]. (On the other hand, patients with abnormal perineal descent may be normally continent and may have no rectal prolapse. A diminished rec-

tal compliance has been shown to contribute to incontinence in patients with abnormal perineal descent [35].)

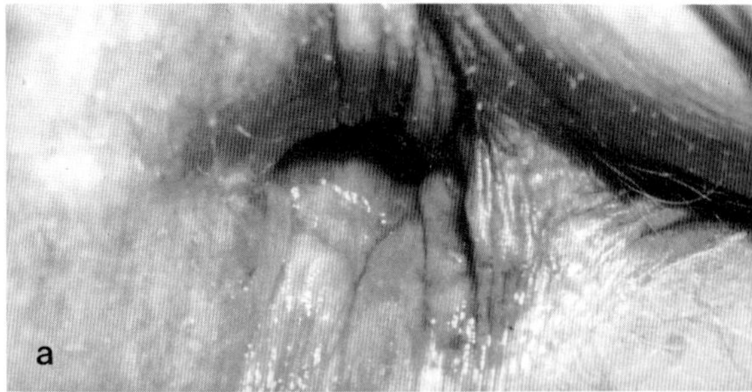

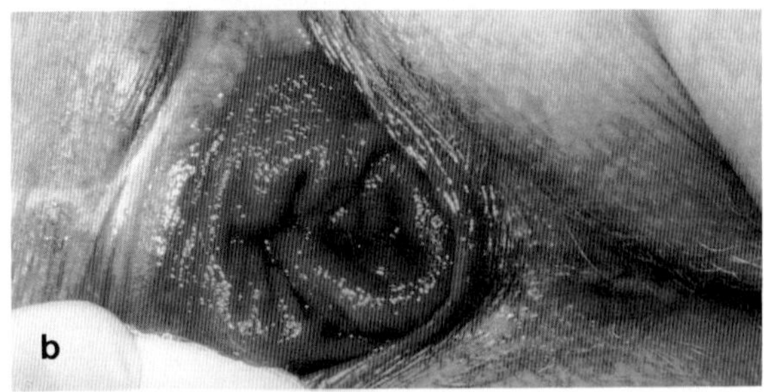

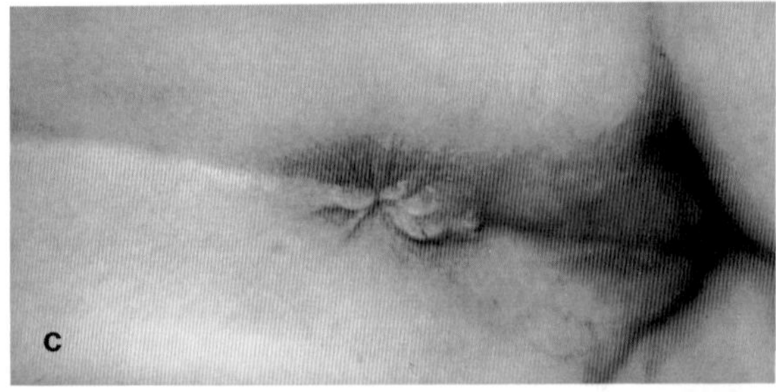

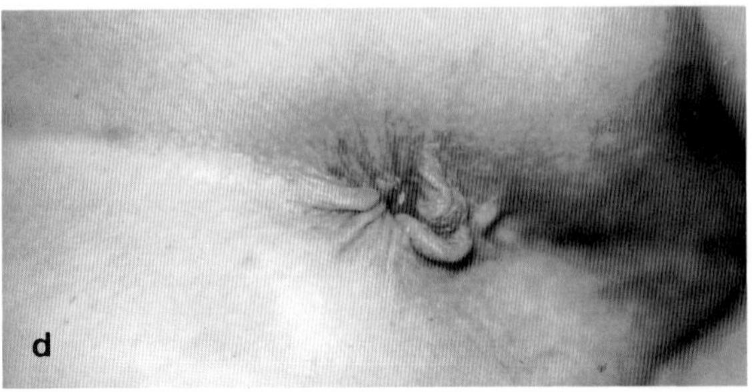

Fig. 23.6a–i. Sphincter function and rectal prolapse. *a, b* Almost permanent prolapse with incontinence in an 82-year-old woman. Lack of basal function of external and internal sphincters, resulting in permanently gaping anus. Repair of prolapse by Wells' procedure; no restitution of anal sphincter function. *c–f* Differentiation between mucosal and rectal prolapse. Fully continent 49-year-old woman with symptoms of occult (internal) prolapse. *c* Normal basal tonus holds anal canal closed and presents resistance to stress. *d, e* On straining a mucosal fold appears anteriorly, representing the lowest part of the descending anterior rectal wall. *e–i* see p. 224

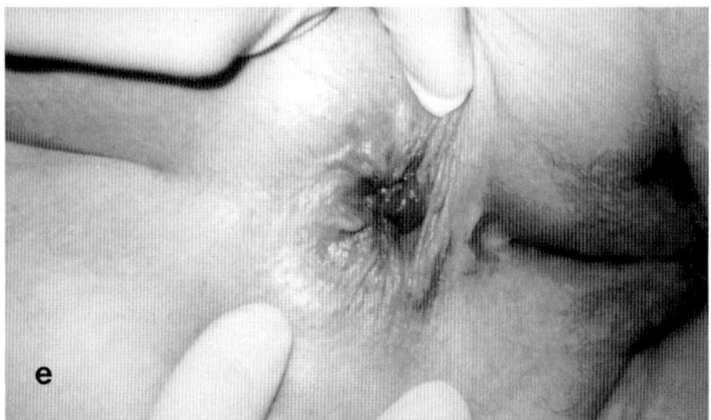

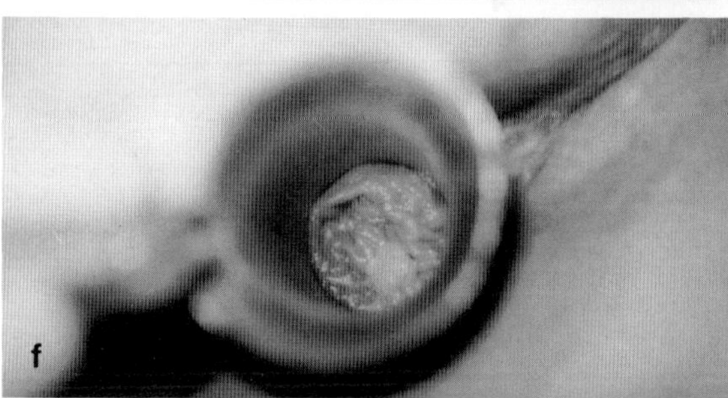

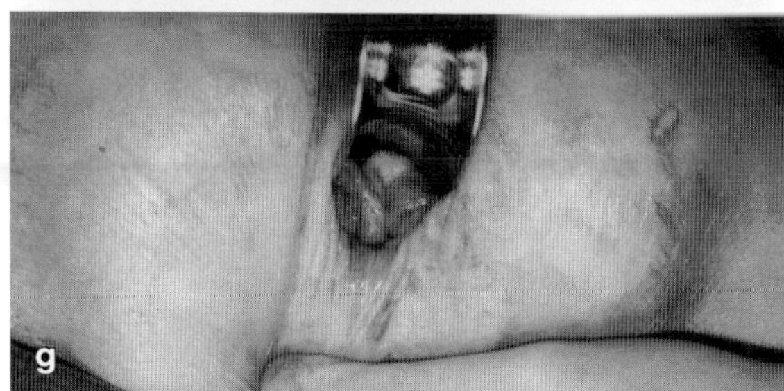

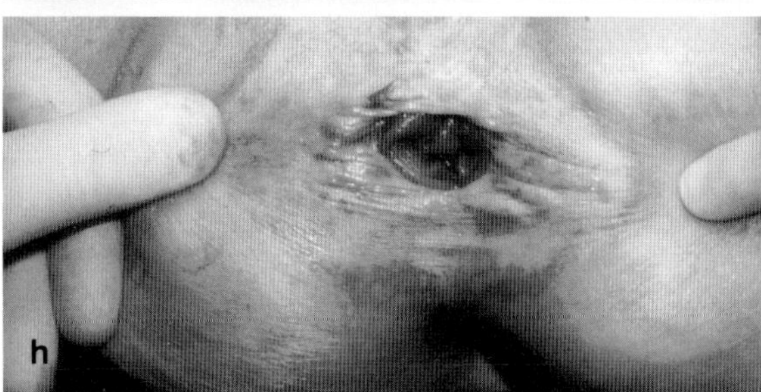

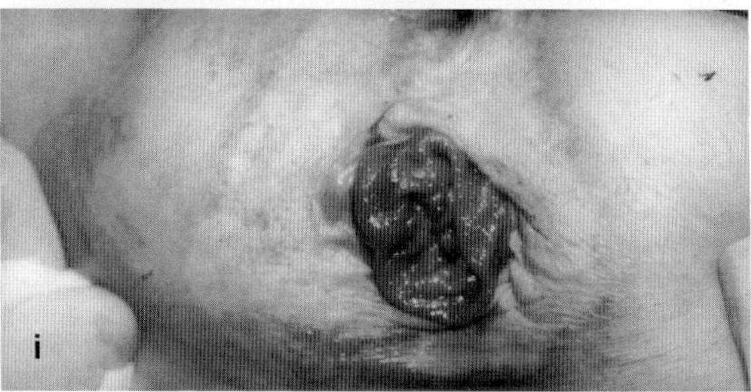

Fig. 23.6e–i. *f* Proctoscopic appearance (same patient as in Fig. 23.10). *g–i* Examination under lumbar anesthesia (relaxation of somatic sphincter muscles) demonstrating permanent internal anal sphincter relaxation and full thickness rectal prolapse (not filled by enterocele). Prior

The *descending perineal syndrome* is suggestive of the presence of an internal rectal prolapse (Fig. 23.4). The symptoms include discomfort and pain in the perineum, discharge of mucus and blood, pruritus and difficulty at defecation, tenesmus, a feeling of partial evacuation, blockage of the passage of stool, downward ballooning (of the perineum) on straining.

Mucosal Prolapse. Internal (Occult) Rectal Prolapse. Rectocele

A bulging or invaginating pouch of Douglas (Fig. 13.1 c) on rectal digital examination and an anterior rectal wall bulge descending into the proctoscope or appearing in and through the anal canal (Fig. 23.4 e–o; 23.6 c–f) are common findings in complete and in internal, occult rectal prolapse. Differentiation from the simple anterior mucosal prolapse may be difficult (Fig. 23.6 g–i; 23.7 a, c, f). On palpation the latter contains only the mucosal layer, no full-thickness wall (Fig. 23.7 b). Mucosal prolapse in patients with rectal prolapse may represent the lower edge of the descending rectal wall (Fig. 23.6 c–f), a concomitant simple mucosal prolapse or prolapsing hyperplastic mucosa (i. e., a variant of the solitary rectal ulcer syndrome (Fig. 23.7 f).
A rectocele may often be palpated or demonstrated by defecography (Fig. 23.4 i–o). It is the result of the herniation of the pouch of Douglas, which – containing intestine – represents an enterocele (Fig. 23.3 c; 23.4).

Solitary Rectal Ulcer Syndrome

This abnormality of the mucosal folds represents traumatic proctitis initiated by chronic intussusception and intraanal or transanal prolapse of the bowel wall. Ulceration is facultative, and there is a nonulcerated form of the condition [24]. The macroscopic appearance consists of thickening, edematous, hyperemic, sometimes hyperplastic nodular or granular, sometimes ulcerated mucosal folds, most often on the anterior aspect (Fig. 23.7 e). The histo-

to this examination, with the somatic sphincter contracted, the presence of a simple mucosal prolapse was considered. An 84-year-old woman, partially incontinent. Good results after Wells' procedure. Same patient as in Fig. 23.8

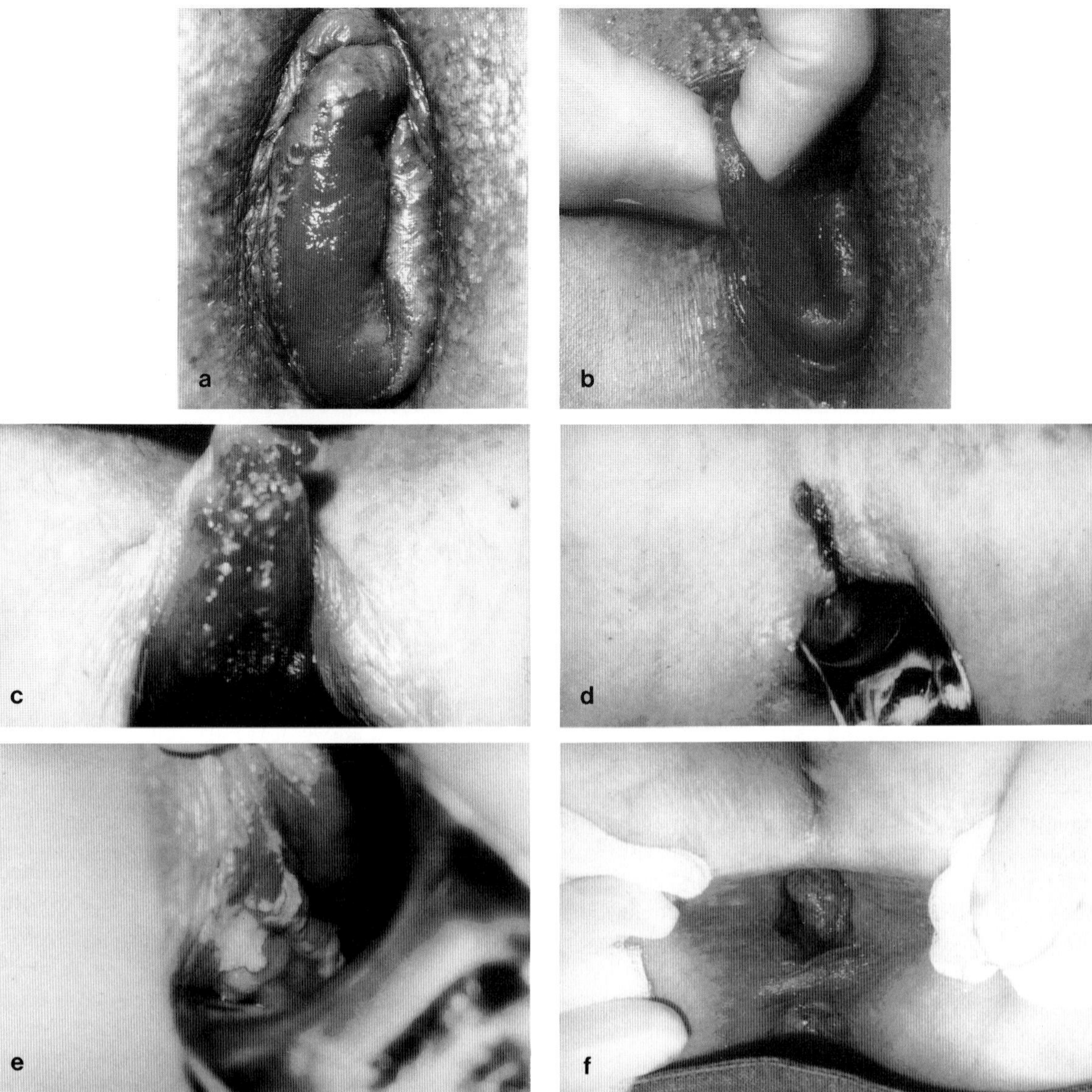

Fig. 23.7a–g. Differentiation between mucosal and rectal prolapse. Solitary rectal ulcer syndrome. *a, b* Circular mucosal prolapse. No intussusception is detectable, no full-thickness rectal wall on palpation, the prolapse does not contain the pouch of Douglas (76-year-old man; cure by transanal circular excision). *c, d* Anterior mucosal prolapse, without symptoms or signs of rectal prolapse (78-year-old woman; cure by transanal excision). *e* Traumatic proctitis of the anterior rectal wall. Hyperplastic, pseudotumorous, nonulcerated form of solitary rectal ulcer syndrome (30-year-old woman, fully continent, severe symptoms of defecation difficulties, perineal pain, mucous discharge. No prolapse detectable. Deep pouch at laparotomy. Cure after proctopexy with resection). *f* Permanent prolapse of anterior hyperplastic mucosa (solitary rectal ulcer syndrome) (61-year-old patient with complete rectal prolapse (reduced on figure), partial incontinence. Cure following proctopexy and resection, with transanal excision of the mucosal prolapse. Same patient as in Fig. 23.9h, i). *g* see p. 226

logical features are an obliteration of the lamina propria by fibroblasts and smooth muscle cells (derived from the greatly thickened muscularis mucosae) and misplaced glands in the submucosa [24]. These features are also encountered in other conditions of chronic mucosal traumatism, such as prolapsing hemorrhoids, mucosal prolapse, and colostomies. The solitary rectal ulcer syndrome must be distinguished in clinically and by means of endoscopic and histological examination from the frequently seen discharge of mucus and blood in proctitis ulcerosa.

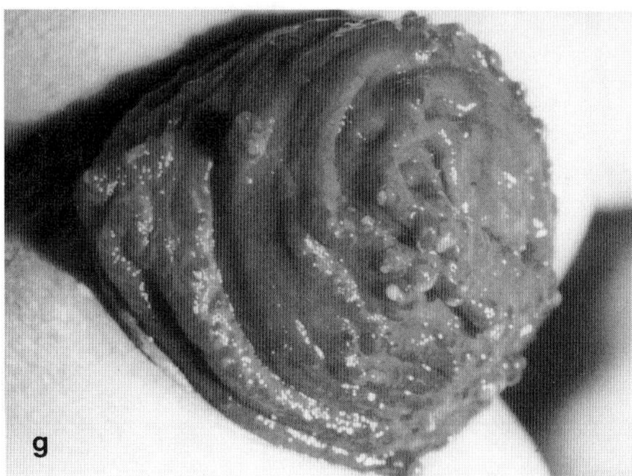

Fig. 23.7. g Complete rectal prolapse with hyperplastic polyps on the prolapsing mucosal folds, representing a variation of traumatic proctitis

Diagnosis, Examination

The clues to the diagnosis of the various forms of rectal prolapse are precise history, clinical anal and pelvic floor examination with digital palpation, proctoscopy and rectoscopy [6–8, 10, 14, 19, 25, 31]. One or several of the associated conditions are frequently observed. Rectal intussusception and internal prolapse are recognized by palpation (also with the patient in the upright position) and by endoscopic visualization with a rigid instrument. The digital examination may reveal a large rectocele which the patient may feel retaining stool on defecation. He or she may give a history of assisting defecation by digitation. Patients with the solitary rectal ulcer syndrome complain of passage of blood and mucus through the anus, and of symptoms of the occult prolapse such as a feeling of tenesmus, difficulty at defecation, and perineal pain. The solitary rectal ulcer syndrome may be suspected by the palpation of thickened mucosal areas and diagnosed in most patients by the macroscopic appearance through the proctoscope or rectoscope.

Difficulty at defecation, straining, perineal descent, and the solitary rectal ulcer syndrome have also been found to be associated with outlet obstruction due to overactivity of the puborectalis muscle (anismus) occurring instead of relaxation during bearing down [24]. However, on the basis of defecographies and clinical examination, the symptoms are much more frequently associated with intussusception and external rectal procidentia [4].

Defecography is frequently not necessary. It may be helpful in some instances to confirm a clinically suspected occult rectal prolapse. The rectocolon should be investigated preoperatively by a barium enema (with respect to colorectal topography and exclusion of other disease), and a lateral proctography can be performed at the same time.

Treatment

Introduction

There are various treatment procedures which are utilized to correct the anatomical abnormalities occurring in rectal prolapse or prevent rectal descent or intussusception. A classification of the procedures was given by Watts et al. [32] according to the approach (transabdominal, perineal, transsacral) and to the type of repair (outlet narrowing, pelvic floor repair, suspension-fixation of the rectum and pelvic colon with or without foreign material or resection, prevention of intussusception, etc.). On the basis of considerable surgical experience and treatment results, a more precise pathophysiological understanding of the disease, and the endopelvic findings mentioned above, it is now quite clear that the essential steps in the successful repair of rectal prolapse are (a) complete mobilization of the rectum down to the pelvic floor; (b) elevation of the rectum including the lower part with the intussuscepting rectal wall segment, and (c) fixation of the elevated rectum, thus preventing further rectal wall descent and invagination. Fixation of the elevated rectum may be performed (a) by wrapping a sheet of material (Ivalon sponge, Marlex, Teflon), which is fixed to the sacrum, around the posterior circumference of the rectum (Wells procedure); (b) by direct suture of the rectum, i. e., by fixing the lateral wings of the prerectal pelvic peritoneum and of the mesorectum and the lateral ligaments, on one or both sides, to the sacrum; (c) resection of the upper rectum and sigmoid colon may be added to the latter procedure, with an end-to-end anastomosis performed between the lower part of the descending colon and the upper, peritonealized part of the ampulla. Indeed, elevation of the mobilized rectal ampulla may result in an abundant, highly mobile pelvic and sigmoid colon on a short mesenteric base (Fig. 23.9 e, f), as already pointed out by Sudeck in 1922 [27]. Resection may prevent volvulus and functional symptoms which can be rather severe [25]. Though in our experience patients without resection may have no bowel management problems, we have observed, in accordance with Watts et al. [32], significant improvement of preoperative functional problems following proctopexy combined with resection. As a consequence, we now prefer proctopexy and resection in patients with functional problems and with diverticular disease.

Shortening the left colon does not contribute per se to the prevention of rectal prolapse, and complete rectal mobilization and fixation remain essential (Fig. 23.9 h, i). This conclusion ensues from the endopelvic findings during operations and also from the rather high recurrence rates after fixation and resection procedures which omit complete rectal mobilization [1, 10, 32].

In cases with concomitant urinary incontinence a Marshall-Marchetti procedure is performed [7, 15). In some patients with an obvious descent of the genital visceral axis (uterus or vaginal stump), an anterior uterus fixation or a plication (shortening) of the round ligaments may contribute to correcting the pelvic descent. A conservative regimen with bulking agents and a high fiber intake may be tried in selected patients with an internal prolapse or a solitary rectal ulcer syndrome.

Technics

Mobilization

After division of the developmental adhesions of the rectosigmoid to the left iliac fossa, the peritoneum is incised on either side along the base of the mesosigmoid and mesorectum, the bowel being pulled straight upward and forward (Fig. 23.8 a–d; 23.9 b). The lateral edges of the peritoneal incision are lifted by forceps, especially when the incision and subsequent mobilization reach the bottom of the pouch and when the incision is completed in front of the rectum (Fig. 23.8 b–c). The uterus is often hitched up using a stay suture. Peritoneal vessels, which may be abundant, are coagulated by diathermy. To open and dissect the presacral space,

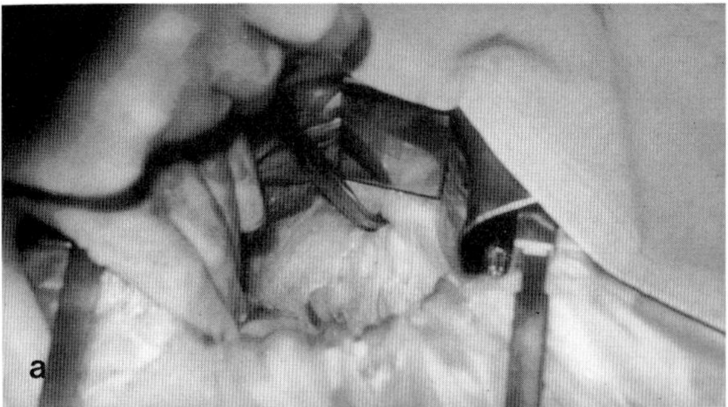
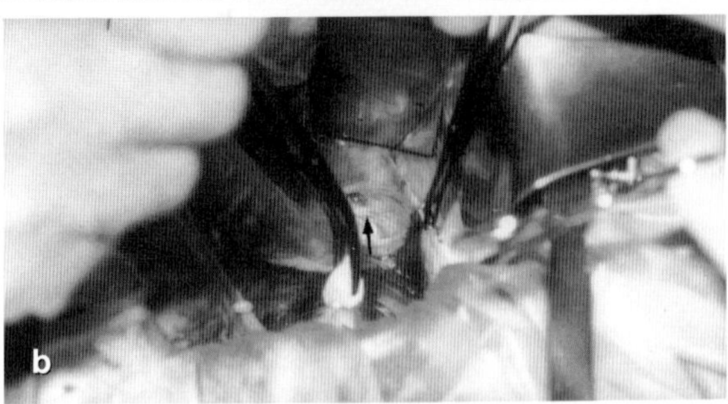
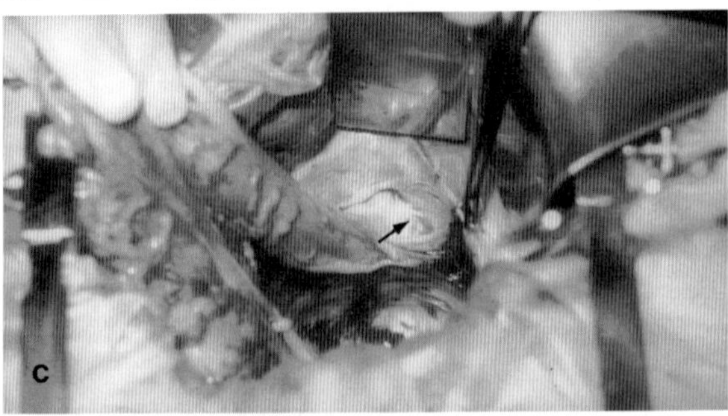
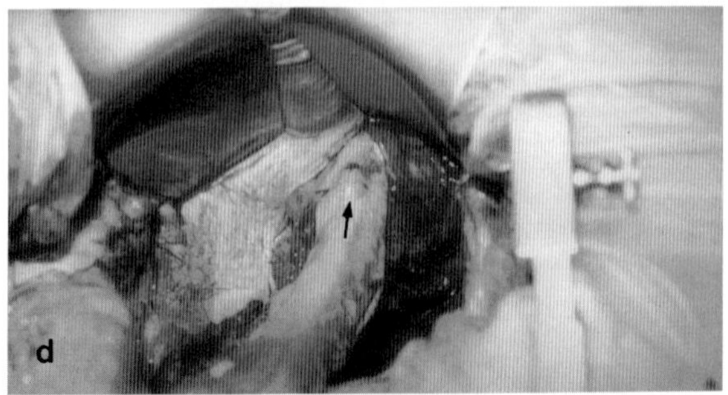
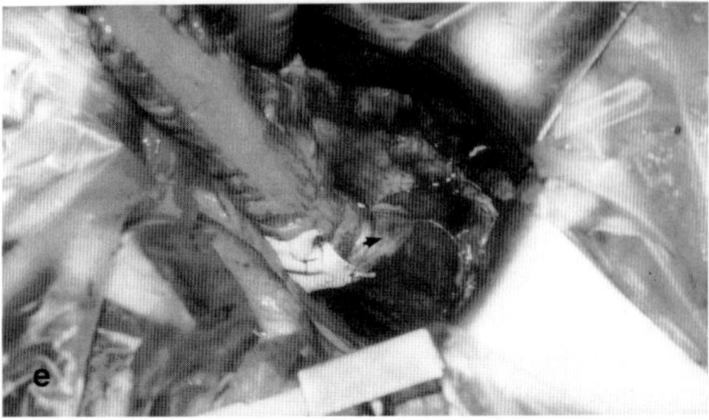

▷

Fig. 23.8 a–e. Mobilization, elevation, fixation of the rectum. *a–d* Successive steps in mobilization and elevation of the rectum. View into the pelvis from cephalad; *a* demonstrates intussusception of the anterior rectal wall. The fibrotic thickening at the area of invagination *(arrows)* is seen in *b–e. e* Fixation of the elevated rectum to the upper sacrum with Teflon sling. Anterior mobilization has contributed to elevation of the crucial point of intussusception (view from right side). (Same patient as in Fig. 23.6 g–i)

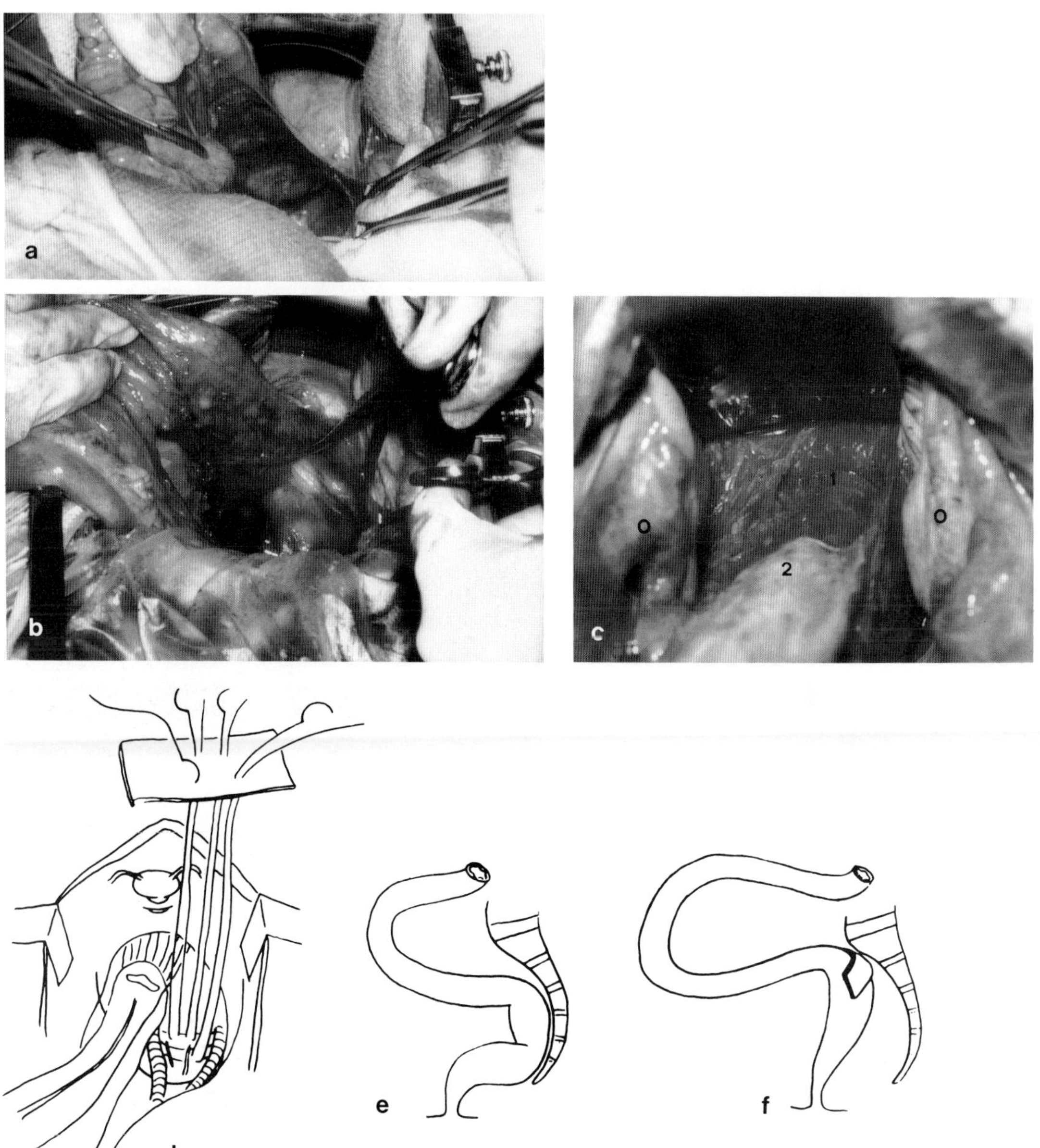

Fig. 23.9 a–i. Steps in mobilization and fixation. *a* Incomplete posterior and lateral mobilization. The subrectal space is not yet opened. Lower rectum still lying on pelvic floor. *b* Sufficient elevation is only achieved after division of the sacrorectal ligament and mobilization down to the pelvic floor. *c* Anterior mobilization raises the anterior rectal wall and the pouch of Douglas by about 4–5 cm (same patient as in Fig. 23.3 b, 23.4). *1*, natural plain of dissection between vagina and rectum; *2*, crucial point of intussusception raised; *0*, ovaries. *d* Fixation of a piece of thin Teflon to the upper sacrum after complete mobilization of the rectum. *e, f* Elevation of the rectum results in a long sigmoid sling on a short mesocolic base. *g–i* see p. 229

the loose connective tissue is incised with scissors near the (visceral) fascia of the mesorectum, leaving intact the visualized hypogastric nerves which, from the sacral promontory, go down along the more lateral aspect of the pelvic wall. Laterally too, the mobilization of the rectum is carried out close to the fascia of the mesorectum. Toward the pelvic floor the rectum turns forward sharply; for complete mobilization the dense connective tissue, the rectosacral fascia [5], must be incised with scissors, and thus the infrarectal space [5] with the pelvic floor at its base is opened. In almost all cases an anterior dissection is also carried out starting at the deepest point of the pouch of Douglas. The rectum

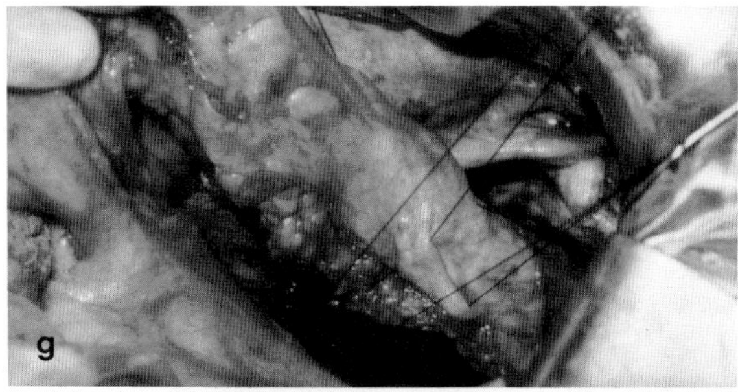

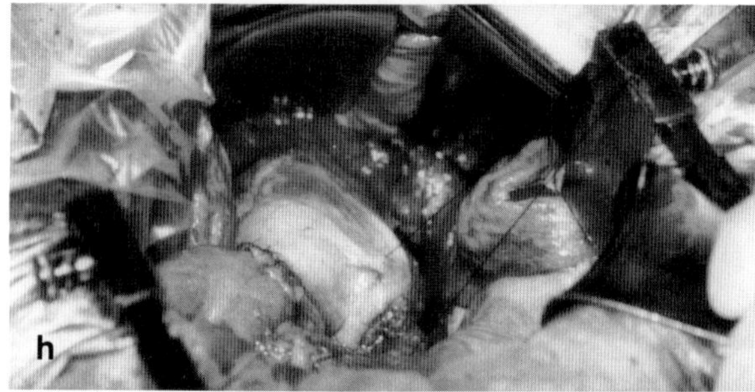

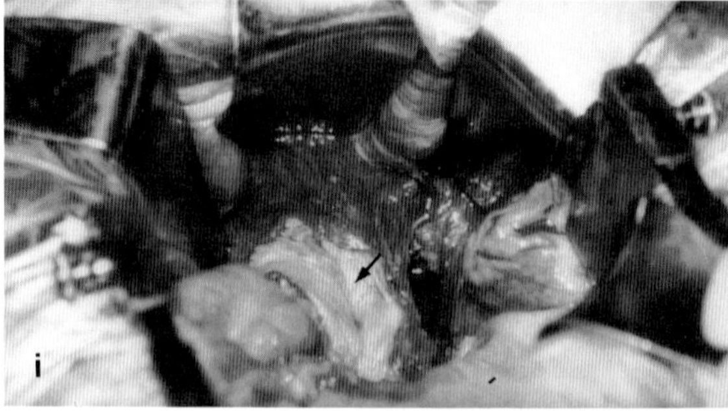

Fig. 23.9. *g* Fixation of the elevated ampulla without implant and without resection: suture of right wing of the elevated visceral Douglas peritoneum with mesorectum and right lateral ligament to the upper sacrum. *h* Fixation of the elevated ampulla after sigmoid and high anterior resection (right side). *i* Slight constriction over rectum *(arrow)* after tightening of the sutures on both sides

is dissected backward from the vaginal wall (or from the fascia of Denonvilliers covering the vesicles) in the natural tissue plane (Fig. 23.9 c) using small gauze pushers and avoiding diathermy on the thin vaginal wall. We feel it necessary – in contrast to some authors [15] – to carry out an anterior dissection; indeed, the invaginating point of the rectum is always elevated by 4–5 cm by this maneuver, which is necessary to lift the anterior aspect of the rectal wall from its critical low position (Fig. 23.9 a–c, g, h).

Elevation of the rectum is now possible without complete transsection of the lateral ligaments which are found quite deep on the pelvic floor. During the

deep posterior and lateral mobilization care must be taken not to incise the low, mobile mesorectum with the upper hemorrhoidal vessels, confusing them with the vessels of the lateral stalks. The extensive posterior mobilization down to the pelvic floor exposes, posteriorly and laterally, the junction of the longitudinal muscular coat of the rectum with the pubococcygeal muscle, without, of course, entering the intersphincteric plane. From its previous deep posterior position, the rectum has now gained, quite an anterior and upward position (Fig. 23.1 e, 23.2 c, 23.9 b, 23.10). (It would be easy to perform a very low anterior resection, which is, however, not carried out because the ampulla should be preserved.)

Fixation of the Elevated Rectum

Fixation is the second essential step in the operative treatment of rectal prolapse. The mobilized rectum, together with the prerectal pelvic peritoneum and the mesorectum, is easily brought up to the upper part of the sacrum and its promontory (Fig. 23.1 e, 23.8 e). The implant (e. g., a rectangular piece of thin Teflon) is fixed to the presacral fascia with four stitches of Nylon or Prolen, while carefully avoiding the middle sacral vessels, the hypogastric nerves, and the common iliac veins (Fig. 23.9 d). The rectum is placed on the Teflon sheet, usually at the level of the lowest peritonealized section, and the Teflon piece is fixed to the mesorectum and the lateral rectal wall by two sutures on either side, leaving the anterior third of the bowel free (Fig. 23.8 e). The peritoneum is closed over the implant.

Some surgeons insert the implant down to the sacrococcygeal level [1, 21, 22]. We avoid this low fixation because it may result in rectal angulation and insufficient elevation. Furthermore, the very low placement of the sheet could interfere with free retrorectal access in the case of a subsequent postanal repair.

Straightening of the ampulla and fixation at the promontory may appear to leave the hollow of the sacrum empty, but in our experience the ampulla always fills the hollow as shown in Fig. 23.10, and as can be observed by digital postoperative palpation along the sacrum from the coccyx up to the implant.

Results with the Wells procedure are favorable (Table 23.3). We have operated on 28 patients with no operative deaths, no infection, and no recurrences. In three patients a subsequent operation became necessary 1–3 years later (one small bowel

Table 23.3. Results of Wells procedure

Reference	(n)	Material	Infection rate (%)	Operative Lethality (%)	Recurrence (%)	Postoperative mucosal prolapse (%)	Improvement in incontinence (%)
Anderson et al. 1981 [2]	39	Ivalon	3	3	3	16	Rare
Keighley et al. 1983 [15]	100	Marlex	0	0	0	5	66
Kupfer and Goligher 1970 [16]	35	Ivalon	11	3	0	–	–
Morgan 1972 [18]	150	Ivalon	3	3	3	9	33
Penfold and Hawley; and Hawley 1972 [21] 1975 [11]	101	Ivalon	1	0	3	33	20–30
Porter 1980 [22]	97	Ivalon	3	0	1	5	50
Schweiger 1983 [25]	77	Dura		3	16	–	Frequent
Stewart 1972 [26]	41	Ivalon	0	0	7	33	66
Wells 1962 [34]	20	Ivalon	0	0	0	0	–
Gemsenjäger 1985 [7]	28	Ivalon 12 Teflon 16	0	0	0	7	33
Average			2.3	1.2	3.3		

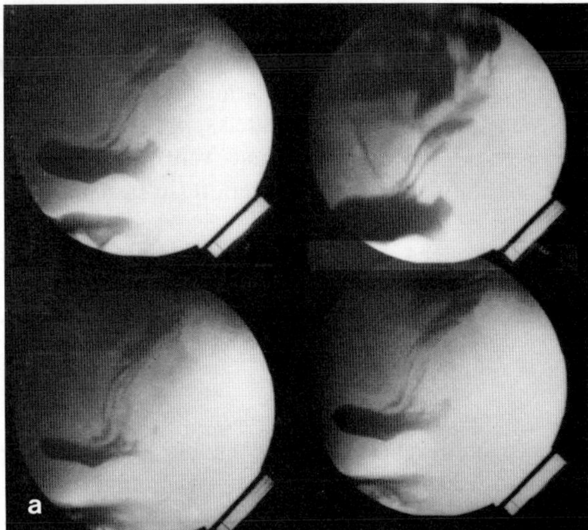
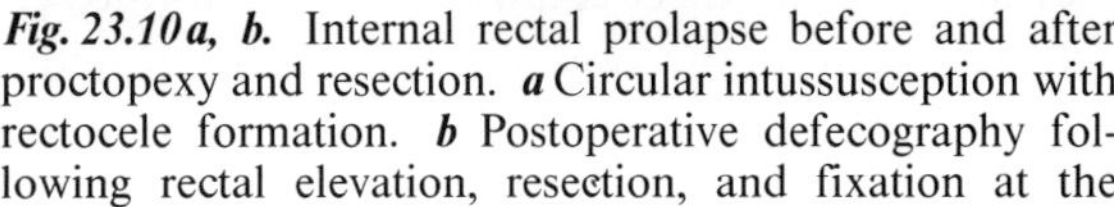
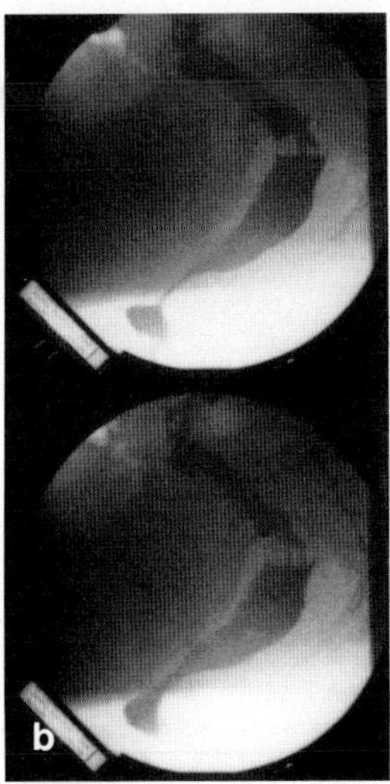

Fig. 23.10a, b. Internal rectal prolapse before and after proctopexy and resection. *a* Circular intussusception with rectocele formation. *b* Postoperative defecography following rectal elevation, resection, and fixation at the upper sacrum. A 59-year-old woman, symptoms of occult rectal prolapse, fully continent (same patient as in Fig. 23.6 c–f)

obstruction; one perforation of the sigmoid sling, possibly due to volvulus or diverticulitis; one patient with persistent presacral pain had the Teflon sheet removed 1 year later – there was no obvious scarring; the patient remained well after rectosigmoid resection with proctopexy).

For several years we have occasionally utilized the lateral *wings of the prerectal pelvic peritoneum and the mesorectum with the lateral ligaments* attach the elevated rectal ampulla to the upper sacrum, namely in patients with diverticular disease or with a very redundant sigmoid who had had a resection performed. We have observed a very good feasiability of this type of proctopexy which has become the procedure of choice, with or without resection, in the last 3 years (Table 23.4). Thirty-eight patients had a proctopexy without an implant, with resection in 28 instances.

The visceral pelvic peritoneal wing and the mesorectum are first fixed to the presacral fascia (by two nonabsorbable sutures) on the right side (Fig. 23.9 g). Fixing is carried out on the left side only if no constricting band is created across the anterior bowel wall (Fig. 23.9 i) and if one or two fingers can be inserted between the rectum and the sacrum with the sutures tied. A constricting effect may also be avoided by longitudinal incision of the prerectal peritoneal band.

Rectosigmoid resection is recommended when there is anatomical gross bowel redundancy, the presence of diverticular disease, and when there is an individual history of irritable colon and functional symptoms. The bowel resection is carried out after the pelvic mobilization of the rectum is completed and before the proctopexy. In most cases the mesosigmoid and the (mobile) mesorectum are divided proximally and distally, respectively. The resection may also be carried out intramesenterically, leaving intact the inferior mesenteric and upper hemorrhoidal vessels. The remaining sling of mesosigmoid and -rectum is than placed down into the hollow of the sacrum, which contributes to its obstruction. The anastomosis is carried out by interrupted extramucosal single-layer sutures. Once the anastomosis is complete, the rectal stump is fixed to the sacrum as described above (Fig. 23.9 h, i). The peritoneum is closed over the anastomosis. Suction drainage is placed below and above the sutured peritoneum.

We have observed an uneventful postoperative course in 27 out of 28 patients treated by resection and proctopexy. One patient of the earlier series had a low anterior resection with a double-layer anastomosis followed by perianastomotic suppuration. It nevertheless healed without colostomy. No instance of recurrence was observed in the 28 patients 6 months to 13 years postoperatively.

Continence, Mucosal Prolapse (Table 23.3). Following abdominal mobilization and fixation of the rectum the results with respect to restoration of continence are reported to be favorable as compared to other procedures [32]. In our series, 24 (36%) out of 66 patients were incontinent preoperatively; following proctopexy eight (33%) regained an acceptable level of continence. In some patients gaping of the anus resolved, indicating cessation of permanent internal sphincter relaxation and improvement of the basal tone of the internal sphincter.

Five (24%) out of our latest series of 21 consecutive patients had a concomitant mucosal prolapse; it inverted spontaneously (by improved sphincter tonus) after abdominal repair in three patients, and was managed by transanal excision in the remaining two.

Clinical and macroscopic evidence of traumatic proctitis (solitary rectal ulcer syndrome) disappeared in 16 out of 18 patients following proctopexy, with or without resection.

Conclusions

Various operative procedures are still utilized for the treatment of rectal prolapse. The operative development and experience with a personal series of 77 patients over a 16-year period are summarized in Table 23.4. Anal (i.e., perilevatoric) encirclement performed with a wire or a Teflon sling may resolve procidentia and improve incontinence in selected patients, but reoperations for adjustment or rupture

Table 23.4. Operative procedures and results in a personal series over a 16-year period

Operative procedure	(*n*)	Years	Complications	Recurrence
Perineal perilevatoric encirclement	7	1970–1976	Three reoperations (rupture, infection, narrowing)	0
Roscoe-Graham procedure	4	1970–1975	–	2
Proctopexy Wells procedure (Ivalon, Teflon)	28	*n* = 27 1970–1984	One small bowel obstruction one sigmoid perforation one patient with pelvic pain, reoperation	0
Lateral ligaments	10	*n* = 5 1985–1986	–	0
Proctopexy and resection Low	3	1970–1975	One anastomotic infection one anastomotic stenosis	0
High	25	*n* = 15 1984–1986	–	0

of the ring may be necessary. Even in the poor-risk patient a Wells-type fixation is currently preferable and usually well tolerated under regional or general anesthesia.

Early in the series we performed the Roscoe-Graham abdominal pelvic floor repair behind the rectum [9], combined with elevation of the Douglas peritoneum. A recurrence developed in two of the four patients. In accordance with Wells [33], we found the operation a difficult one and, furthermore, we noticed that only the upper level of the pelvic floor, i. e., the pubococcygeal muscle, was included in the repair sutures, leaving out the more important level of the underlying puborectalis sling. The Wells procedure proved to be quite satisfactory, but later we realized that an implant was not necessary to fix the rectum to the sacrum and, furthermore, that resection of the abundant sigmoid was safe in the majority of patients.

The conditions for satisfactory results with respect to repair of the procidentia and restoration of continence are:

- The abdominal approach.
- Complete mobilization of the rectum, with resection of the abundant sigmoid and upper rectum in several patients, leaving the elevated ampulla intact, with an end-to-end single-layer anastomosis performed approximately 10-12 cm from the anal verge (on condition that the surgeon is familiar with anterior resection).
- Fixation of the elevated ampulla (below the anastomosis in patients with resection) at the upper sacrum.
- Peritonealization over the pelvic operative field.
- Patients with incontinence lasting beyond 6 months after the correction of the prolapse are offered a postanal repair [20].

References

1. Aminev AM, Malyshev JUI (1964) Rectal prolapse: a comparative evaluation of some operative Methods of treatment concerning late observations made by the surgeons of the Soviet Union. Am J Proctol 15: 355-360
2. Anderson JR, Kennenmonth AWG, Smith AN (1981) Polyvinyl alcohol sponge rectopexy for complete rectal prolapse. J Coll Surg Edinb 26: 292-294
3. Bartolo DCC, Jarratt JA, Read MG, Donnelly TC, Read NW (1983) The role of partial denervation of the puborectalis in idiopathic faecal incontinence. Br J Surg 70: 664-667
4. Bartram CI, Mahieu PHG (1985) Radiology of the pelvic floor. In: Henry MM, Swash M (eds) Coloproctology and the pelvic floor. Butterworths, London, pp 151-186
5. Crapp AR, Cuthbertson AM (1974) William Waldeyer and the rectosacral fascia. Surg Gynecol Obstet 138: 252-256
6. Gemsenjäger E (1981) Klinische und apparative Untersuchung der Kontinenzfunktion. Schweiz Rundsch Med Prax 70: 647-655
7. Gemsenjäger E (1985) Rektumprolaps. Klinik und Therapie. Schweiz Rundsch Med Prax 74: 937-941
8. Gemsenjäger E (1988) Innerer Rektumprolaps. Schweiz Med Wochenschr 18: 814-816
9. Goligher JC (1957) The treatment of complete prolapse of the rectum by the Roscoe Graham operation. Br J Surg 45: 323-333
10. Goligher JC (1980) Surgery of the colon, anus and rectum, 4th edn. Ballière Tindall, London
11. Hawley P (1975) Procidentia of the rectum: Ivalon-sponge repair. Dis Colon Rectum 18: 461-463
12. Henry MM (1985) Descending perineum syndrome. In: Henry MM, Swash M (eds) Coloproctology and the pelvic floor. Butterworths, London, pp 299-302
13. Hiltunen KM, Matikainen M, Auvinen O, Hietanen P (1986) Clinical and manometric evaluation of anal sphincter function in patients with rectal prolapse. Am J Surg 151: 489-492
14. Hoffman MJ, Kodner IJ, Fry RD (1984) Internal intussusception of the rectum. Diagnosis and surgical management. Dis Colon Rectum 27: 435-441
15. Keighley MRB, Fielding JWL, Alexander-Williams J (1983) Results of Marlex mesh abdominal rectopexy for rectal prolapse in 100 consecutive patients. Br J Surg 70: 229-232
16. Kupfer CA, Goligher JC (1970) One hundred consecutive cases of complete prolapse of the rectum treated by operation. Br J Surg 57: 481-487
17. Litschgi M, Käser O (1978) Zum Problem der Enterozelen. Geburtshilfe Frauenheilkd 38: 915-920
18. Morgan CN (1962) The use of Ivalon sponge. Proc R Soc Med 55: 1084-1085
19. Parks AG, Porter NH, Hardcastle J (1966) The syndrome of the descending perineum. Proc R Soc Med 59: 477-482
20. Parks AG, Percy J (1983) Postanal pelvic floor repair for anorectal incontinence. In: Todd IP, Fielding LP (eds) Rob and Smith's operative surgery, 4th edn. Alimentary tract and abdominal wall. 3 Colon rectum and anus. Butterworths, London, pp 433-438
21. Penfold JCB, Hawley PR (1972) Experiences of Ivalon-sponge implantat for complete rectal prolapse at St Mark's Hospital, 1960-70. Br J Surg 59: 846-848
22. Porter N (1980) Results of Ivalon sponge repair for rectal prolapse. In: Pichlmaier H, Grundmann R (eds) Surgery of the colon and rectum. Thieme, Stuttgart, pp 45-49
23. Read NW, Bannister JJ (1985) Anorectal manometry: techniques in health and anorectal disease. In: Henry MM, Swash M (eds) Coloproctology and the pelvic floor. Butterworths, London, pp 65-87
24. Rutter KRP (1985) Solitary ulcer syndrome of the rectum: its relation to mucosal prolapse. In: Henry MM, Swash M (eds) Coloproctology and the pelvic floor. Butterworths, London, pp 282-298
25. Schweiger MC (1983) Rektumprolaps und ulcus simplex recti des Erwachsenen. Klinikarzt 12: 84-96
26. Stewart R (1972) Long-term results of ovalon wrap operation for complete rectal prolapse. Proc R Soc Med 65: 777-778

27. Sudeck P (1922) Rektumprolapsoperation durch Auslösung des Rektum aus der excavatio sacralis. Zentralblatt für Chirurgie 20: 698–699
28. Swash M (1985) Histopathology of the pelvic floor muscles. In: Henry MM, Swash M (eds) Coloproctology and the pelvic floor. Pathophysiology and management. Butterworths, London, pp 129–150
29. Swash M, Snooks SJ (1985) Electromyography in pelvic floor disorders. In: Henry MM, Swash M (eds) Coloproctology and the pelvic floor. Pathophysiology and management. Butterworths, London, pp 88–103
30. Swash M (1985) New concepts in incontinence. Br Med J 4: 290
31. Todd IP (1985) Clinical evaluation of the pelvic floor. In: Henry MM, Swash M (eds) Coloproctology and the pelvic floor. Pathophysiology and management. Butterworths, London, pp 187–191
32. Watts JD, Rothenberger DA, Goldberg SM (1985) Rectal prolapse. B. Treatment. In: Henry MM, Swash M (eds) Coloproctology and the pelvic floor. Pathophysiology and Management. Butterworths, London, pp 308–339
33. Wells C (1959) New operation for rectal prolapse. Proc R Soc Med 52: 602–603
34. Wells C (1962) Polyvinyl alcohol sponge prothesis. Proc R Soc Med 55: 1083–1984
35. Womack NR, Morrison JFB, Williams NS (1986) The role of pelvic floor denervation in the aetiology of idiopathic faecal incontinence. Br J Surg 73: 404–407

24 Anorectal Strictures

M.-C. Marti

Definition and Etiology

A stricture is an abnormal narrowing of a tubular structure like the anorectum. Such narrowings may be classified according their etiology, location, length, and severity. They may be the result of a malignant or a benign process [3]. Malignant lesions may be intrinsic or extrinsic depending on where the primary is located. Intrinsic lesions are caused by anal carcinoma and rectal rumors, whereas extrinsic ones are mainly the result of urogenital tumors in men and women.

Benign strictures may also be intrinsic or extrinsic. Extrinsic lesions are rare and are the result of retrorectal tumors and cysts, endometriosis, hematocele, and pelvic abscess. Intrinsic processes are the most frequent cause of stenotic lesions. They may be the result of inflammatory bowel disease, local infection, abscesses, radiation injury, trauma, and congenital lesions. Inflammatory lesions producing stenosis are caused by Crohn's disease, colitis, amebiasis, lymphogranuloma venereum, gonorrhea, tuberculosis, bilharziosis, and actinomycosis. Anorectal stenosis develops in 4%–9% of patients with colitis [4] and a large percentage of patients with Crohn's disease [5].

Irradiation for carcinoma of the cervix, prostate, and anal canal may occasionally result in a stricture within an area of more or less severe proctitis. The incidence of complications is related to the dosage of irradiation. Most frequently, however, anal stenosis has a posttraumatic and a postoperative origin. Five to ten percent of hemorrhoidectomies result in some degree of stenosis [3]. Stenosis at the anal verge is due to the excess removal of skin below the dentate line leaving bridges which are too small. Stenosis within the anal canal is due to generous inclusion of mucosa and submucosa in the ligation of the hemorrhoidal pedicle.

Various surgical procedures may induce rectal stenosis: low anterior resection with hand suture or stapling, pull-through procedures, rectopexy according to Rippstein with Ivalon sponge implantation.

Fibrotic stenosis occur 2–3 months after surgery.

They result from ischemia, partial anastomotic leakage, and infection. They are more frequent if the anastomosis has been protected by a diverting colostomy. Improper use of the EEA stapler has also been inferred: two small cartridge diameter, extensive devascularization of the bowel, and excessive dilatation of the proximal bowel extremity to allow passage of the stapler. In the immediate postoperative period every anastomosis has a more or less reduced diameter due to local enema. This condition improves spontaneously with stool passage and is usually asymptomatic. After 6 months to 1 year the exact location of an anastomosis can no longer be found by digital examination or sigmoidoscopy. In the case of late stenosis, an anastomotic recurrence should be always suspected.

Clinical Aspects and Diagnosis

Anorectal stenosis results in constipation, difficulties in evacuation, false bowel movements, diarrhea. After colorectal anastomosis the reported incidence of more and less severe stenosis varies from 0% to 50%. Medical records and clinical examination are sufficient to confirm the stricture. Endoscopy, biopsy, extensive X-ray examination, and bacteriological and serological investigations are necessary to confirm the etiology. Endoanal echography and deep biopsy are mandatory in cases of late rectal stenosis in order to exclude tumor recurrence. Multiple biopsies should be performed in cases of narrowing to investigate the various etiologies and to exclude a malignancy.

Treatment of Anal Stenosis

Treatment depends on the nature and extent of the stenosis. Specific measures are required for tumors and infections. Mild stenosis with minimal symptoms may be managed by dietetic measures and repeated dilatation. Severe stenosis should be treated by some form of anoplasty as dilatation would only result in tearing.

Medical and Conservative Treatment

Nonoperative management is based on the administration of laxatives (lubricant and bulk-forming agents), enemas, and repeated instrumental or digital dilatation. A high stenosis, beyond the reach of a Heggar dilator, may be distended with a special balloon dilator.

Anoplasty

If surgery is planned, the following rules must be observed:

- The perianal skin must be healthy and thick.
- Bowel preparation is mandatory to delay the passage of stools.
- Perioperative broad-spectrum antibiotics should be used.
- Meticulous hemostasis must be achieved.
- Suture must be performed only with absorbable material.
- Postoperative care involves repeated local disinfection and dressing, and administration of drugs which reduce bowel motility for 5–7 days.

Lateral sphincterotomy (see Chap. 10) is the most simple surgical treatment of an anal stenosis. It may be used in conjunction with skin flaps, especially if an associated mucosal ectropion is be excised.

Y-V Flap

The incision begins within the anal canal at the level of the dentate line and extends caudally until the mucocutaneous junction or anal margin (Fig. 24.1).

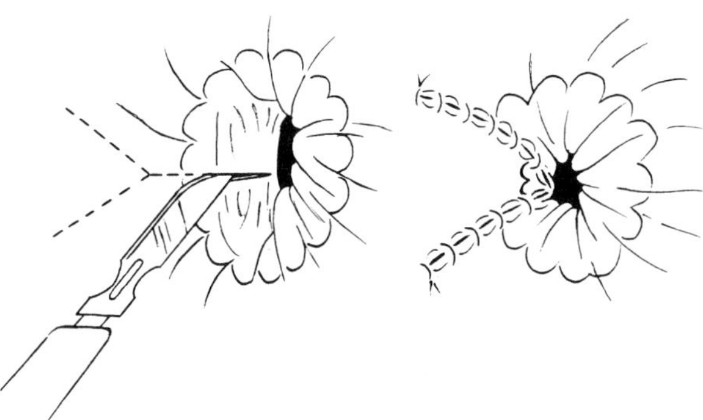

Fig. 24.1. Y-V flap

From this point, two V-shaped incisions into the gluteal skin complete the Y. The full-thickness skin flap should be wide with no subcutaneous tissue or fat. An internal sphincterotomy is performed. The flap is mobilized and advanced into the anal canal. The Y incision is converted into a V and sutured. Lateral edges may be undermined to facilitate suture without tension [7].

Flap Procedure

A lateral radial incision is made at 3 and 9 o'clock through the scarred anal mucosa and scarred adjacent perianal skin. The lower portion of the internal sphincter is incised. A diamond-shaped flap is created [1]. The leading half of the flap must have approximately the same dimensions as the intra-anal portion of the defect that has just been created (Fig. 24.2). The flap is mobilized but undermined as little as possible to prevent a change in the blood supply. The flap is sutured without tension to the

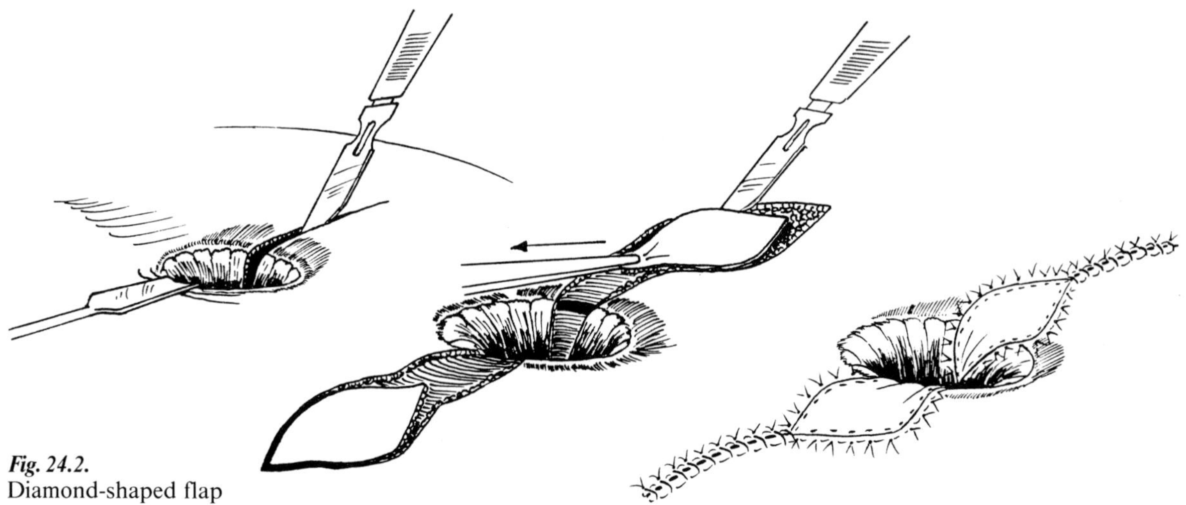

Fig. 24.2.
Diamond-shaped flap

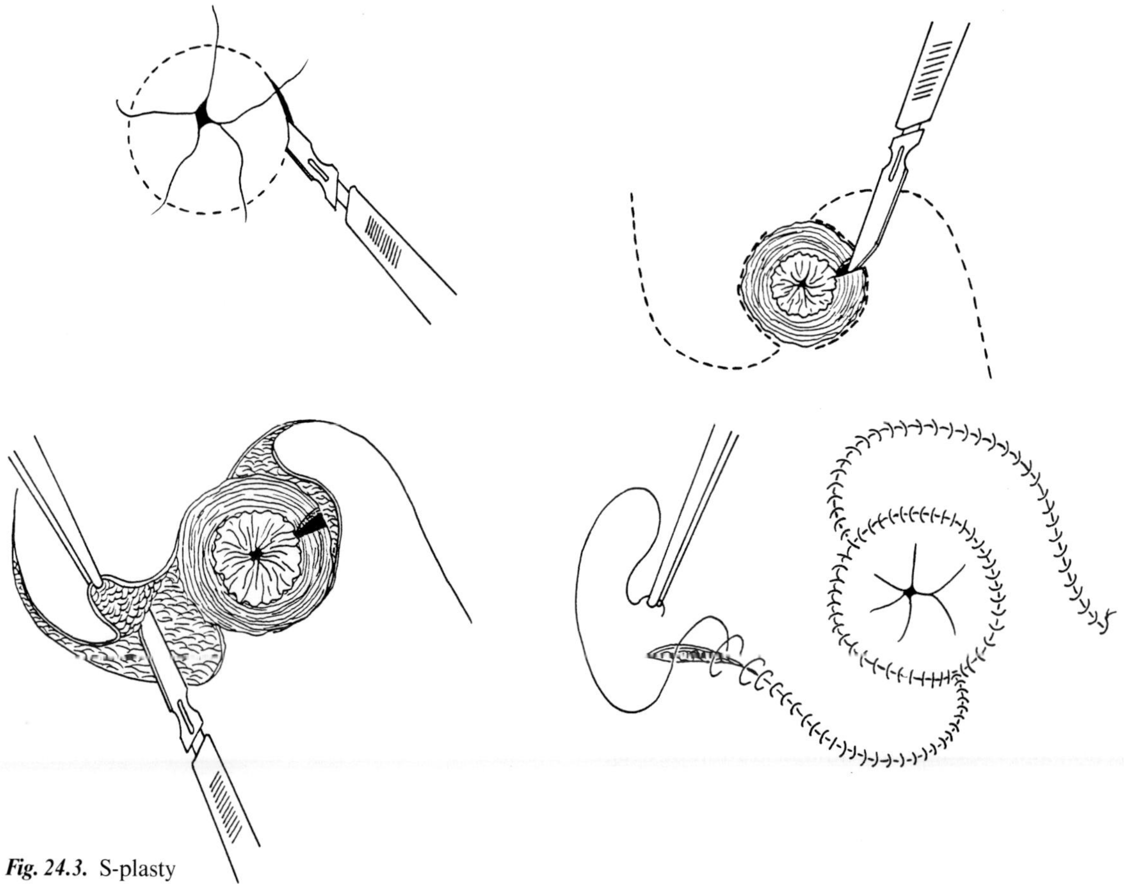

Fig. 24.3. S-plasty

mucosa with absorbable material. The donor defect and the skin are sutured with simple sutures of 4-0 or 5-0 nylon. The same technique may be used if a mucosal ectropion has been excised.

S-Plasty

Fergusson [2] first described a technique to correct a Whitehead deformity with two rotational flaps [6]. This procedure may also be used to treat circumferential anal stenosis (Fig. 24.3). A circular incision is made and all scar tissue or ectropion is excised in a cranial direction until the level of normal and healthy mucosa. Partial internal sphincterotomy is performed. Two or even three wide rotational flaps are created. They are elevated toward their bases and should be lined with as little as possible subcutaneous fat. After careful hemostasis, they are sutured with absorbable material in such a manner that a new 360° mucocutaneous junction is constructed within the anal canal.

The defect at the outer extremities of the flap should be closed only if no tension is created. To prevent abnormal tissue tension, multiple small incisions may be performed. The extremities of the wounds may also be left open for secondary granulation.

Two- and Four-Quadrant Sphincterotomy With or Without Sliding Skin Flaps

In patients with tight anal stenosis in whom sphincterotomy with a sliding graft would not result in an adequate anal canal diameter, Sarner [9] has advocated a two- or four-quadrant sphincterotomy with skin grafts (Fig. 24.4).

Sarafoff Procedure

Excessive tension on the suture line or pulling down of mucosa while performing a Whitehead hemorrhoidectomy results in a so-called Whitehead deformity characterized by stenosis and ectropion formation. Among the various techniques advocated to overcome this lesion, the Sarafoff [8] procedure is very useful in treating particularly the ec-

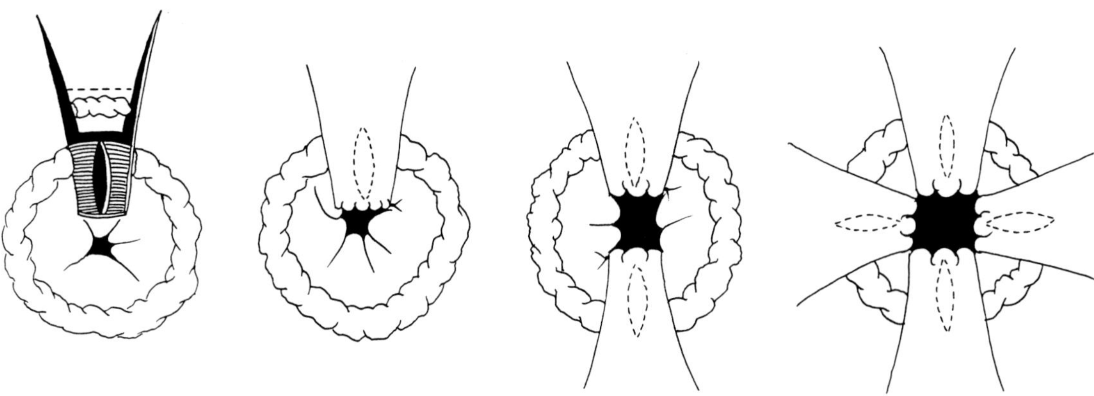

Fig. 24.4. Four-quadrant sphincterotomomy with skin flaps

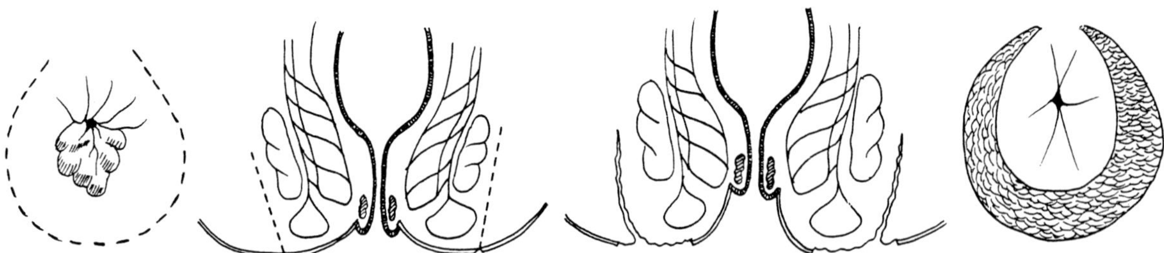

Fig. 24.5. Sarafoff procedure

tropion (Fig. 24.5). A deep circular incision is performed 2 cm away from the anal margin. The skin and the subcutaneous tissue are incised up to the fascia. By retracting the anal canal mucosa and the previous suture line, the ectropion disappears. The wound is left open and heals by secondary granulation in 4–6 weeks.

Treatment of Rectal Stenosis

The best dilatation of a rectal stenosis is obtained by passage of stools. Spontaneous improvement is noticed after closure of a diverting colostomy. If the narrowing is very severe, digital and instrumental dilatation can be performed. In instrumental dilatation, a straight Heggar dilatator or the more recently available curved ones can be used. The instrument is pushed through an anuscope. Dilatation should be performed under general anesthesia or at least sedation. Large bowel preparation and antibioprophyllaxis are required to prevent septicemia. The procedure should be repeated every 2–3 months for 1 year.

Bowel and anastomotic rupture represent the most severe complications of forceful dilatation. In some cases, dilatation may even induce a more severe fibrosis with aggravation of the stenosis. If the fibrotic ring is very stiff and does not allow stretching, partial excision or multiple small incisions may be required.

Resection of the stenosis can be achieved using an EEA stapler; the instrument is introduced through the anal canal and the anal wall is fixed by a short colostomy above the narrowing. In more severe cases, resection of the anastomosis may be necessary.

If none of these measures is successful or if the patient cannot be submitted to major surgery, definitive colostomy should be planned.

References

1. Caplin DA, Kodner IJ (1986) Repair of anal stricture and mucosal ectropion by simple flap procedure. Dis Colon Rectum 29: 92–94
2. Ferguson JA (1959) Repair of "Whitehead deformity" of the anus. Surg Gynecol Obstet 108: 115–116
3. Goldberg SM, Gordon PP, Nivatvongs S (1980) Strictures of the anorectum. Lippincott, Philadelphia, pp 333–341
4. Goulston SJM, McGovern VJ (1969) The nature of benign strictures in ulcerative colitis. N Engl J Med 281: 290–295

5. Greenstein AJ, Sachar DB, Kark A (1975) Strictures of the anorectum in Crohn's disease involving the colon. Ann Surg 181: 207–212
6. Hudson AT (1967) S-plasty repair of Whitehead deformity of the anus. Dis Colon Rectum 10: 57–60
7. Nickell WB, Woodward ER (1972) Advancement of flaps for treatment of anal stricture. Arch Surg 104: 223–224
8. Sarafoff O (1937) Ein einfaches und ungefährliches Verfahren zur operativen Behandlung des Mastdarmvorfalles. Langenbecks Arch Klin Chir 190: 219–232
9. Sarner JB (1969) Plastic relief of anal stenosis. Dis Colon Rectum 12: 277–280

25 Essential Anorectal Pain or Idiopathic Perianal Pain

M.-C. Marti

Essential anorectal pain is characterized by the absence of any anomaly detectable by endoscopy and radiological examinations [10, 12]. Systematization of the pains and their correlation with the patient's medical history and clinical examination are difficult. The term "essential anorectal pain" includes three main diseases which, however, sometimes overlap [3, 10] (Table 25.1):

- Proctalgia fugax
- Coccygodynia
- Anorectal neuralgia

Essential anorectal pain must be distinguished from anorectal or pelvic pain due to identifiable anatomic lesions [3, 10]. This may be done by means of clinical examination and complementary tests. The diagnosis of essential anorectal pain should be made only after having excluded all possibility of an organic lesion.

The medical history of the patient should specify the manner in which these pains appear, their nature, time of appearance, evolution, and intensity. These details help to carry out the clinical examination and arrive at a diagnosis. Additional tests, which are sometimes complex, are also necessary: double-contrast barium enemas, defecography, CAT scan, endoanal ultrasonography, electromyography, and anorectal manometry. However, for most diagnoses, rectal examination, proctoscopy, and the patient's medical history provide sufficient information.

Proctalgia Fugax

Proctalgia fugax was first described by Thaysen [15] in 1935. It is characterized by a short attack of deep rectal pain which almost always comes at night. It occurs repeatedly, but unpredictably and at rather long intervals. Its occurrence is probably more frequent than some statistics would indicate. Because of the brevity of the attacks and the long intervals between them, many patients do not consult a doctor [1, 10, 15]. Proctalgia fugax occurs mostly in men in the 40–60 age group. Some cases in children have been reported.

The pain, which generally occurs in the supra-anal region, is deep, penetrating, and rectal; it is described as gnawing, aching, cramp like, or stabbing; and its location can be described precisely by the patient. In a given patient, it always occurs in the same place. The duration of the attack is extremely short, ranging from several seconds to 30 min, but it is constant for a given person. Patients are woken up by the pain, which may be accompanied by spasms, false bowel movement, painful priapism, and neurovegetative disorders such as paleness, sweating, and lipothymia. It may occur after sexual intercourse. A family medical history is sometimes collected [6]. In general, neither the clinical examination nor the medical history reveal intestinal disorders, alternating diarrhea and constipation, or tenesmus. However, some patients do have symptoms of irritable bowel syndrome [2, 18] or functional colopathy.

Table 25.1. Clinical aspects of essential anorectal pains

Disorder	Mean age at onset	Sex predominance	Nature of pain	Site
Proctalgia fugax	Young adults	Male	Sudden, lasting less than 30 min, ceases spontaneously	Upper anal canal
Coccygodynia	Any age	Female	Continuous with exacerbation	Coccyx, perineum, anal canal
Anorectal neuralgia	Adults	Female	Continuous burning, like a foreign body in the anal canal or pelvis	Well localized in the mid-anal canal

The causes of proctalgia fugax are not understood. Douthwaite [5] has suggested spasms of the levator ani. This disorder has been compared to "rectal angor" resulting from transient mesenteric ischemia, to a muscular spasm in the anorectal junction, or even to a neurovegetative pain factor. Observations have been published demonstrating rectal vascular disorders which respond well to trinitrine treatment [3]. Proctoscopies performed immediately after the peak of an attack, while the pain is still subsiding, have shown an injection of mucus with stenosing edema that gave rise to gaseous distension of the immediately proximal colon. The insertion and withdrawal of a proctoscope allowed the evacuation of the gas, thereby relieving the patient immediately.

In addition, Pilling et al. [13] studied the personality of 48 patients suffering from proctalgia fugax. All of these patients had professional problems, were anxious, tense, and perfectionists, and had frequently shown neurotic symptoms during their childhood. According to Pilling et al., the patients' physical disorders were psychosomatic manifestations of their emotional conflicts.

Treating proctalgia fugax is extremely difficult because of the shortness and unpredictability of the attacks, the lack of knowledge concerning the exact etiopathology of the disorder, and the absence of any organic anomaly after the attacks. After several attacks, many patients find a way of relieving the pain by means of pain-relieving postures, manual pressure on the perineum, endoanal manipulations, enemas, walking, and changing position [3]. These various measures seem to act on the muscles involved in the etiology of the pain. Some authors have found that trinitrine, papaverine, or amyl nitrite [3, 11] give good results, which tends to confirm the vascular origin of this disorder. Venous tonics have sometimes also given good results. Because of the long interval between attacks, it is difficult to claim therapeutic success for the various measures mentioned here.

Coccygodynia

Simpson, in 1859 [14], first described a syndrome he called "coccygodynias". Coccygodynias may present differently according to whether the pain is situated in the coccyx or in the rectum. Coccygodynia is characterized by pain upon movement of or pressure on the coccyx. The patient is usually unable to specify the exact location of the pain. It appears spontaneously and is like a weight in the pelvic region, a burning sensation, a tenesmus that is of average intensity but permanent and anxiety causing. The pain is sometimes punctuated by defecation and exacerbated by prolonged sitting. It thus occurs more frequently in female factory workers, secretaries, or persons who spend long intervals watching television ("television bottom"). Attacks tend to occur at the end of the day and are seen twice as often in women as in men, in all age groups [16, 17].

The patients' medical history often includes past lesions which are often blamed for the occurrence of the coccygodynia:

- Trauma to the sacrococcygeal region including contusion or fracture
- Repeated microtrauma (horseback riders)
- Obstetrical pathologies: forceps births, breech presentation
- Vertebral osteoarthritis and postural disorders of the spine
  Previous history of sciatica pain and radiculopathy
- Multiple rheumatic lesions

The clinical examination is negative even though sometimes small hemorrhoidal lesions are present. Digital examination per rectum, in particular bimanual endoanal and retrococcygeal palpation, reveal painful zones on the coccyx and adjacent structures. The following symptoms should be noted [8]:

- Pain when the coccyx is mobilized
- Pain along the sacrococcygeal junction
- Pain on the anterior surface of the coccyx in the zone of insertion of the anococcygeal ligament
- Pain at the insertion site of the levator ani and on the ischiococcygeal ligaments
- Contractures of the levator ani

Contractures are immediately perceived as a tight cord stretched between the median and the pelvic wall [7, 16, 17]. This contracture is usually unilateral or at least predominates on one side. On the basis of these various clinical findings and indications from medical histories, three causes of coccygodynia have been postulated: past trauma, sacral radiculitis at S4-S5, and postural disorders of the lumbar region with muscular contractures.

Treatment of coccygodynia includes both local and general measures. The local infiltration of lidocaine with or without corticosteroids may relieve the pain [7]. The injection should not be made near the sacrococcygeal joint but through the perineum at the level of the contracture. It is therefore pointless to infiltrate posteriorly. The infiltration is followed by an endoanal massage, as described by Thiele [17], of the contractured zones.

The massage has to be repeated once a day or every 2 days over a period of 5-10 days [16, 17]. The objective is to make the muscular contracture disappear. Even if it lasts no longer than a few minutes, the massage is painful for the patient and tiring for the proctologist. The treatment is to be supplemented by the systemic administration of muscle relaxants and anti-inflammatory drugs for a period of 3-4 weeks. In addition, the patient should undergo physiotherapy to develop the paravertebral muscles, and postural problems should be corrected. Surgery must be avoided. Coccygectomies have usually only aggravated the clinical condition of the patient. Coccygodynia may be considered as the first sign of the degeneration of the lumbosacral intervertebral disc [4].

Supportive psychotherapy may be helpful, in particular in cancerophobic patients. In case these various therapeutic measures are unsuccessful, sacral radicotomy may be considered.

Anorectal Neuralgia

The term "neuralgia" is imprecise and therefore often inadequate, despite its use by most authors. Anorectal neuralgic pain is characterized by its lack of precision. Patients complain of diffuse pain which may radiate in various directions such as the sacrum, thighs, or the anterior part of the vagina. It usually occurs in women over 50 who are often anxious and cancerophobic. The clinical examination is totally negative, but it is noteworthy that almost 60% of these patients have undergone multiple gynecological treatments, in particular hysterectomies, and treatment for discal hernia.

These pains can thus be described as anorectal neuralgia, essentially of genital origin. Some patients present a painless essential contracture of the levator ani at the height of the coccyx, accompanied by tenesmus. These cases can therefore be distinguished from cases of coccygodynia. In some patients, the radiation of the pain follows a partial sciatic distribution and suggests a form of radiculopathy due to compression or fibrosis of a sacral nerve root [3]. Electrophysiological studies suggest that lesions are located on the genital nerve or on a more proximal sacral nerve root [12]. Lastly, some patients who are depressive or even neurotic may develop true psychogenic pain. Some patients present tension headache together with rectal symptoms. This combination of symptoms has been named "top and bottom syndrome" [9].

The diagnosis of anorectal neuralgia should be accepted only once all therapeutic measures have proven unsuccessful. Patients with such a diagnosis have often undergone many medical or even surgical treatments.

The administration of analgesics is useful, but the prescription must be changed frequently. Antidepressants and anxiolytics may be prescribed, and supportive psychotherapy should be undertaken to reassure these patients and teach them how to come to terms with their disorder as there is no truly effective treatment.

References

1. Abrahams A (1935) Proctalgia fugax. Lancet II: 455
2. Bensaude A (1965) Proctalgies fugaces. Acta Gastroenterol Belg 28: 594-604
3. Boisson J, Debbasch L, Bensaude A (1966) Algies anorectales essentielles. Arch Fr Mal Appar Dig 55: 3-24
4. Crenshaw AH (ed) (1971) Campbell's operative orthopedics. Mosby, St Louis
5. Donthwaite AH (1962) Proctalgia fugax. Br Med J 2: 164-165
6. Ewing MR (1953) Proctalgia fugax. Br Med J I: 1083-1085
7. Grant SR, Salvati EP, Rubin RJ (1975) Levator syndrome: an analysis of 316 cases. Dis Colon Rectum 18: 161-163
8. Lievre JA, Attali P (1966) La coccygodynie. Arch Fr Mal Appar Dig 55: 25-38
9. Lovshin LL (1961) Anorectal symptoms of emotional origin. Dis Colon Rectum 4: 399-402
10. Marti M-C (1984) Les algies pelviennes d'origine proctologique. Méd Hyg 42: 3889-3890
11. Mc Ewin R (1956) Proctalgia fugax. Med J Aust 2: 337-340
12. Neill ME, Swash M (1982) Chronic perianal pain: an unsolved problem. J R Soc Med 75: 96-101
13. Pilling LF, Pilling LF, Swenson WM, Hill JR (1965) The psychologic aspects of proctalgia fugax. Dis Colon Rectum 8: 372-376
14. Simpson JY (1859) Clinical lectures on the diseases of women. Lecture XVII. On coccygodynia and the diseases and deformities of the coccyx. M Times and Gaz 40: 1
15. Thaysen EH (1935) Proctalgia fugax. Lancet II: 243-246
16. Thiele GH (1950) Coccygodynia: mechanism of its production and its relationship to anorectal diseases. Am J Surg 79: 110-116
17. Thiele GH (1963) Coccygodynia. Dis Colon Rectum 6: 422-436
18. Thompson WG, Heaton KW (1980) Proctalgia fugax. J R Coll Med 14: 247-248

postoperative clinical signs suggesting infection or a pelvic hematoma require a laparotomy with total diverting colostomy and drainage [24].

In cases of severe extraperitoneal rectal lesions or if signs of infection develop after conservative treatment, emergency laparotomy is necessary. The rectum should be fully mobilized and the lesion repaired. A proximal left end colostomy is established with a distal mucous fistula to allow lavage of the rectal stump [16].

In cases of pelvic fracture with injury to the rectum, severe bleeding and sepsis may occur [7]. The rectum should be repaired, if possible, using an intraluminal approach, and a left iliac colostomy must be performed. This is a compromise as any extensive mobilization of the rectum would increase the risk of bleeding. Clearing of the rectum should be performed through a rigid sigmoidoscope with suction to avoid extravasation of feces [13].

Severe perianal laceration and pelvic fractures can induce massive and uncontrollable bleeding. Ligature of the hypogastric or even iliac artery does not help. If the bleeding is due to a pelvic fracture, the application of a "g-suit" combined with angiographic embolization can be effective [12]. If not successful, an emergency abdominoperineal excision may be necessary to control the bleeding by packing [10].

Drainage

Drainage will be achieved through the anterior abdominal wall in every case. If extensive mobilization of the rectum up to the tip of the coccyx has been necessary, the presacral space should be drained through the perineum. The anococcygeal raphe will be divided longitudinally to avoid nerve damage, and drainage will be exteriorized in front of the coccyx without tearing either the sphincter or the puborectalis sling.

Completion of Laparotomy

Any other intraabdominal lesion should also be repaired. In penetrating trauma, the "rule of two" should be followed. Tangential lesions are rare. Ignorance of a second perforation, even if far away from the first one, results in severe complication and high morbidity and mortality. Injury to the bladder or the vagina should be repaired and drained according to the site of the lesion. Before closing the abdominal cavity, each compartment should be washed and dried to ensure correct hemostasis. If the abdominal wall is contaminated, delayed primary closure may be useful.

Treatment of Sphincter Injuries

Any severe sphincter or pelvic tears should be immediately repaired according to the principles described in Chap. 22.

When Should Continuity Be Restored?

Continuity can be restored after the rectal wounds have healed and the inflammation has disappeared. Sphincter function should be assessed by digital examination, defecography, manometry, and functional examination.

References

1. Abcarian H, Lowe R (1978) Colon and rectal trauma. Surg Clin North Am 58: 519–536
2. Barone JE, Sohn N, Nealon TF (1976) Perforations and foreign bodies of the rectum. Ann Surg 184: 601–604
3. Bartizal JF, Boyd DR, Folk FA (1974) A critical review of management of 392 colonic and rectal injuries. Dis Colon Rectum 17: 313–318
4. Biggs TM, Beall AC (1963) Surgical management of civilian colon injuries. J Trauma 3: 484
5. Black CT, Pokorny WJ, McGill CW, Harberg FJ (1982) Anorectal trauma in children. J Pediatr Surg 17: 501–504
6. Crass RA, Tranbough RF, Kudsk KA, Trunkey D (1981) Colorectal foreign bodies and perforation. Am J Surg 142: 85–87
7. Flint LM, Brown A, Richardson D, Polk H (1979) Definitive control of bleeding from severe pelvic fractures. Ann Surg 189: 709–716
8. Frazer J, Drummond H (1917) A clinical and experimental study of three hundred perforating wounds of the abdomen. Br Med J 1: 321–330
9. Ganchrow MI, Lavenson GS Jr, McNamara JJ (1970) Surgical management of traumatic injuries of the colon and rectum. Arch Surg 100: 515–520
10. Getzen LC, Pollack FW, Wolffmann FF (1977) Abdomino-perineal resection in the treatment of devascularizing rectal injuries. Surgery 82: 310
11. Haas PA, Fox FA (1979) Civilian injuries of the rectum and anus. Dis Colon Rectum 22: 17–23
12. Kusminsky R, Shbeeb I, Makos G, Boland J (1982) Blunt pelviperineal injuries. Dis Colon Rectum 25: 787–790
13. Lavenson GS Jr, Cohen A (1971) Management of rectal injuries. Am J Surg 122: 226–231
14. Lee BJ (1927) Wounds of the abdomen. In: Weed FW, McAfee L (eds) The Medical Department of the United States army in the World War, vol II. US Surgeon General's Office, pp 443–469

15. Marti MC, Garcia J, Cox J (1976) Complications chirurgicales des lavements barytés. Schweiz Med Wochenschr 106: 1182-1187
16. Marti MC, Morel P, Rohner A (1986) Traumatic lesions of the rectum. Colorectal Dis 1: 152-154
17. Maull KI, Sachatello CR, Ernst CB (1977) The deep perineal lacerations - an injury frequently associated with open pelvic fractures: a need for aggressive surgical management. J Trauma 17: 685-696
18. Miller RE, Sullivan FJ (1976) Rectal wounds incurred in Vietnam. Milit Med 141: 764-770
19. Morgan GN (1945) Wounds of the rectum. Surg Gynecol Obstet 81: 56-62
20. Mac Mortensen MJ, Irvin TT (1984) Disembowelment per rectum: a fatal rectal injury. Br J Surg 71: 289
21. Olgilvie WH (1944) Abdominal wounds in the Western Desert. Surg Gynecol Obstet 78: 225-238
22. Pradel E, Baviera E, Juillard F, Terris G (1984) Les ulcérations ano-rectales d'origine sodomique. Med Chir Dig 13: 645-648
23. Reiner SC (1984) Colorectal laceration after manual-anal intercourse. Ann Emerg Med 13: 130-132
24. Robertson HD, Ray JF, Ferrari BT, Bayron J (1982) Management of rectal trauma. Surg Gynecol Obstet 154: 161-164
25. Sohn N, Weinstein MA, Gonchar J (1977) Social injuries of the rectum. Am J Surg 134: 611-612
26. Taylor ER, Thompson JE (1948) The early treatment and results thereof, of injuries of the colon and rectum. Int Abst Surg 87: 209
27. Thal ER, Yeary EC (1980) Morbidity of colostomy closure following colon trauma. J Trauma 20: 287-291
28. Thomas LP (1953) Impalement of the rectum. Lancet II: 704
29. Tournier C, Croguennec B, Pillegand B, Claude R (1981) Ulcères rectaux par sodomisation animale. Nouv Presse Med 10: 1152
30. Wanebo HJ, Hunt TK, Mathewson C (1969) Rectal injuries. J Trauma 9: 721-722
31. Weckesser EC, Putman TC (1902) Perforating injuries of the rectum and sigmoid colon. J Trauma 2: 474-487
32. Witz M, Shpitz B, Zager M, Eliashiv A, Dinbar A (1984) Anal erotic instrumentation. Dis Colon Rectum 27: 331-332
33. Ziperman HH (1970) The management of large bowel injuries in the Korean campaign. US Armed Forces Med J 7: 85-91

27 Foreign Bodies

M.-C. Marti

Anal and rectal wounds may result from ingested foreign bodies and from a variety of objects passed through the rectum. Lesions due to ingested bodies are not common [3], whereas those resulting from foreign bodies introduced into the rectum are becoming more and more frequent [2]. Migration from the peritoneum has been reported on occasion.

Ingested Foreign Bodies

Ingested foreign bodies that occur in natural food, such as pips, thorns, seeds, and soft bones, are normally totally digested by the time they reach the lower intestinal tract. Chicken and rabbit bones, toothpicks, shells, pieces of glass, plastic and metallic clips used in food wrapping can pass through the intestinal tract without being digested and may cause rectal or anal injury.

Infants, children, or mentally deranged adults may ingest foreign bodies of various sizes and forms such as batteries, forks, knives, keys, nails, screws, spoons, etc. Pieces of denture are among the most dangerous foreign bodies as they can easily perforate the bowel.

Narcotics wrapped in condoms have been swallowed to avoid detection by customs authorities and may result in acute obstruction or acute toxicity if absorption occurs after rupture [6].

The signs observed include hemorrhage, mucosal tears, abscesses, bowel perforation, and death [5, 14, 21]. Seventy-five percent of perforations occur at the level of the ileocecal valve and appendix [21], but swallowed objects may lodge in the rectum or in the anal canal and cause trauma such as laceration.

The surgeon should decide whether it is better to wait for the foreign body to pass or to perform an endoscopy to remove it within the first hour or two after ingestion. Even large objects which are 1 cm in diameter and 12 cm long can be spontaneously eliminated. Surgery is required only in 1% of cases. Anorectoscopic removal may be necessary if the foreing body is stuck in the rectal wall or is causing symptoms of impaction.

Migration from the Peritoneum

In cases of gallbladder rupture, stones may be eliminated through the rectum. The peritoneal extremity of ventriculoperitoneal shunts have been spontaneously extruded through the rectum [16, 18].

Introduced Foreign Bodies

As expressed by Goldberg [11], "the variety of objects passed per rectum that become entrapped above the anal sphincter musculature and subsequently require removal is limited only by the imagination of human mind." Injury results from introduction, decubital lesions, penetration of the bowel wall, perforation, and impaction when lost inside the rectum. Various foreign bodies have been introduced into the rectum [2, 8, 13]:

- In diagnostic and therapeutic procedures: thermometers, rectal tubes, enema tips, irrigation catheters.
- To self-treat and to alleviate symptoms of anorectal disease: broomstick handles to relieve itching or to reduce prolapsed hemorrhoids.
- In criminal assault: sticks, glass bottles, tips of air compressors or bicycle pumps.
- For sexual stimulation and autoeroticism (mainly in homosexual men but also in women): vibrators, plastic phalluses and sticks, bottles, baby powder cans, batteries, flashlights, lightbulbs, baseballs, cucumbers, bananas, carrots, grapefruit, oranges, stones, screwdrivers, etc. [2, 7, 9, 10, 13, 19]. Cases of manual anal intercourse resulting in mucosal laceration or even perforation of the rectosigmoid have been reported [20].
- Accidental introduction with loss inside the rectum is very rare.

Treatment

The patients' imagination must be surpassed by the physicians' ingeniousness to withdraw the various foreign bodies inserted into the rectum. Extraction may be difficult for several reasons [4]:

- The foreign body has a smooth surface which is difficult to grasp.
- The foreign body is friable or hard and unyielding.
- Vision may be obscured by mucus and blood.
- The rectal mucosa may be edematous and bulging.
- Negative pressure above the foreign body may hold it by suction and interfere with traction.
- The curve of the sacrum tends to hold the lower end away from the anus.
- The anal sphincter may be in spasm.

The following principles should always be observed:

1. Abdominal and pelvic plain and lateral radiographs should be performed to determine the type, number, size, and location of foreign bodies and to exclude signs of peritoneal perforation.
2. Extraction should always be tried in the lithotomy position to allow simultaneous access to the anorectum and to the abdomen. If surgery is required, the same position is necessary.
3. An intravenous line should be placed to allow adequate relaxation and sedation of the patient if necessary. Local, locoregional, or even general anesthesia may be required to ensure sphincter relaxation or dilatation. Sphincterotomy is rarely necessary.
4. The anal canal should be lubricated. Air should be inflated within the rectum through catheters or sigmoidoscopes to minimize the effect of suction or negative pressure created above the foreign body by withdrawal.
5. Several techniques have been proposed to facilitate extraction:
   - Colonoscopic extraction even for large foreign bodies [22].
   - Use of clamps and various forceps [17].
   - Obstetrical forceps [19].
   - A corkscrew to remove a rubber ball or a corn cob.
   - Slings of mesh placed around the foreign body or stuck to it whith superglue [15].
   - A foley catheter inserted above the object to pull it down and out [23].
   - Insertion of a Stengstaken-Blakemore tube within a hollow object [12].
   - Filling a hollow object with plaster of Paris and gauze: when the plaster sets, extraction is facilitated by the gauze [7].

6. Laparotomy should be used only as the last resort after failure of transanal manipulations [7, 9, 13].
7. Intraabdominal manipulation should help the perineal surgeon without opening the colon. Colotomy should be used only when necessary.
8. Proctosigmoidoscopy should be performed after extraction in each case to ensure that there is no mucosal tear.
9. In cases of perforation or tears, colostomy or Hartmann's procedure may be required [1].
10. A hospital stay of at least 24 h must be organized to rule out bleeding or delayed perforation [7, 13].

References

1. Barone JE, Yee J, Nealon TF (1983) Management of foreign bodies and trauma of the rectum. Surg Gynecol Obstet 156: 453–457
2. Busch D, Starling JR (1986) Rectal foreign bodies: case reports and a comprehensive review of world's literature. Surgery 100: 512–519
3. Classen JN, Martin RE, Sabagal J (1975) Iatrogenic lesions of the colon and rectum. South Med J 68: 1417
4. Couch CJ, Tan EGC, Watt AG (1986) Rectal foreign bodies: Med J Aust 144: 512–515
5. Crass RA, Tranbaugh PF, Kudsk KA, Trunkey DD (1981) Colorectal foreign bodies and perforation. Am J Surg 142: 85–88
6. Dassel PM, Punjabi E (1979) Ingested mariruanafilled balloons. Gastroenterology 76: 166–169
7. Eftaiha M, Hambrick E, Abcarian H (1977) Principles of management of colorectal foreign bodies. Arch Surg 112: 691–695
8. French GWG, Sherlock DJ, Holl-Allen RTJ (1985) Problems with rectal foreign bodies. Br J Surg 72: 243–244
9. Froidevaux A, Marti MC (1977) Les corps étrangers du rectum et de la vessie. Méd Hyg 35: 2330–2331
10. Fuller RC (1965) Foreign bodies in the rectum and colon. Dis Colon Rectum 8: 123–127
11. Goldberg S, Gordon PH, Nivatvongs S (1980) Essentiel of anorectal surgery. Lippincott, Philadelphia
12. Hughes JP, Marice HP, Gathright JB (1976) Method of removing a hollow object from the rectum. Dis Colon Rectum 19: 44–45
13. Kingsley AN, Abcarian H (1985) Colorectal foreign bodies. Dis Colon Rectum 28: 941–944
14. Levy A (1985) Corps étrangers ingérés chez l'adulte. Thèsis, Faculté de Médecine, University of Geneva
15. MacPherson DS, Wyatt R (1978) Cyanoacrylate adhesive for foreign body removal. Br Med J [Clin Res] 2: 476–477
16. Miserocchi G, Sironi VA, Ravagnati L (1984) Anal protrusion as a complication of ventriculoperitoneal shunt. J Neurosurg Sci 28: 43–46
17. Peet TND (1976) Removal of impacted rectal foreign body with obstetric forceps. Br Med J [Clin Res] 1: 500

18. Prabhu S, Cochran W, Azmy AF (1985) Wandering distal ends of ventriculo-peritoneal shunts. Z Kinderchir 40: 80-81
19. Sachdev YY (1967) An unusual foreign body in the rectum. Dis Colon Rectum 10: 220-221
20. Sohn N, Weinstein MA, Gonchar J (1977) Social injuries of the rectum. Am J Surg 134: 611-612
21. Schwartz GF, Polsky HS (1976) Ingested foreign bodies of the gastrointestinal tract. Am Surg 42: 236-238
22. Troy MR (1985) Colonoscopic removal of large bowel foreign bodies: an alternative to laparotomy. Milit Med 150: 146-148
23. Vadlamundi K, van Bockstaele P, McManus J (1972) Foley catheter in removal of a foreign body from the rectum. JAMA 221: 1412

28 Anal Venereology

M. Harms

Most sexually transmitted diseases (STD) are also commonly localized in the anal and perianal area. Despite the rapid progress in the knowledge of STD, we have maintained the classic classification which includes:

- Syphilis
- Gonorrhea
- Chancroid
- Lymphogranuloma venerum
- Granuloma inguinale

Numerous other infectious disorders may also be transmitted by close contact:

- Herpes simplex
- Scabies
- Pediculosis pubis
- Warts - Condylomata acuminata
          - Bowenoid papulosis
- Candidiasis
- Molluscum contagiosum

A large number of other infectious agents may cause anorectal and enteric infections in homosexual men. For this reason, this group of patients needs a speczial approach in investigation and management [6]. Since this category of patients is at greatest risk of developing acquired immunodeficiency syndrome (AIDS), these persons need to be particulary aware of infectious dermatoses such as herpes, candidiasis, dermatophytosis, human papilloma virus (HPV) infections, and especially STD and hepatitis. These infections often anticipate AIDS [3].

Syphilis

Syphilis continues to be one of the major STD worldwide. If untreated, it may continue as a chronic long-term infection which eventually invades all the organ systems.

Etiology. The causative agent is *Treponema pallidum,* a spirochete that penetrates the body through broken skin. Three weeks later a painless ulceration called a chancre develops at the site of inoculation. This lesion is accompanied by regional lymphadenopathy. The second stage, which occurs at about the 8 week after infection and which is due to hematogenous dissemination of *Treponema pallidum* is characterized by a multitude of lesions on the skin and the mucosa. General symptoms such as fever, headache, and sore throat may accompany these lesions. The third stage represents the destruction of tissues and the formation of granulomatous tissue reaction as an immunological response to the spirochetal infection. Any tissue or body organ may be affected.

Clinical Aspect. The typical chancre is an indolent ulceration of 1–2 cm diameter with indurated borders. In the anal localization, regional adenopathy is not always detectable. Atypical primary manifestation may consist of smaller or multiple lesions which may be painful. Herpetic lesions may also serve as inoculation sites, and then the syphilitic infection resembles herpes. Signs of secondary syphilis develop about 6 weeks later (average 9 weeks after inoculation), but may be seen as late as 3–6 months after infection. Macular or papular lesions varying in number and extent appear on the skin and the mucosa. They may join to from larger infiltrative plaques. Even an indurated anal fold or hemorrhoid should be considered as a possible syphilitic lesion. The anogenital area is a preferred site of these lesions, which are called condylomata lata. They can proliferate considerably and are particulary rich in *Treponema pallidum.*

Skin manifestations of tertiary syphilis such as gumma, which is a granulomatous tumor of varying size, is nowadays extremely rare and *usually* not localized in the anal region. Patients with AIDS or human immunodeficiency virus (HIV)-positive serology may present extraordinary atypical lesions (nodular) or signs which are normally not seen any more, such as malignant syphilis with necrotic cutaneous lesions.

Epidemiology. The incidence of syphilis, particulary anal chancre, is high in the homosexual male population.

Assessment

Microscopy. Visualization of the spirochete is performed by dark-field microscopy in specimens from primary and secondary syphilitic lesions.

Serological Tests

- *Nonspecific test* with nontreponemal antigen: the Venereal Disease Research Laboratory (VDRL) test uses cardiolipin, a lipoidal antigen. This test is very sensitive, easy to perform, and decreases in positivity after treatment. It is therefore the best indicator of whether therapy has been efficient and whether a new infection has been contracted.
- *specific tests* use treponemal antigen.
- Fluorescent treponemal antibody test (FTA): Nichol strain treponema is used as an antigen. For the FTA absorption (ABS) test, the patient's serum is absorbed with Reiter strain treponema, to eliminate false-positive reactions, before performing the test. With this specific test antibody classes can be specified (IgM, IgG, IgA). FTA-ABS IgM will indicate a recent infection. This is the first specific test which is positive several days after the chancre has appeared.
- The *Treponema pallidum* hemagglutination assay (TPHA test) uses *Treponema pallidum* as antigen and this is fixed on erythrocytes. This test is not as sensitive as the FTA test and will remain positive for a very long time or even forever.

Therapy. Penicillin is the best treponemicidal treatment. *Early syphilis* (primary and secondary syphilis of less than 1 year's duration) should be treated with:

- Benzathine penicillin G, 2.4 million units i. m. once a week for 2 successive weeks.
- Procaine-penicillin, 1.2–2.4 million units i. m. per day plus probenecid 1.5 g p. o. for 2 successive weeks.

The latter, more aggressive treatment modality is indicated for all patients who are HIV positive or who have a compromised immune status, as treatment failure (neurological relapse) has been reported after benzathine penicillin [1].

In cases of allergy to penicillin the following treatments are recommended:

- Erythromycin: 500 mg p. o. four times a day for 2 weeks.
- Tetracycline: 500 mg p. o. every 6 h for 2 weeks.
- Doxycyline: 200 mg p. o. per day for 2 weeks.

In late syphilis the following treatments are recommended:

- Benzathine penicillin: 2.4 million units i. m. once a week for 3 weeks.
- Erythromycin, tetracycline, or doxycyline is to be taken for 3 weeks (daily dosage as for early syphilis).

To avoid a toxic reaction (Herxheimer's reaction), administration of corticosteroids can be useful in very florid syphilis when a large quantity of treponema is present. Prednisone 0.5 mg/kg is given for the first 5 days of treponemicidal treatment, or 100 mg soluble cortisone i. m. is given with the first penicillin injection. No topical treatment of the skin lesions is necessary. The lesions will disappear within 1 week after the beginning of treatment. Serological tests (VDRL) are necessary after treatment (at 3,6 and 12 months) to establish the efficacy of the treatment. A two-fold decrease of the titer dilution in the VDRL test is considered to be a sufficient response. Serological tests should be continued annually in homosexual patients as the primary lesion – the chancre – is often not visible because of its hidden localization in the rectum. A four-fold increase of the titer dilution in the VDRL test is considered to be a new infection.

Gonorrhea

Gonorrhea is one of the most common STD in the world.

Etiology. The infectious organism is *Neisseria gonorrhoeae,* a Gram-negative Diplococcus. The incubation period is 2–8 days. *Neisseria gonorrhoeae* initially affects the lower urogenital organs in males and females (urethra, cervix uteri). Extragenital primary sites are the rectum, pharynx, and conjunctiva. If untreated, the infection may cause more extensive diseases such as epididymitis, prostatitis, pelvic inflammatory disease, tubo-ovarian abscess, and it can even take disseminated forms such as arthritis and septicemia.

Clinical Aspect. Anorectal gonorrhea is less symptomatic than urethritis. It is therefore important to suspect it in the presence of non specific rectal symptoms [3]. In acute cases, thick yellow pus is discharged from the anus. In more chronic cases, the secretion is thinner and mucous, and is only visible with an anoscope.

Epidemiology. Anal gonorrhea occurs in 40% of infected homosexual men by direct transmission during rectal intercourse. In contrast, anal gonorrhea is seen in women also after an endocervical infection of long duration.

Assessment

- Gram-stained smears show intracellular Gram-negative diplococci.
- Cultures on specific media (chocolate agar) and oxidase reaction.
- Enzyme-linked immunoadsorbent assay (ELISA; Gonozyme).

Differential Diagnosis. All anorectal diseases which are accompanied by mucous secretion have to be considered. Infectious and noninfectious diseases have to be included [6].

Therapy [7]

- Aqueous procaine penicillin G 4.8 million units i. m. with probenecid 1 g p. o.
- Amoxicillin: single dose 3 g p. o. with 1 g probenecid.
- In cases of allergy to penicillin spectinomycin 4 g i. m. (beta-lactamase stable).
- Tetracycline 500 mg p. o. four times a day for 7 days.
- Doxycycline 100 mg p. o. twice a day for 7 days.
- Ceftriaxone 250 mg i. m. (beta-lactamase stable).
- Erythromycin 500 mg p. o. four times a day for 7 days.

It is recommended that patients be checked after treatment in order to detect treatment failures which can include:

- Beta-lactamase-producing gonococcus treated with penicillin for example.
- Insufficient dosage of the chosen drug.
- Insufficient drug absorption insufficient mixing of the penicillin in the solution.
- Reinfection.

Serology for syphilis should be done at the time of treatment and 4–6 weeks after every attack of gonorrhea.

Chancroid

Chancroid is a STD which was prevalent in Africa but which today is not exceptional in western Europe.

Etiology. Chancroid is caused by the Gram-negative bacillus *Haemophilus ducreyi.*

Clinical Aspect. After an incubation time of 3–8 days, a small red papule appears which develops first into a pustule and later into a ulcer. This tender ulcer has undermined edges and is usually surrounded by an erythematous halo. Often multiple lesions are present. Regional adenopathy can be observed in about 50% the cases. The glands tend to suppurate and to break down. Simultaneous infection with *Treponema pallidum* is characterized by the *ulcus mixtum.* It first appears with the characteristic features of chancroid and later develops into the typical indurated form of a syphilitic infection.

Epidemiology. Men are more often affected than women. European cases are commonly found in the large ports.

Assessment

- Direct examination of smears from the pus of the ulcer shows the Gram-negative bipolar bacillus in typically short chains. The bacillus is not always easy to recognize.
- Culture has to be performed in a special laboratory on a specific medium containing human or rabbit blood.

Therapy. It is recommended that antibiotics which are not active for treponemal infection are used.

- Co-trimoxazole: sulfamethoxazole 800 mg and trimethoprim 160 mg once a day for 14 days
- Streptomycin 1 g i. m. a day for 10 days
- Erythromycin 500 mg every 6 h for 1 week

Penicillin is not effective. Topical treatment is not necessary but could comprise antiseptic measures with:

- Chlorhexidine 0.1% solution
- povidone-iodine, solution or ointment
- potassium permanganate solution 1:4000–1: 16000

Lymphogranuloma Inguinale (Durand-Nicolas-Favre Disease)

Etiology. Lymphogranuloma inguinale is a widespread, chronic, infectious STD in the tropics which has also been introduced into temperate regions. It is caused by *Chlamydia trachomatis* serotypes L1–L3.

Clinical Aspect. Different stages characterize this chronic disease. After an incubation time of about 13 weeks, a primary lesion appears but this is seldom seen as it is a very small erosion or ulceration in the anogenital region [5]. This initial lesion can be localized in the rectum or in the vagina as well. The buboes appear 15 days–1 months later. These regional glands are hard and tender, they adhere to each other and may finally break down forming fistulas and sinuses.

The third stage is characterized by chronic procitis or rectitis which is accompanied by general symptoms and followed by rectal strictures. Abcesses and vegetative formations (pseudotumoral) may also be observed. A late complication is anal carcinoma. Differential diagnosis depends on the stage:

1. All erosions and ulcerations (see Table 29.2, p. 254).
2. The bubo must be distinguish from the large number of other diseases with this symptom.
3. Fistulating processes (see Table 29.2, p. 254).

Assessment. Chlamydia can be directly visualized as elementary bodies with the Giemsa stain and with electron microscopy. Culture is possible (McCoy cell culture). In practice these methods are reserved for specialized laboratories. An immunfluorescene test is possible but not specific for *Clamydia trachomatis*. It only indicates group antigen. A serological test with fixation of the complement is also not specific but highly suggestive if there are titers of 1 : 16–1 : 64. The Frei test, which is an intradermal test, is no longer available.

Therapy
- Co-trimoxazole: sulfamethoxazole 400 mg and trimethoprim 80 mg p. o. four times a day for 10–20 days
- Tetracycline 500 mg p. o. four times a day for 10–20 days
- Erythromycin 500 mg p. o. four times a day for 10–20 days

Granuloma Venereum
(Granuloma Inguinale, Donovanosis)

Etiology. Granuloma venereum is a chronic, granulomatous, infectious disease of the anogenital skin. It is caused by *Calymmatobacterium granulomatis,* a Gram-negative bacterium related to the *Klebsiella* group.

Clinical Aspect. After an incubation time of 8 days to 3 months a papular lesion appears which breaks down rapidly. The resulting ulceration is not painful, the edges are not undermined, and the floor is granulomatous. This lesion is not accompanied by adenitis.

Epidemiology. This infection is commonly seen in the tropics and subtropics. It is seen only exceptionally in Europe. Donovanosis is only mildly contagious necessitating repeated exposure for it to develop.

Assessment. Giemsa-stained smears of granulation tissue show the typical Donovan bodies in the mononuclear cells. The Donavan bodies are vacuoles filled with the pathogenic organism with the appearance of a safety pin. Cultures are difficult and can only be done in specialized laboratories.

Therapy. Many broad-spectrum antibiotics are effective. This efficacy must be evident within 7 days [4].
- Tetracycline 2 g a day for 2–3 weeks.
- Co-trimoxazole: sulfamethoxazole 400 mg and trimethoprim 80 mg, two tablets twice a day for 2 weeks; sulfamethoxazole 800 mg and trimethoprin 160 mg, one tablet twice a day for 2 weeks.

Other antibiotics such as erythromycin, streptomycin, chloramphenicol, and gentamycin have been reported to be successful.

References

1. Berry CD, Hooton TM, Collier AC, Lukeehart SA (1987) Neurologic relapse after benzathine penicillin therapy for secondary symphilis in a patient with HIV infection. N Engl J Med 316 (25): 1587–1589
2. Handsfield HH (1984) Gonorrhea and uncomplicated gonococcal infection. In: Holmes KK, Mardh PA, Sparling PF, Wiesner PJ (eds) Sexually transmitted diseases. McGraw-Hill, New-York, p 205
3. Harms M, Mérot Y (1987) Signes cutanés du SIDA. Schweiz Runds Med Praxis 76 (9): 220
4. Hart G (1984) Donovanosis. In: Holmes KK, Mardh PA, Sparling PF, Wiesner PJ (eds) Sexually transmitted diseases. Mc Graw-Hill, New-York , p 393
5. Marchand C, Granier F, Cetre JC, Brutzkus A, Perrot H (1987) Lymphogranulomatose vénérienne anale avec erythème noueux (à propos d'une observation). Ann Dermatol Venereol 114: 65–69
6. Quinn TC, Holmes KK (1984) Proctitis, proctocolitis, and enteritis in homosexual men. In: Holmes KK, Mardh PA, Sparling PF, Wiesner PJ (eds) Sexually transmitted diseases. Mc Graw-Hill, New-York, p 672
7. Rein MF, Caine V, Grossmann JH et al. (1986) 1985 STD treatment guidelines. J Am Acad Dermatol 14: 707–726

29 Dermatological Anal Diseases

M. Harms

Numerous cutaneous diseases (Table 29.1) are localized in the perianal and perineal area. This may be partly explained by the fact that many external irritative and infectious factors increase the probability of dermatosis becoming established in this *intertrigous* area. Other dermatoses are very often situated in this region for unknown reasons, and finally dermatoses may be localized in the perianal area *by chance*. This last group will not be discussed here. Differential diagnosis is made difficult by the great number of diseases and by their similar appearance, as external factors may transform the characteristic signs of many of them. However, only an exact diagnosis allows the correct treatment to be chosen and avoids the use of combined topical treatments which are often responsible for chronic diseases. Table 29.2 should be used for differential diagnosis.

Erythematous Dermatosis

Dermatitis (Eczema)

The different forms of inflammatory diseases of the anal region represent the most common pattern seen in this localization (Table 29.2).

Etiology. The same factors as those causing anal pruritus are often responsible for anal dermatitis [1] (see Chap. 30). Scratching of the anal area will lead to erosion, and infection cannot be avoided. Furthermore, topical treatments with antibiotics and corticosteroids may favorize growth of *Candida*. Finally, it is nearly impossible to detect the primary cause [27].

Clinical Aspect. The earliest changes are *Erythema* and *edema*. These may progress to *vesiculation* and *oozing* and *erosion*. If the process becomes chronic, the skin will be *lichenified* (thickened) with prominent skin marking, excoriated, and either hyper- or hypopigmented. Itching is the main symptom and leads to the itch-scratch-lichenification cycle.

Table 29.1. Cutaneous diseases of the perianal and perineal region

Dermatitis (eczema)		Irritant
		Allergic
		Infectious
Infections	Viral	Herpes
		Condylomata acuminata
		Bowenoid papulosis
	Bacterial	Venereal diseases
		Tuberculosis
		Actinomycosis
	Mycologic	Candidiasis
		Dermatophytosis
	Protozoal	Amebiasis
Dermatosis		Psoriasis
		Bullous diseases
		Hidradenitis
		Lichen sclerosus et atrophicus
Systemic diseases		Crohn's disease
Tumors	Benignant	
	Malignant	
Congential diseases		Acanthosis nigricans
		Darier's disease

Different Categories of Perianal Dermatitis:
1. Irritant dermatitis
2. Contact dermatitis
3. Infectious dermatitis
Frequently different factors act simultaneously or sequentially.

Assessment. Exact anamnesis is very important. The possible contact allergen has to be identified by patch testing. Table 29.3 shows the main allergens in this localization. In the presence of pustules, their content should be examined by Gram's stain. Cultures for *Candida* sould be performed on fungal media. Bacterial cultures are not necessary because infection is not specific. Viral examination should be done particularly if erosion is visible. In cases of well-delimited plaques, a biopsy specimen is neces-

Table 29.2. Differential diagnosis of anal and perianal dermatosis: clinical aspect

Erythematous	Erosive	Ulcerous	Tumerous-vegetative	Fistulous
Dermatitis ————→		Syphilis I ←————	Syphilis II	Hidradenitis suppurativa
Candidosis ————→		Chancroid		
Dermatophytosis		Granuloma inguinale ————→		Lymphogranuloma venerum
	Herpes ————→		Condyloma accuminatum	
			Bowenoid papulosis	
Erythrasma	Behçet's disease			
Acrodermatitis enteropathica	Pemphigus vulgaris	Crohn's disease ————————→	————→	————→
		Pseudomembranous ulceration	Pemphigus vegetans	Actinomycosis
Fixed drug eruption ————→				
Psoriasis	Chronic familial pemphigus ————————→	————→		
Bowen's disease		Ergotism	Acanthosis nigricans	
Paget's disease ————→		Decubitus		
Lichen sclerosus et atrophicans ————→		Tuberculosis		
Darier's disease		Amebiasis		
		←———————— Carcinoma		

sary to eliminate dermatoses, as mentioned in Table 29.2.

Therapy. Table 29.4 shows all the things which have to be avoided and the measures which have to be undertaken. The best cleaning is achieved with water (hip bath). The beneficial effect of this is demonstrated by the observation that Greek babies do not get diaper dermatitis because these infants are cleaned under running water [3]. The patient should try to defecate at home. To avoid moisture the patient should not wear nonporous clothing and garments that keep the buttocks held tighly together. Instead of rubbing with toilet paper, drying can be done with a hair dryer. Instead of ointment only lotions should be used. Every attack of pruritus should be "treated" by a cool hip bath. The use of topical steroids, which is the most important therapeutic tool for dermatitis, is not indicated in the anal region except in cases of acute allergic contact dermatitis. It is better to employ lotions or possibly

Table 29.3. Main allergens responsible for perianal dermatitis

Benzocaine	Lanolin
Peroubalsam	Cocoabutter
Hamamelis	Iodine
Camphor	Resorcinol
Camomile (concentr.)	Antihistamines
Neomycin	Phenol
Turpentine	

Table 29.4. Treatment of perianal dermatitis

To avoid	To recommend
Toilet paper	Cleaning with cool water or disinfecting lotion (hip bath)
Soap	
Rubbing	Drying gently with a cotton towel or a hair dryer
Moisture	
Ointments, creams	Astringent or disinfecting lotions
Allergens	

Table 29.5. Side effects of topical steroids

Exacerbation of infections (viral, bacterial, fungal)
Atrophy: epidermis and dermis (particularly frequent in the anal area)
Slow healing of wounds
Pigmentation troubles
Topical hypersensitivity
Systemic effects

Table 29.6. Topical antibaterial agents for the anal area

Erythromycine 2% (lotion)
Silver sulfadiazine [Silvadene cream (Marion); Flammazine cream (Philips-Duphar)]

creams, but not ointments. Fluorine steroids should be avoided. If they are absolutely necessary, their use should be limited to a strict minimum, and the rules of treatment with topical steroids must be strictly observed [16]. The potency of topical steroids varies a great deal, a fact which has to be taken in account. They should be applied once a day because of the phenomenon of *tachyphilaxis of the skin.* Abrupt discontinuation of topical steroids will be followed by a *flare-up.* Table 29.5 shows the main side effects of topical steroids. In the case of bacterial superinfection only two topical antibiotics are recommended (Table 29.6). If *Candida* is present (which frequently occurs after prolonged application of topical corticoids) topical imidazole (see "Dermatophytic Infection"), nystatin, or Naftifin (Wander) should be prescribed.

Erythrasma

Erythrasma is a superficial infection involving the intertriginous areas.

Etiology. The pathogenic organism is the *Corynebacterium minutissimum.* This dermatosis is not very contagious and is seen mainly in elderly male patients. Humidity (tropical climate) is the most predisposing factor.

Clinical Aspect. Sharply marginated red-brown and slightly scaly plaques occupy the inguinal folds and may extend to the entire anogenital region.

Assessment. A coral-red fluorescence under Wood's light (UVA) is characteristic but may be lacking if the patient has washed before because the color-

giving substance, a porphyrin, is water soluble. The organism may be seen as a Gram-positive filamentous and coccoid bacterium in affected scales.

Therapy. Topical imidazole derivates [17] (see "Dermatophytic Infection") are the best treatment. Topical erythromycin as used in acne therapy [Ery Derm (Abbott), carinamide] and systemic erythromycin (1 g a day for 2 weeks) constitute another effective treatment [4].

Dermatophytic Infection (Ringworm, Tinea)

Fungal infections of the inguinal, genital, and gluteal region fequently occur in adult humans.

Etiology. The fungus is a dermatophyte which is parasitic on the keratin (superficial layers of the skin, nails, hair). In this localization it does not penetrate deeper into epidermis or dermis.

Clinical Aspects. Erythematous macules and papules develop forming symmetric, arciform, and sharply delimited areas. The centers heal spontaneously while the borders advance.

Epidermiology. Heat (tropics), friction, and maceration are predisposing factors. Inguinal tinea is often associated with tinea pedis. Infections can be caused by direct or indirect contact (common bathroom, towels) or by autoinoculation from the interdigital tineas.

Assessment. The hyphae and spores can be microscopically identified in the scales. Fungal cultures are necessary for exact determination.

Therapy. In the treatment of superficial mycosis topical drugs play a central role. Old preparations such as Whitfield's ointment are no longer in use because of the unpleasant properties of soiling and staining the underwear or the skin itself. All the imidazole derivates are excellent broad-spectrum antifungal therapeutics: *clotrimazole, econazole, miconazole* [17]; clotrimazole is perhaps the best tolerated. They should be applied in lotions or creamy preparations twice daily for about 3 weeks, but in any case at least 2 weeks after the disappearance of clinical lesions. Their action is only fungistatic. A new class of antifungal substances are the allylamines. They too have a broad action but are fungicidal for dermatophytes and fungistatic for *Candida.* Naftifin (Exidril) is the only derivate available as a cream and as a lotion [12].

In cases of acute, oozing, inflammatory lesions wet compresses or a hit bath [see "Dermatitis" (Eczema)] are indicated before specific antifungal topics. Systemic treatment should be given if the tinea recurs often, if tinea pedis is also present, or if exceptionally furuncoloid forms are observed. In these cases griseofulvin, 0.75-1.5 mg a day should be given for a least 1 month. Ketoconazole is indicated only if griseofulvin cannot be given or if chronic complicated candidosis is present (200 mg a day for at least 1 month).

Psoriasis Vulgaris

Psoriasis vulgaris is a frequent, chronic, inflammatory, proliferative dermatosis which may affect both sexes at any age.

Pathophysiology. The pathophysiology is not clear, but it has been well established that psoriasis vulgaris is a hereditary disease with variable penetrance. Exogenic (humidity, friction) and endogenic factors are likely to provoke psoriasis.

Clinical Aspect. The typical lesion of psoriasis is an asymptomatic, erythematous, sharply defined plaque covered with loosley adherent scales which appear especially after scratching. There are no scales in the intriginous localizations, instead there is a homogenous dark red plaque.

Assessment. The medical history and circumstances of onset or exacerbation may reveal the disease. Examination of the entire skin surface is necessary to detect other localizations with more specific lesions. Biopsy can be useful, particularly if no other psoriatic lesions are present.

Therapy. In the acute phase the same measures should be undertaken as in simple dermatitis. It is essential to promote drying and to avoid irritants. Specific treatment of psoriasis is generally not possible in the anal area because it is too irritating in association with the humidity and friction. For this reason dithranol, the main topical antipsoriatic agent, cannot be applied in the anal and perianal region. Imidazole derivates (miconazole as a lotion) are useful to combat acute inflammatory sign. Imidazoles seem to have not only an antifungal and an antibacterial effect, but also a real antipsoriatic action. Alphosyl (lotion; Stafford-Miller) containing

allantoin 2% and coal tar 5% is the only antipsoriatic agent which may be applied in the perianal area. In the case of widespread extension in the whole inguinal and perigenital area, systemic treatment with retinoids is helpful. This treatment has to be discussed with a dermatologist [20].

Chronic Benign Familial Pemphigus (Hailey-Hailey Disease)

Benign familial pemphigus is a rare hereditary dermatosis mostly localized in the inguinal region.

Pathophysiology. This autosomal dominant disorder with variable penetrance is not related to the autoimmune bullous dermatosis of the pemphigus group. It can be provoked and exacerbated by external factors such as humidity and infections.

Clinical Aspect. Well-defined erythematous plaques are localized especially in the inguinal region but may also appear in the anal and perianal area. They are characterized by linear fissures. Vesiculous and squamous lesions may be seen as well.

Assessment. Histological examination showing acantholysis is necessary for exact diagnosis.

Therapy. It is very important to keep the area as dry as possible. After antiseptic topical measures (Table 29.7), potent corticosteroids can be used. If there is no response, dapsone (100 mg a day) or surgery are further possibilities [13]. In surgery the whole affected area must be excised. When sufficient granulation tissue has developed, the wound is covered in a second step with a Thiersch transplant.

Table 29.7. Antiseptic agents for cleaning the anal region

Potassium permanganate 1:4000-1:16000 diluted
Silver nitrate 0.1%-0.5% diluted
Chlorhexidine 0.1% (Hibitane; Ayerst, ICI)
Triclocarban (Septivon-Lavril; Porche-Lavril)

Dyskeratosis Follicularis (Darier's Disease)

Etiolgoy. Dyskeratosis follicularis is a chronic autosomal dominant disorder of keratinization which is mainly seen in adults.

Clinical Aspect. When localized in the intertriginous area, the lesions of this diseae are very similar to those in benign familial pemphigus. Brownish follicular papules may form large plaques. Fissures are seen but these are less regular than in benign familial pemphigus.

Assessment. Other localizations such as the head, trunk, neck, palms, and nails can be helpful for diagnosis. Mucous membranes are often involved. Histological features are characteristic.

Therapy. Antibacterial and antiviral topical treatment is often necessary to overcome secondary infection. Topical treatment with retinoic acid can be tried on other localizations but not in the intertriginous regions. Systemic retinoids such as etretinate 1 mg/kg a day may give a very good response [11].

Bowen's Disease

Etiolgoy. Bowen's disease, a form of intraepidermal carcinoma, is seen in the anogenital area of males and females at an advanced age. Carcinogenic factors such as age and arsenic probably play a leading role.

Clinical Aspect. Generally a solitary, rarely multifocal, erythematous, slightly infiltrated, and well-defined plaque can be localized anywhere on the skin surface, but the anogenital region is implicated more often. The plaques can be covered with scales and crusts resembling dermatitis.

Assessment. Histological examination is diagnostic.

Therapy. Surgical excision with safety margins is the therapy of choice. Cryotherapy, electrocoagulation, or laser therapy can be used as well, but must be followed up regularly to avoid relapses.

Paget's Disease

Paget's disease, a rare dermatosis generally seen in the mamilla but which can exceptionally be localized in the anogenital region of aged women.

Pathophysiology. The mammary and extramammary forms are linked to the apocrine glands. It is a carcinoma of the ductal part of these glands.

Clinical Aspects. The characteristic feature is a very slowly advancing erythematous patch which is always well defined.

Assessment. Histological examination is diagnostic.

Therapy. Surgery with safety margins is the treatment of choice.

Acrodermatitis Enteropathica

Etiology. Acrodermatitis enteropathica is a very rare disorder which is caused by a lack of zinc absorbtion.

Clinical Aspect. This dermatosis is seen in young children. It begins in the periorificial zones as erythematous plaques with vesicles and crusting. Secondary infection with *Candida* is common. The same symptoms may be seen in patients (alcoholics) receiving parenteral hyperalimentation, in which case they indicate a zinc deficiency [24].

Assessment. Typical localization is associated with malnutrition. Histological examination is not relevant. Evaluation of the zinc level in a blood test is diagnostic.

Therapy. Zinc substitution with zinc sulfate (50–300 mg a day p.o. with food) rapidly resolves all symptoms but this has to be continued for life.

Lichen Sclerosus et Atrophicans

Etiology. Lichen sclerosus et atrophicans is a rare dermatosis which predominates on the genital mucosa in females after menopause. The etiology is unknown.

Clinical Aspect. Small bluish-white macules form larger irregularly defined plaques. The skin in these plaques is thickened at the beginning and is later atrophic. Erosion fissures and scars are often observed. Severe pruritus is very common.

Assessment. The typical clinical aspect and other localizations beside the genital area are mostly diagnostic. Histological examination is of help.

Therapy. Small lesions can be excised surgically. Topical treatment with potent corticosteroids or intralesional injection with steroids will decrease the pruritus. Regular follow-up is indicated as transformation into spinocellular carcinoma is possible. Testosterone (2%) in a steroid ointment can be tried [5].

Erosive and Ulcerous Dermatosis

Any erosive or ulcerous lesion in the anal or perianal localization is susceptible to being a *venereal disease*. This possibility must be excluded even if the clinical aspect is not characteristic. All erosive lesions might develop into ulcerous lesions due to secondary infection which can hardly be avoided in the anal area.

Herpes Simplex

Herpes simplex is a worldwide, especially cutaneous infection in humans. Beside labial manifestation, genital lesions are also very common. Anal localization is rare.

Etiology. Herpes simplex virus is a DNA virus which infects only humans. It has a universal distribution. Two types of herpes virus, can be distinguished but this is of no practical significance. Direct contact is the most obvious way of infection as the virus does not survive in dry environments.

Clinical Aspect. Primary infection can involve the entire genital area and extend to the anus. It is most frequently seen in girls and young women. This very painful eruption is characterized by an erythema with vesicles, erosions, and edema. *Chronic and recurrent* herpes consists of small vesicles clustered together and followed by erosive and crusted lesions. Patients with acquired immune deficiency syndrome (AIDS) may also show a very extended, even ulcerous involvement including the anal mucosa [22].

Epidemiology. Anal manifestation of herpes simplex is mostly seen in homosexual men and especially in immunocompromised persons (AIDS).

Assessment. Cultures, electron-microscopic identification, and antibody titer evaluation are possible procedures. The most rapid and easy identification is the immunofluorescent method on a smear of the vesicule content. It can be examined for giant cells and inclusion bodies as well.

Table 29.8. Topical antivirals agent

Substance	Remarks
Iodoxyuridine 0.2%	Rare allergy, insufficient concentration
Iodoxyuridine 10%	
Tromantadine	Allergy
Acyclovir 5%	

Therapy. Specific potent antiviral substances are available for topical treatment (Table 29.8). Systemic treatment is necessary in the case of primary infection and of very extended forms.

In the very beginning (first 2 days) herpes should be treated with specific topical treatment (Table 29.8). Creams or ointment should be applied six times a day for 3 days. Acyclovir administered i.v. is indicated in all severe or primary infections especially in immunocompromised persons: 5 mg/kg perfusion of 1 h repeated every 6 h. Oral administration (200–400 mg) should be started as soon as possible after the earliest signs and repeated every 5 h for 3 days. It is not useful for the treatment of established lesions [26]. Immunostimulating medication, e. g., with methisoprinol (50 mg/day for 5 days), has shown to decrease the duration of relapsing herpes [21]. These specific treatments do not prevent recurrences. Older lesions will be easily superinfected and therefore need antiseptic treatment (Tables 29.6 and 29.7). Caution has to be used in the application of topical corticosteroids.

Behçet's Disease

Etiology. Behçet's disease is a systemic disease with multiple cutaneous sings of unknown etiology. There may be ocular, articular, vascular, and neurological manifestations but not always simultaneously in the same patient.

Clinical Aspect. Anal localization of Behçet's disease is not frequent. The appearance of the lesions is absolutely identical to any other erosive onset. These simple erosions may develop into sharply demarcated ulcerations with a yellow base and a inflamed border. They are very painful.

Epidemiology. The disease predominates in males and usually begins between the ages of 10 and 30 years. Genetic transmission is probable since 60%–80% of the patients belong to HLA B5.

Assessment. In the presence of oral and genital aphtosis and ocular lesions, the diagnosis of Behçet's disease is generally accepted. If symptoms are sparse, cutaneous sensitivity (provocation of an aphtoid lesion at the point of injection) constitutes a useful aid. Histology is not specific.

Therapy. No specific treatment is known. In the presence of ocular lesions or extensive aphtoid lesions, treatment with systemic corticosteroids is indicated (1 mg/kg a day) [29]. Heparin is given in the case of venous thrombosis. Colchicine has been tried successfully in erythema nodosum associated with Behçet's disease. It has no influence on the aphtoid lesions. Sulfones have been tried with some success. Immunosuppressive treatment is limited to severe cases. The only therapy which has given satisfactory results in the painful aphtoid lesions is thalidomide (50–300 mg a day for 2–3 months, beginning with the high dosage) [8]. Topical management consists of antiseptic measures (see Table 29.7).

Fixed Drug Eruption

This is an unusual reaction to a drug or food additive. It can be seen anywhere on the skin but is often localized in the anogenital region.

Etiology. The exact allergic mechanism has not yet been fully explained.

Clinical Aspect. An erythematous, well-defined solitary or multiple patch shows rapid pigmentation. The lesions are fequently bullous and erosive. Relapses always occur in exactly the same places.

Assessment. Anamnesis with drug ingestion followed by eruption in the same localization will give the diagnosis. Drugs often implicated are: barbiturates, acetylsalicylic acid, nonsteroidal antiinflammatory agents, allopurinol, antibiotics, phenolphthalin-containing drugs, laxatives, wine.

Therapy. The first step is the elimination of the drug. In the acute phase topical steroids can be used. In the case of erosives lesions antiseptic measures (see Table 29.7) should be undertaken to avoid superinfection.

Pemphigus Vulgaris

Pemphigus vulgaris a chronic autoimmune, bullous, cutaneous disease which often begins on the mucous membranes. The anal mucosa is not often solely affected as is the buccal mucosa.

Pathophysiology. Autoantibodies fixed on the surface of the keratinocytes are responsible for the dissociation in this layer called acantholysis.

Clinical Aspect. Because of mechanical friction no blisters are seen in the anal region, but there are superficial erosions with a tendency not to heal.

Assessment. Direct immunofluorescence of a biopsy specimen is necessary for the detection of antikeratinocyte antibodies.

Therapy. Systemic corticosteroids are the most efficient treatment. Initial dosage must be sufficiently high (prednisone 100–120 mg a day) and the treatment should be continued for as long as the lesions are present. When the lesions have disappeared, the dosage is decreased until the lowest dosage preventing lesions is found. Azathioprine (100–200 mg a day) or cyclophosphamide (50–150 mg a day) may be used to enable lower doses of corticosteroids to be used. Topical prevention of the infection should be provided by antiseptic measure (Table 29.7).

Crohn's Disease

Anal manifestation may be present in about 25% of patients with Crohn's disease, a chronic inflammatory disease of the gut. It is important to underline that these manifestations may precede all other signs by months or even years.

Clinical Aspect. Single or multiple nonindurated fissures and small or large ulcers and fistulas may be present. They are indolent and poorly granulating. Sometimes the borders are undermined [14].

Assessment. Histological examination shows a characteristic granulomatous infiltration.

Therapy. No specific treatment is known. Management with topical antiseptic agents is indicated (Table 29.7).

Ulcers After Use of Suppositories

Two groups of drugs (ergotamine and the morphomimetics) habe been shown to provoke anorectal and vaginal ulcers after prolonged use [10, 28].

Etiology. While ergotamine-provoked ulcers could be explained by local vasoconstriction, there is no hypothesis for the other group.

Clinical Aspect. Large and deep ulcerations on the anorectal mucosa have been described. They are indolent and can reach the sphincter ani.

Therapy. No specific treatment is necessary because healing will occur spontaneously after the use of suppositories is stopped. Antiseptic dressings are useful.

Decubitus Ulcer

Decubitus ulcers frequently occur in pressure areas in elderly, immobile, or paraplegic patients.

Etiology. The determining factor of these trophic ulcers seems to be the loss of sensitivity which leads to lessened mobility and vascular stasis, especially in pressure areas.

Clinical Aspect. Inital erythema and blistering lasting a few days precede ulceration. There is often a deep destruction beneath the ulceration leading to characteristic undermined edges and sinuses. Periostitis and osteomyelitis may develop as well.

Therapy. The best treatment is prevention. Positioning, frequent bedmaking, use of special sheets, and frequent turning of immobile patients are essential. The sitting position is unsatisfactory, the prone position is ideal but difficult to maintain. Beside these mechanical measures, correction of anemia, the nitrogen balance, and hypoalbuminuria is necessary. Caution with hyponoetic agents and tranquillizers is important. Once a sore is established, all further pressure has to be removed. Disinfection with a solution of potassium permanganate (see Table 29.7), or chlorhexidine (diluted, 0.5%) should be performed after every stool. The best disinfection for very large areas of ulceration is a hip bath for several hours per day, a procedure which simultaneously contributes to elimination of pressure. The use of antibiotic ointments and soaked dressings is not well tolerated and does not accelerate the healing process. The use of modern dressings with adhesive plastic films [Opsite (Smith and Nephew), Varihesive (Convatel, Squibb), Comfeel (Coloplast)] is very efficient and practical in use. The most appropriate dressing for deep ulcers is Silastic (Merck), a foam which can be shaped to exactly the necessary dimensions and applied directly into the ulcer cavity. Within several minutes the substance stabilizes and forms a rubber-like model which can be easily removed several times a day for cleaning and disinfection. As the ulcer diminishes, the model has to be remade weekly. Surgical excision is sometimes recommended [2].

Tuberculosis

Different cutaneous forms of the infectious disease tuberculosis are possible. A *primary chancre* in the anal region is exceptional. It is accompanied by unilateral lymphadenopathy. *Lupus vulgaris* and *verrucous tuberculosis* can spread widely over the buttocks and the anal region. The most likely form of tuberculosis seen in the anal localization is the *orificial tuberculosis* occurring particularly in patients with advanced pulmonary or intestinal disease.

Etiology. Orificial tuberculosis is a form of autoinoculation. The lesions are the result of direct inoculation or lymphatic extension around the anus.

Clinical Aspect. Small red papules or nodules break down to shallow and very painful ulcers with undermined edges. The ulcers are generally small less than (2 cm) and do not tend to heal spontaneously.

Assessment. There is always evidence of tuberculous disease, and bacterial confirmation is not difficult.

Therapy. No topical therapy is effective. Routine antituberculous therapy has to be employed.

Amebiasis

Etiology. Infection with the protozoon *Entamoeba histolytica* can provoke anal ulceration by extension of an underlying amebic disease of the bowel or by direct inoculation.

Clinical Aspect. The ulcers either invade deeply, destroy the surrounding tissue rapidly, and have serpiginous underminded edges, or they are filled with granulomatous tissue. Very painful adenosis usually accompanies the ulcer.

Epidermiology. Direct inoculation may occur in endemic countries. Recent cases of this rare anal infection have been reported in human immunedeficiency virus (HIV)-positive individuals [15].

Assessment. Finding of *Entamoeba histolytica* in a biopsy specimen from an edge of the lesion is diagnostic.

Therapy. Appropriate treatment of the bowel infection is necessary (see Chap. 32).

Tumerous, Vegetative and Fistulous Dermatosis

In cases of vegetative and proliferating lesions of the anal area, syphilitic infection must be excluded as a first step (see Chap. 28).

Condyloma Acuminatum

Condylomata acuminata (Ca) are intrepithelial benign tumors caused by infection with human papilloma virus (HPV).

Etiology. A variety of clinical warts is provoked by different HPVs but a specific virus type does not necessarily correspond with a distinct clinical picture. Some types (16, 18, 31, 33) are oncogenic.

Clinical Aspect. The clinical aspect of condylomata acuminata is very typical. These warts are elongated and pedunculated, sometimes with cauliflower-like excrescences localized on the genitalia and in the perianal region. They have to be looked for in the anal canal as well. They are painless and can grow to voluminous formations. Carcinomatous degeneration is possible if they persist for a very long time.

Epidemiology. Ca belong to the sexually transmitted diseases. Partners must be examined and treated simultaneoulsy. Anal localization is particularly frequent in homosexual men. In HIV-positive patients infection with HPV is very common.

Assessment. The clinical aspect is typical and sufficient for diagnosis. If the infection is long standing and tumorous masses are present, histological examination is indispensable to exclude a malignant process.

Table 29.9. Treatment modalities in condylomata acuminata

		Form of application
Podophyllin		Topical
Liquid nitrogen		Topical
Curettage and electrosurgery		
Laser		
5-Fluorouracil		Topical
Immuno-therapy:	Isoprinosine (Newport)	Peroral
	Interferons	Sublesional or subcutaneous injections

Therapy. Many therapeutic modalities are known (Table 29.9). Spontaneous remission, as is common in warts localized elsewhere, generally does not occur with Ca. Therefore it is recommended not to wait before starting treatment even if the signs are minimal. Inspection of the anal canal is always necessary.

Podophyllin in 15%–20% dilution is most effective if the lesions are few and small. A twice weekly application is recommended but large areas should not be treated and excessive amounts should not be applied to the mucous membranes as this substance can be absorbed producing systemic side effects. The surrounding skin should be protected by covering it with a basic ointment. At the beginning of the therapy the liquid should be left on for 1–2 h and then washed off because severe irritation is possible. Later podophyllin can be left for several hours. Cryosurgery will not produce scars if carefully executed. Electrosurgery, curetage, and laser have to be performed under local anesthesia. Laser therapy executed under magnification seems to give better results as recurrences are observed less frequently, and the healing is faster [23].

Various interferons (alpha, gamma) are in clinical trials and promise to give an alternative treatment for HPV infections which are resistant to other treatment.

Bowenoid Papulosis

Etiology. Bowenoid papulosis a new HPV infection caused by types 16 and 18, as well as possibly others [6, 7].

Clinical Aspect. Multiple, flat, sometimes verrucous, reddish-brown to violescent papules are characteristic. They tend to group and coalesce, and may occupy the entire anogenital region.

Epidemiology. As is the case with condyloma acuminatum, this infection is often seen in young adults who are sexually very active. Women may be affected in a particularly extensive way including the whole genital and anal region. Cervical infection with the same virus is often observed.

Assessment. Contrary to condyloma acuminatum, a biopsy specimen has to be taken for histological examination and typing of the virus by the hybridization technic. Application of acetic acid (5%) is useful for visualization of subclinical lesions.

Therapy. Essentially, the same measures are used as for condyloma acuminatum (Table 29.9). It has been noted that recurrences are very frequent, and really effective treatment is not yet available. Repeated laser treatment associated with inferferons [6, 7] will perhaps give better results in the future.

Pemphigus Vegetans

Pemphigus vegetans is a rare variant of pemphigus vulgaris and belongs to the group of autoimmune bullous dermatoses.

Pathophysiology. See "Pemphigus Vulgaris."

Clinical Aspect. Blisters are rarely seen in pemphigus vegetans, only sometimes at the edges of the lesions. Instead vegetation occupies the periorificial areas.

Assessment. See "Pemphigus Vulgaris".

Therapy. In resistant or localized cases surgical excision may be a good treatment.

Acanthosis Nigricans

Acanthosis nigricans is a rare inhomogenous condition characterized by cutaneous hyperkeratosis and pigmentation in the axillae, the neck, the anogenital region, the groins, and the intertriginous folds.

Etiology. An unidentified peptide secreted by the neoplasm or by the pituitary gland is assumed to provoke the lesions.

Clinical Aspect. Brown verrucous lesions develop mainly on intertriginous folds. They are associated with hyperkeratosis of the palms and soles. Extension over the entire skin is possible.

Epidemiology. A benign form may be familial with irregular autosomal dominant inheritance. Another benign form, also called "pseudoacanthosis nigricans," is seen in obese young adults. The malignant form is always associated with a malignant disease.

Assessment. Clinical features are obvious, differentiation between benign and malignant forms is possible by considering genetic factors, age at onset, and association with malignancies.

Therapy. No specific treatment is known. Malignant forms disappear when the tumor is excised or treated efficiently.

Carcinomas (see Chap. 19)

Hidradenitis Suppurativa and Acne Tetrad

Hidradenitis suppurativa is an inflammatory and often very chronic disease causing a furunculoid appearance of the perianal region. It is often widespread over the buttocks. This fistulating, abscessing, and scarring process is seen more often in men.

Etiology. The etiology is not yet well established, but it seems clinically evident that two diseases have to be distinguished [25]. First, hidradenitis suppurativa is a disease of the apocrine glands (Verneuil's disease); and secondly, acne tetrad is clinically identical but is less severe and affects the sebaceous glands and is therefore considered to be a particular form of acne.

Clinical Aspect. All degrees of inflammation, torpid nodules, abscesses, and fistulating processes with draining sinuses are seen. Severe scarring, with frequent tunneling formations, is regular.

Assessment. The distinction of the two entities is clinical: Verneuil's disease is localized only in the axillae and the perigenital-inguinal region. Acne tetrad is present in the same places and also on the neck and the scalp; it is often associated with pilonidal cysts.

Therapy. The treatment of the two entities differs in one respect: while acne tetrad responds extremely well to p. o. isotretinoin [4], this is far less evident with the Verneuil's disease. Isotretinoin is given at a dosage of 0.5–1.0 mg/kg a day for 4–6 months with contraception for women of child-bearing age). After this period surgical treatment is often necessary. Verneuil's disease responds well to p. o. antibiotics. Abscesses have to be drained. Surgical treatment provides the only definitive healing. Topical acne treatment is of no use for these severe forms and is also not tolerated in the anal region.

Actinomycosis

Actinomycosis is a chronic infectious desease which is localized near an orifice and provokes a suppurative and fistulating process.

Etiolgy. Actinomyces isreali is the most common filamentous bacterium which causes actinomycosis. Other bacteria such as *Actinobacillus actinomycetemcomitans* may be associated.

Clinical Aspect. As the more frequent cervicofacial form, the anal localization is charactcrized by indurated nodules which break down forming fistulas, sinuses and constricted scarring.

Epidemiology. The distribution of the infection is worldwide. It rarely occurs in infancy. Adults between the ages of 15 and 20 years are usually affected.

Assessment. Detection of typical sulfur granules in the pus is not always possible. Cultures on a specific medium and detection of antibodies in the serum by immunofluoresence is diagnostic.

Therapy. Beside surgical drainage, high-dosage antibiotics (aminopenicillin) is the best treatment [19]. Although many antibiotics are effective, they have to be applied for a very long period (up to 6 months) because their penetration through the dense fibrotic areas surrounding the colonies is not optimal.

References

1. Alexander-Williams J (1983) Pruritus ani. Br Med J [Clin Res] 287 (2): 159–160
2. Buchanan DL, Agris J (1983) Gluteal plication closure of sacra pressure ulcers. Plast Reconstr Surg 72: 49–54
3. Dafforn-Ierodiaconou E (1983) Greek babies' bottoms. Br Med J 287: 764
4. Dicken C, Powell S, Spear KL (1984) Evaluation of isotretinoin treatment of hidradenitis suppurativa. J Am Acad Derm atol 11: 500–502
5. Flynt J, Gallup DG (1979) Childhood lichen sclerousus. Obstet Gynecol 53 [Suppl 3]: 79S–81S
6. Gross G, Gissmann L (1986) Urogenitale and anale Papillomvirusinfektion. Hautarzt 37: 587–596
7. Gross G, Roussaki A, Schoepf E (1986) Successful treatment of condylomata acuminata and bowenoid papulosis with subcutaneous injections of low-dose recombinant interferon Arch Dermatol 122: 749–750
8. Grosshans E (1986) Thalidomide. In: Saurat JH, Grosshans E, Laugier P, Lachapelle JM (eds) Précis de dermatologie et vénérologie. Masson, Paris, p 640
9. Habif TP (1985) Clinical dermatology: a color guide to diagnosis and therapy. Mosby, St Louis, p 214–215
10. Laplance G, Grosshans E, Heid E, Jaeck D, Welsch M (1984) Ulcérations ano-rectovaginales par suppositoires contenant du dextropropoxyphène. Ann Dermatol Venereol II: 347–355
11. Löwenhagen GB, Michaelsson G, Mobacken H et al. (1982) Effect of etretinate (RO 10-9359) on Darier's disease. Dermatologica 165: 123–130
12. Maibach HI (1985) Naftifine: dermatotoxicology and clinical efficacy. Mykosen 28 [Suppl 1]: 75
13. Michel B (1982) Commentary: Hailey-Hailey disease. Familial benign chronic pemphigus. Arch Dermatol 118: 781–783
14. Neiger A (1985) Manifestations anales et périanales de la maladie de Crohn. Hexagone Roche 13 [Suppl 1]: I–IV
15. Penneys NS, Hicks B (1985) Unusual cutaneous lesions associated with acquired immunodeficiency syndrome. J Am Acad Dermatol 13: 845–852
16. Poffet D, Harms M (1983) Pratique de la corticothérapie locale. Praxis 72: 721–726
17. Raab WPF (1980) The treatment of mycosis with imidazole derivatives. Springer, Berlin Heidelberg New York 122
18. Reuler JB, Cooney TG (1981) The pressure sore: pathophysiology and principales of management. Ann Intern Med 94: 661–666
19. Richtsmeier WJ, Johns ME (1979) Actinomycosis of the head and neck. CRC Crit Rev Clin Lab Sci 11: 175–202
20. Saurat JH (1986) Le psoriasis. In: Saurat JH, Grosshans E, Laugier P, Lachapelle JM (eds) Précis de dermatologie et vénérologie. Masson, Paris, p 149
21. Saurat JH (1986) Inosine, acédobène, dimépranol (Isoprinosine). In: Saurat JH, Grosshans E, Laugier P, Lachapelle JM (eds) Précis de dermatologie et vénérologie. Masson, Paris p 636
22. Seigal TB, Lopez C, Hammer GS, Brown AE, Kornfeld SJ (1981) Severe acquired immunodeficiency in male homosexuals manifested by chronic perianal ulcerative herpes simplex lesions. N Engl J Med 305: 1439–1444

23. Silva PD, Micha JP, Silva DG (1985) Management of condyloma acuminatum. J Am Acad Dematol 13: 457–463
24. Steger JW, Izuno GT (1979) Acute zinc depletion syndrome during parenteral hyperalimentation. Int J Dermatol 18: 472–479
25. Stein E (1986) Proktologie. Lehrbuch und Atlas. Springer, Berlin Heidelberg New York
26. Strauss SE (1985) Herpes simplex virus infection: biology, treatment, and prevention. Ann Intern Med 103: 404–419
27. Wienert V (1985) Diagnose und Therapie des Analekzems. Hautarzt 36: 232–233
28. Wienert V, Grussendorf EI (1980) Anokutaner Ergotismus gangraenosus. Hautarzt 31: 668–670
29. Wong RC, Ellis CN, Diaz LA (1984) Behçet's disease. Int J Dermatol 23: 25–32

30 Pruritus Ani

B. Hammer

Definition

Pruritus ani denotes an unpleasant itching sensation in the anal region that induces an irresistible urge to scratch.

Pathogenesis and Pathophysiology

Both pruritus and pain occur at the dermo-epidermal junction in response to stimulation of the same plexuses of free nerve endings. The point of itching can be demonstrated by neurohistologic means [12]. Physiologically this point is characterized by a reduced threshold for chemical, mechanical, thermal, and electrical stimuli. These stimuli trigger the release of chemical mediators such as histamine, proteolytic enzymes, kinins, and prostaglandins, which stimulate the receptors. The sensation is transmitted to the lateral spinothalamic tract by centripetal neurons and from there is relayed through synapses to the thalamus. It appears that a low-level stimulus leads to the symptom of pruritus while a higher-level stimulus elicits pain. Histamine is a principal mediator of itching. If histamine is introduced into the epidermis by scarification, itching occurs. But if histamine is injected deeply into the dermis, it causes pain [6].

The threshold to pruritus varies greatly in different individuals, as Shelly and Arthur [12] were able to show in "normal" experimental subjects. Pruritus may arise from the perianal skin or from the distal anal canal, which is not covered by cornified squamous epithelium. It is common to refer to the "anal mucosa" when speaking of pruritus ani, when in fact, unlike the skin, irritation of the mucous membranes does not lead to pruritus. There are several reasons why the anus is a site of predilection for pruritus:

- Due to its location in a kind of "pocket" between the gluteal folds, the anus is subject to mechanical irritation. This is compounded by the increased moisture often present in individuals who are overweight, engage in strenuous exercise, or perspire heavily, or by excessive dryness like that encountered in atrophic geriatric skin.
- Stool induces mechanical and chemical skin irritation in individuals who do not or cannot maintain satisfactory anal hygiene. Predisposing factors are a deep-set anus, heavy pilosity, and sphincter incompetence.
- The anal region is subject to many contact inflammations and neoplastic or non-neoplastic tissue changes leading to the drainage of pus, mucus, or other secretions that predispose to pruritus.
- In women, diseases or secretions may spread from the vagina and vulva to involve the anal region.

Classification

Pruritus ani may be classified as primary (idiopathic) or secondary.

Primary Pruritus Ani

Primary pruritus ani occurs in the absence of an apparent etiology, i. e., there is no detectable local disease, and the pruritus is not caused by any known systemic illness. Verbov [15] uses the term "constitutional" pruritus ani, meaning that the individual has a reduced threshold for anal itching. Thus, stimuli having no effect in persons with normal responses (e. g., slight fecal soiling or a very mild hemorrhoidal condition) would cause itching in persons who are constitutionally susceptible. The presence of a psychological conflict appears to have causal significance in many cases [3]. However, psychologists do not believe there is a specific personality type that is predisposed to primary pruritus ani. The anorectal region is a very sensitive zone that is the focus of myriad positive and negative feelings and attitudes that may include sexual eroticism, rejection, guilt, and fear. Usually an underlying sexual problem relating to frustration can be identified in heterosexuals and homosexuals alike. In women, primary pru-

Table 30.1 Main etiology of secondary pruritus ani

Affected organs
Skin ⎫
Bowel ⎬ Including sexually transmitted diseases
Female genitalia ⎭

ritus ani is often associated with vulvar pruritus or "widow's itch," which in some cases is precipitated by masturbation. Job-related stress is believed to be a common predisposing factor in males [10].

Although earlier authors [5, 11] estimated that 45%–70% of pruritus ani cases were idiopathic, we find that virtually all of our cases have a discernable cause and are amenable to effective treatment.

Secondary Pruritus Ani

In secondary pruritus ani a specific etiology for the anal itch can be identified (Table 30.1).

Evolution of Pruritus Ani

In the absence of a sexually transmitted disease or frank dermatosis affecting the perianal skin, a skin lesion cannot be identified initially *(pruritus ani without skin changes)*. Scratching or the action of chemical or infectious agents subsequently evokes a skin reaction characterized by redness, excoriation, weeping, and possibly suppuration. This stage is called *perianal dermatitis*. With sensitization to chemical or infectious agents comes the stage of *acute perianal eczema* with the formation of papules and vesicles. This may progress to *chronic perianal eczema* with lichenification of the skin. Terminology in this area is often imprecise, and it is common to apply the collective term "perianal eczema" to all the cutaneous reactions to pruritus.

Epidemiology

The anus is one of the most common sites for the occurrence of nongeneralized pruritus [1]. Pruritus ani is unquestionably the most common symptom in proctology. In affects males predominantly by a ratio of four to one (see references in [8]). Most patients are between 30 and 60 years of age.

Differential Diagnosis of Secondary Pruritus Ani

As shown in Table 30.1, secondary pruritus can mainly result from skin diseases, bowel diseases, diseases of the female genitalia, including sexually transmitted diseases and others. The most important of these conditions are listed in Table 30.2.

Dermatoses are a common cause of secondary pruritus ani, the most common causative disease being psoriasis. In typical cases the condition can be recognized by a gastroenterologist, especially if psoriatic plaques are found elsewhere on the body. But a large percentage of anal skin diseases are iatrogenic, and many are caused by self-medication leading to contact dermatitis. Common offending substances are locally applied hemorrhoidal creams and suppositories, antibiotics, and even corticosteroids. The latter can lead to sensitization of the skin or atrophy resulting in increased susceptibility to damage. The breakdown products or unabsorbed portions of many orally administered medications act as contact allergens. This applies particularly to laxatives, especially those containing phenolphthalein and anthraquinone glycosides. Rufli ([9] p. 131) mentions barbiturates, pyrazolones, and sulfonamides as the most common orally administered pruritogenic drugs. Quinine, hydantoin, and metronidazole can also incite contact dermatitis, as can the dyes and perfuming agents used in toilet tissue. If a fungal infection is suspected (*Candida,* dermatophytes), a smear should be taken and dissolved in 20% potassium hydroxide for microscopic examination. Culture studies require special nutrient media.

Sexually transmitted diseases have fortunately become a less frequent cause of pruritus ani owing to increased vigilance in AIDS prevention.

In patients with bowel disease, it is essential that history taking include questions about self-medication (including laxatives), deodorant use, food allergies and intolerances, anal hygiene, and characteristics of clothing and undergarments. A number of spices and beverages can cause pruritus ani, especially when consumed in large amounts. Friend [4] lists coffee (regular and decaffeinated), tea, cola, beer, chocolate, and tomatoes (including ketchup) as the principal offenders. Patients can vary greatly in their tolerance to these food items, and some patients are unable to tolerate them at all. The mechanism involved in this etiology of pruritus ani is unknown.

The proctologic examination may have to be repeated several times. Small fistulous tracts, for example, may close temporarily and be missed on ini-

Table 30.2 Etiology of secondary pruritus ani

Skin diseases
  Psoriasis
  Moniliasis and other mycoses
  Neurodermatitis (lichen chronicus simplex)
  Lichen sclerosus
  Contact dermatitis and eczema
  Benign and malignant tumors

Sexually transmitted diseases
  Gonorrhea
  Syphilis (itching very rare!)
  Herpes simplex
  Chlamydia trachomatis
  Lymphogranuloma venereum
  Condylomata acuminata

Bowel diseases
  a) Anorectal diseases
    Hemorrhoids
    Skin tags
    Anorectal prolapse
    Anorectal incontinence
    Hyperhidrosis, especially in obese persons
    Deep-set anus
    Excessive perianal hair
    Proctitis
    Rectal ulcer
    Anal cryptitis
    Anal fistula
    Anal fissure
    Pinworm infestation
    Benign and malignant tumors
  b) Diseases above the rectum
    Colitis of any etiology
    Malignant and benign tumors
    Chronic constipation
    Diarrhea of any etiology, especially in laxative
    abusers
    Irritable colon with excessive mucus production
    Food intolerances and allergies

Diseases of the female genitalia
  Monilial vulvitis
  Vaginal discharge
  Lichen sclerosus
  Uterine prolapse
  Estrogen deficiency in menopausal women

Systemic diseases
  a) Endocrine and metabolic
    Diabetes mellitus
    Hyper- and hypothyroidism
    Uremia
  b) Chronic cholestasis
    Intrahepatic, e. g., primary biliary cirrhosis
    Extrahepatic
  c) Malignant disease
    Lymphoma
    Leukemia
    Multiple myeloma, paraproteinemia
    Carcinoids and carcinomas
    Polycythemia rubra vera
  d) Iron deficiency anemia

Allergic diseases
  Drug reactions
  Parasitic infestations (trichinosis, schistosomiasis, etc.)
  Food allergies

Miscellaneous diseases
  Senile pruritus
  Psychiatric disorders (depression, psychoneurosis)
  Radiodermatitis

tial examination. Occasionally the documentation of an incompetent anal sphincter will require special manometric studies in addition to history taking and digital palpation.

Evaluation for pinworm infestation is most easily accomplished by affixing a strip of transparent adhesive tape to the anal border in the early morning and then removing and examining the tape under a microscope to check for any eggs deposited during the night.

Diarrhea is a more frequent cause of pruritus ani than constipation. There is both a chemical irritation to the anal skin from the frequent passage of stool and a mechanical irritation due to frequent wiping of the area with tissue. Constipation can lead to pruritus by aggravating a hemorrhoidal condition with the development of anitis and by fecal soiling of the anus. Many patients with skin tags are not susceptible to pruritus ani and experience no complaints. However, if anal itching is present and no other cause can be found, excision of the tags will relieve the pruritus in most patients. If disease of the female genitalia is suspected or identified, prompt gynecologic consultation is advised.

Systemic diseases are very rarely associated with pruritus ani as an isolated symptom, and the pruritus is usually generalized. Even so, the anal component may be perceived as particularly distressful. Pruritus limited to the anus and possibly to the vulva is seen most commonly in frank diabetes mellitus, in which case the hyperglycemia and moist environment combine to promote fungal or bacterial infection.

Diagnostic Procedures

It is a classic rule of internal medicine that every patient undergoes a thorough examination before a diagnosis is made and treatment prescribed. However, practical demands place limits on this approach, and I have devised a simple but pragmatic evaluation scheme which is outlined below:

- If the patient presents with several complaints including pruritus ani, a general clinical assessment is done before proceeding to a proctologic examination and, if necessary, a gastroenterologic examination.
- If the patient presents with anal itching as an isolated symptom but is otherwise well, the scheme in Fig. 30.1 is followed.

Most causes of pruritus ani can be recognized and treated by the gastroenterologist or proctologist. These include hemorrhoids, simple fistulas, cryptitis, pinworm infestation, laxative abuse, all forms of colitis, and contact dermatitis. Systemic diseases such as diabetes mellitus and cancer will be detected in the course of the clinical and laboratory evaluation. Greater difficulties are encountered in patients with food allergies or intolerances, which may not be obvious. These cases can be managed by prescribing an elimination diet or by seeking the help of an allergologist.

If evidence of a gynecologic disorder is found in a female patient, or if the patient has a perianal lesion that cannot be readily classified, prompt referral to a gynecologist or dermatologist is advised. The proctologist untrained in dermatology does not have the experience necessary to evaluate, say, contact dermatitis of unknown cause (history, skin tests, serologic studies). A program of interdisciplinary consultation like that practiced at the University of Basel ([9] p. 119) is ideal but cannot always be implemented. Lesions that overtax the capabilities of the proctologist-internist are an indication for surgical consultation with appropriate further evaluation and treatment.

Sullivan and Garnjobst [14] estimate that approximately 5% of patients with pruritus ani require the help of a dermatologist, while Jackson [7] states that an equal percentage require surgical consultation.

The need for psychiatric referral should be carefully deliberated, since the suggestion is likely to be upsetting to the patient. By posing sensitive questions concerning the patient's occupational history, family situation, sexual behavior, etc., even the physician untrained in psychosomatic medicine can

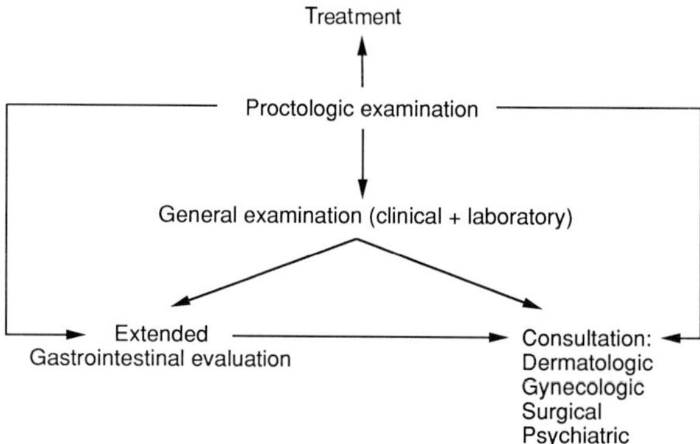

Fig. 30.1. Diagnostic evaluation of pruritus ani

make the patient aware of possible connections and may even offer therapeutic benefit. If these efforts are of no avail and it is suspected that the pruritus ani is "idiopathic" or secondary to depression or psychoneurosis, there should be no difficulty, following several weeks or months of observation, in convincing the patient of the need for psychological or psychiatric evaluation and treatment.

Conservative Treatment

Primary Pruritus Ani

Even when a specific cause for the pruritus cannot be found, the patient should receive instruction in anal hygiene (see below), since even slight fecal residues or other mild irritations of the perianal skin will cause pruritus in certain individuals. Some who are fanatical about anal cleanness may have to be restrained rather than motivated! Rufli ([9] p. 122) recommends cleaning the affected area with pads soaked in 3% boric acid solution twice daily for 10 min. The solitude of this regimen can also be beneficial in terms of stress reduction. Commercial products such as crotamiton lotion or Anal-Gen (BCL Company, Zürich) may also be tried, as can oral antihistamines or sedatives such as benzodiazepine. A trial elimination diet (see "Food Allergies and Intolerances" below) may be worthwhile, since food sensitivities and allergies can have causal significance in pruritus. Some patients benefit from infiltration of the perianal region with a corticosteroid (e. g., triamcinolone 1–4 ml) employing the same technique used for injecting a local anesthetic. As a last resort the patient may be referred to a psychiatrist or psychosomaticist.

Secondary Pruritus Ani

Principle of Treatment

Whenever a likely or potential cause of pruritus ani is identified, it should be eliminated if possible. This may involve the eradication of a hemorrhoidal condition, a dermatosis, or a gynecologic disorder.

Anal Hygiene

Major emphasis is placed on meticulous anal hygiene. The importance of this can be imparted simply by telling the patient to keep the anus as clean as his or her face. Following defecation the anus should first be cleaned with soft, white toilet tissue or facial tissue, which may be moistened with water before use. The area is then cleansed again with wet cotton. If this is not sufficient, final cleansing should be done with a moist medicated pad such as Tucks. Some patients can clean themselves better with a bidet or removable shower head or by using an automatic closet (Closomat). Dryness can be maintained by wearing a cotton against the anus, and this is especially recommended in obese individuals or in other patients who are apt to have excessive intergluteal moisture. The cotton pledget should be just large enough not to be perceived as a foreign body, and it should be changed several times daily. Talcum powder may be shaken onto the pledget to improve the absorption of moisture.

Some patients will require more detailed instructions, and these should be provided in the form of a printed guide. One such guide, drawn from Alexander-Williams [2] and Sullivan and Garnjobst [14], is illustrated below:

1. Use soft white toilet paper or facial tissues to clean the anus. Cleaning may be more effective if the tissue is first moistened with water.
2. For final cleaning, avoid rubbing the anus with a washcloth. Instead, use white cotton soaked in cold water. Clean the anus in this way in the morning and evening, even if you have not had a bowel movement.
3. For difficult cleaning use a soap solution; do not rub bar soap on the anal area. Moist, medicated pads such as Tucks may be used for final cleaning. Many patients obtain better results using a hand-held sprayer, a bidet, or an automatic closet (Closomat).
4. Keep the anal area dry. If necessary, dry the cleaned area with an electric hair dryer and place a strip of cotton in the cleft between the buttocks. Talcum powder may be shaken onto the cotton to help absorb moisture.
5. Wear cotton underclothing instead of nylon. Avoid tight-fitting garments such as corsets and leotards. Avoid wearing tight trousers, and do not wear jeans.
6. Do not apply deodorants to the anus, and use only soft toilet tissue.
7. Avoid constipation by consuming a high-fiber diet (lots of vegetables, whole grain bread). Supplement if necessary with wheat bran and/or mucilage. Small amounts of mucilage are also helpful in relieving diarrhea.
8. If itching is worse following bowel movements, do a rectal irrigation using a 50- to 100-ml bulb syringe and warm water.
9. If you tend to scratch the affected area at night, put on light cotton gloves before retiring.
10. Do not use ointments, creams, suppositories, hip baths, or other products unless told to do so by your doctor.

For the occasional patient who becomes obsessive about cleanliness and practices too much anal hygiene rather than too little, a balance can often be struck by reducing the cleaning procedures. These patients tend to belong to the group with primary (idiopathic) pruritus ani.

Pruritus Ani in Elderly Patients and Menopausal Women

The fissuring that occurs in atrophic geriatric skin can perpetuate anal pruritus. In these cases it is beneficial to follow cleaning by the application of a mild cream such as cold cream, Decoderm base cream Merck, Darmstadt, or dexpanthenol cream. Pruritus ani or pruritus of the anus and vulva in menopausal women may result from an estrogen deficiency and will respond to hormonal replacement therapy.

Anti-Inflammatory and Astringent Hip Baths

For acutely inflamed skin we prescribe hip baths with camomile (e. g., Kamillosan; Degussa, Frankfurt) twice daily. When acute inflammation has subsided, the resistance of the skin to various types of injury can be increased by prescribing astringent hip baths once or twice daily, e. g., with tannin solutions (Lohtannin; Wolo, Zürich) or potassium permanganate (0.1–0.2 ppt).

Bacterial and Fungal Superinfection

When superinfection is suspected, the physician concerned with an accurate diagnosis will prepare a smear and, if necessary, will culture for fungi and bacteria so that a specific antimicrobial therapy can be prescribed. This may be supplemented by the application of a corticosteroid cream. The busy proctologist or gastroenterologist generally prefers to treat empirically by prescribing a trial of Decoderm trialolent (fluprednylidenacetat, gentamycin, Chlorhydroxychinolin), Mycolog (Triamcinolon, Neomycin, Gramicidin, Nystatin) or other trivalent cream for a maximum of 3 weeks. These products contain a corticosteroid, an antibiotic, and a fungicide. This therapy may be used adjunctively in the presence of a causally treated disease to promote more rapid healing.

Weight Reduction

Weight reduction is a desirable measure in overweight patients. Obesity promotes sweat secretion and leads to increased mechanical irritation of the skin between the buttocks.

Hemorrhoids

Second and third degree hemorrhoids are managed by sclerotherapy or rubber band ligation. Infrared coagulation may be used for first degree hemorrhoids. Hemorrhoidal creams and suppositories have their place in these cases for the temporary relief of anitis and perianal dermatitis.

Food Allergies and Intolerances

Evaluation for a presumed food allergy requires the help of an allergologist (epicutaneous and scratch tests, serologic studies). The distinctions between food allergies and intolerances are ill-defined and in any case have little relevance in terms of therapy. Thus, even when the precise etiologic mechanism is unknown, an elimination diet may be prescribed to see whether the pruritus will disappear. As noted in "Differential Diagnosis of Secondary Pruritus Ani" above, the elimination of coffee (including decaffeinated), tea, cola, beer, chocolate, and tomatoes (including ketchup) may suffice. Smith et al. [13] extended this list and were able to achieve partial or complete relief of pruritus in 27 of 56 patients. Their elimination diet includes nicotine abstinence (Table 30.3).

If the elimination diet is successful in stopping the

Table 30.3. Elimination diet for patients with pruritus ani. (From [13])

Coffee
Tea
Cola
Alcohol
Chocolate
Tomatoes (including ketchup)
Citrus fruits
Pork
Milk
Nuts
Spices
Smoking

pruritus, individual items may be reintroduced after about 3 weeks so that the offending item can be identified (exposure diet). Some patients on this regimen who have a food intolerance rather than an allergy report finding a threshold for the pruritogenic effect. For example, 6 or 9 dl beer may evoke anal itching while 3 dl does not.

Surgical Treatment

Primary Pruritus Ani

Classic surgical procedures involving partial resection of the anal skin and subcutaneous nerve division are no longer practiced today.

Secondary Pruritus Ani

Surgical referral is indicated in cases where secondary pruritus ani overtaxes the abilities of the attending internist-proctologist. This is the case, for example, in patients with surgically treatable anorectal incontinence, large condylomata acuminata, large cutaneous and colorectal tumors, complicated fistulous lesions, and occasionally in patients with large hemorrhoids. The appropriate surgical procedures are described elsewhere in this book.

References

1. Achten G, De Maubeuge J (1975) Le prurit anal. Arch Fr Mal App Dig 64: 561–572
2. Alexander-Williams J (1983) Causes and management of anal irritation. Br Med J 287: 1528
3. Duret-Cosyns S (1975) Prurit anal et psychosomatique. Arch Fr Mal App Dig 64: 601–608

4. Friend WG (1977) The cause and treatment of idiopathic pruritus ani. Dis Colon Rectum 20: 40–42
5. Fromer JL (1955) Dermatologic concepts and management of pruritus ani. Am J Surg 90: 805–815
6. Greaves MW (1982) The nature and management of pruritus. Practitioner 226: 1223–1225
7. Jackson CC (1974) Surgical indications in pruritus ani. Rocky Mt Med J 61: 29–32
8. Pecorella G, Pepe G, Pepe F, Gula A, Cannamela G, Calabrese C, Pecorella S (1985) Attuali orientamenti di diagnosi e terapia del prurito anale. Minerva Med 76: 1221–1226
9. Rufli T (1976) In: Buchmann P (ed) Lehrbuch der Proktologie. Huber, Bern
10. Schuppli R (1959) Über den Pruritus vulvae. Schweiz Med Wochenschr 89: 425–426
11. Shapiro AL, Rothman S (1945) Pruritus ani: a clinical study. Gastroenterology 5: 155–168
12. Shelley WB, Arthur RP (1970) The neurohistology and neurophysiology of the itch sensation in man. Arch Dermatol 76: 296–323
13. Smith LE, Henrichs D, McCullah RD (1982) Prospective studies on the etiology and treatment of pruritus ani. Dis Colon Rectum 25: 358–363
14. Sullivan ES, Garnjobst WM (1978) Pruritus ani: a practical approach. Surg Clin North Am 58: 505–512
15. Verbov J (1984) Pruritus ani and its management – a study and reappraisal. Clin Exp Dermatol 9: 46–52

31 Resurfacing the Perineal Area in Soft Tissue Defects

R. Gumener and D. Montandon

Introduction

Soft tissue defects of the perineum may result in significant anatomical and functional anomalies. Every effort has to be made to restore contour and function, the psychological impact of such a problem being disastrous. Skin defects in this area may result from infection, burns, skin tumor surgery, pressure sores, trauma, or radiodermatitis. Congenital anomalies will not be discussed here.

Soft tissue defects in this particular area, as in all cases of plastic surgery, can be repaired by primary closure, spontaneous wound healing, skin grafting, regional flaps (random, axial, myocutaneous or distant flaps). The most suitable technique should be chosen according to the sex and age of the patient and the precise location, depth, and extent of the defect. The major problems for reconstruction in this area are fecal contamination, difficult immobilization, and the problems associated with urethral or rectal repairs [4].

Wound Healing

Wound healing is achieved by contraction of the granulation tissue and migration of epithelial cells after fibroblasts from the granulation tissue and epithelial cells from the wound edges acquire contractile properties [14]. In the perineal area, this phenomenon plays an important role in closing soft tissue defects. Small raw areas after trauma or tumor excision can thus permit "controlled" wound healing! Frequent dressings with local steroids will inhibit granulation tissue, while dressings with hypertonic solutions or a tulle gras type of dressing will activate it.

If distortion or stenosis as a result of the contraction phenomena of wound healing is likely to have functional repercussions, then a skin graft or a skin flap technique should be used. While skin grafting results in some contraction, a flap should prevent it.

Primary Closure

When the skin defect is small, a direct closure can be performed if no significant retraction is anticipated. This is possible by undermining and mobilizing the surrounding well-vascularized cutaneous tissue, particularly the mobile scrotal skin and, to some extent, the labial skin [4].

Skin Grafts

Coverage of a large, uncomplicated, raw, uninfected area is best achieved by split-thickness skin grafting, the external lateral side of the thighs and buttocks being the ideal donor sites. A manual, electric or air-driven dermatome (Brown) is used to take long strips of split-thickness skin. For larger pieces, drum dermatomes (Rees-Paget) are preferred. The thickness of the grafts will vary between 0.2 mm and 0.4 mm [1].

Grafts can be meshed, which means that tiny multiple slits are made to allow the graft to expand to 1.5 or three times its original size. The slits also facilitate drainage of the wound. The graft is applied to the wound and stretched over the area, then sutured to its border. For large grafts, a spray of biological glue will help the immobilization of the graft and the healing. A tie-over dressing will complete the operation. The dressing is to be removed after 48–72 h to permit direct control of the position of the graft and avoid maceration and infection. Hematoma or a serous accumulation of fluid can then be evacuated. Postoperative care is very important: the site must be cleaned and dried at least twice a day. A dry dressing will avoid maceration and infection or movement at the graft-host interface [12].

Flaps

When the defect is too large or too deep, or is surrounded by a significant area of scarred or irradiated tissue with poor vascularization, the simple procedure described above is not feasible and the surgeon will have to use skin or myocutaneous flaps.

The thighs and the buttock will give regional skin flaps of the random type. Z-plasty flaps, advancement, transposition or rotation random flaps will solve many problems, restoring contour and usually permitting direct closure at the donor site [4, 5, 8, 10, 16, 18, 20]. These random flaps lack a recognized anatomical arteriovenous system and survive on dermic and subcutaneous circulation: they must therefore be of the classic length-to-width ratio of 2.5 : 1.

For an axial skin flap only, the groin is available in this area. It is vascularized by an axial arteriovenous system, i.e., the superficial iliac circumflex vessels. It can be used for defects in the suprapubic and anterioperineal area.

When the defect is larger, or the circulation in the area of the wound is impaired, e. g., due to radiotherapy, or the defect is deep, it is useful to bring in a bulky, well-vascularized tissue. This can be best achieved by myocutaneous flaps [4, 10, 11, 13]. The skin in such flaps is transferred on a muscle pedicle which is a vessel carrier. Perforating vessels from the muscle vascularize the skin. The best myocutaneous flaps for perineal reconstruction are the gracilis, the semimembanous, the tensor fasciae latae, the inferior thigh flap, the rectus femoris, the biceps femori, the gluteal thigh myocutaneous flap, and, in some particular cases, the rectus abdominus fan flap. The advantages of such flaps are: optimal wound healing because of the rich vascularization of these flaps, good filling of deep defects, and, in some cases, functional reconstruction as in the treatment of anal incontinence [4, 6, 7, 9, 11, 17].

Pre- and Perioperative Care

When good and safe control of an infected perineal wound is obtained and when a relatively short time (10–12 days) is planned for good healing after reconstruction, patients are given a low-residue diet. In some particular cases, to avoid long contamination of the wound or of the reconstructed area with faces, a provisory colostomy is performed. Local preparation is by frequent dressings and baths, keeping the area as clean as possible. An indwelling urethral catheter is inserted, and a systemic antibiotic therapy should accompany the treatment.

Patients are usually operated on in the lithotomy position. Anesthesia is local, caudal, or general according to the extent of the surgical procedure, as well as the age and the wishes of the patient. Local

infiltration with a vasoconstrictor helps to diminish the bleeding. Hemostasis is performed very carefully.

Infections

Infection in this area often results in skin loss. Resurfacing by split-skin grafts or local flaps should take place only after the end of the infectious course.

Hidradenitis Suppurativa

Recurrent folliculitis or skin irritation can result in hidradenitis suppurativa [2–10]. This disease of the apocrine gland areas can develop draining sinus tracts and thick scar tissue after developing multiple abscess-like swellings. Surgery is indicated in the chronic forms: limited areas can be excised and closed directly, whereas after excision of large areas resurfacing is achieved by either split-thickness skin grafts or local flaps. A systemic antibiotic therapy accompanies the treatment. (The importance of the postoperative dressings has already been stressed.)

Fournier's Gangrene

Fournier, in 1883 [3], described an idiopathic gangrene of the penile and scrotal skin. Other authors have described a perineal or ischiorectal abscess, a perineal fistula, necrotizing fasciitis, or gangrenous erysipelas resulting in a variable extent of necrosis of the perineum (Figs. 31.1, 31.2) [5, 16, 20].

Systemic antibiotic therapy, antitetanus immunization, control of underlying debilitating conditions, and thorough debridement precedes surgical treatment. For small areas of scrotal loss, spontaneous epithelialization is allowed. Healing can be rapid and the final aspect good. Larger areas of necrosis can be resurfaced after debridement with a split-thickness skin graft or with the remaining scrotal skin. For still larger areas, when the testes are denuded and the spermatic cord exposed, resurfacing with cutaneous or musculocutaneous flaps from the thigh will give the best results. The testes and cord may be buried in a subcutaneous medial thigh pocket (Fig. 31.1).

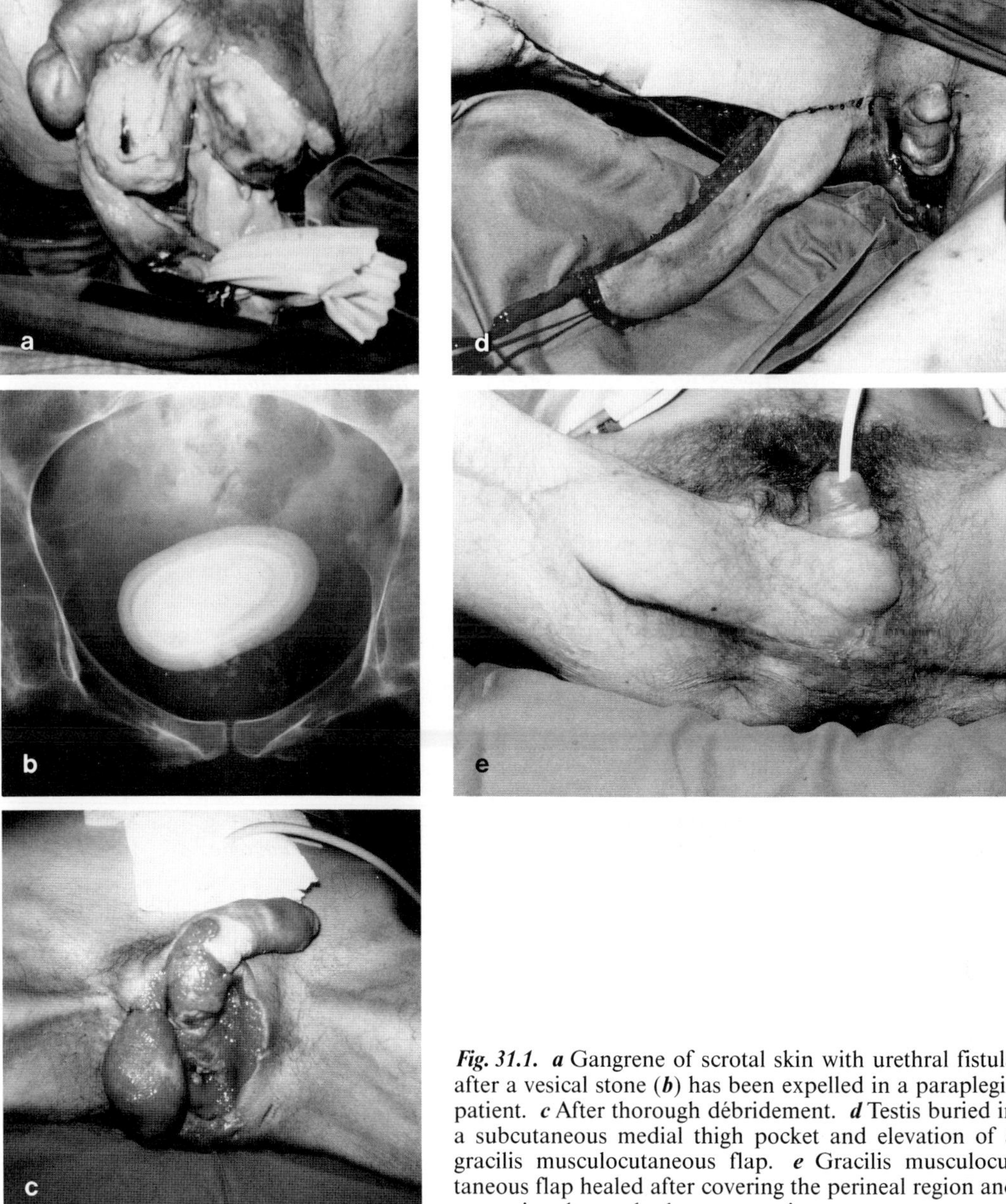

Fig. 31.1. *a* Gangrene of scrotal skin with urethral fistula after a vesical stone (*b*) has been expelled in a paraplegic patient. *c* After thorough débridement. *d* Testis buried in a subcutaneous medial thigh pocket and elevation of a gracilis musculocutaneous flap. *e* Gracilis musculocutaneous flap healed after covering the perineal region and protecting the urethral reconstruction

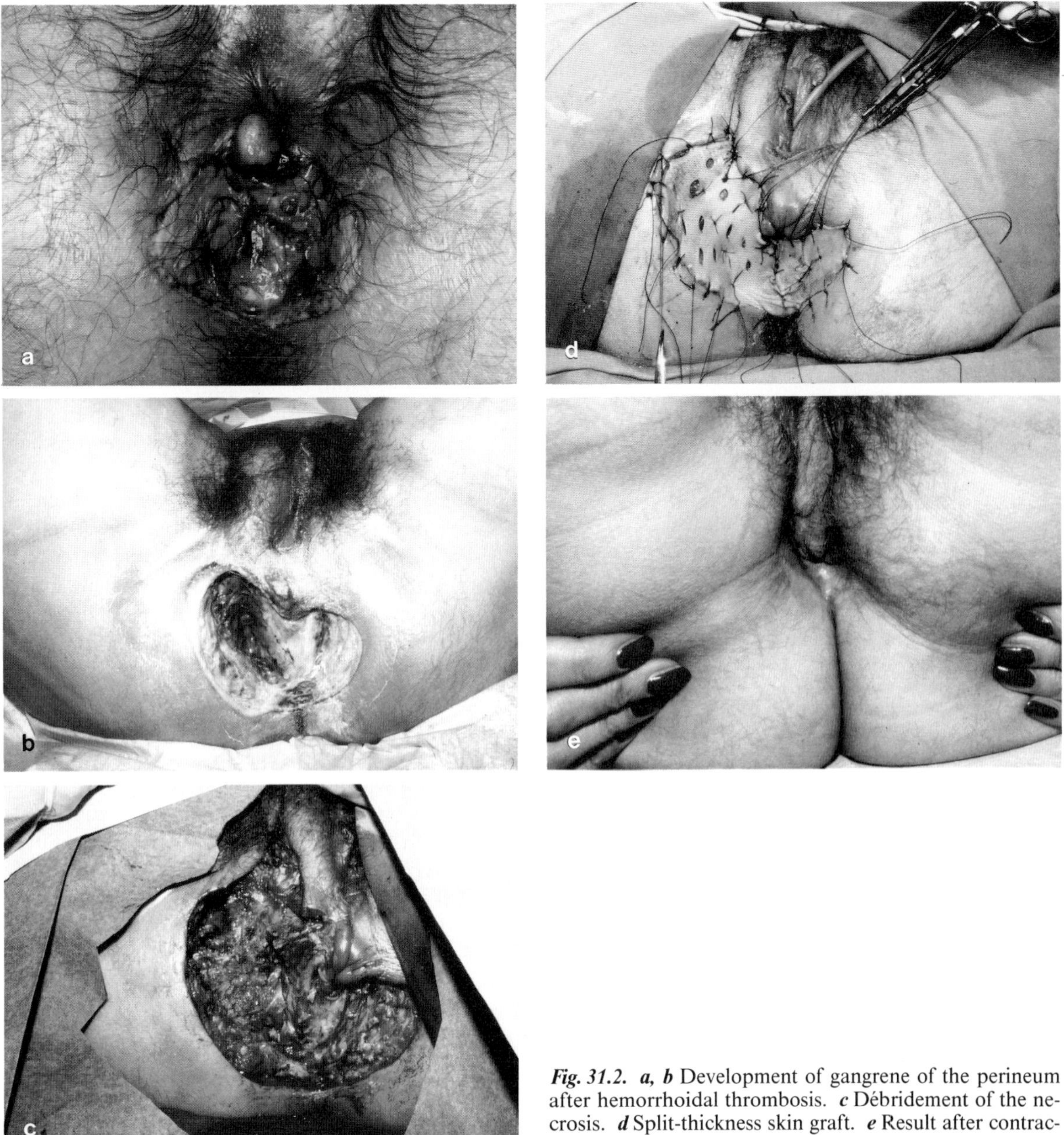

Fig. 31.2. *a, b* Development of gangrene of the perineum after hemorrhoidal thrombosis. ***c*** Débridement of the necrosis. ***d*** Split-thickness skin graft. ***e*** Result after contraction of the wound

Burns (Fig. 31.3)

Treatment must take into account the lapse of time since the original accident. In a freshly burned area, early diagnosis of the depth of the burn is very important. A second-degree burn will heal spontaneously with little or no distortion. Good local wound cleaning and appropriate dressings will prevent infection and allow proper healing.

A full-thickness burn will need rapid, special treatment to avoid retraction of the tissues. Daily bathing is of great importance in keeping the site as clean as possible. Early excision and grafting, i. e., on the 3rd–5th day, will avoid any significant distortion. When healing is achieved, a Jobst-type compression will help to prevent hypertrophy of scars and later deformity.

Tumors

The type of reconstruction will depend not only on the depth and width of excision, but also on whether or not surgical excision can be considered curative and whether or not the tissue has been irradiated.

For superficial skin and mucosal tumors, such as Bowen's disease (Fig. 31.4) (carcinoma in situ), Paget's disease, pseudo-malignancies such as giant condyloma acuminatum (Buschke-Loewestein) (Fig. 31.5), bowenoid papulosis, and radiodermatitis, total excision has to be performed with electrocautery [19] or laser. Peroperative frozen sections are requested in cases of doubt regarding the extension of the tumor so as to avoid recurrence. Direct closure is performed when possible.

Resurfacing with a skin graft is recommended for wider excisions such as an extensive superficial vulvectomy. In this particular case, the postoperative care is very important as has been mentioned before ("Skin Grafts") (Figs. 31.4, 31.5).

Nevus, blue nevus, and giant hairy nevus should be excised because they are subject to irritation and thus have a tendency to transform into melanoma. Excision with a margin of a few millimeters and direct closure will be possible in most cases. Otherwise, particularly for giant hairy nevus, serial excision or excision and a skin graft will be necessary. For this kind of tumor, surgery should commence at an early age.

Nonregressing hemangioma and lymphangioma which obstruct or destroy any important structure should be excised and resurfaced by a skin graft or skin flap if direct closure is not possible.

For cancer involving the skin, mucosa, and deeper structures, large and deep excision, in some cases

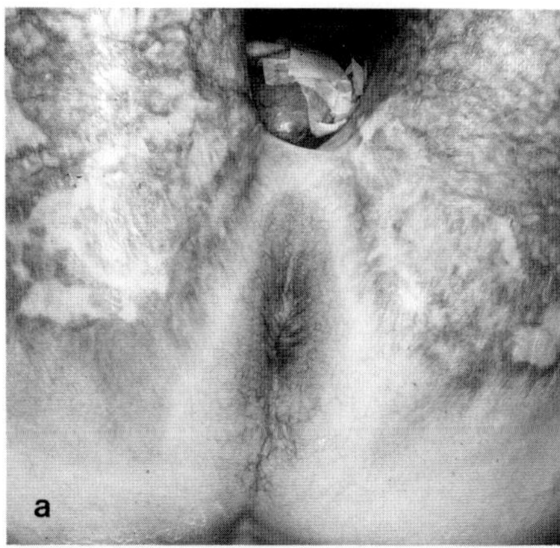
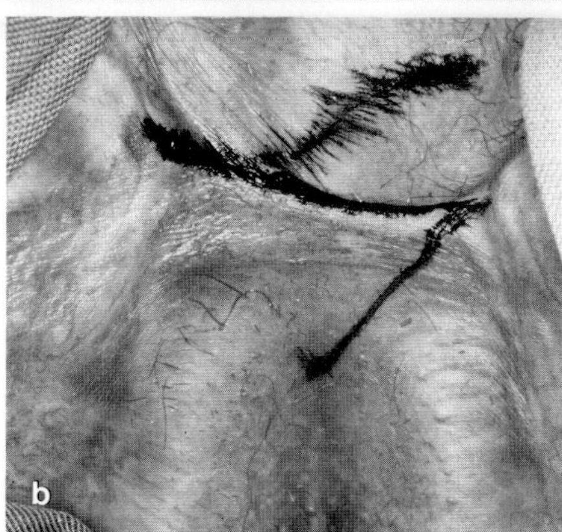
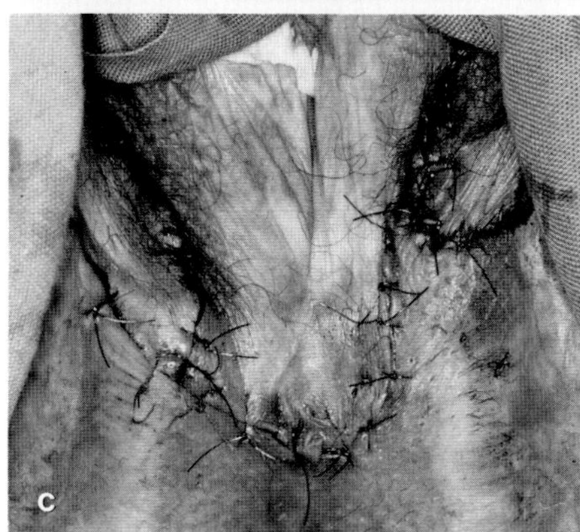

Fig. 31.3. a Burn contraction. *b* Combination of a Z and advancement flap using scrotal skin. *c* Advancement of scrotal skin

Fig. 31.4. a Perineal bowenoid lesion. *b* Excision. *c* Split-skin graft. *d* Early result

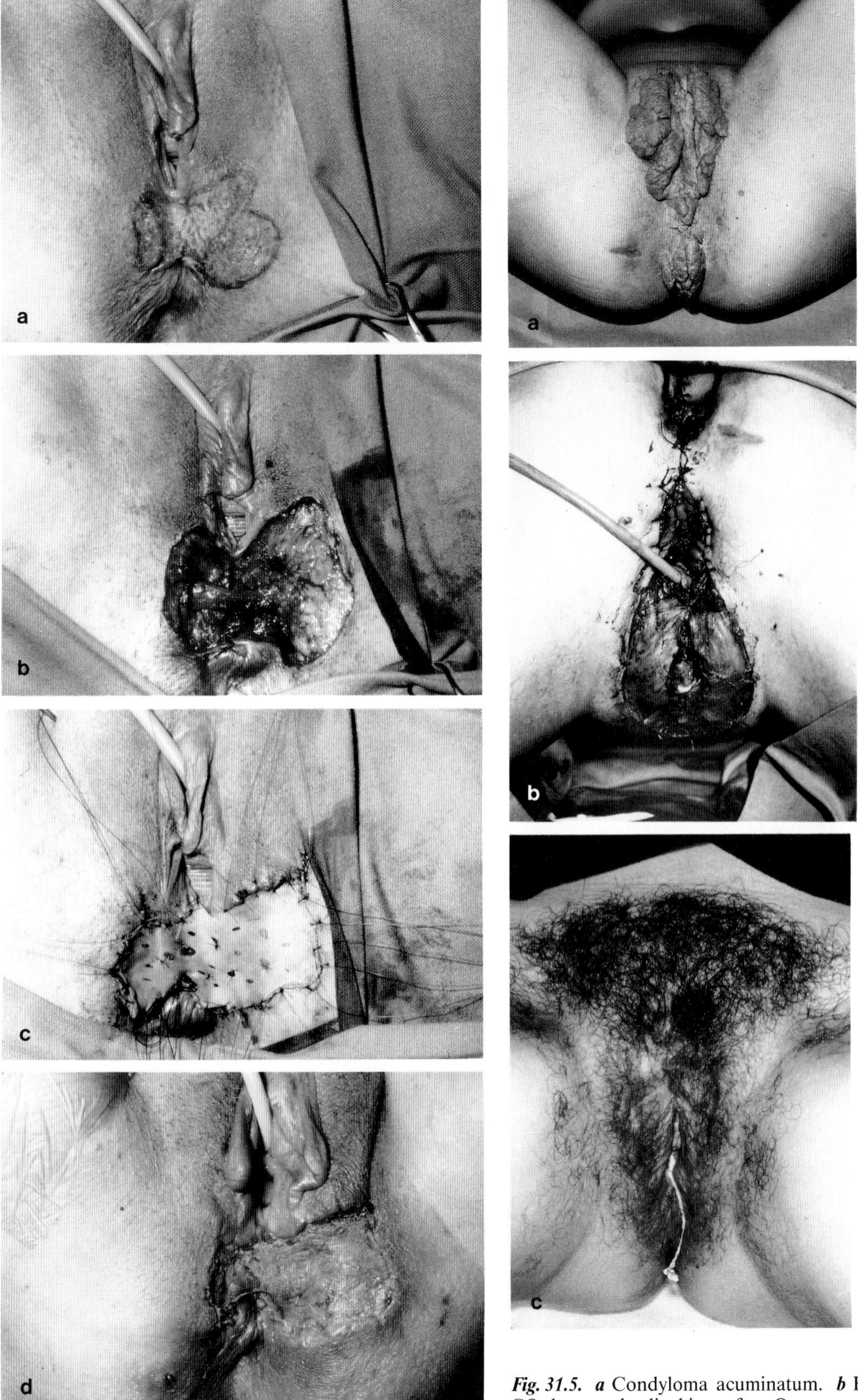

Fig. 31.5. *a* Condyloma acuminatum. *b* Excision with a CO_2 laser and split-skin graft. *c* One year after operation

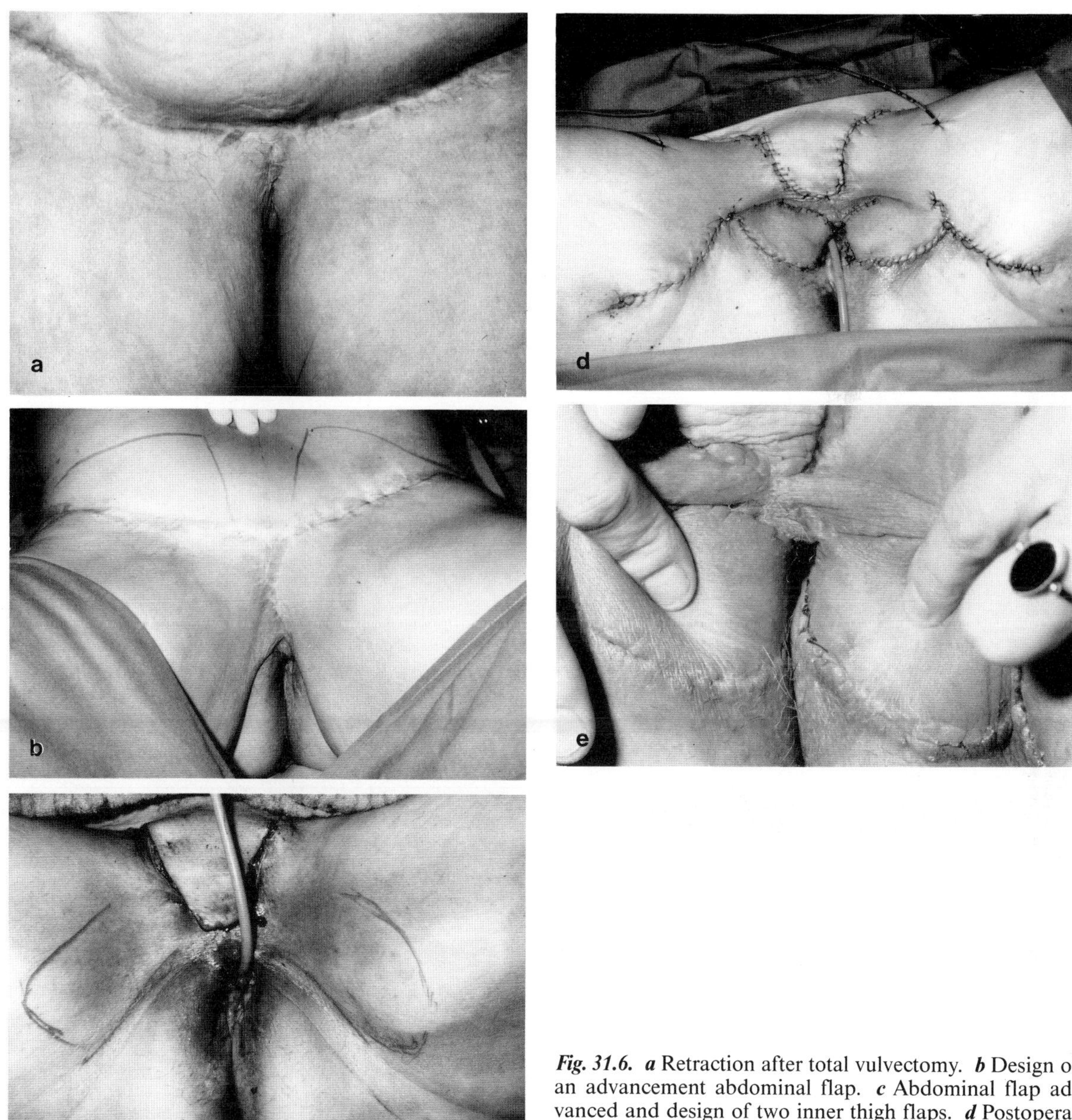

Fig. 31.6. *a* Retraction after total vulvectomy. *b* Design of an advancement abdominal flap. *c* Abdominal flap advanced and design of two inner thigh flaps. *d* Postoperative result. *e* Final vagina reconstruction with non-hair-bearing tissue

followed by radiotherapy, is necessary. For these more complex reconstructions, distant flaps may be necessary (Fig. 31.6). The gracilis musculocutaneous flap is very useful in reconstructing the vagina [4], a competent anus, or for closing some rectovaginal and rectovesical fistulas [4, 6, 7, 9, 10, 13, 17]. A tensor fasciae latae is an alternative with the rectus femori musculocutaneous flap, but it must be stressed that large free skin grafts can often help to solve definitively or apparently difficult coverage problems.

Pressure Sores

Pressure sores are special and real surgical problems, particularly in para- or tetraplegic patients. These patients should be cured as rapidly as possible so as to allow a fast socioprofessional reintegration. The majority of the pressure sores are localized in the pelvic region, the most frequent one being the ischiatic pressure sore (Fig. 31.7). In this location, surgical treatment is always necessary, conservative therapy will only delay the final heal-

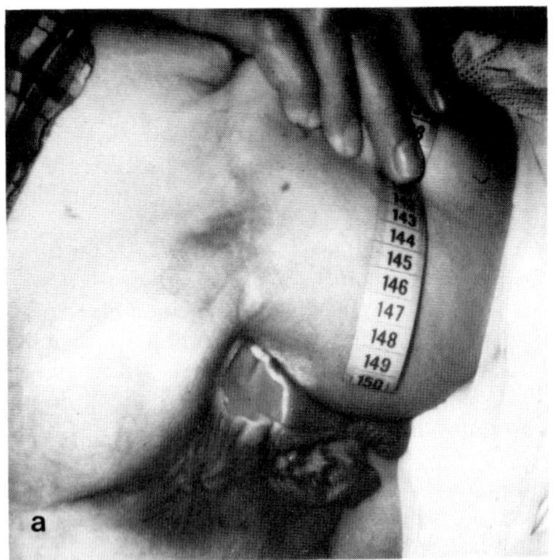

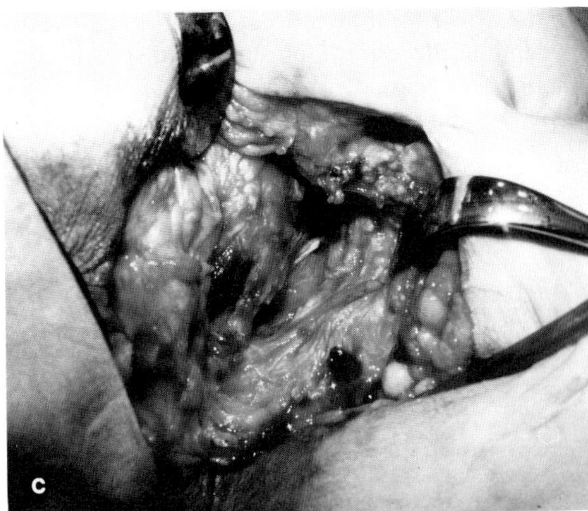

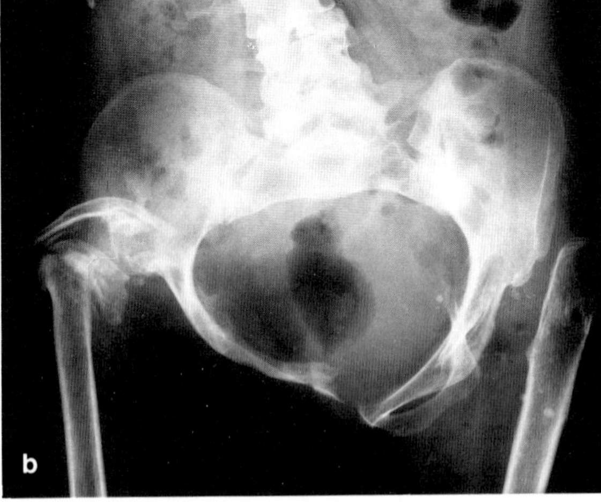

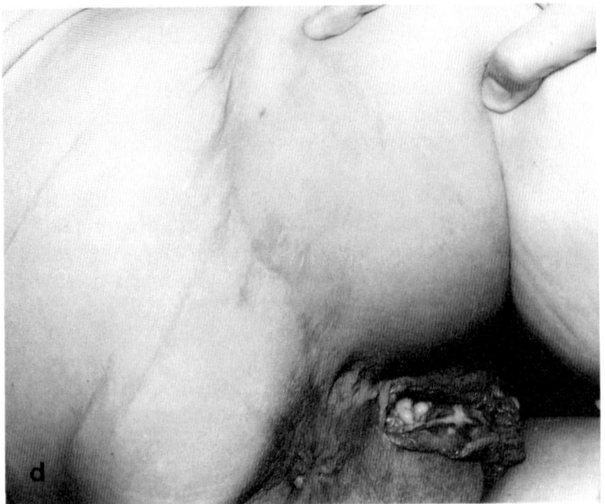

Fig. 31.7. a Paravulvar pressure sore in a paraplegic patient. **b** X-rays of this patient showing the total ischiectomy on the right side. **c** The biceps femori muscular flap was used to fill the cavity along the remaining pubic bone. **d** Result at 1 year

ing. The planning of the surgical procedure is delicate because it has to take into account the possibility of a recurrence [13].

The use of the musculocutaneous flap and a fluidized bed (Clinitron) have dramatically improved the results of surgery. The musculocutaneous flap provides bulky, well-vascularized tissue for the soft tissue defect and guarantes good defense against infection and better healing. The fluidized bed which distributes pressure equally all over the body immediately allows the patient to lie on the flap. After 3 weeks in this bed, a normal sitting pressure is permitted progressively.

For the pressure sore in the ischiatic region, our first choice is the V–Y gluteal musculocutaneous flap, followed by the V–Y biceps femori musculocutaneous flap. The tensor fasciae latae musculocutaneous flap is particularly indicated for patients with low paraplegia. These patients can gain a protective sensitivity in this area using the sensitivity of the skin of the anterolateral thigh, given by the lateral femoral cutaneous nerve which is a branch of T-12 [15].

Perineal Wounds

In persistant perineal sinus following removal of the rectum, surgical treatment using a low-string muscle graft (semimembranous muscle) to fill the cavity seems to be very effective [11].

Traumatic industrial accidents, road accidents, war wounds, penetrating injuries, and self-inflicted injuries can result in different soft tissue defects. The treatment will be chosen according to the size and the depth of the lesion. Colostomy and systemic antibiotic therapy are considered only in cases of rectal perforation (see Chap. 26).

References

1. Converse JM, McCarthy JG, Brauer RO, Ballantyne DL Jr (1977) Transplantation of skin: grafts and flaps. In: Converse JM (ed) Reconstructive plastic surgery, vol 1. Saunders, Philadelphia, pp 152–239
2. Converse JM, Popkin GL, Paletta FX, Casson PR, Robins P (1977) Tumors of skin. In: Converse JM (ed) Reconstructive plastic surgery, vol 1. Saunders, Philadelphia, pp 2879–2880
3. Fournier JA (1883) Nécrose du scrotum. Méd Prat 4: 589
4. Furnas DW, McCraw JB (1980) Resurfacing the genitalia area. Clin Plast Surg 7: 235–258
5. Giladi A, Hurwitz P, Wexler MR, Neuman Z (1973) Gangrene of peno-scrotal and perineal skin as complication of ischiorectal abscess. Chir Plast (Berl) 2: 57–61
6. Grim M, Ditterova L, Vejsada R, Hnik P, Smetana K Jr, Haninec P (1981) Experimental and anatomical basis for reconstruction of anal sphincter musculature employing gracilis muscle grafts with intact neurovascular supply. In: Freilinger G, Holle J, Carlson BM (eds) Muscle transplantation. Springer, Vienna
7. Hakelius L (1981) Treatment of anal and urinary incontinence with free muscle transplants. In: Freilinger G, Holle J, Carlson BM (eds) Muscle transplantation. Springer, Vienna
8. Hirshowitz B, Moscona R, Kaufman T, Pnini A (1980) One-stage reconstruction of the scrotum following Fournier's syndrome using a probable arterial flap. Plast Reconstr Surg 66: 608–612
9. Holle J (1981) Myoplastic operations for anal sphincter reconstruction. In: Freilinger G, Holle J, Carlson BM (eds) Muscle Transplantation. Springer, Vienna
10. Maillard GF, Gumener R (1985) The genitalia. In: Harahap M (ed) Skin surgery. Green, St Louis
11. Mann CV, Springall R (1986) Use of a muscle graft for unhealed perineal sinus. Br J Surg 73: 1000–1001
12. Marchac D (1973) Extensive superficial vulvectomy with primary skin grafting for premalignant lesions. Br J Plast Surg 26: 40–43
13. Mathes SJ, Nahai F (1982) Clinical application for muscle and musculocutaneous flaps. Mosby, St Louis, pp 388–422
14. Montandon D, d'Andiran G, Gabbiani G (1977) The mechanism of wound contraction and epithelialization. Clin Plast Surg 4: 325–346
15. Nahai F (1980) The tensor fascia lata flap. Clin Plast Surg 7: 51
16. Parkash S, Gajendran V (1984) Surgical reconstruction of the sequelae of penile and scrotal gangrene: a plea for simplicity. Br J Plast Surg 37: 354–357
17. Pickrell KL (1954) Rectal sphincter reconstruction using gracilis muscle transplant. Plast Reconstr Surg 13: 46
18. Pickrell KL, Peters C, Neale H (1975) Construction of the perineal body in the female. Plast Reconstr Surg 55: 529–532
19. Robinson JK (1980) Extirpation by electrocautery of massive lesions of condyloma acuminatum in the genito-perineo-anal region. J Dermatol Surg Oncol 6: 733–738
20. Tripathi FM, Khanna N, Venkateshwarlu V, Sinha JK (1978) Gangrene of the scrotum: a serie of 20 cases. Br J Plast Surg 31: 242–243

32 Parasitology of the Human Colorectoanal Tract

A. A. Poltera

Introduction

In this chapter some common parasitic diseases of the colorectoanal tract (CRAT) are discussed. The term "parasite" is strictly used for protozoa (unicellular organisms) and metazoa (helminths) [4]. There are special chapters in this book for infections caused by bacteria, fungi, and viruses (Chaps. 4, 28, 29).

Classification [1]

Protozoa

Unicellular parasites of interest in this chapter may be located in the small intestine and cause either lesions or interference at this level of the human host *(Cryptosporidia, Giardia lamblia)*. These parasites are then eliminated via the CRAT and may therefore be subject to laboratory microscopic detection during examination of the stools.

Similarly, there are unicellular parasites which can be found in the stools but which are generally considered to be noninfectious (e. g., *Entamoeba coli* or *Entamoeba hartmanni, Chilomastix mesnili, Iodamoeba butschlii,* and others). The protozoon which may cause a variety of lesions in the CRAT is *Entamoeba histolytica.* The disease it causes is called amebiasis.

Helminthic Metazoa

Helminths are grouped into:

- Trematodes (flat worms with suckers)
- Nematodes (round worms)
- Cestodes   (tapeworms)

Lesions in the CRAT are primarily caused by some trematodes (five types of *Schistosoma*) and to a lesser extent by nematodes *(Strongyloides stercoralis, Trichuris trichiura, Enterobius vermicularis)* all of which will be mentioned briefly.

Some other members of these two foregoing groups are either detected by the presence of their eggs in the stools *(Fasciola hepatica, Clonorchis sinensis, Opistorchis viverrini)* or by the adult worms in the stools *(Ascaris lumbricoides, Ankylostoma duodenale/Necator americanus* = hookworm) or both *(Ascaris,* hookworm). These worms do not cause lesions in the CRAT, but exceptionally there may be mechanical obstruction or ectopic localizations. The adults of *Angiostrongylus costaricensis* live intravascularly and cause lesions in the CRAT. In addition there are larvae of nematodes *(Anisakis, Oesophagostomum)* which can affect parts of the gastrointestinal tract (GIT) and also the colon.

Similarly, the adult cestodes are usually not located in the CRAT, but they are detected by the presence of their eggs in the stool *(Hymenolepis nana, Taenia saginata, Taenia solium, Diphyllobothrium latum)* or portion(s) of the adult worm *(Taeniae, Diphyllobothrium)* or the cystic stage (*Echinococcus granulosus,* cysticercosis) which can be detected by direct (e. g., sonography, laparotomy) or indirect methods (e. g., circulating antibody detection).

Amebiasis

Epidemiology [6, 8, 10]

Although *Entamoeba histolytica* (Eh) was discovered in St. Petersburg (Russia), it is now mainly restricted to tropical and subtropical regions – but patients with nonimported amebiasis have been reported from central Europe. The parasite persists in the soil or on plants in an encysted form which is spread by contamination with human feces. This encysted form must be swallowed to have access to the human colon where it will excyst to the motile and potentially invasive trophozoitic stage.

Pathophysiology and Clinical Presentation [1, 2, 4, 6, 7]

The trophozoites of Eh may enzymatically cause ulcers in the colonic mucosa which can, although rarely, lead to perforation (high mortality rate), but they may also have access to the blood stream and then cause localized parenchymatous destruction in various organs (so-called amebic abscesses mostly occurring in the right lobe of the liver). In some instances the host may react with proliferation of the skin (mucocutaneous amebiasis) and/or with granulation tissue (ameboma of the colon) or with fistula formation.

In the case of colonic ulcers, the patient will suffer from mucohemorrhagic dysentery – called amebic dysentery – and have abdominal pain/cramps, tenesmus, and usually mild fever.

On the other hand, in the case of ameboma, mucocutaneous amebiasis or amebic liver abscess, there is usually no concomitant amebic dysentery, and the local condition must be differentiated from a malignancy.

Diagnostic Procedures [3, 4, 6, 7]

Amebic dysentery is directly diagnosed by the presence of trophozoites of Eh in the patient's stools. The sole presence of cysts of Eh is not sufficient to establish a parasite-disease relationship – such a person may only be a disease-free carrier.

Warm, fresh stools from a patient with amebic dysentery are *examined immediately or fixed.* In the former case, the fresh preparation will show motile *trophozoites* with continuous pseudopodia formation, while in the latter case a merthiolate -iodine-formaldehyde (MIF) mixture is best used for fixation and staining as it allows examination after considerable delay. In such preparations it is possible to observe the characteristic features of the trophozoite, i.e., a single nucleus with a prominent nucleolus and nuclear membrane, possibly ingested red blood cells or their fragments, irregular form of cytoplasm.

The *cysts* are always round in shape and must have up to four nuclei – but not more – which distinguishes them from cysts of the nonpathogenic *Entamoeba coli* with four to eight nuclei.

On *rectosigmoidoscopy,* suggestive – but not pathognomonic – patterns for amebic dysentery may be present, e.g., friable mucosa, hyperemia, small ulcerations with a hemorrhagic and often undermined border. If Eh is searched for in biopsies, it is best found in the mucus surrounding the excised tissue. Eh stains brilliantly with periodic-acid-schiff stain (PAS), and its use is recommended in pseudomalignant lesions. For cellular details of Eh Heidenhain's iron hematoxylin stain is best. Immunofluorescent methods can be very helpful provided they have the appropriate specificity.

Circulating *antibody* determination of Eh in amebic dysentery is of little interest since the titers may only be weakly positive or even negative. This contrasts with amebic liver abscesses were antibody determination is vital for the diagnosis (90%–95% positive). Preparations for antigen detection of Eh in stools are not used in general, and their value has not been fully established.

Chemotherapy [2, 4, 6, 9]

Today's treatment for amebic dysentery is medical, but the choice of drug(s) and regimen(s) varies according to different authors. The effective agents are mostly 5-nitroimidazoles and they are all available in oral formulations. The recommended dosage varies according to the package instructions and so does the treatment duration (from 1 to 10 days). The more commonly used products are tinidazole, secnidazole, metronidazole, and ornidazole. In the rare instance of perforated amebic colitis, parenteral tinidazole, metronidazole, or ornidazole may be administered in association with supportive antishock therapy including steroids. Some authors still recommend the use of emetine or 2-dehydroemetine. Oral suspensions for children are available for tinidazole (very bitter) and for metronidazole (acceptable taste). Rectal suppositories (metronidazole) appear not to be indicated in amebic dysentery.

The "treatment" of patients who are passing cysts is controversial. In endemic areas it appears impossible from the economic point of view. A recent study indicates that these patients eliminate the cysts spontaneously provided sufficient follow-up time for observation is accorded [7]. To terminate the passage of cysts, additional diloxanide treatment of all patients with amebic dysentery is recommended [2, 4, 6, 9, 10]. However, a nonabsorbable arsenical (diphetarsone) is also effective [4]. There is some evidence that a high-dosage, short-course therapy of 5-nitroimidazoles is highly effective in clearing cysts of Eh in patients with amebic dysentery.

Balantidiasis [1, 2, 4, 8–11]

The ciliated, soil-transmitted protozoon called *Balantidium coli* has, like Eh an invasive trophozoite and an encysted form. In tropical and subtropical regions it has a reservoir in wild and domestic pigs where it causes little damage. However, in man, although the disease is rare, it presents as severe hemorrhagic dysentery. Deep mucosal ulcerations are often found, and the parasites may penetrate the blood vessels of the CRAT. Perforation of the colon has been reported. The clinical picture may resemble amebic dysentery. The motile trophozoites are best found in a fresh and warm stool preparation, but these big forms even impress in a fixed preparation (MIF). Chemotherapeutically, contact amebicides or tetracyclines are recommended, but metronidazole has also been effective.

Schistosomiasis

Epidemiology [4, 5, 9, 11]

The causative agent of urinary schistosomiasis or bilharziasis was discovered by T. Bilharz in the last century, but the disease has been endemic along the river Nile for thousands of years as evidenced by eggs found in mummies. In this century the causative agents of intestinal and hepatic schistosomiasis have been progressively identified. The life cycle of schistosomes involves a snail for multiplication of the asexual stages and a vertebrate host for the sexual stages. For man there are different endemic areas:

- Africa with three species: *Schistosoma mansoni* (Sm), *Schistosoma haematobium* (Sh), *Schistosoma intercalatum* (Si). There is considerable overlap of the former two, but each of them has its own transmission areas. Si is mainly seen in focalized areas of Central Africa.
- Asia with two species: *Schistosoma japonicum* (Sj) mainly in Japan (now under control), the Philippines, the mainland of China, and parts of Indonesia, and *Schistosoma mekongi* along the river Mekong.
- Latin America with Sm in Brazil, Venezuela, and in some of the Caribbean islands.

Pathophysiology and Clinical Presentation [1, 2, 4, 8]

Cercaria leave the snails and are aquatic. When man has contact with water, these cercaria penetrate through the skin or mucous membranes and reach a vascular compartment by migration and maturation. Male and female worms unite intravascularly, and the female produces eggs with given characteristics for each species which may remain at the periphery of their vascular compartment or move with the blood stream toward a parenchymatous organ.

For Sm and Sj the vascular region is the territory of the portal system and the draining organ is the liver. The deposition of the eggs at the periphery results in changes of the CRAT, mainly of a granulomatous and/or polypoid nature. When the egg is actively passing through the mucosa, it may cause a small focus of bleeding. There is associated lower abdominal pain, and irregular fever may occur. In the blood there is concomitant eosinophilia and circulating specific antibodies can be detected. If the egg is passively moved to the liver, it will induce granulomatous changes along the intrahepatic ramifications of the portal veins and finally lead to portal hypertension. The degree of pathology is basically dependent on the number of eggs deposited. For Si the same principles apply, but the granulomatous reaction is particularly intense in the CRAT.

For Sh the localization of the adult worms is the territory of the inferior vena cava, particularly the vessels surrounding the urinary bladder. The eggs deposited in the periphery reach mainly the urine via the bladder, and their passage causes hematuria and dysuria. Occasionally, eggs are also deposited in the rectum. If the eggs are passively transported in the blood stream, they will reach the lung and, rarely, the spine.

Other organs may show egg involvement, and the occurrence of ectopic adult worms has been reported.

Diagnostic Procedures [3, 4, 8]

The *free eggs* can be collected in the stools (Sm, Si, Sj) or in the urine (Sh). In the former, the Kato technique [3, 4] is most suitable, whereas in the latter centrifugation followed by the hatching test is more appropriate. The eggs are identified by the position of a surface spine and the size and shape of the egg. Lateral spines are found in Sm and Sj, the two are distinguishable by their shape and size. Terminal spines are seen in Sh and Si, again the egg form permits differentiation and the site where the eggs were collected gives further help. The viability of the egg is assessed by observing the movements of the miracidia inside the egg.

The *tissue-bound eggs* are found in biopsies and identified by their spine and shape. Their viability is assessed by the transparency of the egg. Dark eggs are dead and usually calcified. In advanced granulomata, the egg may be reduced to shell, and sometimes blackish pigment is present. Among the inflammatory cells many eosinophils can be seen.

Rectoscopy is a routine procedure in many Sm and Si areas. The fine granulomatous pattern with occasional polypoid formation is suggestive of schistosomiasis and best verified by snipping of the rectal mucosa with a small curet. The mucosal snips are immediately placed on a glass slide and compressed with another glass slide for examination under a microscope. Again, gross viability is indicated by the transparency of the eggs: if they are opaque they are considered dead; if they are translucent, they may still be alive.

The determination of specific circulating *antibodies* is helpful in the three major species. In hepatic and intestinal schistosomiasis *liver biopsy* may be indicated. In urinary schistosomiasis ultrasound, pyelography, and cystoscopy may all be indicated.

Chemotherapy [2, 4, 5, 10]

The treatment of schistosomiasis has been simplified by the introduction of single day therapy with praziquantel. The dosages involved vary with the age of the patient and the species involved. For adults the package instructions recommend the following:

- For Sh and Sm, 40 mg/kg as a single dose or twice 20 mg/kg 4 h apart with food
- For Sj, 20 mg/kg three times a day with food at intervals of 4 h.

The occurrence of abdominal cramps after praziquantel has been reported, and, rarely, bloody diarrhea has been noted.

Therapy with older agents involved a repeated administration, be it of oxamniquine (Sm), metrifonate (Sh) or niridazole (Sm, Sh, Sj).

Miscellaneous

S. stercoralis [1, 3, 4, 8, 10, 11]

The nematode *S. stercoralis* is now considered to be pathogenic since it may cause death in naturally or chemotherapeutically immunosuppressed patients. The distribution of this soil-transmitted worm is mainly tropical and subtropical, but autochtonous infections have been reported in temperate zones. The adult worms are localized in the mucosa of the upper intestine and the rhabditiform larvae leave

the patient with the stools. Under normal circumstances a different larval stage – the filariform larvae – invades man through the skin. However, in immunosuppressed patients there is continuous reinfection through the mucosa of the GIT of the host by *S. stercoralis* ending in a fatal overload. In such patients the CRAT may show at rectosigmoidoscopy shallow band-like ulcerations in which filariform larvae can be seen by the microscopist. The rhabditiform larvae of the stools are best detected by using the Baermann method [3, 4], and this should be specified to the laboratory. Eosinophilia is a constant feature of strongyloidiasis, and circulating antibodies are detectable in the serum. Duodenal probing may yield the parasite as well. Thiabendazole was the drug of choice, but in some countries this product has been withdrawn by some manufacturers. At present albendazole seems to be the alternative (15 mg/kg for 3 days in adults).

T. trichiura [1, 3–5, 8, 10, 11]

The whipworm *T. trichiura* is generally not considered to be a very pathogenic nematode of man since the infection is usually mild in adult patients. The distribution is mainly subtropical and tropical. The adult worm is located in the colon and produces characteristic bipolar eggs which are eliminated in the stools. In children, however, the infestation often involves the CRAT and it can be heavy. Rectal prolapse with parasites burrowed in the mucosa is not unusual. The treatment consists of a course of mebendazole as the drug of choice (for adults 100 mg bd for 3 days).

E. vermicularis [1, 2–4, 8, 9, 11]

The pinworm *E. vermicularis* may cause intense anal pruritus. Its geographical distribution is cosmopolitan. The adult worm may be found in the rectal ampula. The characteristic eggs can be found in the stools, but they are discovered more efficiently on a transparent adhesive tape pressed to the perianal region and then mounted on a glass slide for microscopic reading. Rarely, appendicitis may be caused by the adult pinworm, which has also been discovered in ectopic localizations such as the omentum. The usual treatment consists of administering mebendazole (100 mg single dose, to be repeated after 2 weeks), in treating the whole family, and in insisting on hygienic measures. Other anthelminthics are also in use.

A. lumbricoides [1, 2–4, 10, 11]

The soil-transmitted round worm *A. lumbricoides* has a cosmopolitan distribution. The single adult worm may give rise to clinical symptomatology by its localization in the bile duct, pancreatic duct, or appendix. Rarely, the adult can perforate the GIT and therefore cause peritonitis. In massive *A. umbricoides* infestation, particularly in childhood, a number of worms may become entangled within the lumen and hence cause partial obstruction, volvulus, or incarceration of hernia. The treatment of such rare complications is usually surgical, but chemotherapy has occasionally proven successful in cases of partial obstruction, and the delivery of such a worm bolus will delight the noninvasive gastroenterologist. The blockage often takes place at the beginning of the CRAT. There are several anthelminthics for ascariasis: pyrantel pamoate (750 mg) and albendazole (400 mg) can be recommended as single doses for adults, but other drugs are also in use (piperazine, levamisole, mebendazole).

Taeniae [1, 2–4, 8–10]

The beef tapeworm is the most common tapeworm, and its segments are eliminated in the stools. The patient sometimes report anal irritation on passing these segments and occasionally they recover them from the stools. In the laboratory, the differentiation between beef *(T. saginata)* and pork *(T. solium)* tapeworm is possible by counting the uterine ramifications within the segment and, in the case of totally expelled worms, by their heads; the eggs, however, are alike. The tapeworms can be treated by a single dose of chewable niclosamide (2 g single dose), mebendazole (300 mg bd for 3 days), or by praziquantel (10 mg/kg single dose). Some doctors prefer to administer simultaneously a purge and an antiemetic to avoid regurgitation of *T. solium* eggs from the duodenum into the stomach where such eggs can hatch and lead to cysticercosis, a potentially fatal condition.

A. costaricensis [1, 2, 10, 11]

The adults of the soil-transmitted nematode *A. costaricensis* live in the mesenteric arteries, preferably in the ileocecal region and therefore may affect the upper part of the CRAT. The parasite leads to a local granuloma formation which may lead to mechanical obstruction. Deposited eggs can be found in the granulation tissue. The intravascular adult worm may lead to thrombosis, infarction, and ileus. The clinical presentation is therefore variable, and the diagnosis is initially clinical since no larvae or eggs are detected in the stools. Pain and eosinophilia are usually present. On rectal examination the intraabdominal mass is sometimes palpable near the appendix.

In the past the treatment was mainly surgical and consisted in resecting the affected part. Chemotherapy with thiabendazole was successful in some patients.

This abdominal angiostrongyloidiasis is prevalent in Central and South America. It has to be distinguished from the meningoencephalitic angiostrongyloidiasis caused by *Angiostrongylus cantonensis* in Asia.

Anisakis [1, 2, 4, 8, 11]

The larva of the marine nematode *Anisakis* is ingested by eating raw parasitized fish (herring worm disease) and may cause a variable symptomatology depending upon the location of the invasive larva(e). Usually the location is the upper GIT and only rarely the CRAT. It may present as a pseudotumoral mass which consists of eosinophilic granulation tissue. Determination of circulating antibodies in the serum has become possible. There is no specific chemotherapy available, but removal of an individual larva by gastroscopy has been performed.

Oesophagostomum [1, 4, 11]

The larva of *Oesophagostomum*, a nematode originating from primates, ruminants, and pigs may cause in man a variable symptomatology depending on the localization of the larva, which mainly affects the CRAT. Basically the larva induces an eosinophilic granulation tissue appearing as nodules, which may give rise to intussusception, incarceration of a hernia, or may cause colonic perforation followed by purulent focalized peritonitis. The treatment usually consists in removal of this helminthoma. Diagnosis is based on the biopsy specimen. No chemotherapy has proved effective. The geographical distribution is mainly tropical Africa, but rare cases have been reported from Indonesia and Brazil.

References

1. Binford CH, Connor DH (1976) Pathology of tropical and extraordinary diseases, vols 1, 2. Armed Forces Institute of Pathology, Washington DC
2. Braunwald E, Isselbacher KJ, Petersdorf RG, Wilson JD, Martin JB, Fauci AS (1987) Harrison's principles of internal medicine. McGraw-Hill, New York
3. Dietrich M, Kern P (1983) Tropenlabor. Diagnostik für die ärztliche Praxis mit einfacher Laborausrüstung. Fischer, Stuttgart
4. Gentilini M, Duflo B (1986) Médecine tropicale. Flammarion, Paris
5. Gilles HM (1984) Recent advances in tropical medicine. Churchill Livingstone, Edinburgh
6. Martinez-Palomo A (1986) Amebiasis. Elsevier, Amsterdam. Human parasitic diseases, vol 2
7. Nanda R, Baveja U, Asnand BS (1986) Entamoeba histolytica cyst passers: clinical features and outcome in untreated subjects. Lancet II: 301–303
8. Peters W, Gilles HM (1977) A colour atlas of tropical medicine and parasitology. Wolfe, London
9. Piekarski G (1975) Medizinische Parasitologie in Tafeln. Springer, Berlin Heidelberg New York
10. Rakel RE (1986) Conn's current therapy. Saunders, Philadelphia
11. Stürchler D (1981) Endemiegebiete tropischer Infektionskrankheiten. Karten und Texte für die Praxis. Huber, Bern

33 Pediatric Proctology

A. F. Schärli

Although some conditions of the anorectal region resemble those of adult life, many of them are entirely different in childhood. A presentation of the lesions most frequently encountered is thus meaningful. These include changes of the perianal skin, acquired disorders such as anal fissures, prolapse of polyps, and some of the reasons for rectal bleeding. In addition, malformations and disorders of bowel evacuation will be mentioned.

Lesions of the Perianal Skin

More than any other area of the skin, the perianal skin of the child tends to undergo inflammatory changes of various kinds. Depending on the cause and the stage, any form of dermatitis is characterized by reddening of the skin, blisters, papules, erosions, and scaling. Since there may be a number of possible causes of dermatitis in one and the same child, differentiation of the different types is often quite difficult. A *distinction* should be made between:

- Dermatitis (diaper rash, seborrheic, atopic).
- Skin infections due to viruses, bacteria, fungi, or parasites.
- Effects of topical drugs, contact dermatitits.
- Other dermatoses.

Dermatitis

Diaper Rash

Etiology. Chemical irritants from urine or feces, together with cutaneous friction, lead to intertriginous inflammation [26].
Most Common Site. Initially erythematous and later erosive skin changes develop in the skin folds (buttocks, genitalia, groin) and areas tightly covered by diapers. Secretions and the constant friction together cause localized maceration. If left untreated, the dermatitis spreads to the stomach, back, and thighs.

Seborrheic Dermatitis

The skin manifestations consist of circumscribed erythema covered with solid scales. The affected areas are particularly susceptible to bacterial or mycotic superinfection [7].

Localization. Beside the anal and genital regions, these manifestations are almost always found on the trunk, scalp, and face.

Age. Seborrheic dermatitis is most common in the first 6 months of life which is why it is popularly attributed to allergy to cow's milk ("milk crust").

Atopic Dermatitis

These erythematous, in some cases weeping, lesions often affect infants in the anal region, whereas in older children they are usually in the hollows of the elbows and knees.

Predisposition. There is almost always a family history of eczema.

General Treatment of Dermatitis. In any form of dermatitis the success of treatment depends not on the variety of agents available but on the selective application of tried and tested dermatological specialities.

Causal Therapy. Rubber and plastic diaper coverings should be avoided. The intertriginous areas should be cleansed by means of frequent hig baths. Mildly antiinflammatory or disinfectant additives (chamomile preparations, potassium permanganate in very low concentrations) or bath oils are permitted, but not alkaline foam baths. Fatty ointments are often detrimental on account of their emollient effect on the skin.

Symptomatic Therapy. Zinc pastes and zinc oils have proved valuable after bathing and thorough drying. Uncovered and weeping areas are treated more frequently. In severe inflammation, application of a steroidal cream, alone or as a base, is recommended for 2–3 days.

Perianal Infections of the Skin

Viruses, bacteria, and fungi find a fertile environment in the warm, humid anal folds. However, multiplication of anal pathogens is almost always superimposed on dermatitis (superinfection).

Viral Infections

Two typical viral conditions occur in children.

Molluscum Contagiosum

Etiology. This infection is caused by human papilloma viruses. A single perianal molluscum develops initially. Scratching or direct friction causes granual spread from one buttock to the other. Thus the lesions multiply locally or are transmitted to the trunk, extremities, and face.

Diagnosis. The condition is easy to diagnose. The nodular lesions are characterized by a central, navel-shaped dell, which, when pierced, expresses a semisolid, yellowish bead of matter that contains the viruses (Fig. 33.1).

Condylomata Acuminata (Genital Warts)

Etiology. Genital warts are also induced by papilloma viruses. They are found in groups on both sides of the anal region. They occasionally penetrate the anal canal as far as the dentate line. The humid warmth and friction there can cause them to rupture and bleed.

Diagnosis. The soft, verrucous, light-to-dark brown epithelial lesions can cause pain, itching, and defecation difficulties (Fig. 33.2).

Treatment. Therapy with caustic agents such as podophyllum and dichloroacetic acid is unpleasant for patients with molluscum contagiosum or condylomata acuminata. In children we therefore perform curettage under brief anesthesia. Caustic treatment of the lesion with silver nitrate offers the advantages of immediate staunching of bleeding and almost complete absence of pain. Within a few days the dry crust covering the scarless epithelialized skin is shed. This method minimizes the risk of recurrence.

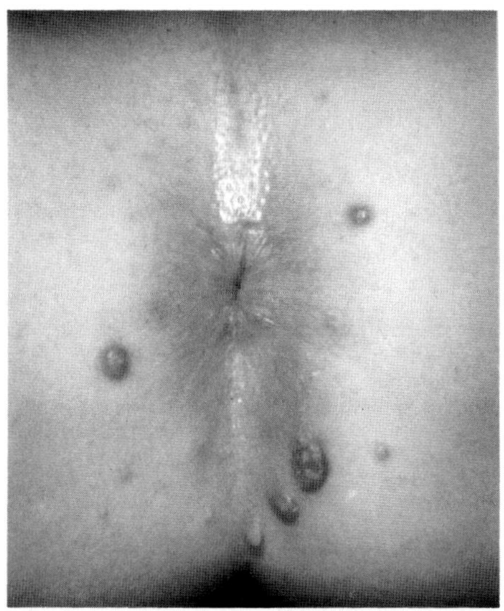

Fig. 33.1. Perianal molluscum contagiosum

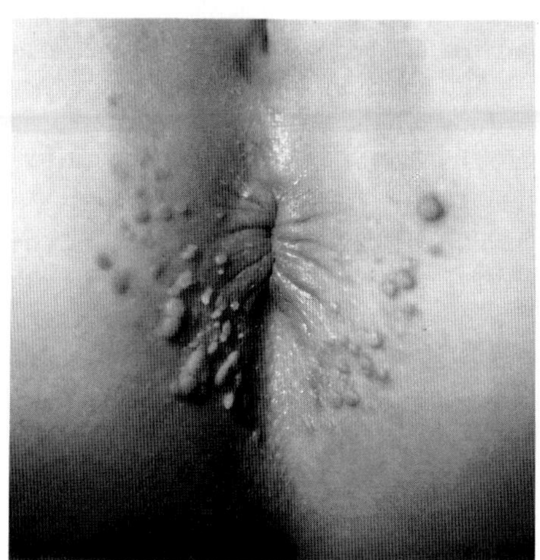

Fig. 33.2. Perianal condylomata acuminata

Bacteria

Etiology. Large numbers of pathogens are constantly present in the anal region. In the presence of dermatitis or weeping eczema, *Escherichia coli,* staphylococci and Pseudomonas multiply rapidly. The superinfection aggravates the underlying condition and makes it more difficult to rectify.

Types of Infection

- Staphylococcal folliculitis is rare in children.
- Localized abscesses are usually confined to the buttocks and are colonized by a mixture of *E. coli,* staphylococci, and anaerobic bacteria.

- Most superinfections are intertriginous.
- One of the most serious complications is exfoliative dermatitis.
- Under the effect of staphylococcal toxins, Lyell's syndrome occurs in predisposed children. These burn-like cutaneous lesions may occur on the trunk, extremities, and face, as well as in the anal region.

Treatment. General dermatological principles are also applied in the treatment of this disease. Systemic administration of antibiotics is necessary in the more severe cases. Lyell's syndrome also calls for intensive medical care.

Perianal Candidiasis

Etiology. As soon as cutaneous defense mechanisms are weakened, the yeast *Candida albicans* is able to take on a parasitic mycelial form. In most cases a *C. albicans* infection is manifested primarily as skin changes. Apart form the local superinfection, oral or gastrointestinal candidiasis is also an important source of infection.

Diagnosis. The intertriginous lesions spread marginally in tongue-shaped form, frequently disseminating into the groin, the fold of the umbilicus, and the neck. Initially salmon pink, they later become dark red and exhibit a blister-like, scaling crust. Diagnosis is based on microscopic investigations and cultures, thus permitting differentiation from bacterial intertrigo (Fig. 33.3).

Treatment. Emphasis should be placed on baths with greatly diluted potassium permanganate solution and application of gentian violet or ointments containing clioquinol, nystatin, or amphotericin. In cases of oral or gastrointestinal involvement, nystatin is also administered by mouth.

Contact Dermatitis

Contact dermatitis with anal involvement is extremely rare in children. Major skin damage can, however, result from excessively high concentrations of antiseptics (necrosis), from fatty ointments (maceration), or from prolonged use of steroids.

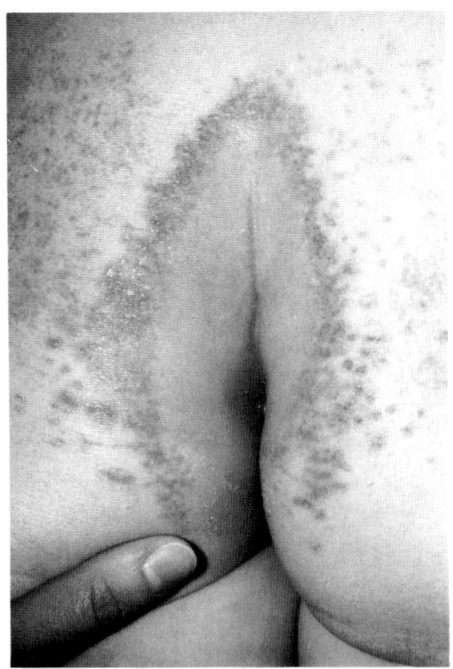

Fig. 33.3. Candida dermatitis

Inflammation of the Anal Canal

Anal Inflammation

Inflammation of the anal mucosa is never an isolated event. Spread of other inflammatory processes results in hyperemia of the mucosa and hypersecretion with spontaneous mucous discharge.

Etiology. Anal inflammation is the result of an anal fissure, mucosal or rectal prolapse, or, most frequently, chronic diarrhea.

Symptoms. Patients complain of a burning feeling or continuous itching, particularly on passing stools. The mucous discharge from the anal canal leaves stains on diapers and underwear.

Endoscopy. The hyperemic and edematous anal mucosa and possibly also erosions are visible in the anoscope. The mucosa is abnormally sensitive and bleeds easily.

Treatment. The cause of the anal inflammation must be eliminated. The symptoms respond well to anesthetizing ointments or suppositories containing steroidal substances.

Inflammation of the Anal Crypts and Papillae

Etiology. The rectal columns continue distally into the papillae which demarcate the mucosal crypts of Morgagni. The anal glands are located in the crypts. In the course of an anal inflammation or of diarrhea the papillae undergo edematous swelling.

Symptoms. Spontaneous pain in the anal canal is rare, but passage of stools is painful. Anoscopic inspection reveals papillary edema or some fibrin in crypts.

Treatment. The treatment is the same as for anal or perianal inflammation.

Perianal Abscess

Anatomy. An anal crypt or anal gland can develop inflammation with formation of an abscess extending into the tissue folds and along the myofascial structures. Eventually an inflammatory lump develops beneath the skin. We have observed perianal abscesses in early infanthood only.

Predisposition. While abscesses in the adult are frequently preceded by hemorrhoids or anal fissures, those in children may occasionally be associated with chronic constipation. In the many abscesses found in infants, however, an already existing condition can rarely be detected.

Course of the Abscess. The abscessing inflammation breaks through near the anus, at the lateral gluteal wall or the perineum. Only two courses have been observed for abscesses in children (Fig. 33.4) [25]:
- Intrasphincteral (subcutaneous anal abscess, submucous anorectal abscess).
- Intersphincteral (perianal abscess).

Symptoms. Initially there is a dull, penetrating pain. Eventually an inflammatory bulge develops in the perianal region, accompanied by doughy edema of the perianal skin. Fluctuation is observed in rare cases. Spontaneous rupture of the abscess leaves a residual watery or purulent secretion which gives rise to perianal dermatitis. Fever and periodic crying are always initially observed in infants, particularly in connection with the passage of stools. Sometimes there is weight loss.

Treatment. Cure can never be achieved with conservative treatment and antibiotics – on the contrary,

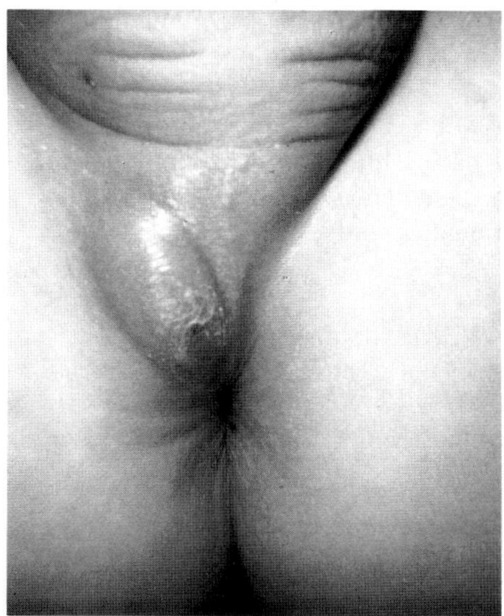

Fig. 33.4. Perianal abscess: typical location in a 4-months-old baby

the abscess may spread and an internal fistula may form. The treatment of choice is complete deroofing of the abscess, preferably with a T-shaped or radial incision. The abscess is cleansed by means of antiseptic dressings (polyvidone-iodine, chlorhexidine) and hip baths. The wound should initially be kept open with a clioquinol tent dressing. It always closes spontaneously after 10–14 days.

Complications. If the incision is inadequate, the wound closes prematurely, and the abscess recurs. Even after proper treatment, a residual secreting perianal fistula is often observed.

Perianal Fistula

After the acute abscess stage, the disease very often progresses to a chronic fistula stage. Initially almost impossible to probe, the chronic inflammation eventually results in a rigid, thick-walled fistular canal.

Pathological Anatomy. Four main courses are known, of which only the superficial forms occur in children (Fig. 33.5) [13, 20, 25]:

- Intrasphincteral or mucocutaneous
- Intersphincteral
- Transsphincteral (only in adults)
- Supralevator (only in adults).

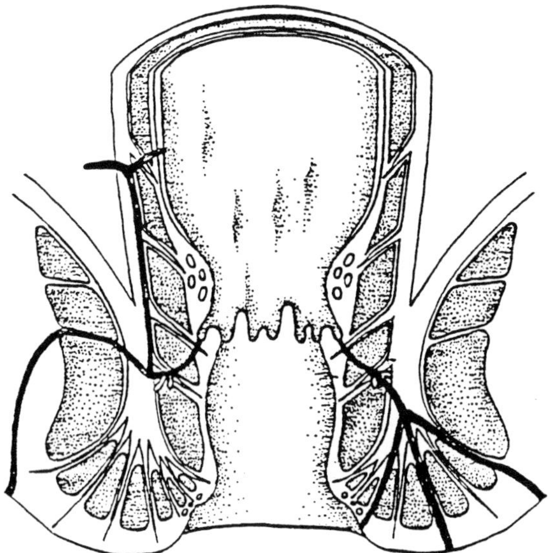

Fig. 33.5. Fistular tracts (*left,* in adults; transsphincteral, supralevator; *right,* in children: subcutaneous, intermuscular)

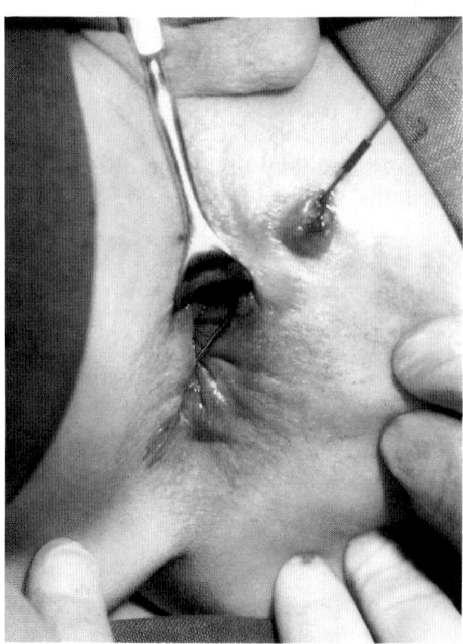

Fig. 33.6. Anorectal fistula with excess granulation tissue and extensive scarring

Symptoms. There is a regular purulent discharge from a small fistular opening with a reddened margin or from the crater of a dyke-like elevation. Passage of stool becomes painful during the development of the abscess. Clinical improvement occurs only after the fistula has been opened up.

Clinical Demonstration. A bulb-headed probe can be inserted into the tract to determine its depth and direction. By spreading the anus apart or using an anoscope, the internal opening originating in a crypt can be seen (possibly following irrigation with a staining solution). X-ray examination is never necessary (Fig. 33.6).

Treatment. Any fistula is an absolute indication for surgery. The tract is probed as far as the opening into the anal canal and filled with methylene blue. The classic thread method has not proved suitable for use in children and should therefore no longer be used. Fresh fistulas must be entirely laid open, the granulation tissue removed by curettage, and a tampon applied to the lesion [4]. Chronic fistulas with marked induration of the tract can be completely resected. When the tract is being laid open or subjected to complete dissection, care should be taken that no side channels are overlooked. These interventions do not impair continence.

Complications. Recurrence of fistulas after use of the thread method was once common and can still be observed today:

- When the fistula is not completely opened up.
- When side channels are missed.
- When follow-up treatment is not carried out consistently.

Pilonidal Sinus

Located in the middle line of the sacrococcygeal region, pilonidal sinus is associated with loose hairs which spread in the corium and subcutis; the fistulas are surrounded by inflamed granulation tissue and can form abscesses.

Etiology. Diverse theories have been postulated. An observation always made in children, however, is of a congenital dermal sinus with connective tissue fixation at the coccygeal bone, which becomes the focal point for infection and abscess formation. Dermoid cysts are found in rare cases.

Symptoms. These begin with the formation of an abscess. In the chronic stage, constant or intermittent purulent discharge from the fistula tracts is observed.

Treatment. In the acute stage the abscess is laid open along its length and the cavity treated with antiseptic dressings. A chronic pilonidal sinus is excised and allowed to develop secondary granulation tissue. Follow-up surgery with wound curettage or marginal excision may often be necessary. A primary suture is not to be recommended in any case. Infections often recur when basic treatment is not carried out with sufficient thoroughness.

Anal Fissure

Anal fissure is a linear ulcer of the sensitive anoderm that can extend as far as the internal sphincter.

Pathogenesis. Usually rupture of the posterior commissure is due to the passage of hard stools. Predisposing factors include anal eczema, intertrigo, infection, scarring; more rarely, sequelae of trauma following introduction of thermometers, suppositories, or enemas.

Typical Triad of Symptoms
- Intense pain during and after defecation.
- Traces of blood on the stools, or bloodstained underwear after defecation.
- Sphincteric spasm.

The result is a vicious circle: the need to defecate triggers anxiety at the prospect of pain, which in turn leads to contraction of the sphincter. Defecation is delayed as a result of the pain, and a large, scybalous mass of retained stools is formed, the passage of which then aggravates the anal fissure.

Examination. Young children in particular tend to offer resistance to inspection of the fissure owing to fear of pain. Application of a local anesthetic spray (lidocaine), as used in ears, nose, and throat procedures, is helpful in these circumstances. Sometimes ketamine anesthesia is necessary. There is notable sphincteric spasm on digital inspection.

Findings. Fissures are located singly or in groups parallel to the axis of the anal canal, mainly in the dorsal anoderm between the dentate line and the external anal ring. At the lower end, the fissure may occasionally be obscured by an external skin tag ("sentinel pile"), while a hypertrophic anal papilla may be located at the upper end. The slightest contact can be extremely painful and easily lead to mild bleeding (Fig. 33.7).

Treatment of Fresh Fissures
- Anesthetizing spray (proctological spray, lidocaine spray) or ointment during the day and particularly before defecation.
- Lubricant to facilitate passage of stool (liquid paraffin).
- Glycerin suppositories as a stool softener.
- Use of mucilage preparations, lactulose, agar (but *not* laxatives) to modify stool consistency.
- Chamomile baths, or manual cleansing of the anus.
- Antiseptic or antimycotic ointments in the event of infection.

Treatment of Chronic Fissures. The risk of scarring and fibrosis of the sphincter make more extensive measures necessary:

- Cauterization of the fissure with silver nitrate.
- Simple dilatation of the sphincter under general anesthesia, though this may have the drawback of deepening the fissure and opening scars.
- Submucosal, posterior myotomy of the internal sphincter soon brings about easier defecation and leads to healing.

Hemorrhoids

Incidence. Though hemorrhoids and their complications account for more than two-thirds of proctological complaints in adults, they are very rarely encountered in childhood.

Etiology. Hemorrhoids originate from enlargement and displacement of the corpus cavernosum recti (superior hemorrhoidal plexus). They are probably a result of:

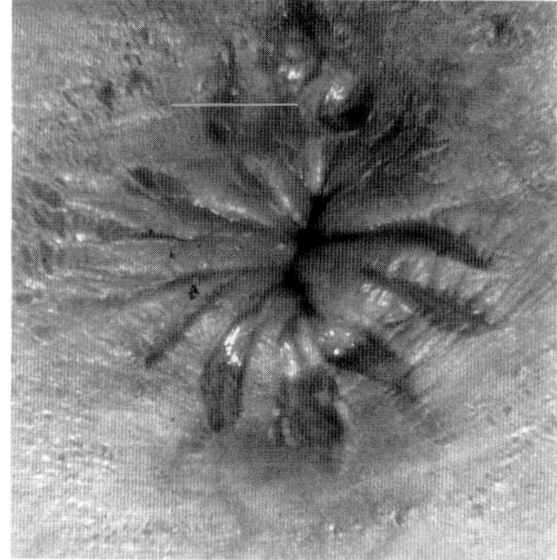

Fig. 33.7. Fresh anal fissures in the circumference of the anus

- Frequent straining owing to chronic constipation.
- Disturbed transsphincteric blood drainage from the hemorrhoidal plexus as a result of sphincter spasm.
- True malformations as seen in lymphangiomatosis (Fig. 33.8).

Symptoms. Bleeding (bright red), pain, and prolapse are the symptoms of hemorrhoids. Pain on defecation leads to the same vicious circle as occurs in anal fissures. Complications include painful thrombi as a result of impeded venous return, considerable spontaneous hemorrhage, ulceration, and perianal dermatitis.

Endoscopy. The degree of the hemorrhoids and complications are established by anoscopy. For this procedure children require brief anesthesia.

Treatment
- Dietary regulation of disturbed intestinal activity (e. g., bran, mucilage preparations, fluids, but *not* laxatives).
- Avoidance of excessive straining.
- Repositioning of prolapsed hemorrhoids.
- Anal hygiene (hip baths, mild disinfectants).
- Local anesthetics.
- Anal dilatation by bougies.
- Submucosal application of sclerosing agents is almost always successful in young patients (sodium tetradecyl sulfate, phenol in almond oil).

So far only five of our patients with prolapsed hemorrhoids have required surgical management. Thrombosed hemorrhoids heal within a few days with bed rest and application of anesthetizing and antithrombotic ointments; surgery is hardly ever necessary.

Rectal Prolapse

Prolapse of the anal mucosa usually occurs after rectal continence-preserving procedures. The mucous membrane is dark red and exhibits longitudinal folds; the prolapse is often only unilateral. In many cases repositioning is not possible (Fig. 33.9). This form is usually referred to as "incomplete prolapse."

Anorectal prolapse (procidentia) is a rosette-like prolapse affecting all layers of the rectal wall, with the anorectal zone remaining relatively firmly fixed. This type of prolapse results from loosening of the connective tissue linking the rectum with the sac-

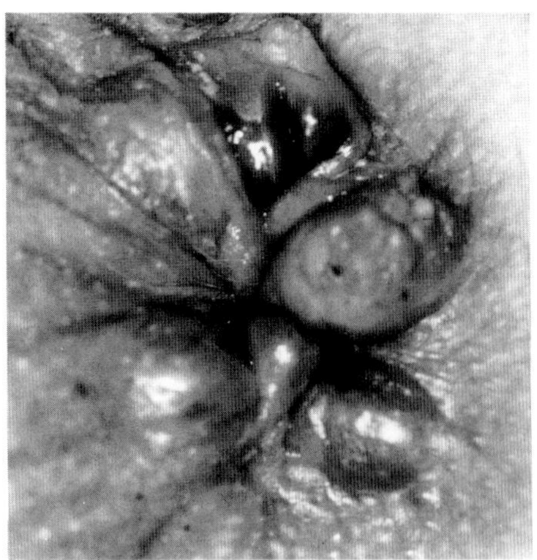

Fig. 33.8. Hemorrhoidal prolapse in a child with lymphangiomatosis

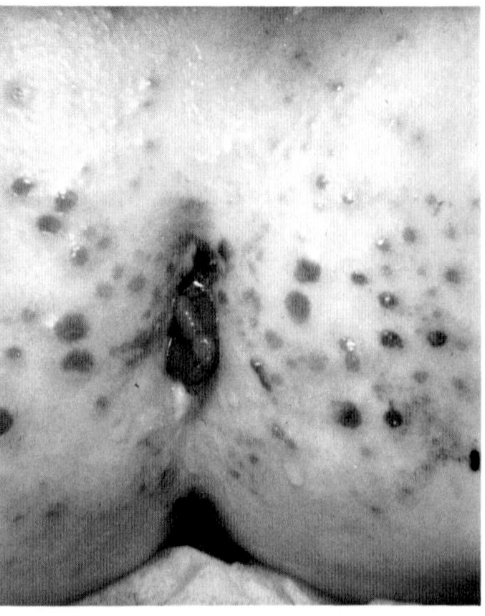

Fig. 33.9. Prolapse of the mucous membrane following surgery for anal atresia. Note local irritation of perianal skin

rum and from elongation of the levator ani muscle (Fig. 33.10). This form is usually referred to as "complete prolapse."

Etiology. Complete rectal prolapse has several possible causes:

- A predisposing factor is the direct sacral course of the rectum in the child.
- Paralysis of the pelvic muscles in myelomeningocele or defective sacral development can lead to elongation of the levator ani muscles.

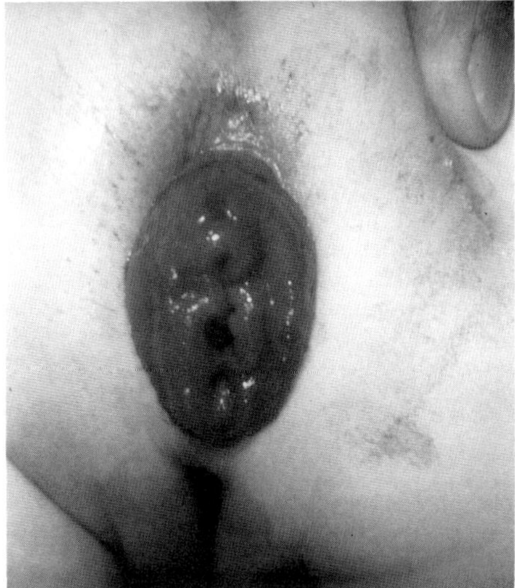

Fig. 33.10. Rectal prolapse

- Malnutrition, marasmus, and possibly also cystic fibrosis cause loosening of the connective tissue, which then gives way under abdominal pressure, particularly in severe constipation.

Any rectal prolapse is preceded by prolonged disturbance of defecation (chronic constipation, in rare cases diarrhea), an important role being played by an unbalanced, mainly liquid diet without bulkage, or by excessive toilet training (prolonged sessions on the "pot"). Prolonged coughing in pertussis is also a major cause of prolapse in infants.

Symptoms. In children aged between 6 months and 4 years there is a rosette-shaped protrusion of the rectum from the anus, initially after prolonged straining, later at every passage of stools. However, it usually resolves spontaneously or can be repositioned by applying slight pressure with the help of Vaseline-impregnated gauze. Recurrent prolapse is accompanied by bleeding, mucous discharge, or perianal dermatitis.

Treatment. Simple prolapse of the mucous membrane after rectal continence-preserving procedures is excised together with the mucocutaneous scar. Anorectal prolapse is treated in five "S" steps:

- Stool evacuation: constipation (the most frequent cause) is eliminated.
- Sitting on the pot: the child must not be kept on the pot for long periods. Short but more frequent sessions are preferable. Covering the pot with a board with a hole in it prevents the buttocks from protruding too far into the pot.

- Sedation: mild sedation and careful psychological handling of the children can often reduce anxiety at the prospect of a bowel movement.
- Sclerosing agents: submucous injection of a sclerosing agent (phenol in almond oil, sodium tetradecyl sulfate, polidocanol) in four quadrants 2 cm above the dentate line has proved valuable provided that the levator muscle and the connective tissue are not yet entirely atonic.
- "Suture":
  1. A circular chromic catgut suture may sometimes be indicated in paralysis of the pelvic muscles.
  2. Suturing of the rectum to the sacral bone (proctopexy): The atonic levator musculature is laid bare by a longitudinal incision from the apex of the coccyx to within 1 cm of the anus. The posterior wall of the rectum is drawn tight and fixed to the interior surface of the sacrum. This intervention is well tolerated by young children and is suitable for correction of short prolapses.
  3. The Delorme-Rehn transanal resection technique should never be used in young children.
  4. Laparotomy and proctopexy by the Ripstein-Wells method in extensive prolapse in older children: a strip of dura mater is fixed by a series of sutures to the posterior wall of the deep rectum and then to the sacral bone.

Polyps of the Anus and Colon

The classification of polyps is based on histological criteria (Table 33.1). Those found in children usually take the form of benign polypoid lesions. Only the neoplastic polyps are considered to be precancerous. The polyposis syndromes deserve particular attention [3, 12, 13, 19].

Nonneoplastic Polyps

Juvenile (Mucous Retention) Polyps

Mucous retention polyps usually occur in children. About 70% are located in the proximal anal canal and distal rectum and can often be detected on digital examination. Multiple polyps are found in 14%–20% of cases. Peak incidence occurs between the ages of 4 and 5 and between 17 and 25 (Fig. 33.11).

Symptoms. The cardinal symptom is painless anal bleeding. In some cases a bleeding of a bluish-co-

Table 33.1. Polyps of the anus, rectum, and colon

Origin	Solitary	Multiple (polyposis syndromes)
Hamartia	Juvenile polyp Peutz-Jeghers polyp	Juvenile polyposis Peutz-Jeghers syndrome Cowden's syndrome
Hyperplasia	Hyperplastic polyp	Hyperplastic polyposis
Inflammation	Fibrous anal polyp Inflammatory polyp	Inflammatory polyposis (e. g., in ulcerative colitis)
	Lymphoid polyp Granulomatous polyp	Lymphoid polyposis
		Cronkhite-Canada syndrome
Neoplasia	Tubular adenoma	Adenomatous polyposis
	Villous adenoma	Gardner's syndrome
	Tubulo-villous adenoma	Turcot's syndrome Zanca's syndrome

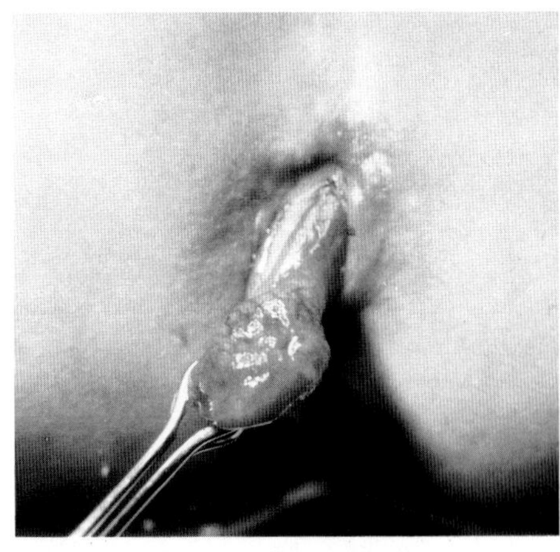

Fig. 33.11. Juvenile polyp of retal mucosa

lored (infarcted) polyp may present at the anus. Colicky pain develops when the polyp is pulled or if it autoamputates.

Morphology. Juvenile polyps are reddish, stalked, in rare cases broad-based protrusions from the mucous membrane. In contrast to adenomas, their surface is smooth. Section reveals mucus-filled cysts (hence "mucus retention polyps"). Histological investigation of the inflammatorily altered stroma reveals irregularly elongated and dilated crypts and even epithelium rich in goblet cells. The polyp is often ulcerated and covered with fibrinopurulent exudate.

Etiology. Juvenile polpys are though to be either developmental malformations containing normal intestinal tissue (hamartomas) or the outcome of chronic inflammation following local injury. There is no justification for classifying them with neoplastic polyps or precanceroses.

Peutz-Jeghers Polyps

Peutz-Jeghers polpys are nonneoplastic and consist of differentiated epithelium. The number of polyps may vary.

Etiology. They are considered to be hamartomas and occur not only in hereditary Peutz-Jeghers syndrome, but occasionally also without any preceding family history.

Morphology. They are usually stalked, sometimes of considerable size, and have a lobulated surface. Histologically, they present as tree-like ramified lamina muscularis mucosae on which densely clustered crypts with an epithelium rich in goblet cells are scattered.

Manifestation. They usually occur in childhood or adolescence. Later in life, new lesions may develop in the stomach, small intestine, and colon.

Prognosis. As with juvenile polyps, excision is unlikely to have any sequelae. The polyps may, however, be the initial manifestation of the syndrome, thus making check-ups indispensable over a period of years (see "polyposis Syndromes", p. 296).

Hyperplastic Polyps

Hyperplastic polyps are small, circumscribed mucosal hyperplasias which are the most common type of polyp found in the colon, rectum, and proximal anal canal.

Morphology. Hyperplastic polyps are pale gray, broad-based (sessile), with a diameter of 3–5 mm. Histological investigation reveals elongated, convuluted crypts with a star-shaped lumen in cross-section. The elongated proliferation zone is located in the basal crypt region. The differentiation pattern is quite distinct from that of adenomas.

Inflammatory Polyps

Inflammatory polyps are localized swellings of the mucosal membrane which are the result of inflammatory edematous and regenerative changes. They

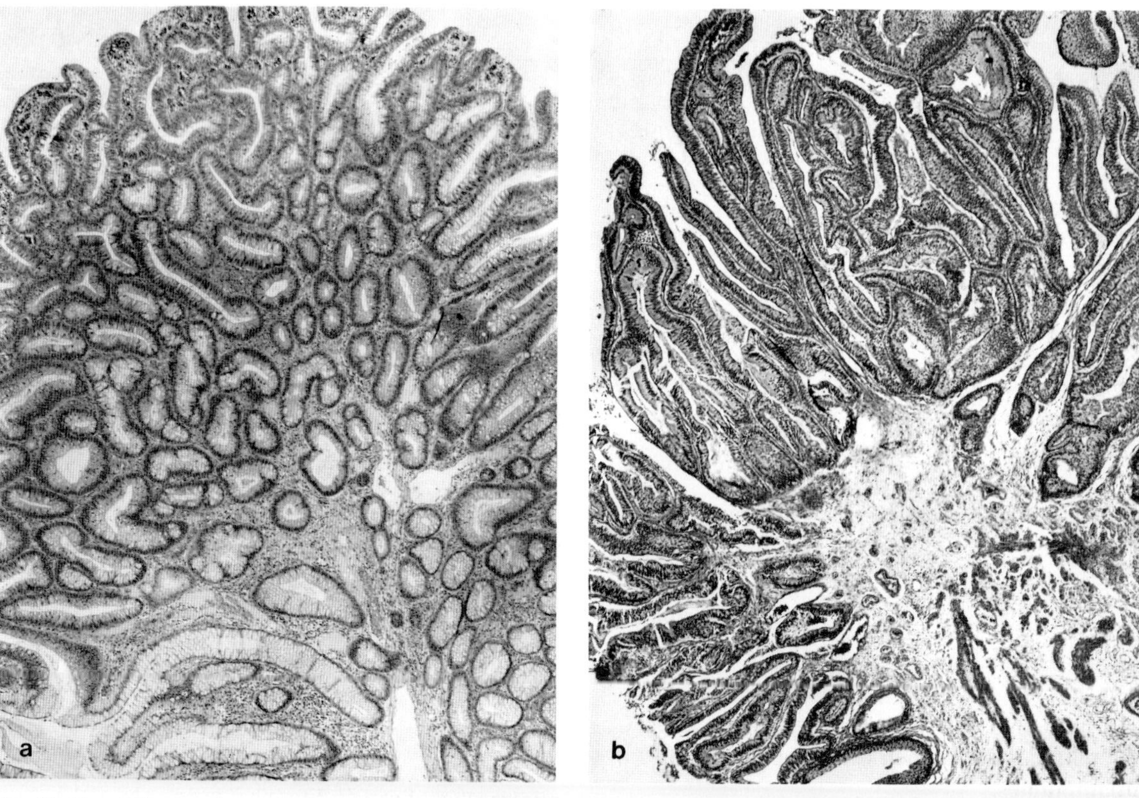

Fig. 33.12. *a* Villous adenoma of rectal mucosa; *b* tubular adenoma. Hematoxylin and eosin; *a* × 50, *b* × 100

may be surrounded by ulcerated zones and usually occur in prolonged, active ulcerative colitis or granulomatous colitis (Crohn's disease). Inflammatory polyps with granulation tissue may also appear in association with injuries to the mucous membrane, for instance in anastomoses.

Neoplastic Polyps (Adenomas)

The category of neoplastic polyps comprises tubular, villous, and mixed tubulovillous adenomas (Fig. 33.12).

Symptoms. Adenomas generally cause bleeding. They may secrete increased amounts of mucus (particularly in the case of villous adenomas) and lead to diarrhea, tenesmus, intussusception, and perianal protrusions.

Treatment. All solitary adenomas should be excised. This is performed endoscopically, particularly in the case of stalked adenomas. Life-long follow-up examinations (endoscopic and radiological) at 2 year intervals are essential.

Polyposis Syndromes

The polyposis syndromes are classified according to the histological polyp type and whether they are solitary or multiple (Table 33.1). Polyposis syndromes usually manifest themselves in the gastrointestinal tract, frequently as early as in childhood.

Juvenile Polyposis

Juvenile polyposis is very rare. The risk of gastrointestinal carcinoma developing is thought to be slight.

Forms
- Nonfamilial, often occurring in association with cardiac defects, malrotation, and hydrocephalus.
- Autosomal recessive, with no additional malformations.

Manifestation. The infantile, nonfamilial form occurs in the 1 year of life and involves the stomach and colon and, in only about half of patients, the small intestine. Complications often lead to a fatal outcome as early as the 2 year of life. The second

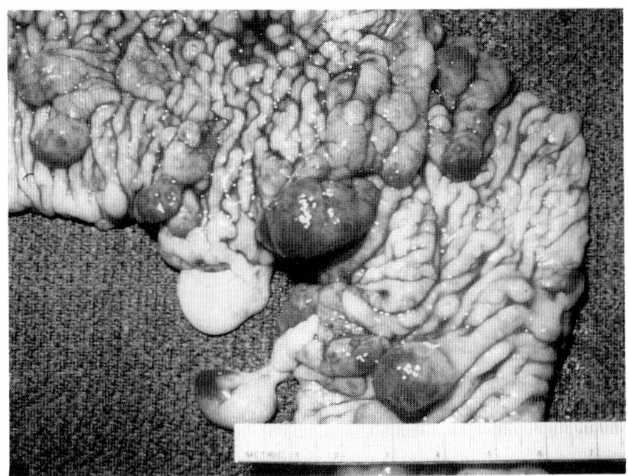

Fig. 33.13. Juvenile familial adenomatous polyposis (adenomatosis)

form develops in older children and in adults. It varies with regard to age at development and the number and location of polyps (Fig. 33.13).

Symptoms. Recurrent bleeding, intussusception, hypochromic anemia, and malnutrition suggest the possibility of juvenile polyposis.

Peutz-Jeghers Syndrome

Peutz-Jeghers syndrome involves multiple Peutz-Jeghers-type polyps, mucocutaneous pigmentation, and a preceding family history.

Pathogenesis. Peutz-Jethers syndrome is due to an autosomal dominant gene of varying penetrance. It appears as a result of mutation in up to 45% of cases.

Manifestation. It usually occurs between the 10th and the 13th years of life. The circumoral and oral pigmentation is usually present at birth. Polyps may develop in the entire gastrointestinal tract.

Morphology. Brown or bluish-brown pigmented nevi 0.5–1.0 cm in diameter are found on the lips and the mucous membrane of the mouth. The polyps may be between a few millimeters and several centimeters in diameter and may be stalked or sessile.

Complications. Intussusception, ulceration, and bleeding are frequent complications. Carcinomas very rarely appear in Peutz-Jeghers polpys.

In familial adenomatous polyposis large numbers of adenomas (100–5000) are found in the colon and rectum. The association with colorectal carcinoma at a relatively early age is extremely high, and a preceding family history can usually be found.

Pathogenesis. This condition is an inherited autosomal dominant disease, which also occurs sporadically.

Manifestation. The condition usually occurs between the ages of 15 and 25, but in isolated cases also toward the end of the 1st decade of life.

Symptoms. Bleeding, frequent passage of stools, and mucus discharge are the symptoms of familial adenomatous polyposis. In about two-thirds of patients a colorectal carcinoma already exists by the time the condition is diagnosed.

Morphology. Dense carpeting of the mucous membrane by polyps is found. Most of the polyps measure less than 0.5 cm in diameter though they can grow to up to 3 cm. Histologically, the polyps are tubular, tubulovillous, and, more rarely, villous adenomas. A characteristic feature is the large number of very small adenomas which can affect only a few of the adjacent crypts.

Prognosis. Familial adenomatous polyposis inevitably develops into a malignant condition.

Therapy. Proctocolectomy is the therapy of choice. The children of patients with familial adenomatous polyposis should be regularly examined every 2 years from the age of 14 up to middle age.

Anorectal Malformations

Classification

In 1970, pediatric surgeons from many countries devised a classification of all forms of anorectal atresia based on the position of the rectal atresia in relation to the levator [16]. The complexity of this classification prompted a complete revision in 1984 [22]. The primary subdivision into high rectal atresia, above the levator (supralevator), and low anal atresia (translevator) is necessary because the two forms are embryogenetically and anatomically distinct. In a number of malformations the rectal pouch (and possibly a fistula) are centrally located, traversing the muscles of the pelvic floor. These are

Table 33.2. "Wingspread" classification of anorectal malformations

A High supralevator malformations

Female	Male
1. Anorectal agenesis	1. Anorectal agenesis
a. With rectovaginal fistula	a. With rectoprostatic urethral fistula
b. Without fistula	b. Without fistula
2. Rectal atresia	2. Rectal atresia

B. Intermediate malformations

Female	Male
1. Rectovestibular fistula	1. Rectobulbar-urethral fistula
2. Rectovaginal fistula	2. Anal agenesis without fistula
3. Anal agenesis without fistula	

C. Low, translevator malformations

Female	Male
1. Anovestibular fistula	1. Anocutaneous fistula
2. Anocutaneous fistula	2. Anal stenosis
3. Anal stenosis	

D. The other types of malformation are rare; they are described according to the position of the rectal pouch (and the fistula).

E. A separate classification has been created for complex anomalies with retained cloaca.

termed intermediate forms. For the sake of simplicity in clinical practice, the new classification includes only the more common types of malformation (Table 33.2).

Diagnostic Procedure

Although clinical examination is sufficient to detect the type of malformation and to determine the therapeutic procedure, there are a number of malformations with an indistinguishable external aspect. A precise differentiation at least between supra- and translevator anomalies is important. Several diagnostic techniques need to be discussed in detail:

- ultrasonography of the pelvis and perineum (Table 33.3);
- Wangenstein-Rice invertogram (Table 33.4 and Fig. 33.14);
- fistulography (Table 33.5 and Fig. 33.15);
- voiding cysto-urethrogram (Table 33.6);
- loopogram of the distal colon and rectum (Table 33.7);
- perineal needle aspiration of the rectal pouch and dye study (Table 33.8);
- endoscopic examinations of urethra, bladder, and vagina.

Table 33.3. Ultrasonography

Techniques	Diagnostic clues	Disadvantages
1. Position of child variable, mostly lateral position	1. Reliable detection of rectal pouch	1. Fistulas may be difficult to find
2. Search for rectal pouch, fistulas	2. Length and width of fistula	2. Examination depends on the experience of the investigator
3. Observation of movements of the pelvic floor	3. Position and activity of pelvic floor musculature	
	4. Changing position of the terminal rectum	

Table 33.4. Invertogram, lateral film of pelvic region (Wangensteen-Rice) [24]

Techniques	Diagnostic clues	Disadvantages
1. Position on child's head	1. Intestinal distension	1. Gas passage to the rectal pouch needs 12 h
2. Right-angle flexion of the legs	2. Malformations of the sacrum	2. Variable position of terminal rectum depending on contraction of pelvic floor
3. Anal dimple to be market (barium paste)	3. Air-fluid level in rectal pouch	3. Incomplete filling of the rectum with air may be misinterpreted as a high lesion
4. True lateral film through trochanter	4. Construction of lines for determination of levator and terminal rectum (Fig. 33.14)	
	5. Gas in bladder signifies rectourethral fistula	

        ▷

Fig. 33.14. a Invertogram of anal agenesis with guide lines, **b** anorectal agenesis with rectourethral fistula. *PC,* midline of os pubis to lower edge of S_5; *I,* parallel to PC through lower edge of os ischii; *M,* parallel midline between *PC* and *I* lines

Table 33.5. Contrast studies of external fistulas

Techniques	Diagnostic clues	Disadvantages
1. Fistulogram with water-soluble contrast	1. Length, course, and caliber of fistula detectable	1. Incomplete filling of fistula may be misleading
2. Complete filling of rectal pouch	2. Position of terminal rectum (Fig. 33.15)	
3. Marking of perineum with barium paste	3. Construction of auxiliary lines helpful	
4. Lateral film		

Table 33.6. Voiding cysto-urethrogram

Techniques	Diagnostic clues	Disadvantages
1. Bladder filled with indwelling catheter or retrograde urethrography	1. Detection of rectourethral, rectovesical, or rectobulbar fistula	1. Narrow fistulas may remain undetected
2. Indicated for all cases of severe hypospadias	2. Position of terminal rectum	

Table 33.7. Loopogram of distal colon through colostomy

Techniques	Diagnostic clues	Disadvantages
1. Use water-soluble contrast	1. Position of terminal rectum and fistulas detectable	1. Misleading interpretation due to contraction of pelvic floor, microcolon, or fecaloma
2. Anal dimple to be marked	2. Construction of auxiliary lines helpful	
3. Anteroposterior and lateral films		

Table 33.8. Puncture of rectal pouch, contrast instillation under ultrasonographic control

Techniques	Diagnostic clues	Disadvantages
1. Insertion of fine needle in rectal pouch under sonographic control	1. Detection of terminal rectum and fistulas	1. Only indicated if other methods fail to clarify the nature of the malformation
2. Injection of water-soluble contrast		
3. Lateral films		

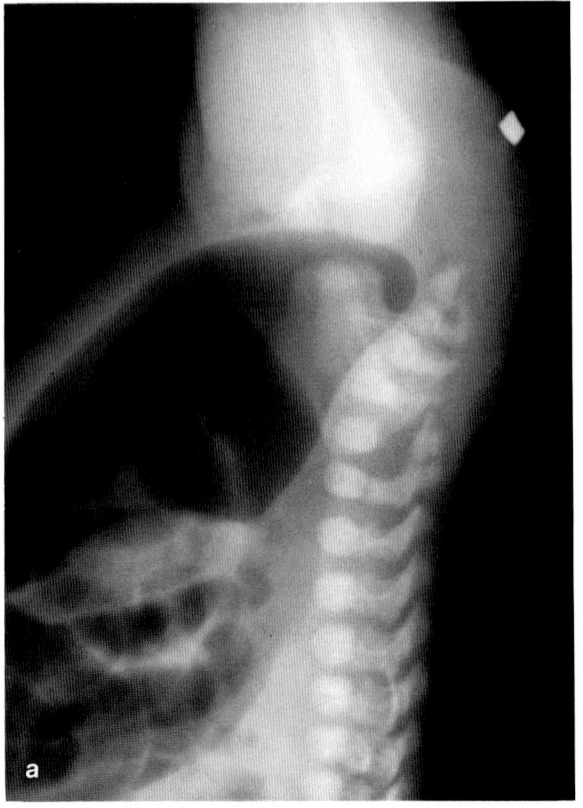

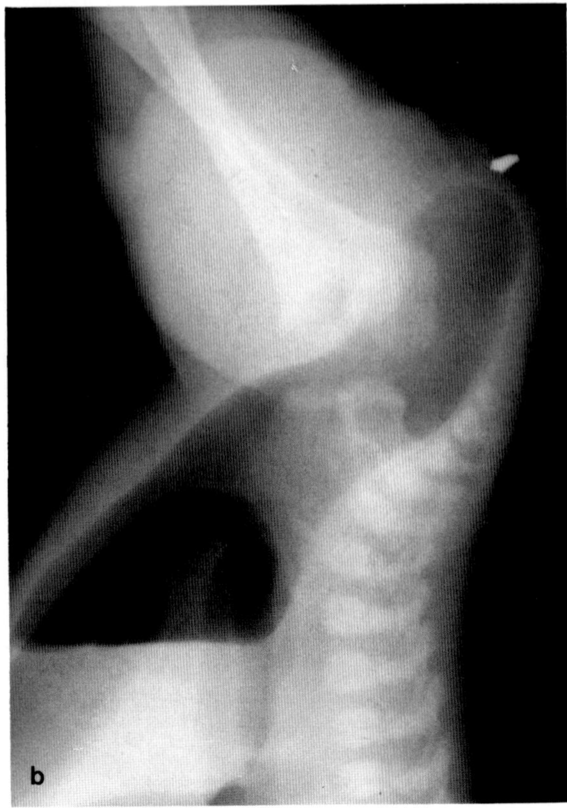

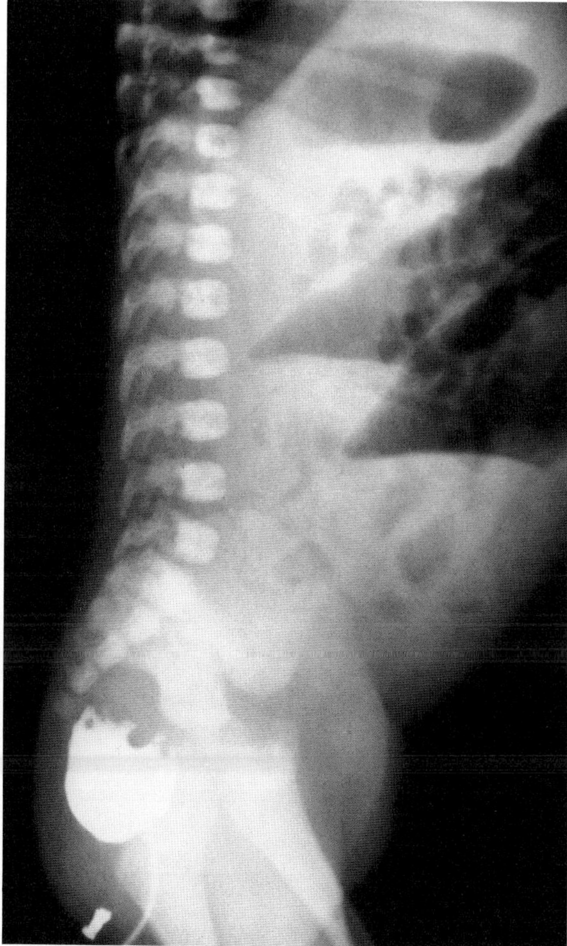

Fig. 33.15. Anorectal agenesis with rectovestibular fistula

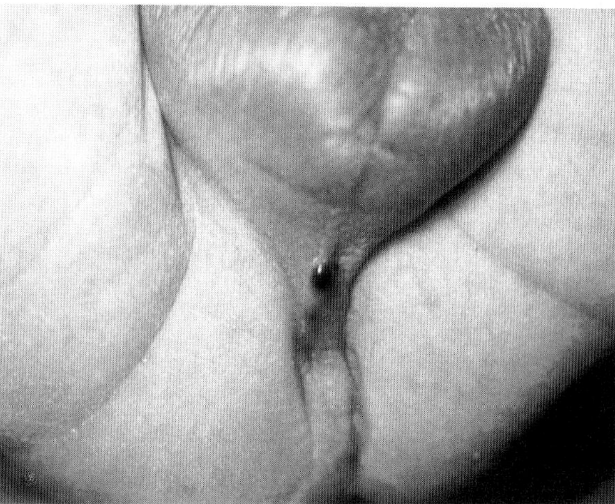

Fig. 33.16. Imperforate anus with anocutaneous fistula

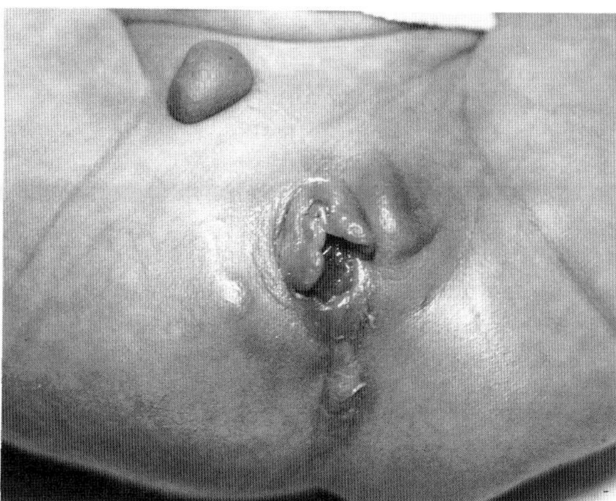

Fig. 33.17. Anorectal agenesis with rectovaginal fistula. Malformation of external genitalia

Interpretation of Diagnostic Procedures

Some auxiliary lines are recommended for the exact determination of the rectal pouch and terminal rectum. The terminal bowel in high anomalies is at the level of the pubococcygeal line (PC line) or just below at the M line (mid-distance of PC line and tuber ossis ischii). In intermediate abnormalities, the bowel descends to the I line (parallel to the PC line through the ischium) [21].

The presence of a single orifice in female patients constitutes a cloacal anomaly. The level of the rectum can be seen endoscopically. Two orifices are present in the case of a rectovaginal fistula. Passage of meconium through the urethra in the absence of an anus denotes a rectourethral or rectobulbar fistula in male patients. Patients with a very flattened hind end, lacking an intergluteal cleft, are likely to have a high anomaly (Fig. 33.16). Fistulas to the perineum or posterior fourchette of the labia minora always represent the group of low anomalies (Fig. 33.17).

Accompanying Congenital Malformations

More than 40% of children with anorectal anomalies suffer from one or more additional malformations. In supralevator forms, the incidence is even over 65%. The chances of survival depend largely on the severity of the concomitant malformation [17].

Urogenital Malformations

The close link between embryonic rectal and urogenital development explains why malformations of the kidneys, ureters, bladder, and genitals account for over half the concomitant abnormalites. Most common are hydronephrosis, vesicoureteral reflux, ureteral stenosis, vesical diverticulum, and hypospadias. In girls, septations of vagina and uterus are found (Fig. 33.18).

Malformations of the Spinal Column

Among the most common spinal abnormalities are partial and complete sacral agenesis and lumbar malformation. They are often accompanied by defective innervation of the pelvic floor and therefore play an important role in the development of incontinence.

Other Malformations

Statistical analysis of pooled data reveals the incidence of esophageal atresia to be 6%, that of other intestinal malformations is 8%, cardiac malformation 9%, and CNS anomalies 10%.

Treatment

A correct operation depends on the type of malformation.

Low, Translevator Anomalies

Stenotic Anomalies

Simple dilatation with Hegar bougies up to Fr 10 is mostly sufficient to achieve a normal anorectal caliber. In some cases, a stricture formation may need Y–V or Z-plasty. Only rarely is a mobilization of the anorectum necessary. For this procedure, it is best to use the sacroperineal route.

Covered Anus

A covered anus with or without fistula is treated using a V-flap of skin in order to achieve retropositioning of the anus. This flap is then inverted and sutured to the posterior half of the anal mucosa. Contrary to some authors, we do not feel that a simple cut-back incision gives an acceptable esthetic (although good functional) result.

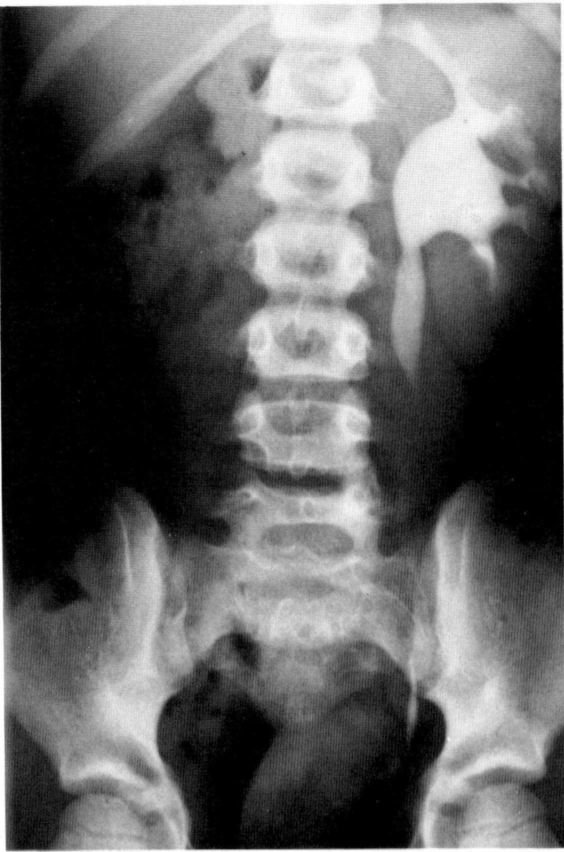

Fig. 33.18. Anorectal agenesis with absent right kidney and sacral malformation

Intermediate Anomalies

For intermediate malformations, three techniques are most frequently used.

Sacroperineal Rectoplasty (Stephens) [22, 23]

Sacroperineal rectoplasty was designed to preserve the puborectalis sling. Through a vertical sacral incision this muscle and the rectal pouch can be isolated. From a perineal incision lying over the center of the external sphincter, a canal is prepared through the center of the striated muscle extending anterior to the puborectalis. Following mobilization of the rectal pouch, a fistula to the urethra, vestibulum, or vagina is divided. The rectum is then pulled through the preformed canal to the perineum.

Anterior Perineal Approach (Mollard) [11]

The anterior perineal procedure begins with a crescent-shaped transverse perineal incision. The upward dissection on the dorsal surface of the urethra extends to above the puborectalis. Following division of a fistula, the rectal pouch is then mobilized and pulled down in front of the puborectalis to the anal site for suture to the skin edges.

Posterior Sagittal Anorectoplasty (Pena de Vries) [14]

Posterior sagittal anorectoplasty is now the most widely used procedure (see below).

High Supralevator Anomalies

Many procedure of the past are no longer recommended, although they all contributed to a better understanding of the morphology and anatomy of high supralevator malformations. Most surgeons advocate primary colostomy rather than an abdominoperineal pull-through procedure in the neonatal period.

Colostomy

Whenever a pull-through procedure in the newborn seems to be inappropriate, we prefer a sigmoid colostomy. The advantage over a transverse colostomy is evident. The entire colon remains functionally intact. The length of the descending colon is preserved. Irrigation and emptying of the rectal pouch is facilitated. If a urethral fistula is present, the risk of contamination of the urinary tract is decreased. Hyperchloremic acidosis does not occur and a two-stage pull-through procedure is feasible.

Sacroabdominoperineal (Mucosa-Stripping) Anorectoplasty (Stephens-Rehbein-Kiesewetter) [8, 9, 15, 21]

Sacroabdominoperineal anorectoplasty starts with the sacroperineal approach according to Stephens as described before. The abdominal portion of the operation is performed through a left paramedian or lower hockey-stick incision. No perirectal dissection is done. Instead, the mucosa of the rectal pouch is dissected free from the muscularis. If a fistula is present, this is ligated after removal of the mucosa.

The pouch is incised onto the top of a Hegar dilator introduced from the perineum. The proximal bowel is brought down through a distal sleeve and guided to the anal site. This operation avoids trauma to the pelvic nerves and preserves the striated muscles.

Posterior Sagittal Anorectoplasty (Pena, de Vries) [1, 14]

With the patient in a prone jackknife position, a midsagittal incision is made from the sacrum to the anal site, as determined by electrostimulation. The midsagittal incision is continued down, and the muscle fibers are split precisely in the midline with continuous use of the electrostimulator. After identification of the rectal pouch, a fistula is divided and oversewn. The terminal bowel is mobilized no more than necessary to bring it down to the anal site. When the bowel is ectatic, a wedge resection is taken, and the rectum is reconstructed in a tubular fashion. The striated muculature is sutured circumferentially in layers so as to create a new anal canal. The anal orifice and canal should accommodate a Hegar 12 dilator.

Sacroabdominoperineal Operation With Skin Flaps (Millard Rowe) [10]

Recognizing the high incidence of anal stenosis and mucosal prolapse, Millard and Rowe introduced the dorsally based trap-door incision at the anal site. Following a pull-through procedure, the bowel is brought down to within 1.5 cm of the perineal skin. The skin flaps are then interdigitated in the terminal bowel and the raw surface of the anal canal is thereby covered.

Smooth Muscle Duplication (Hofmann-von Kap-herr, Holschneider) [5, 6]

Following a pull-through operation, the mucosa of the terminal bowel segment is detached from the muscularis. The seromuscular sleeve is then turned back up over the proximal bowel and the serosal surfaces are sutured to each other. It is hoped that the duplication of circular musculature will act as an internal sphincter.

Intussuscepting Technique (Schärli) [17]

The abdominal part of the operation starts with the preparation of a long vital seromuscular cuff. This is facilitated by injecting saline into the submucous layer. Care is taken to avoid vascular damage. A rectourethral fistula is divided within the rectal pouch. The seromuscular cuff is then intussuscepted, following preparation of the new anal canal within the striated muscles, and sutured to the perianal subcutaneous sheath. The sigmoid colon is then pulled through the intussuscepted seromuscular cuff (Fig. 33.19). The perineal part of the opera-

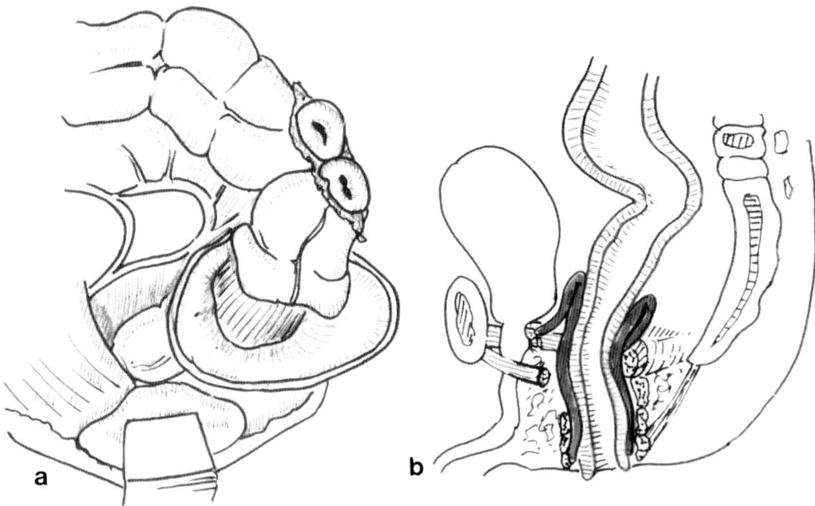

Fig. 33.19. *a* Preparation of seromuscular cuff in anorectal agenesis (mucosa stripping); *b* position of pulled-through sigmoid colon following intussusception of former rectal cuff

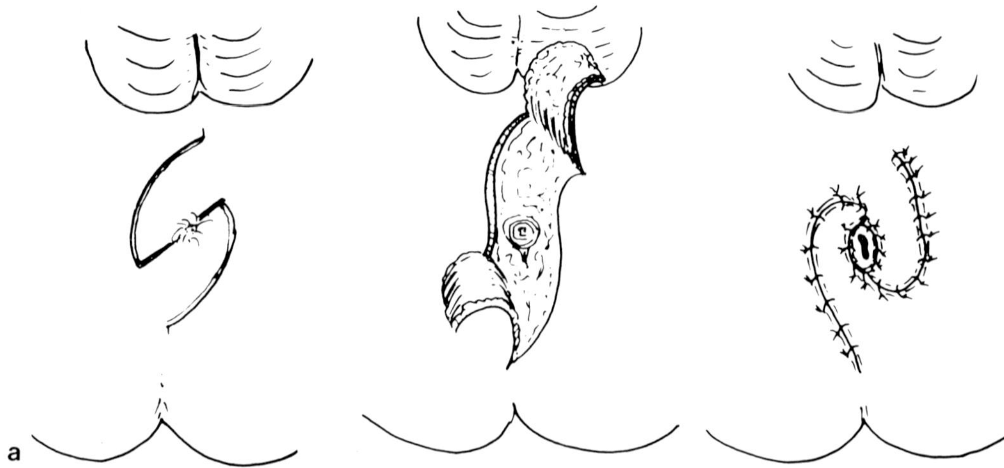

tion can be done according to the surgeon's individual experience (Stephens, Mollard, Pena-de Vries approach).

In the past, pediatric surgeons did not give too much attention to the perineal phase of the operation. Quite often, the anus remained patulous and the mucocutaneous anastomosis became scarred and stenotic.

An S-shaped incision of the perineum gives a far better view of the perineal body, facilitating the identification of the external sphincter and the pull-through procedure. A similar procedure has been suggested by Ferguson [2] for the repair of a Whitehead deformity. The two flaps are placed around the newly created anus and sutured so as to invert the anal orifice. This inverting perineoplasty has the

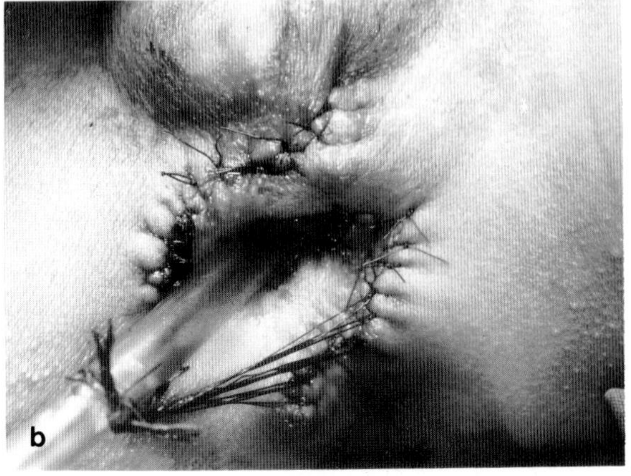

Fig. 33.20. *a* S-shaped incision makes invertoplasty of anal mucosa possible; *b* completion of the operation

advantage of a far better cosmetic appearance and, in addition, it brings sensory elements of the perineal skin into the anal canal (Fig. 33.20). Our experience with this procedure is limited and the follow-up time short. From our cases, we have the impression that regular bowel movements without intermittent soiling will eventually lead to good continence.

Postoperative Assessment

Results of surgery are difficult to compare in the literature. There are too many differences in classification and criteria for evaluation. In spite of various „objective" measures ot determine continence, the only reliable and comparable measure is, on the one hand, the patients' ability to remain clean or, on the other, staining, fecal soiling, or related complications. It is to be hoped that the 1984 Wingspread format will make it possible to compare results of various operative procedures. We can assume that over 90% of patients with low anomalies will be continent, whereas more than 70% of patients with high rectoanal agenesis will have difficulties of some sort, and 25% will be incontinent [18, 22]. Improvement of continence can be achieved by biofeedback training, by just getting older, and in some instances by corrective surgical procedures.

References

1. de Vries PA, Pena A (1982) Posterior sagittal anorecto-plasty. J Pediatr Surg 17: 638
2. Ferguson JA (1959) Repair of "Whitehead deformity" of the anus. Surg Gynecol Obstet 108: 115–116
3. Gebbers JO, Laissue JA (1984) Pathologie der Analtumoren. Praxis 73: 847–862
4. Goligher JC (1980) Surgery of the anus and rectum. Baillière Tindall, London
5. Hofmann-von Kap-herr S, Koltai I (1981) New methods in the treatment of anorectal incontinence. Z Kinderchir 32: 258
6. Holschneider AM, Hecker WC (1981) Reverse smooth muscle plasty: a new method of treating anorectal incontinence in infants with high anal and rectal atresia. J Pediatr Surg 16: 917
7. Jacobs AH (1978) Eruptions in the diaper area. Pediatr Clin North Am 25: 209–224
8. Kiesewetter WB (1976) Imperforate anus. II. The rationale and technique of the sacro-abdomino-perineal operation. J Pediatr Surg 2: 106
9. Kiesewetter WB (1966) Imperforate anus: the role and results of the sacro-abdomino-perineal operation. Ann Surg 164: 655
10. Millard DR, Rowe MI (1982) Plastic principles in high imperforate anus. Plast Reconstr Surg 69: 399
11. Mollard P, Marechal JM, Jeaubert de Beaujeu M (1978) Surgical treatment of high imperforate anus with definition of the puborectalis sling by an anterior perineal approach. J Pediatr Surg 13: 499
12. Otto HF, Gebbers JO (1976) Polypöse Dickdarmläsionen im Kindesalter. Differentialdiagnose und Systematik. Z Kinderchir 18: 357–373
13. Parks AG (1976) Anorektale Chirurgie. In: Von Zenker R (ed) Chirurgie der Gegenwart, vol 2. Urban and Schwarzenberg, Munich
14. Pena A, deVries PA (1982) Posterior sagittal anorectoplasty: important technical considerations and new applications. J Pediatr Surg 17: 796
15. Rehbein F (1959) Operationen der Anal- und Rectumatresie mit Recto-Urethralfistel. Chirurgie 30: 417
16. Santulli TV, Kiesewetter WB, Bill AH Jr (1970) Anorectal anomalies: a suggested international classification. J Pediatr Surg 5: 281–287
17. Schärli AF (1971) Die angeborenen Mißbildungen des Rektums und Anus. Huber, Bern Wien Stuttgart
18. Schärli AF, Kiesewetter WB (1969) Ano-recto-sigmoid-pressure studies as a quantititive evaluation of post-operative coninence. J Pediatr Surg 5: 694
19. Sherlock P, Morson BD, Barbara L, Veronesi U (1983) Precancerous lesions of the gastrointestinal tract. Raven, New York
20. Stelzner F (1976) Die anorektalen Fisteln, 2nd edn. Thieme, Stuttgart
21. Stephens FD, Smith DE (1971) Anorectal malformations in children. Year Book, Chicago, pp 33–211
22. Stephens FD, Smith DE (1986) Classification, identifications and assessment of surgical treatment of anorectal anomalies. Ped Surg Int 1: 200–208
23. Stephens FD (1953) Congenital imperforate rectum, recto-urethral and recto-vaginal fistulae. Aust NZ J Surg 22: 161
24. Wangensteen OH, Rice CO (1930) Imperforate anus: a method of determining the surgical approach. Ann Surg 92: 77
25. Winkler R (1977) Analabszesse und -fisteln. Richtlinien der Diagnostik, operativen Therapie und Nachsorge. Akt Chir 12: 171
26. Wolf HH (1980) Windeldermatitis. Pädiatr Prax (München) 24: 469

34 Pregnancy and Proctological Disease

M.-C. Marti

Introduction

The actual frequency of proctological diseases occurring during pregnancy is poorly documented in the literature. It is estimated [7, 11] that 85% of primi- or multiparae with proctological diseases developed them during or after their first pregnancy. The appearance of proctological diseases in women is related to the menstrual cycle and gravidity. Several physiopathological mechanisms have been suggested:

- The anatomical proximity of the genital organs to the anorectum
- The presence of estrogen receptors in the hemorrhoidal plexuses [13]
- Anatomical and physiological modifications induced by gravidity

The anatomical proximity of the vagina and anus explains why certain urogenital infections spread to the anus and rectum and also why diseases spread in the opposite direction. For example, gonococcal infections of the vagina are complicated by anorectal extension of the disease in 25%–75% of cases even without anal intercourse [8].

The discovery of estrogen receptors in hemorrhoidectomy specimens raises more questions than it answers. These receptors could partly explain why congestive, edematous or even thrombotic hemorrhoidal attacks occur at different phases of the endocrine cycle, during pregnancy, and when oral contraceptives are used [13].

Pregnancy causes the pelvic floor and perineal blood vessels to undergo major changes. The uterus expands, the cervix becomes softer, and the vaginal wall thickens and becomes more supple, longer, and congested. The bladder trigone becomes wider, longer, and raised. A marked tumescence of the pelvic vessels appears. There is hypertrophy of the anal muscles, and the pelvic fascia becomes progressively distended up to the third trimester to enable birth to take place. During the same period, the perineal skin becomes pigmented and tranformed by the higher activity of the sebaceous glands and by the increased secretion of mucus by both the vaginal and the anal glands.

The appearance, extension, and treatment of proctological diseases during pregnancy are dependent on these various changes. Childbirth favors the appearance of thrombotic lesions in hemorrhoids and traumatic lesions on sphincter muscles. Repeated pregnancies and deliveries may result in permanent lesions of the pelvic floor [14]. Several distinct types of proctological diseases are related to pregnancy (Table 34.1).

Proctological Diseases Provoked by Pregnancy

Some proctological diseases may be provoked by pregnancy (Table 34.2). Varices, simple congestion of the anal canal, edema of anal papillae, and acute thrombosis are direct consequences of pelvic venous stasis. Acute thrombosis ist the only case which calls for surgical treatment, namely a simple incision and expulsion of the clot. The other vascular lesions should be treated by lying down frequently for short periods and applying creams containing phlebotrophic and anti-inflammatory substances. Constipation should be treated by frequent and regular intake of mucilaginous substances.

Table 34.1. Proctological disease and pregnancy

Diseases provoked by pregnancy
Diseases aggravated by pregnancy
Diseases resulting from pregnancy
Diseases that threaten pregnancy
Diseases that contraindicate pregnancy
Diseases that contraindicate delivery by the normal route

Table 34.2. Proctological diseases provoked by pregnancy

Anal varices
Simple congestion of the anal canal
Papillary edema
Acute thrombosis
Anal pruritis caused by vaginal mycosis
Anal neuralgias
Changes in stool movements

Pruritus, *Trichomonas* infections, and mycosis spread to the rectum and are promoted by hypersecretion of mucus with modified pH. The result may be vulvovaginitis accompanied by severe proctitis, with a tendency to superinfection by staphylococci and enterococci. The treatment of vaginal mycosis and the endoanal application of mycostatis usually results in regression of the pruritus and the remission of the lesions. Furthermore the lesions usually heal spontaneously – and definitely – after childbirth.

Anal neuralgias are attributed to the stretching of the pelvic nervous plexuses during pregnancy. These lesions are rare but difficult, and even impossible, to threat. They may be aggravated by changes in stool movements, and particularly by periods of constipation with impaction of solid feces. In this case, pressure exerted on the puborectalis sling and the levator ani may be considerable. After treatment during the acute period with enemas, long-term administration of mucilaginous laxatives is most helpful.

Proctological Diseases Aggravated by Pregnancy

Certain pre-existing proctological diseases may be aggravated and give rise to acute complications during pregnancy (Table 34.3). Anal pruritus may also be aggravated. A nearly symptom-free rectal prolapse may decompensate during pregnancy, particularly if a period of constipation arises.

The main anal infections which are aggravated during pregnancy are condyloma acuminatum and herpetic lesions. Vaginal hypersecretions which have a modified pH promote the anal extension of lesions with maceration of the perineum, fetid superinfection, and pruritus.

During pregnancy, the application of podophyllin is proscribed due to the fetal risks incurred by an increased absorption of the drug. Electrocoagulation or electroresection of the lesions should be restricted to the most severe cases, as risks of recurrences cannot be eliminated [17]. Vaginal and vulvar herpes may worsen during pregnancy and spread to the anus, contra-indicating childbirth by the normal route, as will be discussed below.

Table 34.3. Proctological diseases aggravated by pregnancy

Hemorrhoids and their complications
Condylomas
Anal pruritus
Prolapses of the anus and the rectum

Proctological Diseases Resulting from Pregnancy and Childbirth

Many proctological diseases are caused by pregnancy and childbirth and are mainly due to the mechanical and traumatic demands made on the perineum by pregnancy and childbirth (Table 34.4).

Skin tags arise as a result of hemorrhoids in which congestion ceased after parturition. Although they are not very symptomatic, they may reach enormous size, and after the resumption of menstruation it may be necessary to remove them surgically as they hinder local hygiene and defecation.

Although anal fissures are rare during pregnancy, they frequently arise during the postpartum. Martin [10] observed 45 anal fissures (10.7%) after delivery in a group of 425 women. Of these, 21 were multiple and 24 single; in the latter, 15 were located on the anterior commissure.

Postpartum anal fissures are most often located on commissures, either on the anterior commissure or situated in opposition on both commissures, in contrast to the posterior fissures typically found in men or nulliparae. This anatomical tendency arises because of the muscular weakness of the rectovaginal septum and the pelvic floor. It treatment is quite difficult as the classical hypertonia of the internal sphincter, which may be treated by an internal submucosal sphincterectomy, may not be present.

Coccygodynias and anorectal neuralgias are more often observed in women than in men [9] and are especially frequent in multiparae.

Occult pudendal nerve damage can occur without external anal sphincter divison after vaginal delivery, especially in forceps deliveries or after prolonged deliveries [14] resulting in idiopathic inconti-

Table 34.4. Proctological diseases resulting from pregnancy

Skin tags
Fissures
Fissure on the anterior commissure
Mirror fissures on the anterior and posterior commissures
Coccygodynias
Anorectal neuralgias
Sequels of episiotomy and tears
Endometriosis
Rectovaginal fistulas
Fistulas in the scars of previous episiotomies in the case of Crohn's disease
Pelvic nerve damage and idiopathic incontinence
Descending perineum syndrome
Prolapse

nence. Reports of large series have not indicated that episiotomy offers a clear benefit to women in terms of decreased numbers of lacerations [15]. Furthermore Thorr [16] shows in a prospective study that no third – or fourth – degree laceration occurred without antecedent episiotomy in any women. Poorly reconstructed obstetrical tears and episiotomies may give rise to permanent lesions of the sphincter, resulting in incontinence of varying degrees of severity and permanent irritations of the perineum.

Moreover, prolonged delivery, which is rarely seen today in industrialized countries but still occurs in regions of the Third World having little access to medical services, may give rise to widespread destruction of the rectovaginal septum and the appearance of severe rectovaginal fistulas [11]. Foreign body granulomas, which may be mistaken for anal fistulas, are due to the use of nonabsorbable thread in episiotomy sutures which may be spontaneously eliminated several years after childbirth. The incidence of endometriosis is rising and is linked to the increasingly frequent practice of episiotomies [6]. Diagnosing these pseudotumoral, cystic, or fistulous – and sometimes bleeding – lesions may be difficult. Straightforward surgery may become complicated when the lesions are embedded in the sphincter muscles. Endocrine medical treatment to complement surgery may prove necessary.

The descending perineum syndrome is a direct consequence of postpartum distention of the fascia and pelvic musculature resulting in a stretching of the pudendal nerves [14]. This pelvic weakness may be improved by toning exercises and endoanal electrostimulation.

Prolapses of varying degree may arise as a consequence of repeated pregnancies and deliveries, most of which took place without episiotomies. This may involve simple rectal intussusception, exteriorized rectal prolapse, rectocele, or uterine prolapse with or without cystocele. Lesions may vary in complexity and extent and require surgical correction that may prove to be difficult.

Proctological Disease Endangering Pregnancy
(Table 34.5)

Perineal abscesses and suppurations are rare in pregnant women and rarely threaten pregnancy. Incision and drainage of these lesions must be undertaken early and the risk of bacteremia avoided with brief antibiotic prophylactic treatment. Fistulecto-

Table 34.5. Proctological diseases threatening pregnancy

Abscess
Acute attack of Crohn's disease requiring surgery
Acute and complicated ulcerative colitis

my should be undertaken only after menstruation has resumed. Close supervision is necessary to avoid reactivation of the infection.

Contrary to former belief, colitis is now not thought to have a harmful effect on pregnancy, particularly when the proctitis is in remission at the time of conception. The risks of abortion or premature delivery are higher if conception takes place during an active phase of the disease [18]. Aggressive treatment is necessary to reduce the activity of the disease and to allow normal pregnancy. Järnerot [4] published results of 1555 pregnancies in women suffering from colitis who were treated: 83.3% had a normal pregnancy and gestation, 9.1% spontaneous abortion, 4.8% therapeutic abortion, 1.9% dead child delivery, and in 1.1% of deliveries the child suffered from a congenital anomaly.

In contrast, pregnancy

- Is not connected with a higher risk of relapse if the disease is in remission at the time of conception.
- Results in improvement of only a minority of patients if the disease is active, although there is a higher risk of acute attacks after the pregnancy.
- Aggravates the prognosis of a first attack of colitis with the risk of either spontaneous abortion or the development of fulminating lesions during postpartum.

The evolution of proctitis during or after a first pregnancy does not indicate the risks involved in subsequent pregnancies. Crohn's disease does not seem to have a harmful effect on pregnancy; moreover, pregnancy is not linked with particular mortality or morbidity arising from Crohn's disease [2].

Proctological Diseases
That Contraindicate Pregnancy

In some proctological diseases (Table 34.6), pregnancy may be contraindicated for three main reasons.

Eugenic Reasons. The disease may be hereditary and entail the risk of giving birth to a child affected by the disease; this is the case in familial polyposis.

Table 34.6. Proctological diseases contraindicating pregnancy

Carcinoma of the rectum
Carcinoma of the anal canal and the anal margin
Actinic lesions
Familial polyposis
Crohn's disease and colitis in the acute phase or poorly controlled

Table 34.7. Proctological diseases that may contraindicate vaginal delivery

Extensive perineal suppurations
Lymphogranuloma venereum
Anal herpes
Severe traumatic lesions of the perineum
Ileoanal pouches
Sequels of low rectal surgery
Abdominoperineal resection for Crohn's disease, ulcerative colitis, carcinoma
Actinic lesions

Family and Human Reasons. The vital prognosis for the mother may be so poor that even if the pregnancy comes to term, the mother will not survive long to take care of her child. This is the case in cancers of the rectum and of the anus.

Teratogenic Reasons. The patient must undergo radiological examination and radiotherapeutic and chemotherapeutic treatments which may have harmful effects on the fetus. This is the case in neoplasia, and also in Crohn's disease and coloproctitis in the acute phase or poorly controlled, which necessitate aggresive treatment that have teratogenic effects (high doses of steroids) or give rise to fetal lesions due to transplacental passage (kernicterus due to sulfasalazine).

In these situations, which are fortunately infrequent, the parents and the various specialists implicated in the treatment – the gynecologist, proctologist, gastroenterologist, pharmacologist, and pediatrician – must discuss the matter frankly. Contraceptive measures should be planned until the risks have been well assessed and controlled. If necessary, termination of the pregnancy must be considered.

Proctological Diseases That Contraindicate Vaginal Delivery

Various proctological diseases may contraindicate delivery by natural routes and call for a cesarean section (Table 34.7). Extensive perineal suppurations which have developed from anal fistulas, Verneuil's disease, Crohn's disease, or Nicolas-Favre disease may require a cesarean section. Delivery by natural routes involves the risk of bacterial dissemination, an evident superinfection of episiotomy wounds, and even extensive pelvic and perineal lesions due to existing sclerous modifications (Nicolas-Favre). In patients with Nicolas-Favre disease, the appearance of occlusion may impose a cesarean section before term with colostomy being performed during the same operative session [7].

Due to the progress of antibiotic therapy, however, the risks of such complications developing have been reduced.

Extensive anal and vaginal herpes is accompanied by such a high risk of keratitis and fatal encephalitis of the newborn, that delivery by natural routes is formally contraindicated and a cesarean section is absolutely required. Similarly, women who have undergone perineal surgery for sphincteral repair of traumatic or obstetrical lesions should not deliver by natural routes to avoid postoperative results being worsened.

Postactinic and cicatricial perineal sclerosis as after abdominoperineal resection for carcinoma decrease the elasticity of the perineum and may prolong or complicate childbirth. Crohn's disease, ulcerative colitis, and polyposis treated by total colectomy with ileostomy or with ileoanal anastomosis do not seem to interfere wich normal delivery. Ostomates can become pregnant following ostomy. There is an increased risk of miscarriage [12] and premature labor [1]. A major problem during pregnancy in ostomates is intestinal obstruction. The other complications listed by Gopal [3] are stomal dysfunction and obstruction, ileostomy and colostomy prolapse, and nipple valve retraction in the case of Kock's pouches. Kretschew [5] suggests that ostomates should wait at least 1 year following surgery to become pregnant. Recent studies indicate that ostomates can successfully deliver children vaginally.

Results of a larger inquiry published by Gopal [3] show that 75% of women who had previous vaginal births had vaginal births when they became pregnant after ostomy surgery. Of women who were pregnant for the first time following the ostomy surgery, only 50% had a vaginal delivery. The reasons for this disparity have not being explained but may result from the fears of the obstetrician [3]. Out of 119 pregnancies in patients having undergone colectomy with ileostomy [12], 99 came to term and 82 delivered by the vaginal route. Eighteen patients (15%) presented complications with their ileostomy.

In the case of Crohn's disease, vaginal delivery may be complicated by rectovaginal fistulas and fistulas on episiotomy scars, even several years after childbirth [2].

Conclusion

Proctological diseases and pregnancy are interrelated in many ways. These diseases may be due to pregnancy, be aggravated during pregnancy, complicate pregnancy, contraindicate pregnancy, or even contraindicate vaginal delivery. Treatment and the time at which surgery is performed must be chosen with care, taking into consideration the risks involved both for the mother and for the child. In principle, elective surgery should only be undertaken after menstruation has resumed, when pelvic congestion has subsided, and the patient has resumed a normal life.

References

1. Barwin BW, Harley JM, Wilson W (1974) Ileostomy in pregnancy. Br J Clin Pract 20: 256–258
2. Granchrow MI, Benjamin H (1975) Inflammatory colorectal disease and pregnancy. Dis Colon Rectum 18: 706
3. Gopal K, Amshel AL, Shonberg J et al. (1985) Ostomy and pregnancy. Dis Colon Rectum 28: 912–916
4. Järnerot G (1982) Fertility, sterility and pregnancy in chronic inflammatory bowel disease. Scand J Gastroenterol 17: 1–4
5. Kretschew KP (1972) Intestinal stoma. Saunders, Philadelphia, pp 281–283
6. Liebeskind M, Lugagne F, Courtin A, Redelsperger (1981) Aspects proctologiques de l'endométriose. Proct 3: 193–197
7. Marks MM, Thiele GH (1955) Management of proctologia disease in pregnant an parons women. Am J Surg 90: 826–833
8. Marti M-C (1979) Vénéréologie anale. Méd Hyg 37: 280–282
9. Marti M-C (1984) Les algies pelviennes d'origine proctologique. Méd Hyg 42: 3289–3290
10. Martin JD (1953) Postpartum anal fissure. Lancet i: 271–273
11. Pope CE (1952) Anorectal complications of pregnancy. Am J Surg 84: 579–591
12. Rhodes JB, Kirsner JB (1965) The early and late course of patients with ulcerative colitis after ileostomy and colectomy. Surg Gynecol Obstet 125: 1303–1314
13. Saint-Pierre A (1982) Problèmes posés par la présence de récepteurs hormonaux au niveau des hémorroïdes. Ann Gastroentérol Hépatol (Paris) 18: 19–27
14. Snooks SJ, Setchell M, Swash M, Henry MM (1984) Injury to the innervation of the pelvic floor sphincter musculature in childbirth. Lancet ii: 546–550
15. Thacker SB, Banta D (1983) Benefits and risks of episiotomy: an interpretative review of the english language literature 1860–1980. Obstet Gynecol Surv 38: 322–338
16. Thorp JM, Bowes WA, Brame RG, Cefalo R (1987) Selected use of midline episiotomy: effect on perineal trauma. Obstet, Gynecol 70: 260–262
17. Von Krogh G (1981) Podophyllotoxin for condylomata acuminata eradication. Acta Derm Venereol [Suppl] (Stockh) 98: 1–48
18. Willoughby CP, Truelove SC (1980) Ulceratocolitis and pregnancy. Gut 21: 469–474

35 Interference Between Gynecological or Urological Diseases and Proctological Lesions

P. Aeberhard

The intimate anatomical relationship between the anorectum and the uterus, vagina, bladder, prostate, and male urethra and the sharing of the same supporting structures of the pelvic floor by these organs form the basis for the many interrelations between gynecological and urological diseases and anorectal pathology. These interdisciplinary aspects of proctology may conveniently be discussed under the headings of:

- The pelvic floor
- The perineum and anal sphincter
- Anorectal complications of the treatment of pelvic malignancies

The Pelvic Floor: Interrelations of Rectal Intussusception, Vaginal Relaxation, and Pelvic Floor Dysfunction

Definitions

For the definition of *rectal intussusception* and of the syndrome of the *descending perineum* the reader is referred to Chap. 23. For the syndromes of *vaginal relaxation* of interest to the proctologist the following definitions apply to findings when the patient ist not straining and no traction is applied to any structure [2].

Rectocele (Fig. 35.1)

First Degree. When the perineum is depressed, a saccular protrusion of the vaginorectal wall is visible.
Second Degree. The sacculation is visible at the introitus without depressing the perineum.
Third Degree. The sacculation protrudes or extends outside the introitus.

Enterocele

First Degree. The sac is visible in the vagina when the perineum is depressed.
Second Degree. The sac just extends through the introitus.
Third Degree. The total sac extends out of the introitus and generally contains small and/or large bowel.

Prolapse of the Vaginal Apex

Following total or incomplete hysterectomy the apical vaginal scar or remaining cervix can prolapse. This can occur alone or in combination with a cystocele, enterocele, or all three. Grading criteria are analogous to those applied for rectocele and enterocele.

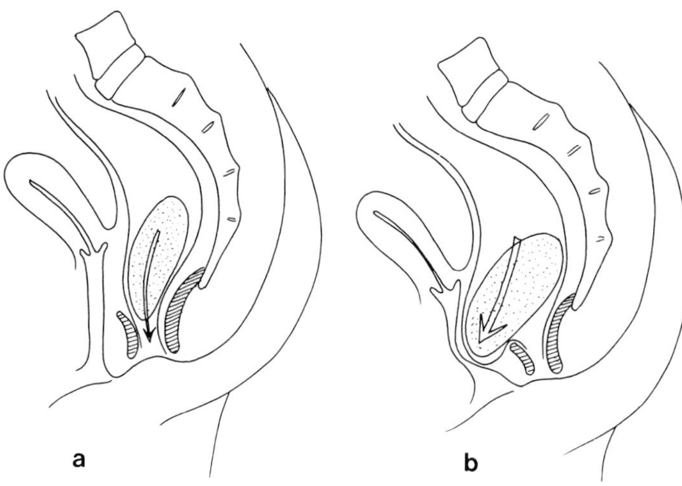

Fig. 35.1. a Normal defecation; *b* the mechanism of "obstructive costipation" in rectocele

Clinical Picture

Patients presenting with a history of severe chronic constipation associated with symptoms of rectal pressure, incomplete evacuation, repetitive defecation, and the necessity to apply manual pressure to achieve evacuation may be identified as suffering from rectal intussusception (first-degree rectal prolapse), the descending perineum syndrome, rectocele, enterocele, posthysterectomy vaginal prolapse, or any combination of these abnormalities. Blood in stools and mucus discharge are complaints frequently mentioned by this type of patients. These symptoms often constitute a severe limitation on the quality of life.

It has been estimated that *rectal intussusception* (RI) is up to ten times more common than external rectal prolapse [4]. RI was associated with rectocele in 26 of 42 patients studied by Mahieu [22], and Berman et al. [4] found perineal descent of more than 4 cm below the ischial tuberosities during straining in 46 out of 58 patients with distal RI. Of 52 patients with distal RI studied by Berman et al. [4], 25 had had previous anorectal procedures including hemorrhoidectomy, hemorrhoidal ligation, and sphincterotomy, and 35 had had previous pelvic or vaginal procedures, mostly hysterectomy and cystocele or rectocele repair. Enterocele is associated with previous abdominal or vaginal hysterectomy with or without colpoperineoplasty in the majority of cases [16].

Management of Vaginal Relaxation Associated With Obstructive Constipation

Conventionally, the repair of *rectocele* has been performed transvaginally by the gynecologist. The posterior repair may be combined with anterior repair of cystocele. In the "low" variety of rectocele, repair may be performed endorectally as described by Sullivan et al. [39], Khubchandani et al. [20] (Fig. 35.2), and Sehapayak [36]. There is still debate about the best method to treat *RI associated with rectocele*. Satisfactory results have been reported with Delorme's operation and modifications, in which the associated rectocele was either dealt with endorectally or repaired using a separate transvaginal approach [4, 40]. The multiplicity of methods advocated for the repair of *enterocele* and posthysterectomy *prolapse of the vaginal apex* testifies to the difficulty of finding a satisfactory solution to this problem. Enterocele may be managed by the Moschcowitz (Fig. 35.3) method of suture obliteration of the hernial sac [13]. Enterocele combined with posthysterectomy prolapse of the vaginal apex is repaired using various methods of fixing the vaginal vault to the sacrospinal ligament, promontorium, or the periosteum of the sacrum [16, 18] (Fig. 35.4). Concomitant rectocele and cystocele must be dealt with separately.

The Perineum and Anal Sphincters

Role of the Perineal Body in the Spread of Infections

Fournier's gangrene [9], the most life-threatening of perineal infections, is discussed in detail in Chap. 31. Fournier's disease is a typical infection of the compromised host, which may originate from various colorectoanal sources including anorectal abscess and fistula, rectal trauma and biopsy, perforated rectal carcinoma, and sigmoid diverticulitis, as well as from genitourinary sources such as ure-

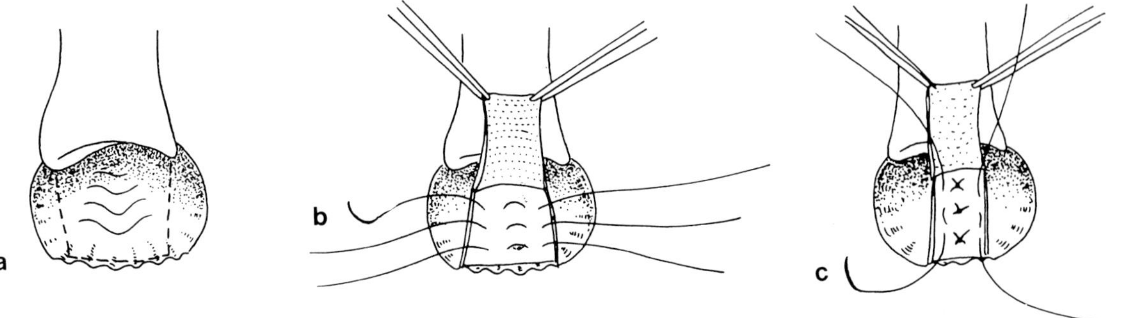

Fig. 35.2 a–c. Endorectal repair of rectocele. *a* Outline of mucomuscular flap starting at the dentate line. *b* Plication of lax rectovaginal septum by three or four transverse sutures. *c* The transverse plication is complemented by vertical plication. The mucomuscular flap is then sutured back in place after appropriate trimming. (Adapted from [20])

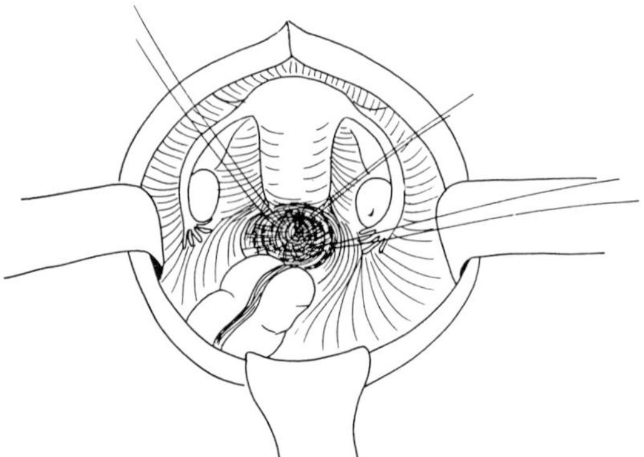

Fig. 35.3. The Moschcowitz repair for enterocele. Obliteration of the enterocele sac by a series of purse-string sutures, starting at the base of the sac. The threads of the second suture are tied to those of the first suture and so on

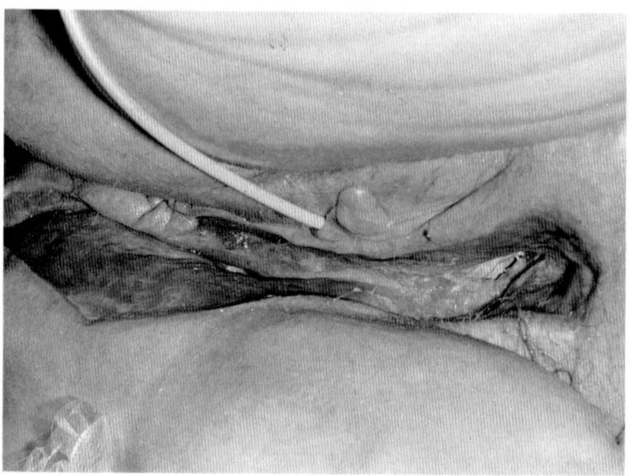

Fig. 35.5. Open granulating wound following incision of Bartholin's abscess in a 53-year-old, very obese diabetic patient (140 kg/155 cm)

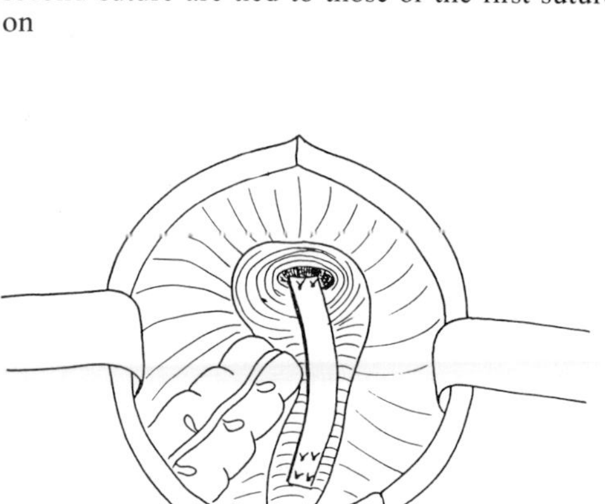

Fig. 35.4. Sacral colpopexy for repair of posthysterectomy prolapse of the vaginal apex. The rectum is displaced to the left. Vertical incision of peritoneum overlying the hollow of the sacrum. Complete removal of enterocele sac. The vaginal apex is fixed to the periosteum of the sacrum using a fascial strip taken from the rectus sheath

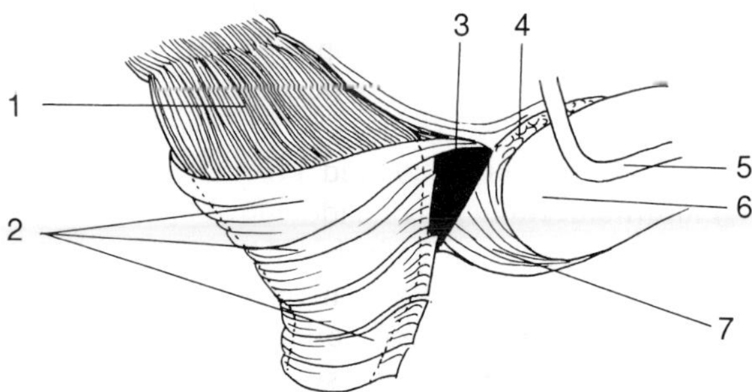

Fig. 35.6. The perineal body. *1,* Rectum (longitudinal muscle); *2,* levator ani, rectourethralal muscle, and anal sphincters; *3,* perineal body; *4,* deep tranversus perinei muscle; *5,* urethra; *6,* bulb of penis; *7,* bulbocavernosus muscle

thral stricture, urethral diverticulum, and traumatic rupture of the urethra.

Bartholin's abscess may spread to the perineum and extend as far as the buttocks, as we have seen in a very obese patient (Fig. 35.5). The anatomical basis for the spread of infections in this area has been discussed by Khan et al. [19]. The *perineal body* or central tendon of the perineum (centrum tendineum perinei) is a solid, wedge-shaped or rectangular mass of connective tissue and muscle fibers located between the anorectal junction and the posterior membranous urethra above the bulbocavernous muscle. Superiorly, it is limited by Denonvilliers' fascia and caudally by the deep external sphincter (Fig. 35.6). By its relationship to the ischiorectal fossae, perirectal space, and superficial perineal pouch (spatium perinei superficiale) the perineal body forms a "traffic center" which may direct and facilitate the spread of infections in various directions, including the propagation of retroperitoneal and intrapelvic suppurative processes to the superficial perineal pouch and external genitalia.

Obstetrical Trauma to the Anal Sphincters

Obstetrical trauma to the anal sphincters, which may result in anal incontinence and rectovaginal fistula, will be discussed only briefly in this chapter. For more details, the reader is referred to Chaps. 16 and 22.

Ectopic location of the anus too close to the introitus and outside the center of the typical skin pigmentation has been identified by Corman [6] as an important predisposing factor for obstetrical sphincter injury. He reported on 28 patients referred for repair of obstetrical sphincter lesions, 20 of whom had had midline episiotomy. An ectopic position of the anus was found in all of these patients.

Perineal Endometrioma

Endometriosis is by definition the ectopic location of functional endometrial glands and stroma. The most common locations of endometriosis include the ovaries, uterine ligaments, rectovaginal septum, and the pelvic peritoneum covering the uterus, tubes, rectum, sigmoid, and bladder. Perianal endometriosis is so rare as to represent no more than a surgical curiosity [11]. The foci of endometriosis undergo cyclic menstrual changes with periodic bleeding. The irritative effect of blood stimulates a marked fibroproliferative response which may progressively obliterate recognizable features. Endometriosis of longer standing will often form cysts filled with chocolate-colored material. These nodules are referred to as "endometrioma." Perianal endometrioma has usually been found in old episiotomy scars at intervals ranging from 45 days to 14 years ofter delivery and perineal trauma [28]. Endometrioma presents as an asymptomatic nodule or as a painful mass which may cause discomfort only at the time of menstruation. The differential diagnosis includes perianal fistula and abscess, thrombosed hemorrhoids, sebaceous cyst, suppurative hidradenitis, melanoma, and squamous or basal cell carcinoma of the perianal skin. Perianal endometrioma is best treated by surgical excision. The intimate relationship of the nodule to the anal sphincter may necessitate plastic repairs or reinforcement of thinned-out parts of the sphincter muscle.

Anorectal Complications of the Treatment of Pelvic Genitourinary Malignancy

General Remarks on Morbidity of Pelvic Surgery and Radiotherapy

Tumors of the bladder an prostate comprise 26.6% of male malignancies [37], and tumors of the bladder, uterus, and ovary comprise about 16.5% of female malignancies. The localized stages of these tumors are managed by surgery or radiotherapy or by combined surgical and radiooncological treatment as described below. Radiation therapy to pelvic

Table 35.1. Radiation tolerance of normal abdominal and pelvic structures. (From [27])

	cGy
Small bowel	4500
Colon and rectum	6000
Bladder	7000
Ureter	7500

malignancies may be administered in the form of external beam megavoltage therapy or as brachytherapy using implants of cesium 137, iridium 192, iodine 125, or gold 198, or as a combination of external beam and interstitial therapy. Neighboring pelvic organs may be affected by radiotherapy as "innocent bystanders." The radiation tolerance of normal abdominal and pelvic structures is listed in Table 35.1.

The probability of radiation damage occurring is enhanced by coexisting conditions such as marked obesity, arteriosclerotic vascular disease, and diabetes. Morbidity due to pelvic irradiation includes radiation cystitis, ureteritis, procitis, and enteritis which may all progress to fistula formation. Fistulas usually appear within 2 years of radiotherapy. Vesicovaginal, vesicoenteric, rectovesical, and rectovaginal fistulas occur more frequently after treatment of gynecological malignancies, whereas rectourethral fistula is mainly a complication of radiotherapy for cancer of the prostate. The clinical picture of *radiation proctitis* is characterized by tenesmus, diarrhea, rectal bleeding, fecal urgency, and incontinence. Radiation proctitis may progress to anal stenosis and rectal stricture, or to full-thickness necrosis with fistulization to the vagina, bladder, or urethra.

For the classification of morbidity of radiation therapy, several *grading systems* have been introduced [23, 29, 30]. The grading system published by the Radiation Therapy Oncology Group (RTOG) [28,

Table 35.2. Morbidity grading system for radiotherapy

Grade I	Minor symptoms requiring no treatment
Grade 2	Symptoms responding to simple outpatient management; lifestyle (performance status) not affected
Grade 3	Distressing symptoms altering patient's lifestyle (performance status). Hospitalization for diagnosis or minor surgical intervention (e. g., urethral dilatation) may be required
Grade 4	Major surgical intervention (such as laparotomy, colostomy, cystectomy) or prolonged hospitalization are required
Grade 5	Fatal complications

33] seems ot be the most appropriate (Table 35.2). Grades 1 and 2 are classified as anticipated treatment reactions. They are listed as complications only if they persist for more than 1 month after completion of therapy or if they progress to a higher grade.

Overall, the incidence of severe complications of pelvic radiation therapy has decreased considerably. The incidence of radiation-induced fistula is now below 1% [35]. The decrease in morbidity has resulted from several advances: CT provides more precise information of the anatomical relationship of the tumor to adjacent organs. Most centers utilize computerized dosimetry systems which measure the radiation distribution and allow the limitation of the dose to the tolerance of surrounding normal pelvic structures.

Cancer of the Prostate

Treatment Concepts

Localized disease amenable to curative treatment by surgery, radiation therapy, or a combination of both is present in less than half of the patients in whom cancer of the prostate is diagnosed [7, 24, 26]. Carcinoma confined to the prostate may be treated surgically by radical perineal prostatectomy [8, 10], or by radical retropubic prostatectomy combined with bilateral pelvic lymphadenectomy [3, 15] or by radiotherapy which may be delivered as external beam radiation or brachytherapy with interstitial implants alone or in combination [1, 14, 23, 30, 34]. Radical surgery may be combined with adjuvant radiotherapy [32, 33]. Radiation may be used as salvage therapy for local failure after radical surgery [31], and salvage surgery has been applied for local failure of definitive radiotherapy [21].

Complications of Surgical Treatment

There are anorectal complications of *surgery alone:* in a series of 692 patients who underwent bilateral pelvic lymphadenectomy and radical prostatectomy for stages A–DI adenocarcinoma, there were nine intraoperative rectal injuries (1.3%), six of which were treated with layered closure and three with colostomy [15]. Of 215 consecutive patients, 207 of whom underwent radical perineal prostatectomy and eight retropubic prostatectomy, ten (5%) suffered rectal injuries which were closed in layers and healed primarily, whereas another four (2%) developed rectal abscess requiring drainage and two

(1%) additional patients had to be managed by colostomy [10]. In a smaller series of 30 patients reported by Elder et al. [8], no rectal injuries occurred.

Complications of Radiotherapy and Combined Treatment Modalities

Radiotherapy to prostatic cancer is administered at dosages of 6000–7000 cGy to the prostate volume and as an extended field dose of 4000–4500 cGy to the pelvis [35]. In radiotherapy for prostatic carcinoma, the anterior wall of the rectum is included in the treatment volume. A standard dose of 6500–7000 cGy of external radiation or an equivalent dose of interstitial radiation can exceed the radiation tolerance of the rectum. A dose of 6500 cGy is efficacious in the management of small tumors, but doses of more than 7000 cGy have been advocated for the treatment of stage C lesions. Treatment of extensive tumors with more than 7000 cGy of external radiation alone or combined with interstitial radiation constitutes a serious risk of injury to the rectum [12, 14]. About 15% of patients having radiotherapy for prostatic carcinoma suffer chronic rectal symptoms that are mild and managed easily by diet and medication [34]. Severe rectal injury requiring hospitalization and major medical or surgical treatment was observed in six out of 348 patients (1.7%) reported by Green et al. [12]. In this series, the highest complication rates were found in patients having 7000–7500 cGy external radiation (5%), and in those having a combination of gold 198 brachytherapy and external radiation (14%). In two RTOG trials in which the patients received minimal total doses of 6500 cGy external beam radiation to the prostate and 4500 cGy to the pelvis, proctitis and/or rectal ulcer was observed in 8.2%, rectal bleedng in 1.4%, and rectoanal stricture in 0.6% of 487 patients treated [30]. Mazeron et al. [23], using exernal beam radiation of a total dose of 6500 cGy in 60 patients, reported four serious gastrointestinal complications including two cases of severe proctitis.

Iodine 125 brachytherapy is efficacious in stage B prostatic carcinoma. The low-energy gamma emission of iodine 125 has a short tissue penetration resulting in only a small volume of the rectum receiving a high dose. Severe rectal complications occur less frequently with iodine 125 than with external radiation, and ulcers resulting from interstitial therapy have a better tendency to heal than those due to external radiation [12, 35]. Of 152 patients who had interstitial implanation of iodine 125 combined with bilateral pelvic staging lymphadenectomy as definitive treatment of localized prostatic carcinoma from 1975 to 1983, two suffered rectal ulcers and three developed prostatic rectourethral fistulas, a severe complication rate of 3.3% [17]. In a similar protocol using a combination of external beam and interstitial iodine 125 radiation and bilateral pelvic lymphadenectomy in 104 patients, 7% suffered prolonged distressing proctitis, and 4% developed rectal ulceration or rectourethral fistula necessitating colostomy. Prolonged proctitis was only observed in patients in whom less than a 0.5 cm space had been maintained between the closest seed and the rectal mucosa [1].

In *salvage radiotherapy* for residual or recurrent local tumor following radical prostatectomy, a higher complication rate has been reported than in the case of primary definitive irradiation [39]. Likewise, salvage surgery after failure of radiotherapy has been fraught with a higher complication rate than primary radical surgery [21].

Cancer of the Bladder

Treatment Concepts

Invasive transitional cell carcinoma of the bladder may be treated by preoperative radiotherapy followed by cystectomy or by radical cystectomy alone [35, 38]. Definitive radiotherapy may be followed by radical cystectomy in patients whose tumors do not respond initially or recur subsequent to radiotherapy. Salvage cystectomy performed after definitive radiotherapy provides the highest potential for the development of complications, many of which can be prevented by careful selection of a bowel segment outside the radiation field for conduit formation.

Treatment Morbidity

As radiotherapy for carcinoma of the bladder encompasses a higher field than that used for cancer of the prostate, rectal complications have not been as prominent as those reported after radiotherapy for cancer of the prostate. The main gastrointestinal complications of radiotherapy of bladder cancer include strictures of the small bowel and colon [35].

Carcinoma of the Uterus

Treatment Concepts

Localized cancer of the *endometrium* is treated by total abdominal hysterectomy and bilateral salpingo-oophorectomy. Radiotherapy may form part of the treatment concept. Over the last few years, preoperative implants have been progressively abandoned in favor of postoperative radiotherapy which is given in patients who have a depth of infiltration of more than one-third of the myometrium. Vaginal implants of cesium 137 are used as a safeguard against vaginal stump recurrence.

The Fédération Internationale de Gynécologie et Obstétrique (FIGO) stages I and IIA carcinoma of the *uterine cervix* may be treated with either irradiation or radical hysterectomy, with a recent trend in favor of surgical treatment. Definitive radiotherapy is used in patients with stages IIB, III, and IV tumors [25]. Adjunctive extrafascial hysterectomy may be used following radiotherapy in bulky stage I and stage II lesions of the cervix. Anterior, posterior, or total pelvic exenteration have been used to treat persistent or recurrent tumor following radiotherapy. As the local failure rate of modern radiotherapy is quite low, the indications for pelvic exenteration are decreasing.

Complications of Radical Hysterectomy

Pelvic abscess, pelvic cellulitis, pelvic lymphocyst, and vesicovaginal and ureterovaginal fistulas are rare complications of radical hysterectomy. In a collective review of complications of radical hysterectomy by Nagell et al. [27], no rectal complications were reported.

Complications of Radiation Therapy

Rectal ulceration and rectovaginal fistula occur almost exclusively at the level of the highest dose from an intracavitary implant. In a collective series of 9373 patients having radiotherapy for cancer of the uterine cervix, Nagell et al. [27] reported an 8.2% incidence of sigmoiditis, 0.9% rectal strictures, and 1.2% rectovaginal fistulas. This review was based on papers published between 1970 and 1977. In a report on complications of radiotherapy based on 811 patients with carcinoma of the cervix treated by definitive radiation therapy from 1959 to 1977, Perez et al. [29] found 39 colorectoanal complications corresponding to RTOG grades 3–5, including 17 cases of proctitis, seven rectal ulcers, eight sigmoid strictures, and seven rectovaginal fistulas. Of patients with complications of radiotherapy, 75% had only one organ affected, whereas 25% had a combination of two or three complications; 80% of rectosigmoid complications occurred within 30 months of initial therapy. With maximal total doses $\leqslant 8000$ cGy, the incidence of severe complications was below 5%, but increased to 10%–15% with higher doses. Combes et al. [5] reported a 7.2% incidence of severe complications including obstructing rectosigmoiditis (3.1%) and rectovaginal fistula (1.4%) in 581 patients with stage II carcinoma of the uterine cervix treated with external beam radiation and intracavitary cesium 137 between 1976 and 1978.

Management of Radiation Proctitis

Radiation proctitis is managed conservatively using steroid-containing medications, a low-residue diet and appropriate stool softeners. A classically presenting radiation ulcer should preferable not be biopsied as this may worsen symptoms. Failure to improve on conservative measures and progression of the ulcer in size and depth under therapy are indications for fecal diversion.

The surgical treatment of rectal strictures and rectovaginal and rectourethral fistulas are dealt with elsewhere in this volume (see Chaps. 16, 17, and 24).

References

1. Abadir R, Ross G Jr, Weinstein S-H (1984) Carcinoma of the prostate treated by pelvic node dissection iodine-125 seed impant and external irradiation: a study of rectal complications. Clin Radiol 35: 359–361
2. Beecham C-T (1980) Classification of vaginal relaxation. Am J Obstet Gynecol 2: 957–958
3. Benson RC Jr, Tomera KM, Zincke H, Fleming TR, Utz DC (1984) Bilateral pelvic lymphadenectomy and radical retropubic prostatectomy for adenocarcinoma confined to the prostate. J Urol 131: 1103–1106
4. Berman IR, Manning DH, Dudley-Wright K (1985) Anatomic specificity in the diagnosis and treatment of internal rectal prolapse. Dis Colon Rectum 28: 816–826
5. Combes PF, Daly NJ, Horiot J-C, Achille E, Keiling R, Pigneux J, Pourquier H, Rozan R, Schraub S, Vrousos C (1985) Results of radiotherapy alone in 581 patients with stage II carcinoma of the uterine cervix. Med J Radiat Oncol Biol Phys 11: 463–471
6. Corman ML (1985) Anal incontinence following obstetrical injury. Dis Colon Rectum 28: 86–89
7. Donohue RE, Mani JH, Whitesel JA, Mohr S, Scanavino D, Augsburger R, Biber RJ, Fauver HE, Wettlaufer JN, Pfister RR (1982) Pelvic lymph node dissection. Guide to patient management in clinically locally confined adenocarcinoma of prostate. Urology 20: 559–565
8. Elder JS, Gibbsons RP, Correa R Jr, Brannen GE (1984) Morbidity of radical perineal prostatectomy following transurethral resection of the prostate. J Urol 132: 55–57
9. Fieve G, Laprevote-Heully MC, Brice M, Lambert H, Frisch R, Larcan A (1978) Les gangrènes périnéales. Ann Med Nancy-Est 17: 1515–1518
10. Gibbsons RP, Correra R Jr, Brannen GE, Mason JT (1984) Total prostatectomy for localized prostatic cancer. J Urol 131: 73–76
11. Gordon PH, Schlotter JL, Balcos EG, Goldberg SM (1976) Perianal endometrioma. Report of five cases. Dis Colon Rectum 19: 260–265
12. Green N, Goldberg H, Goldmann H, Lombardo L, Skaist L (1984) Severe rectal injury following radiation for prostatic cancer. J Urol 131: 701–704
13. Haest JWG, Broeders GHB, Hoogeveen AJA (1979) Abdominal surgical treatment of enterocele. Eur J Obstet Gynecol Reprod Biol 9 (1): 55–56
14. Hanks GE, Leibel SA, Krall JM, Kramer S (1985) Patterns of care studies: dose-response observations for local control of adenocarcinoma of the prostate. Int J Radiat Oncol Biol Phys 11: 153–157
15. Igel TC, Barrett DM, Segura JW, Benson RK, Rife CC (1987) Perioperative and postoperative complications from bilateral pelvic lymphadenectomy and radical retropubic prostatectomy. J Urol 137: 1189–1191
16. Jaisle F (1981) Die operative Behandlung der Enterozele und des Scheidenblindsackvorfall. Geburtshilfe Frauenheilkd 41: 777–780
17. Jordan GH, Lynch DF, Warden SS, McCraw D, Hoffmann GC, Schellhammer PF (1985) Major rectal complications following interstitial implantation of 125 Iodine for carcinoma of the prostate. J Urol 134: 1212–1217
18. Kauppila O, Punnonen R, Teisala K (1986) Operative technique for the repair of posthysterectomy vaginal prolapse. Ann Chir Gynaecol 75: 242–244
19. Khan SA, Smith NC, Gonder M, Ravo B, Siddharth P (1985) Gangrene of male external genitalia in a patient with colorectal disease. Dis Colon Rectum 28: 519–522
20. Khubchandani IT, Sheets JA, Slasik JJ, Hakki AR (1983) Endorectal repair of rectocele. Dis Colon Rectum 26: 792–796
21. Mador DR, Huben RP, Wajsman Z, Pontes JE (1985) Salvage surgery following radical radiotherapy for adenocarcinoma of the prostate. J Urol 133: 58–60
22. Mahieu P, Pringot J, Bodart P (1984) Defecography II. Contribution to the diagnosis of defecation disorders. Gastrointest Radiol 9: 253–261
23. Mazeron JJ, le Bourgeois JP, Abbou CC, Lusinchi A, Lipinski F, Auvert J, Pierquin B (1985) Téléradiothérapie des adénocarcinomes prostatiques non métastatiques. J Eur Radiother 6: 139–146
24. Mc Millan SM, Wettlaufer JN (1976) The role of repeat transurethral biopsy in stage A carcinoma of the prostate. J Urol 116: 759–760
25. Mendenhall WM, Thar TL, Bova FJ, Marcus RB Jr, Morgan LS, Million R (1984) Prognostic and treatment factors affecting pelvic control of stage IB and IIA–B carcinoma of the intact uterine cervix treated with radiation therapy alone. Cancer 53: 2649–2654

26. Murphy GP, Natarja N, Pontes JE, Schmitz RL, Smart CR, Schmidt JD, Mettlin C (1982) The national survey of prostate cancer in the Unites states by the American College of Surgeons. J Urol 127: 928–934
27. Nagell JR Jr, Donaldson ES, Hanson MB (1983) Curr Probl Cancer 815: 1–41
28. Paull T, Tedeschi LG (1972) Perineal endometriosis at the site of episiotomy scar. Obstet Gynecol 40: 28–34
29. Perez CA, Breaux S, Bedwinek JM, Madoc-Jones H, Camel HM, Purdy JA, Walz BJ (1984) Radiation therapy alone in the treatment of carcinoma of the uterine cervix. II. analysis of complications. Cancer 54: 235–246
30. Pilepich MV, Pajak T, George FW, Asbell SO, Stetz J, Zinninger M, Plenk HP, Johnson RJ, Mulholland SG, Walz BJ, Kalish L (1983) Preliminary report on phase III RTOG studies of extended-field irradiation in carcinoma of the prostate. Am J Clin Oncol 6: 485–491
31. Ray GR, Bagshaw MA, Freiha F (1984) External beam radiation salvage for residual or recurrent local tumor following radical prostatectomy. J Urol 132: 926–930
32. Robey EL, Schellhammer PF (1987) Local failure after definitive therapy for prostatic cancer. J Urol 137: 613–619
33. Rosenberg SJ, Loening SA, Hawtrey CE, Narayana AS, Culp DA (1985) Radical prostatectomy with adjuvant radioactive gold for prostatic cancer: a preliminary report. J Urol 133: 225–227
34. Schellhammer PF, El-Mahdi AE, Ladaga LE, Schultheiss T (1985) 125-Iodine implantation for carcinoma of the prostate 5-year survival free of disease and incidence of local failure. J Urol 134: 1140–1145
35. Schellhammer PF, Jordan GH, El-Mahdi AM (1986) Pelvic complications after interstitial and external beam irradiation of urologic and gynecologic malignancy. World J Surg 10: 259–268
36. Sehapayak S (1985) Transrectal repair of rectocele: an extended armamentarium of colorectal surgeons. Dis Colon Rectum 28: 422–433
37. Silverberg E, Lubera J (1987) Cancer statistics. CA 37 (1): 2–19
38. Skinner DG, Lieskovsky G (1984) Contemporary cystectomy with pelvic node dissection compared to preoperative radiation therapy and cystectomy in management of invasive bladder cancer. J Urol 131: 1069–1972
39. Sullivan ES, Leaverton GH, Hardwick CE (1968) Transrectal perineal repair: an adjunct to improved function after anorectal surgery. Dis Colon Rectum 11: 106–114
40. Uhlig BE, Sullivan ES (1979) The modified Delorme operation: Its place in surgical treatment for massive rectal prolapse. Dis Colon Rectum 8: 513–521

J. Nicholls, FRCS, St. Mark's Hospital, London;
R. Glass, FRCS, The London Hospital, London

Coloproctology

Diagnosis and Outpatient Management

1985. 236 pp. 49 figs. Softcover
ISBN 3-540-15240-0

Coloproctology is a concise, authoritative guide to the diagnosis and outpatient management of anal and colorectal disease. It offers an up-to-date yet simple and safe approach to the subject for those training in surgery, gastroenterology and proctology. The book contains a detailed account of the organisation of outpatient services, anorectal examinations and the diagnosis of common clinical presentations using suitable flow charts. Each disease is then discussed individually, and where relevant, the results of various outpatient treatments are compared. Also included are sections on stomas and medications used in coloproctology as well as 200 references for further reading. The illustrations and text are carefully integrated to provide a clear and didactic approach.

Springer-Verlag Berlin
Heidelberg New York London
Paris Tokyo Hong Kong

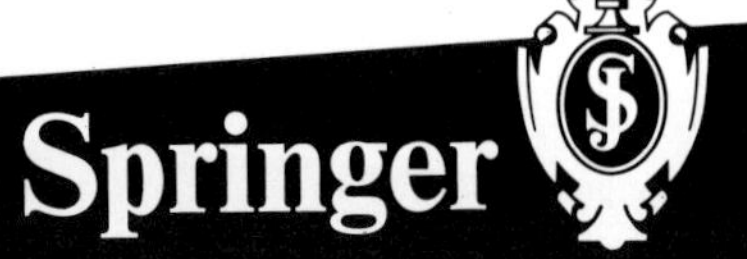

E. Stein, Ludwigshafen

Proctology

1990. Approx. 500 pp. Approx. 300 figs., mostly
colored, in approx. 600 sep. illus.
Hardcover ISBN 3-540-17755-8

This comprehensive work combines the advantages of
a textbook with the lucidity of an atlas, offering unified
presentation of text and illustration. It is undoubtedly a
milestone in the literature on the subject.

First, the topographic anatomy, the physiologic and
pathophysiologic locomotor system of the ano-rectum
together with proctologic examination techniques are
described. Then follows the systematic and practice-
oriented approach to the etiology, clinical findings,
diagnosis, differential diagnosis, therapy and prognosis
of all diseases belonging or extending to proctology.
The individual chapters, consistently constructed
according to a unified scheme, contain extensive details
of the literature and are remarkable for their precise
text conveying the latest state-of-the-art in diagnosis
and therapy.

The abundant colored illustrations provide the reader
with an instant guide to accurate differential diagnostic
evaluation. Similar findings that frequently occur are
also depicted for comparison; in this way, the reader
can acquire sound insight into the wide variety of
proctologic conditions that may confront him.

Springer-Verlag Berlin
Heidelberg New York London
Paris Tokyo Hong Kong

Springer